Diagnostic Cytopathology Essentials

Content Strategist: Michael Houston
Content Development Specialists: Rachael Harrison, Joanne Scott
Content Coordinator: Sam Crowe, Humayra Rahman Khan
Project Manager: Julie Taylor
Design: Charles Gray, Miles Hitchen
Illustration Manager: Jennifer Rose
Illustrator: Antbits Ltd
Marketing Manager(s) (UK/USA): Gaynor Jones/Abigail Swartz

Diagnostic Cytopathology Essentials

Gabrijela Kocjan, MD, MB BS,
Specialist in Clinical Cytology (Zagreb),
FRCPath(London)
Head of Diagnostic Cytopathology,
Consultant Cytopathologist
University College London
London, UK

Winifred Gray, MB BS, FRCPath
Consultant Cytopathologist/Histopathologist (retired)
John Radcliffe Hospital
Oxford, UK

Tanya Levine, MA(Oxon), MB BS,
RCDipPath(Cyto), FRCPath
Director
London Regional Cytology Training Centre
Consultant Cellular Pathologist
North West London Hospitals NHS Trust
London, UK

Ika Kardum-Skelin, MD, PhD, Specialist in
Clinical Cytology (Zagreb)
President
European Federation of Cytology Societies
Assistant Professor and Consultant Cytologist
Specialist in Medical/Clinical Cytology
Head of Department of Clinical Cytology and Cytogenetics
Merkur University Hospital
School of Medicine
University of Zagreb
Zagreb, Croatia

Philippe Vielh, MD, PhD
Pathologist, Director of Cytopathology
Department of Medical Biology and Pathology
Institut de Cancérologie Gustave Roussy
Villejuif, France

**For additional online content visit the expertconsult
website**

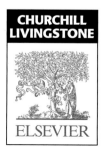

**CHURCHILL
LIVINGSTONE**

ELSEVIER

Edinburgh   London   New York   Oxford   Philadelphia   St Louis   Sydney   Toronto   2013

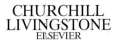

CHURCHILL LIVINGSTONE
ELSEVIER

an imprint of Elsevier Limited

© 2013, Elsevier Limited

First published 2013

The rights of Gabrijela Kocjan, Winifred Gray, Tanya Levine, Ika Kardum-Skelin and Philippe Vielh to be identified as authors of this work has been asserted by them in accordance with the Copyright, Designs and Patents Act 1988.

Notices

Knowledge and best practice in this field are constantly changing. As new research and experience broaden our understanding, changes in research methods, professional practices, or medical treatment may become necessary.

Practitioners and researchers must always rely on their own experience and knowledge in evaluating and using any information, methods, compounds, or experiments described herein. In using such information or methods they should be mindful of their own safety and the safety of others, including parties for whom they have a professional responsibility.

With respect to any drug or pharmaceutical products identified, readers are advised to check the most current information provided (i) on procedures featured or (ii) by the manufacturer of each product to be administered, to verify the recommended dose or formula, the method and duration of administration, and contraindications. It is the responsibility of practitioners, relying on their own experience and knowledge of their patients, to make diagnoses, to determine dosages and the best treatment for each individual patient, and to take all appropriate safety precautions.

To the fullest extent of the law, neither the Publisher nor the authors, contributors, or editors, assume any liability for any injury and/or damage to persons or property as a matter of products liability, negligence or otherwise, or from any use or operation of any methods, products, instructions, or ideas contained in the material herein.

ISBN: 978-0702-04450-2
E-ISBN: 978-0702-05033-6

†The following figures are taken from Gray, W., Kocjan G. (eds). *Diagnostic Cytopathology*, 3rd edition. 2010, Churchill Livingstone.

Working together to grow libraries in developing countries

www.elsevier.com | www.bookaid.org | www.sabre.org

ELSEVIER   BOOK AID International   Sabre Foundation

The publisher's policy is to use **paper manufactured from sustainable forests**

ELSEVIER   your source for books, journals and multimedia in the health sciences

www.elsevierhealth.com

Printed in China
Last digit is the print number: 9 8 7 6 5 4 3 2 1

Contents

	Foreword	vii
	List of contributors	ix
	Dedication	xi
	Acknowledgements	xi
1	Introduction	1
2	Female genital tract	3
3	Respiratory	59
4	Serous effusions	103
5	Urine cytology	135
6	Thyroid gland	147
7	Haemopoietic	173
8	Breast	245
9	Salivary gland	279
10	Liver, biliary tree and pancreas	309
11	Childhood tumours	351
12	Miscellaneous	359
	Cerebrospinal fluid	360
	Skin	366
	Malignant tumours	369
	Soft tissue and musculoskeletal system	372
	Synovial fluid	387
13	Techniques	391
	Routine procedures — John E. McGloin	392
	Immunocytochemistry — Nataša Nolde	398
	Polymerase chain reaction — Tim Diss	404
	In situ hybridisation (ISH) — Alexander Valent	410
14	Self-assessment questions	415
	Subject Index	443

Foreword

It gives me great pleasure to see that the idea born at a meeting of European Federation of Cytology Societies (EFCS) in October 2010 in Split, where European Cytology Education and Training were discussed, has come into being in the shape of *Diagnostic Cytopathology Essentials*. It is a product of the EFCS' ambition to have a comprehensive, 'official' textbook, the contents of which represent a minimum requirement for a competent cytopathologist.

Cytopathology is a diagnostic discipline which has been used for more than 150 years, since Walshe in the middle of the 19th century demonstrated that cells from lung cancer can be detected in sputum. Another milestone was the introduction of aspiration cytology in 1926 by Ellis and Martin, while in 1928, Papanicolaou published that cells of cervical cancer could be identified by microscopy. However, cytopathology was finally accepted in 1943 when its importance in cervical screening was recognised. From then on, both exfoliative and aspiration cytopathology continued to be recognised as essential in diagnosis and clinical patient management.

In the 21st century, in the era of modern techniques and shortage of pathologists, does cytopathology still remain an appropriate diagnostic tool? An answer to this question can be found in the Training Charter for Pathology, first published in 2012 by the Union Européenne des Médecines Spécialistes (UEMS), Board of Pathology. The Charter defines cytopathology as an integral part of pathology and its competency has to be trained. It is left to the pathologist to decide under which conditions to use cytopathology, histopathology, or a combination of both, to obtain a correct diagnosis and to evaluate if the respective sample material should be used for additional methods concerning prognosis and therapy. The UEMS and the EFCS agree that only structured training will result in the mandatory qualifications fulfilling the set criteria.

This book is aimed predominantly at junior pathologists and technical staff ambitious for education in cytopathology. It is concise and well illustrated with important morphological features highlighted through bullet points. Particular attention has been given to the 'diagnostic pitfalls' and 'further investigations' which are highlighted for every entity. In addition to the common organ systems, the book contains chapters on haemopoietic and paediatric cytopathology, otherwise not part of traditional textbooks. Also notable is a technical chapter which outlines in brief, illustrated by schematic drawings, the routine cytopathology staining, immunocytochemistry and molecular techniques. The book contains many useful tables, important weblinks and up-to-date classifications. Lastly, the self-assessment chapter contains the images from the book put into diagnostic context, for candidates to test their knowledge.

As an advocate of harmonisation of cytopathology training in Europe, I am convinced that the book forms a sound basis for a comprehensive pan-European teaching programme and a prospective European Cytopathology Diploma examination. Moreover, given that cells are universal, I anticipate that it will be used throughout the world as a standard guide to cytopathological diagnosis.

Martin Tötsch
Secretary General
European Federation of Cytology Societies
Member of the UEMS Board of Pathology
Graz, February 2013

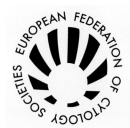

This publication has been produced to act as the official textbook to support the European Training Curriculum in Pathology recommended by the European Federation of Cytology Societies (EFCS) (www.efcs.eu/) and endorsed by the Union Européenne des Médecins Spécialistes (UEMS) Board of Pathology (www.uems.net/).

Ika Kardum-Skelin (EFCS President)
Martin Tötsch (EFCS Secretary General)

List of contributors

Tim Diss, PhD
Clinical Scientist
Histopathology Department
University College London Hospital
London, UK

Winifred Gray, MB BS, FRCPath
Consultant Cytopathologist/Histopathologist (retired)
John Radcliffe Hospital
Oxford, UK

Ika Kardum-Skelin, MD, PhD, Specialist in Clinical Cytology (Zagreb)
President
European Federation of Cytology Societies
Assistant Professor and Consultant Cytologist
Specialist in Medical/Clinical Cytology
Head of Department of Clinical Cytology and Cytogenetics
Merkur University Hospital
School of Medicine
University of Zagreb
Zagreb, Croatia

Gabrijela Kocjan, MD, MB BS, Specialist in Clinical Cytology (Zagreb), FRCPath(London)
Head of Diagnostic Cytopathology
Consultant Cytopathologist
University College London
London, UK

Tanya Levine, MA(Oxon), MB BS, RCDipPath(Cyto), FRCPath
Director
London Regional Cytology Training Centre
Consultant Cellular Pathologist
North West London Hospitals NHS Trust
London, UK

Teresa Marafioti, MD, FRCPath
Department of Cellular Pathology
University College London Hospital
London, UK

John E. McGloin, BSc, MSc, MBA
Head Biomedical Scientist
Cytology Laboratory
University College London Hospital
London, UK

Nataša Nolde, PhD
Institute of Oncology Ljubljana
Department of Cytopathology
Ljubljana, Slovenia

Martin Tötsch, MD
Secretary General
European Federation of Cytology Societies
Institute of Cytology
University Hospital of Graz
Medical University of Graz
Graz, Austria

Alexander Valent, RNDr, PhD
Research Cytogeneticist
Molecular Pathology, Cytogenetics
Department of Medical Biology and Pathology
Institut de Cancérologie Gustave Roussy
Villejuif, France

Philippe Vielh, MD, PhD
Pathologist, Director of Cytopathology
Department of Medical Biology and Pathology
Institut de Cancérologie Gustave Roussy
Villejuif, France

Dedication

To our children and grandchildren:
Adili
Alexander
Alice
Arabella
Benjamin
Elizabeth
Hazel
Hugo
Iva
Jake
Matko
Max
Rosalind
Tom

Acknowledgements

We wish to acknowledge the help and dedication of the Elsevier team, in particular that of Michael Houston who was the driving force to get this project through the publishing process. We would also like to acknowledge Rachael Harrison, Joanne Scott and Julie Taylor whose meticulous attention to detail played such an important part in the creation of this book.

Dr Vielh is indebted to Dr Felipe Andreiuolo for his help in making photomicrographs. Dr Kocjan wishes to thank Dr Ruma Saraswati, Dr Ian Proctor, Dr Priya Mairembam and Mrs Bridgette Smith for their help with the manuscript.

CHAPTER 1

Introduction

The practice of cytopathology is based on the microscopic identification of individual cells and cell arrangements in samples taken from tissues suspected of abnormality. Through pattern recognition gained by experience, this identification can provide diagnostic information for the clinician. Historically, cytology preceded the use of histological techniques on actual tissue sections; however, with improvements in histological techniques and staining methods during the nineteenth century, the diagnostic use of cytology was largely restricted to the study of exfoliated cells in readily available samples such as sputum and urine. With the advent of the Papanicolaou stain in the early twentieth century, interest in broader aspects of cytology was aroused, particularly the possibility of preventing cervical cancer by recognition of a premalignant phase of the disease.

By the 1950s, cervical screening programmes were under development in Europe. Cytodiagnosis was also enjoying a renaissance, not just for examination of urine and sputum, but also for samples such as cerebrospinal and serous effusion fluid. It was regarded as a rapid, simple and economical method, providing information prior to histological diagnosis and in some cases obviating the need for surgery when metastatic spread of malignant tumours could be established without further intervention. Diagnosis was not confined to tumours, as many infections and other disease processes could be suggested, particularly with the use of special stains. New techniques to enhance exfoliative sampling such as bronchial washings and brushings taken at bronchoscopy became available; in some specialties cytopathology was a necessary step in the diagnostic work-up of cases, for example, in patients suspected of having lung cancer.

In the latter part of the twentieth century several factors led to an upsurge in the use of cytology for diagnosis, a trend that continues today. The first was a rapidly growing interest in fine needle aspiration (FNA) sampling, initially for thyroid disease, then very soon from an increasing range of internal sites – it is said that no organ is safe now from the exploring needle! Cytopathologists who took the FNA samples themselves saw the added benefit of being able to examine the patient, get a full history and ensure adequacy of sampling when on-site assessment of samples could be included. Today, rapid on-site evaluation of specimens (ROSE) is advocated as best practice in cytopathology. The reliability of FNA diagnosis has come to be accepted by clinicians generally, and the pathologist has an important role within the multidisciplinary teams that decide on patient management strategies.

A further factor that has contributed to the increasing diagnostic use of FNA has been the recent emergence of numerous technical improvements in both sampling and cell processing. These include image guidance techniques for FNA, improved antibody staining with a wider repertoire of antibodies, and the use of new ancillary techniques such as flow cytometry and in situ hybridisation. All of these procedures have improved the accuracy of cytology and increased the confidence of clinicians in the contribution of cytodiagnosis to better patient management. Alongside the diagnostic applications of cytology, its role in preventive medicine in the cervical and breast screening programmes is well established, controversial though these programmes have been. Again, new developments such as liquid-based cytology for sample handling have enhanced the accuracy of cell recognition in cervical screening, which is now, thanks also to proper training and quality control, accepted as a successful programme for the reduction of mortality and incidence of cervical cancer. A full account of the history of both diagnostic and screening applications of cytology can be found in the introduction to the third edition of *Diagnostic Cytopathology*. It makes fascinating reading.

It is hardly surprising, given such a history, that the practice of cytodiagnosis requires appropriate specialist training. Nowadays, it is considered essential for pathologists to undergo training in all aspects of cytopathology. Specialist organisations such as the European Union of Medical Specialists (www.uems.net), in association with the European Federation of Cytology Societies (http://www.efcs.eu/), are aiming to harmonise cytopathology postgraduate training in Europe. The EFCS advocates a general training in all aspects of cytopathology as a core component of pathology training. The work of standardising medical training and practice in the European Union is acknowledged by the allocation of grants and resources towards projects that promote educational training platforms, including cytology, while allowing for national differences in the provision of service. To this end, this book has the imprimatur of the EFCS as part of the cytopathology training syllabus, eventually enabling formal assessment of such training.

Rationalisation of pathology services through centralising cytology laboratories, particularly those performing cervical screening, may appear to diminish the demand for specialist cytopathologists who have had a broad-based training. However, cervical cytology diagnostic skills are still expected from pathologists within the multidisciplinary meetings where histological, cytological and colposcopic correlation determines patient management. Pathologists therefore need to acquire the necessary experience so as to be able to review complex cytology cases to guide treatment.

Following the publication in 2010 of the third edition of *Diagnostic Cytopathology*, with its comprehensive systems-based approach to the subject, we, as editors and contributors to the book, agreed with the publishers that a shorter training manual would be a more easily accessible version for daily use. It should serve as an introduction to the field, a bench book with a reminder of the important differential diagnoses and ancillary tests available, and, not least, as an entrée to the 'big book', from which much of the material here is derived, for further reading in areas of interest.

To this end, we have compiled for each system a series of bullet-point facts about the cytological features of the major common entities encountered in everyday practice, accompanied by a range of illustrative figures, with indications of the differential diagnosis and appropriate further investigations to avoid pitfalls. A chapter with sections on the technical aspects of sample preparation and ancillary testing is included. Our intention is to provide the essential information for all levels of training and experience, of use to both technical and medical staff working in cytology laboratories worldwide.

The layout of the book is intended to be user-friendly. Different entities occupy a clearly defined space, usually one or two pages for each, with text aligned as far as possible to extensive high-quality images. The 'self assessment' chapter at the end of the book contains examples from within the book to reinforce some of the points made throughout. There are very few histological images, but a sound awareness of histopathology is a precondition for gaining full benefit from the book, as is the case for practising cytopathology in general.

We hope the reader of this book, will find that cells, as well as tissues, can provide definitive answers to important clinical questions, thus achieving maximum information from minimal intervention.

CHAPTER 2

Female genital tract

Contents

Normal anatomy of the gynaecological tract   3

Cytology of normal cells from the cervical transformation zone   6

Cytological findings in cervicitis/vaginitis   14

Common cervical/vaginal microorganisms   16

Common viral infections   18

Iatrogenic changes in cervical cytology   20

Repair and regeneration in the cervix   23

Cervical sample adequacy   24

Cytology of CIN and cervical squamous cancer   25

Borderline nuclear changes in cervical cytology   38

Glandular neoplasms in cervical cytology   40

Management of women with abnormal cervical cytology   46

Cytology of the vulva and vagina   47

Uterine cytology   50

Ovarian cytology   52

Normal anatomy of the gynaecological tract (Fig. 2.1)

- Screening for pre-cancerous changes of the cervix provides the bulk of the workload for many cytology laboratories
- Crucial to this process is an understanding of the morphology of cells from the normal cervix, vulva, vagina, and endometrium as they appear in cytological preparations
- The morphology of these cells is similar whether assessing conventional direct smears or liquid-based preparations

Knowledge of the physiology of the normal cervical transformation zone is important in understanding the development of the pre-cancer – cancer sequence, as the labile cells from this area are particularly susceptible to oncogenic 'hits'.

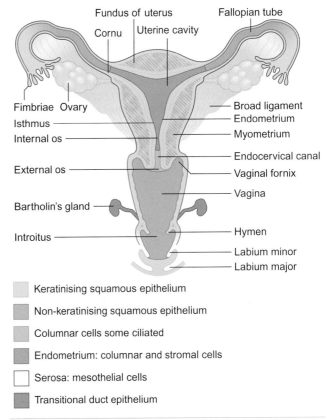

Keratinising squamous epithelium

Non-keratinising squamous epithelium

Columnar cells some ciliated

Endometrium: columnar and stromal cells

Serosa: mesothelial cells

Transitional duct epithelium

Fig. 2.1[†] Diagram of the female genital tract demonstrating the main structures and the types of epithelium covering the surface accessible to sampling directly, or indirectly by exfoliative cytology. (Courtesy of Professor D. Coleman and Mrs P. Chapman, with permission from Butterworths, London.)

Transformation zone (Figs 2.2–2.4)

- Before puberty the 'original' squamocolumnar junction is level with the external os
- At puberty the cervix increases in size
- The lower endocervix now protrudes into the vaginal canal. This is lined by a single layer of mucinous epithelium
- The 'original' squamocolumnar junction moves circumferentially outwards onto the ectocervical aspect of the cervix
- The exposed endocervix appears red, if examined visually, reflecting the rich vascular supply under the single cell layer (ectropion)
- Under the acid pH of the vagina, this mucinous layer undergoes squamous metaplasia and is termed the 'transformation zone' Squamous metaplasia is important as the fragile, single-cell mucinous layer is replaced by a more resistant multi-layered epithelium. The first step in squamous metaplasia in the transformation zone is reserve cell hyperplasia. Reserve cells proliferate as a row of small, round cells beneath the columnar epithelium. These cells gradually mature via immature squamous metaplastic cells into mature squames. Over time, these multi-layered cells become indistinguishable from normal, mature squamous epithelium. Histologically the only clue to the origin of these cells is the presence of mucinous/endocervical crypt epithelium beneath.

    This process of squamous metaplasia continues throughout a woman's reproductive life. As this is centred on a labile cell population, this normal physiological pathway can be diverted to neoplastic change with the acquisition of high-risk human papilloma virus (see later)
- After the menopause, the cervix reduces in size and the 'original' squamocolumnar junction migrates back into the endocervical canal

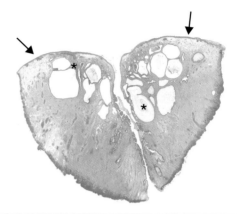

Fig. 2.2 Whole-mount histological section of the cervix including transformation zone from a 35-year-old woman. Note the Nabothian follicles (*) caused by the plugging of endocervical crypt openings by squamous metaplastic epithelium, and the location of the original squamocolumnar junction (*arrows*).

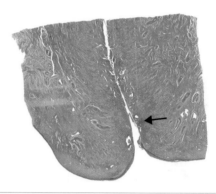

Fig. 2.3 Whole-mount section of cervix from a post-menopausal woman. Note the original squamocolumnar junction now lies within the endocervical canal (*arrow*).

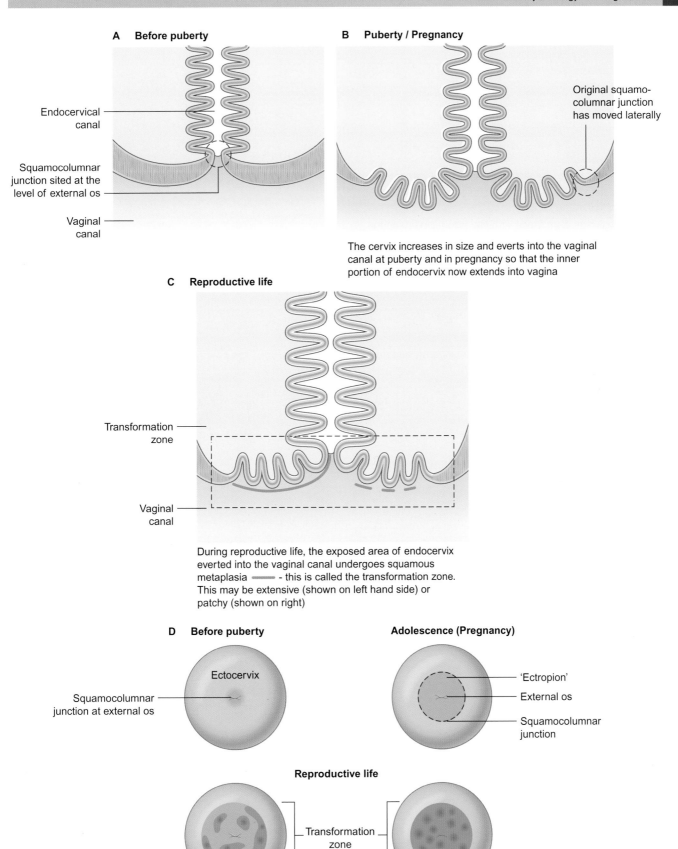

A   Before puberty

Endocervical canal

Squamocolumnar junction sited at the level of external os

Vaginal canal

B   Puberty / Pregnancy

Original squamo-columnar junction has moved laterally

The cervix increases in size and everts into the vaginal canal at puberty and in pregnancy so that the inner portion of endocervix now extends into vagina

C   Reproductive life

Transformation zone

Vaginal canal

During reproductive life, the exposed area of endocervix everted into the vaginal canal undergoes squamous metaplasia ▬▬▬ - this is called the transformation zone. This may be extensive (shown on left hand side) or patchy (shown on right)

D   Before puberty

Ectocervix

Squamocolumnar junction at external os

Adolescence (Pregnancy)

'Ectropion'

External os

Squamocolumnar junction

Reproductive life

Transformation zone

Incomplete squamous metaplasia

Complete squamous metaplasia

Fig. 2.4 (A–D) Schematic diagrams of the cervical transformation zone.

Cytology of normal cells from the cervical transformation zone

Squamous cells (Figs 2.5–2.8)

- Most numerous epithelial type
- Superficial cells are large, polygonal cells with small and pyknotic nuclei
- May be single or aggregated with 'pearl' and 'raft' formation
- Intermediate cells are large, polygonal cells with cytoplasm often folded at the periphery
- Their nuclei are round/oval with fine vesicular chromatin
- In the second half (progesterone-rich) of the cycle, the cells can appear ragged with many Döderlein bacilli ingesting the cytoplasmic glycogen

Metaplastic cells (Figs 2.9–2.11)

- Normal constituent of samples from the transformation zone
- When immature, do not exfoliate spontaneously and may have 'spidery' cytoplasmic processes reflecting forceful detachment from other cells during sampling
- Recognisable metaplastic cells are similar in size to parabasal or early intermediate cells
- Some may resemble endocervical cells reflecting their immaturity
- May have delicate cyanophilic cytoplasm or maybe be prematurely keratinised. When fully mature they are indistinguishable from normal squamous epithelial cells from the ecotcervix

Anucleate squames (Figs 2.12, 2.13)

- Presence indicates hyperkeratosis which may be secondary to prolapse or HPV infection
- Identification of low diagnostic predictive value

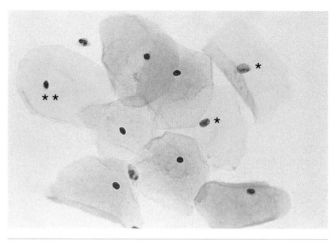

Fig. 2.5[†] Normal intermediate (*) and superficial cells (**).

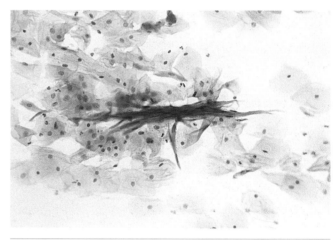

Fig. 2.6[†] An epithelial spike/raft of parakeratotic squamous cells.

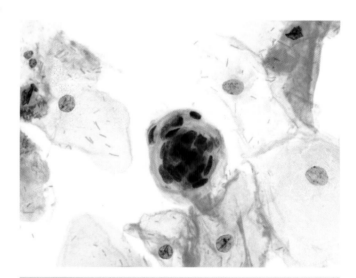

Fig. 2.7[†] Concentric epithelial pearl found in a normal cervical cytology sample.

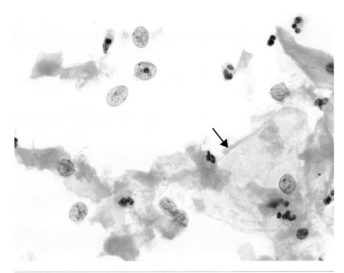

Fig. 2.8 Degenerating intermediate cells surrounded by Döderlein bacilli. Note extruded bare nuclei. Glycogen evident in the cytoplasm of a viable intermediate cell (*arrow*).

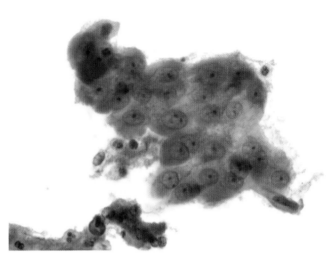

Fig. 2.11 Immature squamous metaplastic cells resembling endocervical cells.

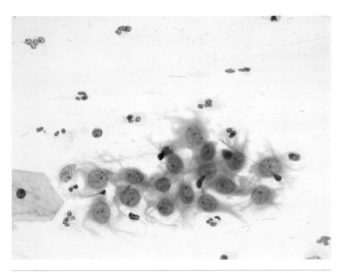

Fig. 2.9 Normal metaplastic cells with 'spidery' cytoplasmic processes.

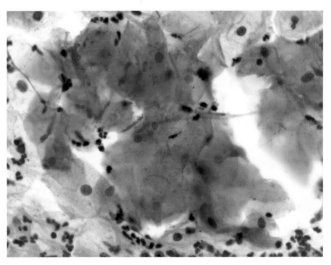

Fig. 2.12 Abundant anucleate squames with highly keratinised cytoplasm.

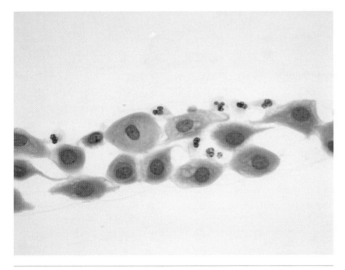

Fig. 2.10 Metaplastic cells are immature cells which are similar in size to parabasal cells.

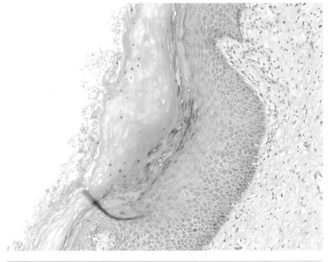

Fig. 2.13 Corresponding histology of Fig. 2.12 from the hysterectomy specimen showing marked hyperkeratosis of the ectocervix secondary to prolapse.

Endocervical cells (Figs 2.14–2.19)

- Columnar cells with regular nuclei in the middle to basal third of the cell
- Nuclei have a fine and even chromatin pattern with one or more small nucleoli – often near the nuclear membrane
- There may be variation in nuclear size within a group, although the polarity is always maintained
- Cells arranged in a honeycomb or picket-fence sheet depending on orientation
- Ciliated columnar cells may also be seen as a normal component – particularly if origin from upper endocervical canal/low isthmic portion

Endometrial cells (Figs 2.20–2.22)

- Usually seen up to day 12 of cycle
- After this, consider, depending on age of patient:
  - irregular cycles
  - dysfunctional uterine bleeding
  - exogenous hormones (combined oral contraceptive/ hormone replacement therapy)
  - IUD carriage
  - endometrial pathology
- Appear as tightly formed three-dimensional clusters ± dense stromal cores
- May appear degenerate along with associated histiocytes

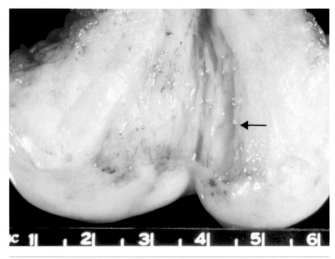

Fig. 2.14 Normal cervix sliced open to reveal endocervical canal (*arrow*). Note glistening appearance due to presence of mucus.

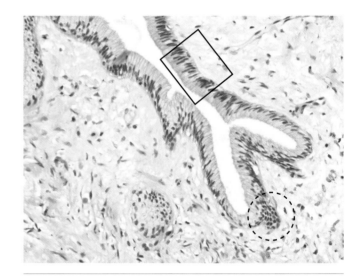

Fig. 2.15 Normal histology of endocervix including picket-fence arrangement (*box*) and 'honeycomb' arrangement of cells (*circled*).

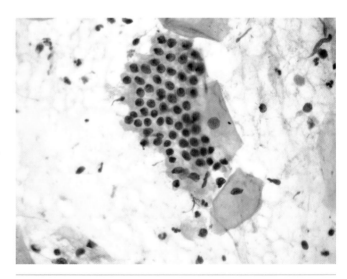

Fig. 2.16 Honeycomb pattern of normal endocervical cells. Note the similarities in cellular arrangement to the circled area in Fig. 2.15.

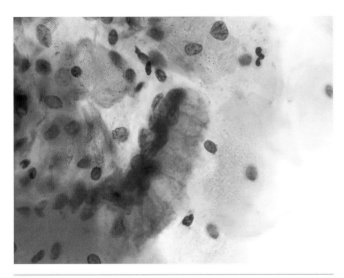

Fig. 2.17 Picket-fence arrangement of normal endocervical cells – compare to boxed area in Fig. 2.15.

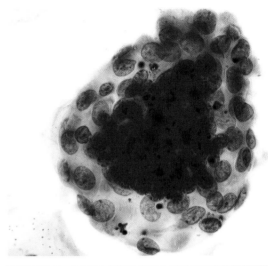

Fig. 2.20 Well-preserved endometrial group with dense stromal core surrounded by a covering layer of endometrial epithelial cells.

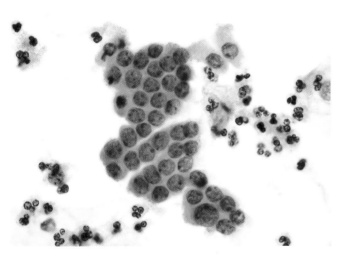

Fig. 2.18 Variation in nuclear size of endocervical cells but maintained polarity.

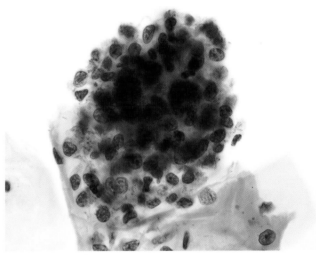

Fig. 2.21 Degenerate endometrial cells (day 10 of cycle).

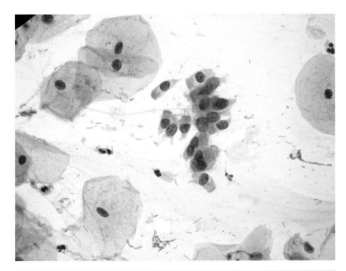

Fig. 2.19 Normal ciliated endocervical cells.

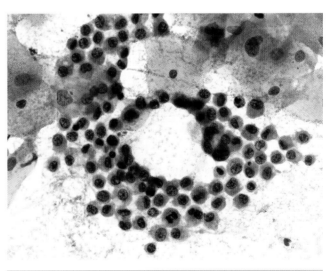

Fig. 2.22 Dispersed and mitotically active histiocytes day 10.

Reserve cells (Figs 2.23, 2.24)

- Rarely identified in cervical samples *de novo*
- When confidently identified, represent reserve cell hyperplasia in which three-dimensional groups of small and darkly staining cells are present in syncytial groups from the endocervical/transformation zone
- Distinguished from endometrial cells as no stromal cores
- Different from endocervical dyskaryosis due to lack of architectural pattern and chromatin abnormalities found in the latter

Inflammatory cells

Neutrophils

- Very common
- Origin may be physiological from the cervical canal mucus plug or pathological (inflammation)
- If present in large numbers may obscure underlying epithelial cell morphology, rendering it unsuitable for further assessment

Other inflammatory cells (Fig. 2.25)

- Macrophages: Commonly seen around day 10 of cycle and in post-menopausal samples
- May be singly dispersed or in loose sheets
- Identify reniform nucleus and delicate cytoplasm
- May aggregate as giant cells – particularly in post-menopausal samples (see Fig. 2.25)
- Lymphocytes, plasma cells, eosinophils and mast cells may be identified (see follicular cervicitis)

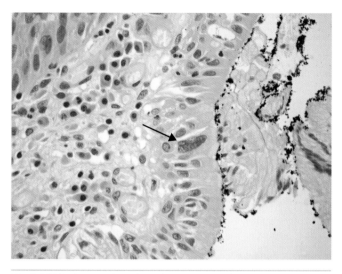

Fig. 2.23 Histology section of transformation zone showing reserve cell hyperplasia with endocervical cell multinucleation (*arrow*).

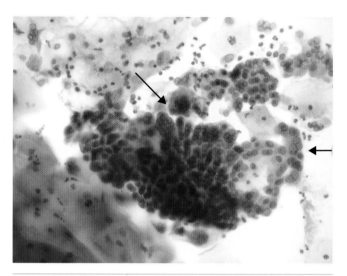

Fig. 2.24 Reserve cell hyperplasia. Note multinucleated endocervical cells (*arrows*). Note correlation with histology section in Fig. 2.23.

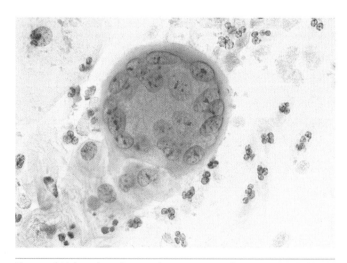

Fig. 2.25[†] Multinucleated macrophages or giant cells are a non-specific finding, especially after the menopause. They are also seen in granulomatous inflammation or repair and after radiotherapy.

Other findings in cervical samples

Spermatozoa (Fig. 2.26)

- Post-coital samples
- Up to several days following intercourse

Infestations (Figs 2.27–2.29)

These may represent cervical infection *per se* or contaminants due to poor personal hygiene from the lower GI tract or skin and include:

- *Enterobius vermicularis*
- Schistosomiasis

External/atmospheric contaminants (Figs 2.30–2.32)

- Much more common in direct smears than liquid-based preparations
- Include: plant particles, pollen, insect parts, fungi from atmosphere and laboratory contaminants, cotton fibres from tampons and starch granules

Artefacts in processing (Figs 2.33, 2.34)

- Cornflake artefact: commoner in direct smears than liquid-based samples
- Results from air-trapping during cover-slipping or inadequate removal of spray fixative containing carbowax
- At times it may obscure the nuclear detail completely
- Fragments of dried paint from surface marking of some LBC slides may be evident in samples after processing

Pregnancy and post-partum (Fig. 2.35)

- Progesterone levels increase (from placenta)
- Predominance of intermediate cells
- Variable numbers of navicular cells
- Rarely Arias–Stella and decidualised cells may be seen

Post-menopausal changes (Figs 2.36–2.40)

An atrophic pattern gradually evolves:
- Early atrophy: large numbers of intermediate cells
- Late/well-developed atrophy: parabasal cells predominant
  - endocervical cells are few or absent
  - often inflammatory changes coexist
  - direct smears may contain 'blue blobs', possibly degenerate inspissated mucin in origin
- Continued oestrogenisation in the post-menopausal state may reflect:
  - obesity: adipose tissue acts as a depot for steroid hormone production (common)
  - drugs: HRT (common), digitalis
  - steroid-producing ovarian tumours, e.g. Sertoli–Leydig cell and granulosa tumours (rare)

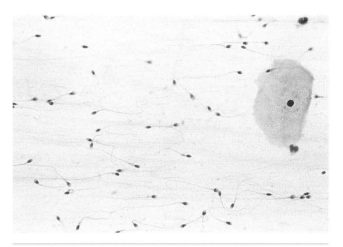

Fig. 2.26† Spermatozoa identified by darkly staining ovoid heads and preserved tails.

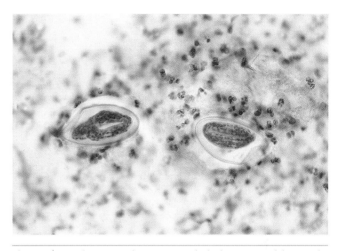

Fig. 2.27† *Enterobius vermicularis* ova. Note thick glassy eosinophilic capsule around the internal larva.

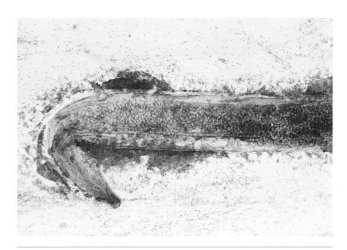

Fig. 2.28† Adult *Entoerobius vermicularis* in direct smear – far less common than ova above.

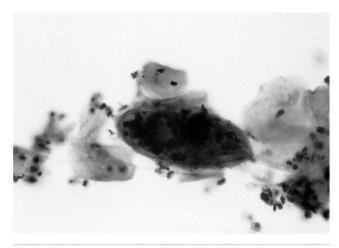

Fig. 2.29† Schistosomal subtypes may be difficult to identify. *S. haematobium* has a terminal spine (see above), *S. japonicum* has a lateral spine.

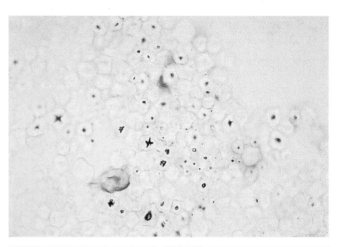

Fig. 2.32† Talc/glove powder in a direct smear.

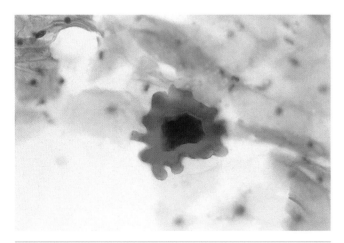

Fig. 2.30† Plant particle (scleroid) seen in a direct smear.

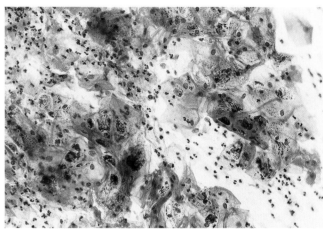

Fig. 2.33† 'Cornflake' artefact noted as a brown, slightly refractile deposit overlying nuclei.

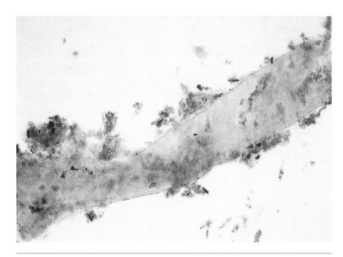

Fig. 2.31† Cotton fibres in a direct smear.

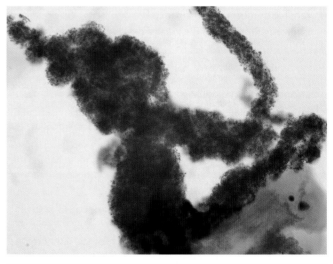

Fig. 2.34 LBC artefact circle paint (Hologic/ThinPrep sample).

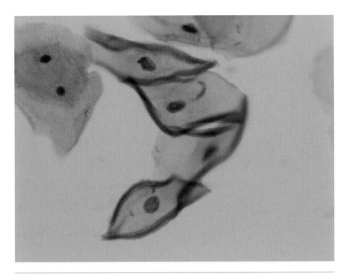

Fig. 2.35 Navicular cells in pregnancy are boat-shaped intermediate cells with rolled cytoplasmic edges containing glycogen.

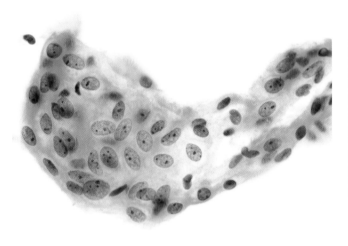

Fig. 2.36 A sheet of parabasal cells in an atrophic sample.

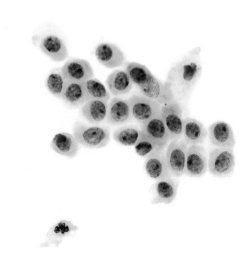

Fig. 2.37 Parabasal cells may appear to simulate the honeycomb pattern of endocervical cells.

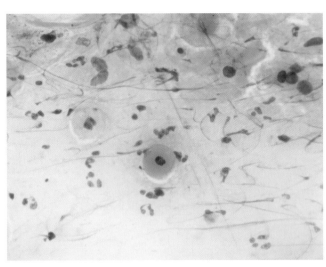

Fig. 2.38 Atrophic parabasal cells are often degenerate with orangeophilic cytoplasm and small pyknotic nuclei.

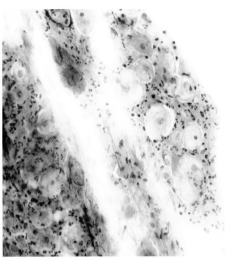

Fig. 2.39 Inflammation in an atrophic cervical sample.

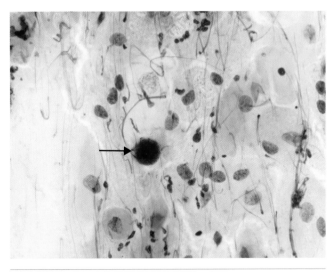

Fig. 2.40 'Blue blob' (*arrow*) in a direct cervical smear.

Cytological findings in cervicitis/vaginitis

Non-specific changes (Figs 2.41–2.45)

- Numerous neutrophils
- 'Dirty' fibrinous exudate
- Squamous and endocervical cells show inflammatory/degenerative changes:
  - cytoplasmic vacuolation, orangeophilic staining and perinuclear haloing
  - nuclear enlargement, membrane wrinkling, multinucleation ± karyolysis and karyorrhexis

Specific types (Figs 2.46–2.49)

- Follicular cervicitis
  - lymphocytes, tingible body macrophages and plasma cells present
- Atrophic cervicitis
  - very common due to post-menopausal thinning of vaginal and cervical epithelium
  - degenerate orangeophilia of parabasal cells with pyknotic nuclei
  - numerous background neutrophils

Differential diagnosis

- Lymphocytes in follicular cervicitis misdiagnosed as severely dyskaryotic cells if lymphoid and plasma cell chromatin overlooked
- Degenerate parabasal cells in atrophic cervicitis may simulate keratinised severely dyskaryotic cells but nuclei are pyknotic with normal nuclear:cytoplasmic ratios

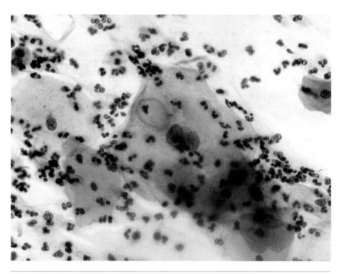

Fig. 2.41 Acute cervicitis with many neutrophils in the background and within squamous epithelial cells.

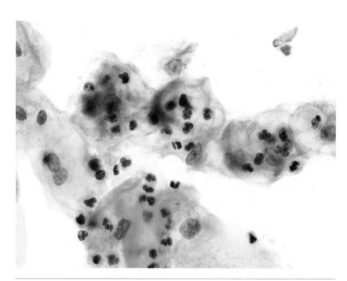

Fig. 2.42 Numerous neutrophils within the degenerate cytoplasm of squamous epithelial cells.

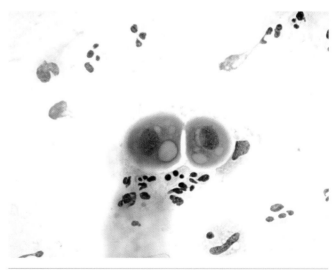

Fig. 2.43 Inflammatory cytoplasmic changes with vacuolation in metaplastic cells.

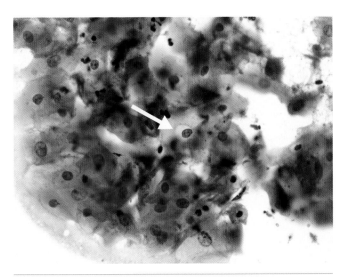

Fig. 2.44 Perinuclear inflammatory halo (*arrow*).

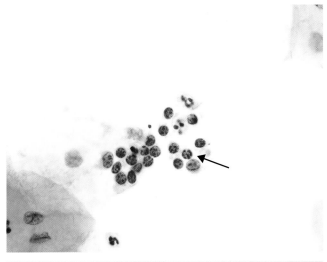

Fig. 2.47 Small mature lymphocytes simulating severe dyskaryosis if lymphoid and clock-face chromatin pattern of plasma cells (*arrow*) not appreciated.

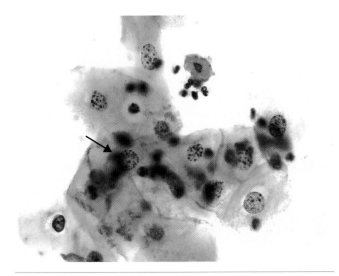

Fig. 2.45 Degenerative karyolysis in squamous epithelial cells secondary to inflammation. Note nuclear membrane dissolution (*arrow*).

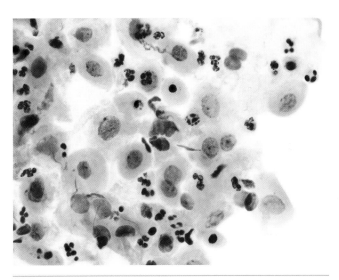

Fig. 2.48 Atrophic cervicitis.

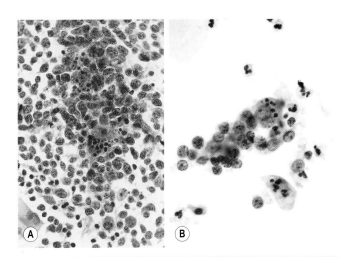

Fig. 2.46† Follicular cervicitis. An aggregate of lymphocytes present (A) in association with a tangible body macrophage (B).

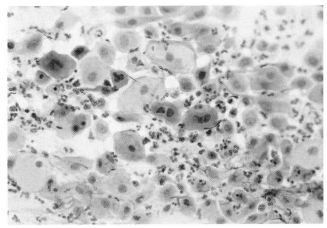

Fig. 2.49† This atrophic sample is from a 59-year-old post-menopausal woman in which there are scattered and degenerate parabasal cells. Follow-up smears were normal after application of local oestrogen cream.

Common cervical/vaginal microorganisms

Bacteria (Figs 2.50–2.52)

Endogenous flora include:

* Döderlein's bacilli/lactobacilli
  - Rod-shaped organisms
  - Common in progesterone-rich states
  - Secrete enzymes that dissolve intermediate cell walls to release glycogen for their nutrition
* *Leptothrix* spp.
  - Non-pathogenic thread-like bacteria
  - May be associated with *Trichomonas* spp.

Exogenous flora include:

* Staphylococci, streptococci and *Gardnerella* spp.
* Require microbiopsy for formal identification

Protozoa (Figs 2.53–2.55)

* *Trichomonas vaginalis* (TV)
  - Venereal infection
  - Common female symptom is offensive vaginal discharge
  - Unicellular tear-shaped organism with slate-grey cytoplasm
  - Crescentic nucleus faintly visible
  - Detached squamous cytoplasmic fragments may appear similar but lack nuclear details of TV

Fungi (Figs 2.56–2.58)

* *Candida* spp.
  - Dimorphic fungus
  - White curdy non-odorous discharge and pruritus vulvae

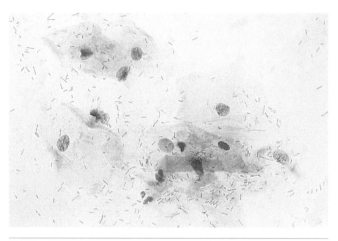

Fig. 2.50[†] Lactobacilli. The background of this sample shows numerous rod-shaped organisms, arranged singly and in short chains. Cytolysis of intermediate cells is also apparent, leaving bare nuclei and wisps of cytoplasm.

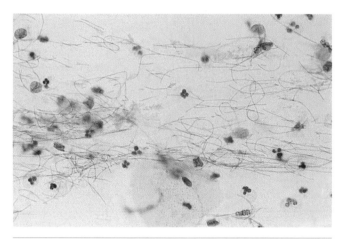

Fig. 2.51[†] Leptothrix organisms are seen in this sample in long strands and loops. Note the absence of any significant inflammatory infiltrate.

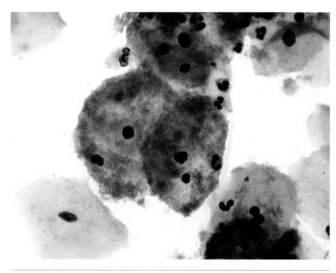

Fig. 2.52[†] Coccoid overgrowth creating a bacterial haze over a superficial cell.

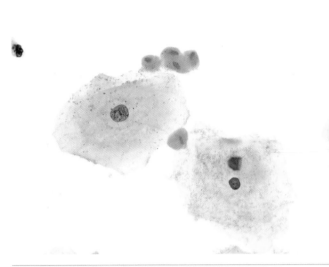

Fig. 2.53 *Trichomonas* sp. with crescentic-shaped nuclei.

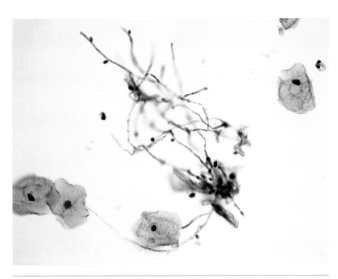

Fig. 2.56 *Candida* sp. pseudohyphae and spores.

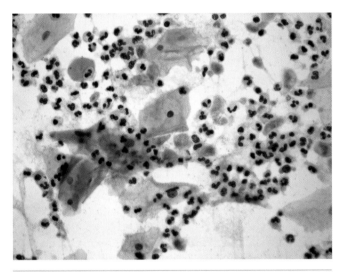

Fig. 2.54 *Trichomonas vaginalis* with associated acute inflammatory reaction.

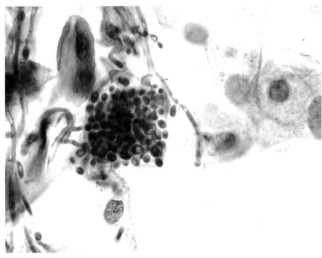

Fig. 2.57 *Candida* sp. spores.

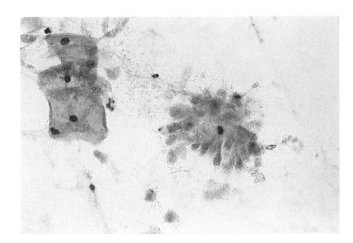

Fig. 2.55[†] *Trichomonas vaginalis* surrounding and invading a degenerate squamous epithelial cell.

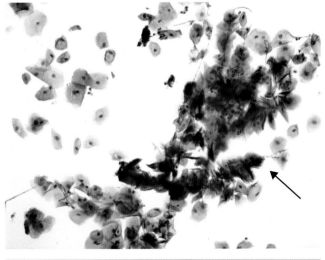

Fig. 2.58 Characteristic appearance of squamous epithelial cells in liquid-based cytology samples with 'skewering' of squamous cells through *Candida* sp. pseudohyphae (*arrow*).

Common viral infections

Human papillomavirus (HPV)

- Very common sexually acquired infection
- Some 40 subtypes of the > 150 strains can infect the female genital tract
- 'Low-risk' types (include HPV 6, 11) associated with condylomata
- 'High-risk' types (includes HPV 16, 18) associated with pre-cancer–cancer pathway (see CIN and CGIN section)
- Most infections, whether low or high risk, will regress within 2 years

Microscopic appearances (Figs 2.59–2.61)

- Koilocytosis in squamous cells shows well-defined perinuclear cytoplasmic clearing with a surrounding dense peripheral cytoplasmic rim
- Variable nuclear enlargement and hyperchromasia (see low-grade dyskaryosis section)
- Bi- and multinucleation common
- Cytoplasmic keratinisation

Diagnostic pitfalls

Koilocytes need to be distinguished from:

- Cytoplasmic glycogen: characteristic yellow glycogen deposits distinct from HPV-related clearing
- Perinuclear inflammatory halos: typically smaller than in koilocytosis and not surrounded by a dense peripheral cytoplasmic rim

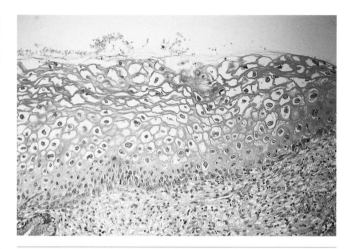

Fig. 2.59† Flat condyloma with surface koilocytosis.

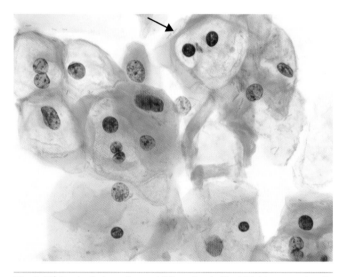

Fig. 2.60† Cytological corollary to H&E section in Fig. 2.59. Note cytoplasmic clearing and thickening of cytoplasm beyond this to cell membrane (*arrow*).

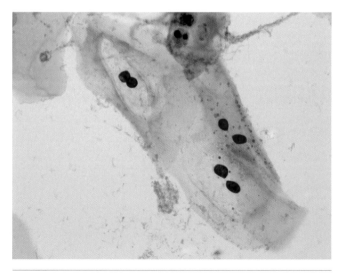

Fig. 2.61† Koilocytes with borderline nuclear changes and near-normal nuclei.

Herpes simplex virus infection (HSV)

- HSV infection of the genital tract commonly caused by HSV II (herpes genitalis) rather than HSV I (herpes labialis)
- 90% of primary genital tract HSV infection of external genitalia is associated with HSV cervicitis ± systemic symptoms
- Infection is self-limiting with, in some women, recurrent milder episodes (reflecting antibody response)

HSV infection may affect the cervix alone without involving the external genitalia.

Cytological findings (Figs 2.62 A, B and C)

- Swollen nuclei and multinucleation
- Ground-glass chromatin with prominent nuclear membranes
- Nuclear inclusions

Differential diagnosis

- Multinucleation and nuclear swelling may be non-specific and found in various inflammatory and repair processes
- Ground-glass nuclear chromatin changes and intranuclear inclusions are most-specific pointers to infection

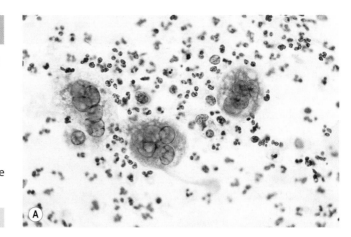

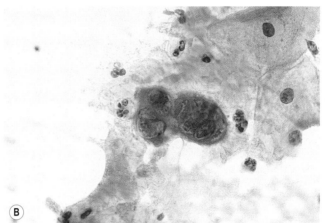

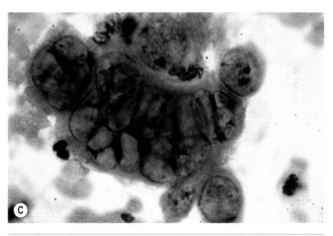

Fig. 2.62[†] HSV changes within epithelial cells. (A) Nuclear ground-glass pattern develops. (B) Nuclear inclusion bodies appear as cells start to degenerate. (C) High-power view of infected multinucleated cell with ground-glass chromatin and nuclear inclusions.

Iatrogenic changes in cervical cytology

Hormonal therapy

- Oral contraceptives (COC)
  - cytolysis (progesterone-only types)
  - normal endometrial cells out of cycle (breakthrough bleeding)
- Hormone replacement therapy (HRT)
  - variable oestrogenisation
  - ± exfoliated endometrial cells
- Tamoxifen
  - clean background with variable oestrogenisation
  - screen for endometrial cells as increased risk of endometrial pathology in long-term use

Endometrial cells in post-menopausal patients should always warrant further investigation irrespective of morphology.

Intrauterine devices (IUD) (Figs 2.63–2.65)

- Endometrial cells shed throughout cycle
- Endometrial cells may appear atypical as groups and single cells
- Variable increase in inflammatory cells
- Inflammatory changes in endocervical cells
- ± actinomyces colonies
- Psammoma bodies (very rare)

Diagnostic pitfalls

- Single atypical endometrial cells distinguished from severely dyskaryotic cells by homogeneous nuclear features and lack of three-dimensionality to nucleus
- Atypical endometrial cells in women over 40 years may not only be attributable to IUD carriage and repeat sampling after removal of the device and/or gynaecological referral maybe advised

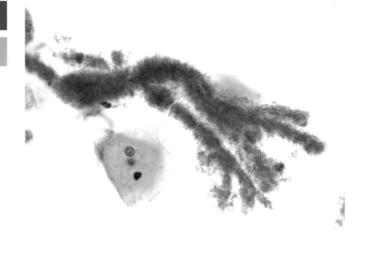

Fig. 2.64 Actinomyces colonies with typical 'bottle brush' appearance may be associated with IUD carriage.

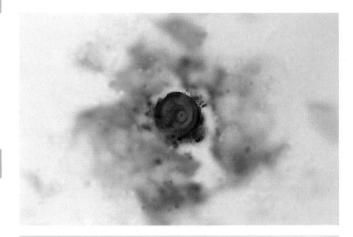

Fig. 2.65[†] Psammoma body in a cervical sample associated with IUD carriage.

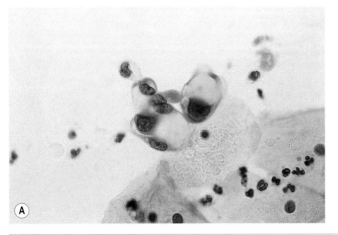

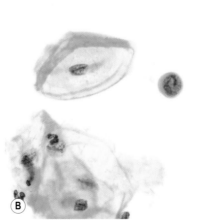

Fig. 2.63[†] (A) IUD changes in a three-dimensional endometrial cluster with enlarged nuclei and prominent cytoplasmic vacuolation. (B) Single atypical endometrial cell mimicking severe dyskaryosis.

Iatrogenic changes – surgical intervention

- Repair and metaplastic changes may be seen following various surgical procedures, e.g. biopsy and conisation

Cytological findings (Figs 2.66–2.68)

- Repair changes
- Inflammation
- Tubo-endometrioid metaplasia (TEM)
  - crowded hyperchromatic cell groups
  - ± ciliated cell borders
- Lower uterine segment sampling
  - intact glands from the lower uterine segment
  - particularly common in sampling following conisation due to shortening of the endocervical canal following treatment
  - Characterised by large microbiopsies containing uniform and crowded glandular cells with crisp anatomical borders
- Often with adherent surface stromal cells and capillary fragments

Differential diagnosis

- TEM and LUS may be mistaken for cervical glandular intraepithelial neoplasia (CGIN)
- LUS lacks abnormal chromatin and architectural features of CGIN
- TEM can be difficult to categorise precisely, particularly if ciliated cells not apparent and pseudostratified endometrioid cells predominate
- Clinical history of previous conisation useful

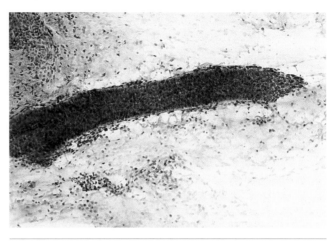

Fig. 2.67[†] Lower uterine segment. Note central fibrovascular core around which bland cells with uniform oval nuclei are arranged.

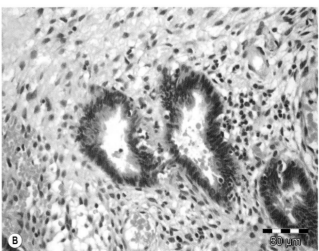

Fig. 2.68 Lower uterine segment sampling following previous conisation.

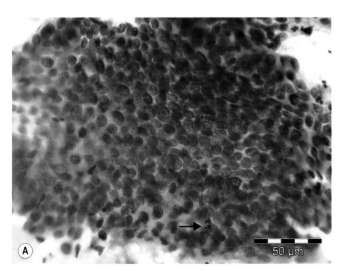

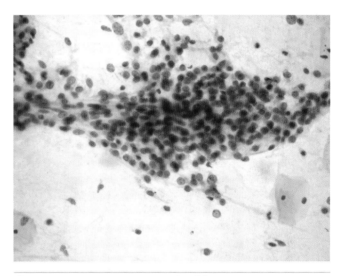

Fig. 2.66 (A) Hyperchromatic crowded group in woman of 35 years. Note mitosis (*arrow*). Initially diagnosed as possible CGIN, on conisation was tuboendometrioid metaplasia. No history of previous conisation given. (B) Tubo-endometrioid metaplasia on subsequent cone.

Iatrogenic changes – radiation

- Radiotherapy commonly used in treatment of female genital tract malignancies
- May be very difficult to interpret in cytological preparations such that cytology is not usually advocated as a means of patient follow-up/surveillance

Cytological findings (Figs 2.69, 2.70)

- Swelling and enlargement of cells but with maintained nuclear:cytoplasmic ratios
- Bizarre cell shapes
- Altered cytoplasmic staining between and within cells
- Extreme nuclear degenerative changes

Diagnostic diagnosis

In recurrent/residual malignancy the neoplastic cells will have unequivocal malignant cytology with raised nuclear:cytoplasmic ratios.

- A 'two cell population', if present, is helpful in identifying neoplastic from non-neoplastic populations
- Follow-up cytology ± colposcopy and biopsy may be advisable in equivocal cases

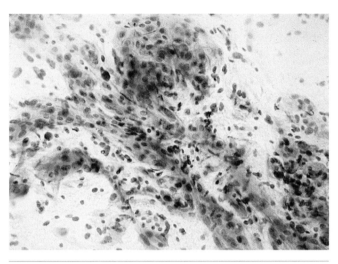

Fig. 2.69[†] Vaginal direct smear 6 months after cervical carcinoma radiotherapy. Note marked variability of nuclear size and eosinophilia of cytoplasm.

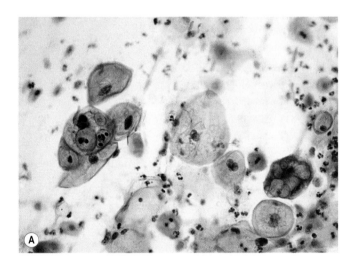

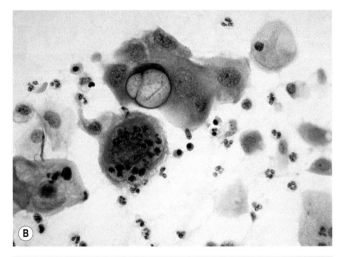

Fig. 2.70[†] **A & B** Radiation damage in vaginal direct smear from a post-menopausal woman treated for carcinoma of the ovary by surgery and radiotherapy. The cells and nuclei are swollen and deeply stained but the nuclear:cytoplasmic ratio is normal. Fine and coarse vacuolation of cytoplasm has occurred and degenerate polymorphs are seen within cells. Note also some binucleation and the prominent nucleoli.

Repair and regeneration in the cervix

- Epithelial repair and regeneration occurs following cervical damage and/or ulceration
- Causes include: cervicitis, surgical intervention, ablative treatment and irradiation and maybe centred on the endocervix, transformation zone and/or ectocervical mucosa

Cytological findings (Figs 2.71, 2.72)

- Immature population of parabasal, metaplastic and reserve cells
- Epithelial cells arranged in flat syncytial sheets with enlarged nuclei and nucleoli across all the cells and with even chromatin distribution
- Typically abundant cytoplasm with ragged margins ± leucophagocytosis
- ± mitoses
- Fibroblasts/stromal cells with oval nuclei and poorly defined cytoplasm also present
- ± background acute inflammation, red blood cells and cellular debris

Differential diagnosis

- Dyskaryosis and invasive carcinoma may appear similar due to nuclear enlargement and prominent nucleoli
- In repair, there is uniformity of nuclear features across a group of cells with maintained uniform chromatin pattern, unlike dyskaryosis/carcinoma

Further investigations

- Usually, the diagnosis of repair is straightforward
- Occasionally, particularly in the presence of heavy inflammation, distinction from dyskaryosis or worse may be difficult and a borderline category of reporting justified, with repeat sampling and/or biopsy depending on the clinical setting

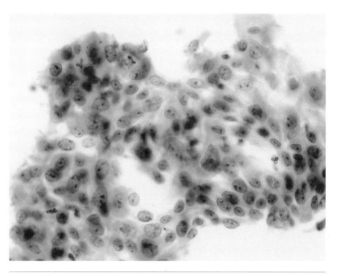

Fig. 2.71[†] Repair changes in a flat sheet of metaplastic squamous cells. Note nuclear enlargement and prominent nucleolation but with even chromatin and maintenance of polarity.

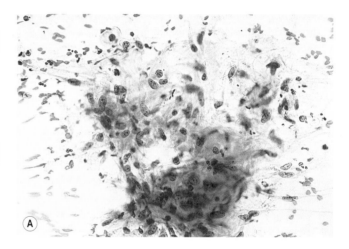

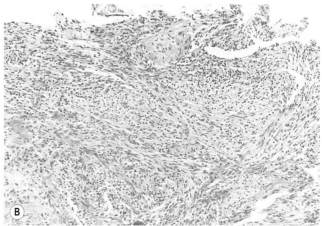

Fig. 2.72[†] (A) Repair changes in stromal cells in a cervical smear. Note elongation of nuclei but with even chromatin and indistinct cell borders. (B) Subsequent biopsy reveals immature granulation tissue.

Cervical sample adequacy

Conventional/direct smears

- Clearly displayed epithelial cellular material covering at least ≥ one-third of the cover-slipped area

Liquid-based cytology samples (Figs 2.73, 2.74)

- The Bethesda System: ≥ 5000 cells/sample
- In the UK, currently no nationally agreed criteria but likely to be based on a quantitative assessment of cell numbers
- Although, with any numerical system, strict objective criteria may not be applied to every case due to cellular clustering, atrophy and cytolysis requiring a degree of subjective judgement too

Reasons for inadequate samples

- Insufficient epithelial material due to poor sampling/poor transfer of material onto the slide (the latter in direct smears)
- Air-drying and/or cornflake artefact (direct smears)
- Excess of neutrophils obscuring the underlying cell morphology
- Excess of blood and mucus obscuring the underlying cell morphology
- Excess of bacteria ± cytolysis

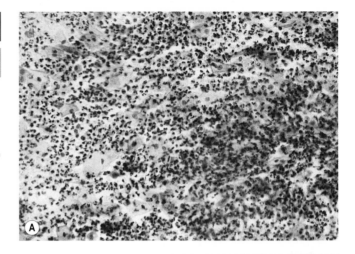

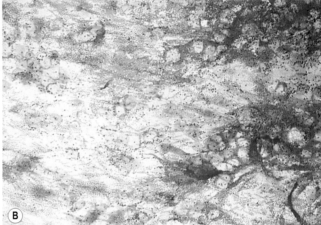

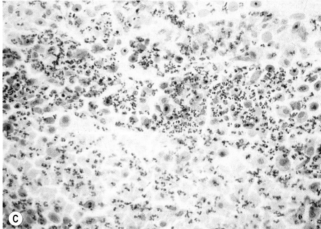

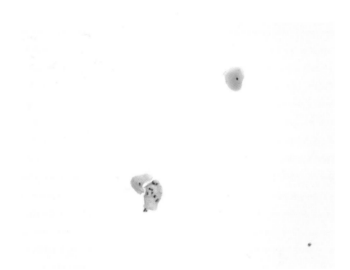

Fig. 2.73 Inadequate hypocellular sample.

Fig. 2.74[†] Unsatisfactory samples due to: (A) an excess of polymorphs, (B) an excess of blood in a direct/conventional smear. (C) An unsatisfactory post-menopausal sample due to an excess of acute inflammatory cells and small numbers of diagnostic epithelial cells.

Cytology of CIN and cervical squamous cancer

- Invasive squamous cell carcinoma is preceded by pre-cancerous changes in the epithelium of the transformation zone: cervical intraepithelial neoplasia (CIN)
- Histologically, CIN is subdivided into CIN I, II and III, reflecting increasing atypia of the epithelial thickness from the basal third (CIN I) to full thickness (CIN III)
- Any grade of CIN may regress within 2 years of development but 30% of women with CIN III, if left untreated, may develop squamous cell carcinoma within 15 years

Dyskaryosis and abnormal chromatin (Figs 2.75–2.80)

- Cytological diagnosis of CIN lesions requires recognition of dyskaryotic/abnormal nuclei
- Abnormal chromatin pattern is the single most important discriminator in recognition of dyskaryotic cells
- Normal chromatin pattern is described as 'vesicular' and has fine and evenly distributed chromatin
- Abnormal chromatin is coarse, uneven and stippled
- Dyskaryotic nuclei may appear hyperchromatic but, particularly in LBC preparations, also hypochromatic (pale cell changes), both representing an abnormal spectrum of chromatin distribution

Other features of dyskaryotic cells

- The nuclear membrane may be irregularly thickened due to submembranous chromatin condensation
- In LBC preparation, nuclei may be three-dimensional with ridges and clefts ('squashed raisin' appearance)
- Variable nuclear enlargement ± bi- and multinucleation
- ± abnormalities in number and size of nucleoli

Grading of squamous dyskaryosis (Table 2.1)

- Grading was based on nuclear:cytoplasmic surface area ratio of dyskaryotic cells
- Recent morphometric data indicate mean nuclear:cytoplasmic diameter ratios are more robust discriminators
- The chromatin pattern and degree of hypo- and hyperchromasia do not influence the grading
- Comparison of grading systems shown in Table 2.1

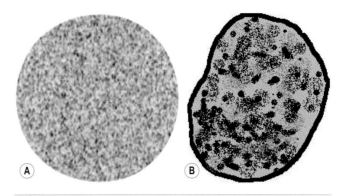

Fig. 2.75 (A) Even, finely stippled normal vesicular chromatin pattern. (B) Dyskaryotic abnormal chromatin pattern characterised by coarse and uneven stippling with irregular and thickened nuclear membrane.

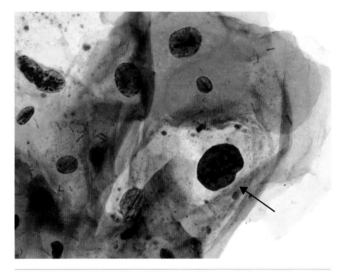

Fig. 2.76 Hyperchromatic dyskaryotic nucleus (*arrow*).

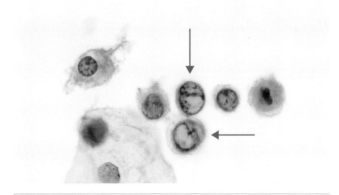

Fig. 2.77 Pale cell dyskaryosis (*arrows*).

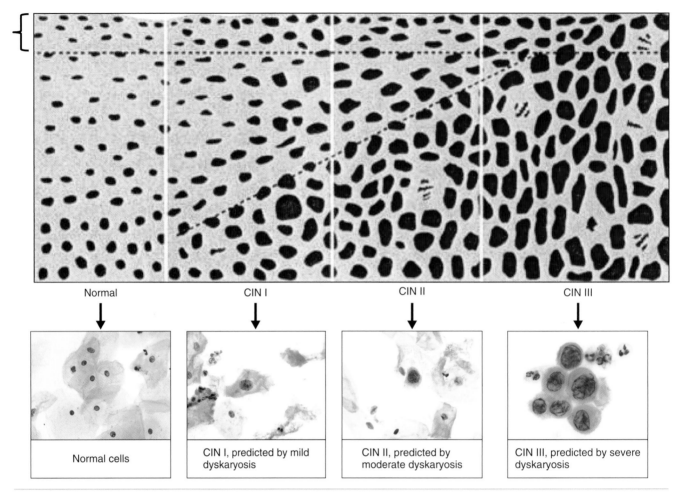

Normal CIN I CIN II CIN III

Normal cells | CIN I, predicted by mild dyskaryosis | CIN II, predicted by moderate dyskaryosis | CIN III, predicted by severe dyskaryosis

Fig. 2.78 Note: Even in CIN I, subtle cytological abnormalities are noted in the superficial layers (*bracketed*) allowing cytological prediction of the grade of CIN by microscopic examination of these superficial layers.

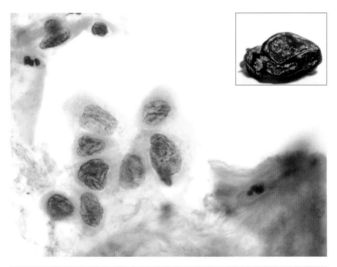

Fig. 2.79 Severely dyskaryotic cells with nuclei similar to a 'crushed raisin' (*inset*).

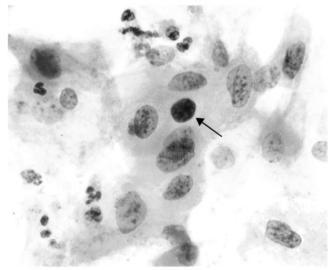

Fig. 2.80 Dyskaryosis. Note variation in chromasia of cells with, in arrowed cell, dense hyperchromasia evident.

Table 2.1 Comparison of different terminology systems for abnormal cervical cytology

BSCC 1986	BAC and NHSCSP new terminology (2013)	The Bethesda System 2001	ECTP terminology	AMBS 2004
Negative	Negative	Negative for intraepithelial lesion or malignancy	Within normal limits	Negative
Inadequate	Inadequate	Unsatisfactory for evaluation	Unsatisfactory due to…	Unsatisfactory
Borderline nuclear change	Borderline change, in squamous cells	Atypical squamous cells of (ASC-US) undetermined significance	Koilocytes (without changes suggestive of intraepithelial neoplasia) Squamous cell changes (not definitely neoplastic but merit early repeat)	Possible low-grade squamous intraepithelial lesion
		ASC-H (cannot exclude HSIL)		Possible high-grade sqamous intraepithelial lesion
	Borderline change in endocervical cells	Atypical endocervical, endometrial or glandular (NOS or specify in comments)	Atypical glandular cells (quality)	Atypical endocervical cells of undetermined significance
		Atypical endocervical or glandular cells, favour neoplastic		Atypical glandular cells of undetermined significance
Mild dyskaryosis	Low-grade dyskaryosis (includes all cases of koilocytosis provided that no high-grade dyskaryosis is present)	Low-grade squamous intra-epithelial lesion (LSIL)	Mild dysplasia (CIN I)	Low-grade squamous intraepithelial lesion
Moderate dyskaryosis	High-grade dyskaryosis (moderate)	High-grade squamous intra-epithelial lesion (HSIL)	Moderate dysplasia (CIN II)	High-grade squamous intraepithelial lesion
Severe dyskaryosis	High-grade dyskaryosis (severe)	HSIL	1. Severe dysplasia (CIN III) 2. Carcinoma in situ (CIN III)	
Severe dyskaryosis? invasive	High-grade dyskaryosis? Invasive squamous cell carcinoma	Squamous cell carcinoma	1. Severe dysplasia? invasive 2. Invasive squamous cell carcinoma	Squamous cell carcinoma
? Glandular neoplasia	? Glandular neoplasia Endocervical Non-cervical	1. Endocervical carcinoma in situ 2. Adenocarcinoma Endocervical Endometrial Extrauterine NOS	Adenocarcinoma AIS Endocervical Endometrial Extrauterine NOS	Endocervical adenocarcinoma in situ Adenocarcinoma

BAC, British Association of Cytopathology; ECTP, European Commission Training Programme; AMBS, Australian Modified Bethesda System. (Reproduced with permission of Wiley-Blackwell, from Denton KJ, Herbert A, Turnbull LS, et al. The revised BSCC terminology for abnormal cervical cytology. Cytopathology 2008; 19:137–57.)

Mild dyskaryosis/low-grade dyskaryosis (Figs 2.81–2.88)

- Abnormal chromatin patterns as outlined previously
- Nuclear:cytoplasmic diameter ratio increased but < 50%
- Typically mature superficial and intermediate cells
- ± koilocytes: may have near-normal nuclei and are reported as low-grade dyskaryosis provided no high-grade cells are identified
- If molecular testing for high-risk HPV is being employed in the sample, do not report the morphological presence of koilocytes in the text as this may introduce confusion depending on the HPV result

Differential diagnosis

- Reactive/inflammatory changes although nuclei may be enlarged and ± irregular in outline, chromatin pattern is normal
- Navicular cells may mimic koilocytes
- Glycogen in the former helps distinction

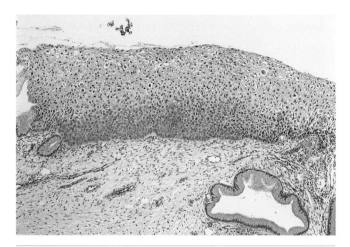

Fig. 2.81[†] Section of cervical squamous mucosa showing CIN I. There is crowding of the cells in the basal third of the epithelium, so that the basal layer is no longer distinct. Nuclei in this area are enlarged and hyperchromatic and show some loss of polarity. The middle and upper layers show persistence of nuclear enlargement, but the changes are less marked and the epithelium matures normally. Koilocytes are visible towards the surface (H&E).

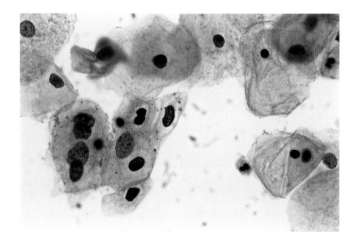

Fig. 2.82[†] Low-grade (mild) dyskaryosis. Nuclear enlargement and hyperchromasia are seen in the enlarged nuclei on the left of the field. The small abnormal pyknotic nuclei have visible chromatin structure and amount to borderline nuclear change. The binucleated cells and cytoplasmic clearing may indicate HPV infection but do not amount to classic koilocytosis.

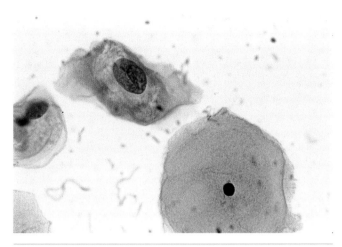

Fig. 2.83[†] Low-grade dyskaryosis (mild dyskaryosis and koilocytosis). The cell in the upper part of the field is a koilocyte with a broad cytoplasmic perinuclear halo and condensed cytoplasm at its margin. The nucleus has a simple fold and slight coarsening of the chromatin but is grossly enlarged, amounting to mild dyskaryosis.

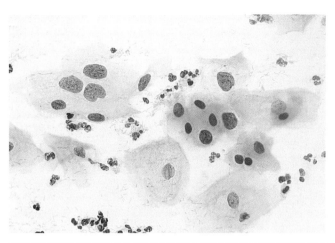

Fig. 2.86[†] Low-grade (mild) dyskaryosis. Abnormal chromatin pattern and irregularity of nuclear outline are seen in the upper part of the field, as well as nuclear enlargement and hyperchromasia.

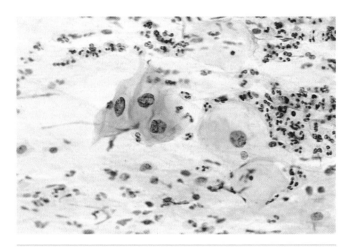

Fig. 2.84[†] Low-grade (mild) dyskaryosis. The abnormal chromatin pattern clearly distinguishes the low-grade dyskaryosis from inflammatory nuclear change.

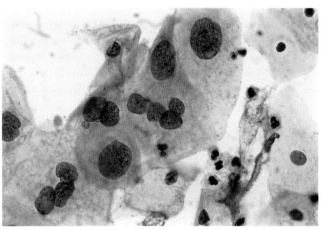

Fig. 2.87[†] Low-grade (mild) dyskaryosis. The dyskaryotic cells show varying nuclear enlargement, abnormal chromatin pattern, mild irregularities of outline and multinucleation. Normal superficial and intermediate squamous cells are seen on the right of the field.

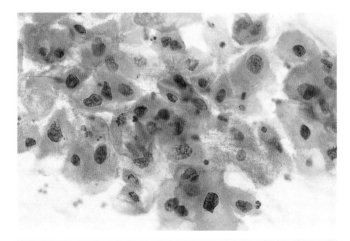

Fig. 2.85[†] Low-grade (mild) dyskaryosis. A florid example, showing some binucleation and orangeophilia of keratin associated in this case with HPV infection.

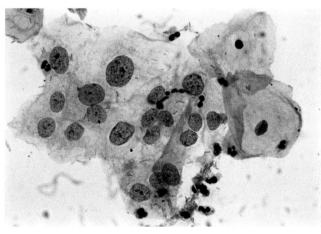

Fig. 2.88[†] Low-grade (mild) dyskaryosis. The abnormal nuclei are not hyperchromatic, and are an example of 'pale' dyskaryosis.

Moderate and severe/high-grade dyskaryosis (Figs 2.89–2.105)

- Abnormal chromatin pattern as previously described
- Nuclear:cytoplasmic diameter ratios increased in small/immature cells and >50%:
  - distinguishing between moderate and severe may be difficult
  - if nuclear:cytoplasmic ratio >50% but <75% = moderate, if >75% = severe
- Other features include:
  - ± irregular nuclear membranes
  - ± three-dimensional complex membrane folding
  - ± bizarrely shaped keratinocytes, including spindle and tadpole types and some necrosis, indicating at least keratinising CIN III (see also Squamous cell carcinoma section)
  - ± pale cell/hypochromatic severe dyskaryosis
  - ± prominent nucleoli
  - ± small cell variant (same size or smaller than neutrophils)
  - ± bland cell variant (described in ThinPrep) characterised by chaotic aggregation of severely dyskaryotic cells with subtle chromatin abnormalities that may be mistaken for endocervical metaplastic groups

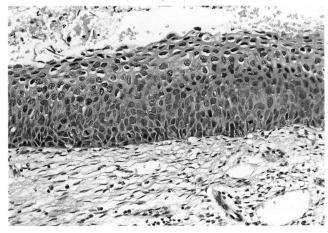

Fig. 2.89[†] Section of cervical squamous mucosa showing CIN II. The squamous cells show nuclear crowding, enlargement, hyperchromasia and disorganisation extending into the middle third. Above this, the cells are maturing, but abnormality persists to the surface.

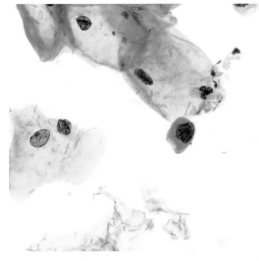

Fig. 2.90 Single moderate dyskaryotic cell.

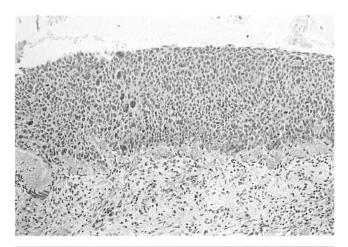

Fig. 2.91[†] Section of cervical squamous mucosa showing CIN III. There is complete replacement of normal squamous cells by crowded abnormal cells with marked nuclear pleomorphism, hyperchromasia and loss of polarity. No evidence of cell maturation can be seen. Note that the basement membrane is intact. The underlying stroma shows non-specific inflammation and marked vascular engorgement.

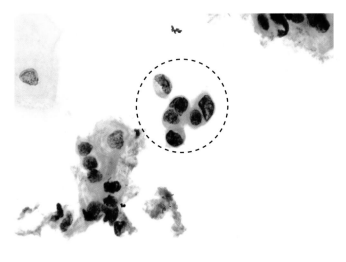

Fig. 2.92 Severely dyskaryotic cells (circled area). Note irregular nuclear membranes and variation in chromatin pattern.

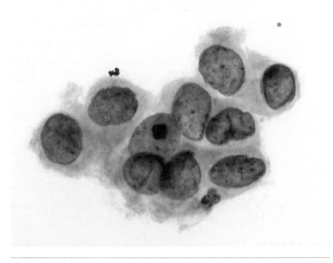

Fig. 2.93 Pale cell, severely dyskaryotic cells. Abnormal chromatin pattern and irregular nuclear membranes still evident.

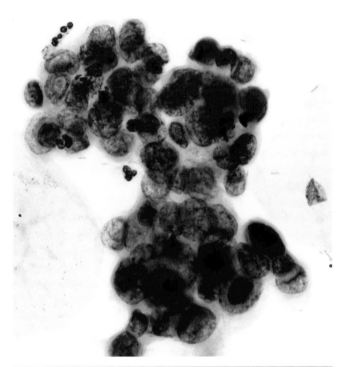

Fig. 2.94 Microbiopsy of severe dyskaryosis.

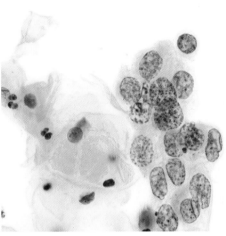

Fig. 2.97 Microbiopsy of severe dyskaryosis. Note loss of polarity, abnormal chromatin pattern and irregular nuclear contours of the cells.

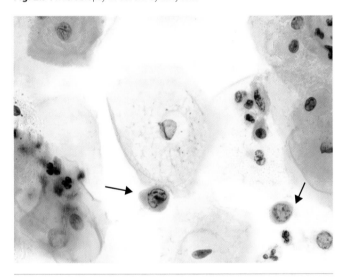

Fig. 2.95 Scattered small severely dyskaryotic cells (arrows).

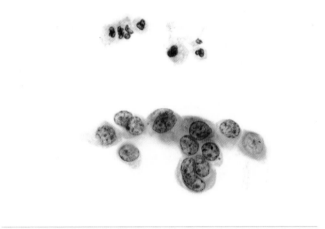

Fig. 2.98 Severe dyskaryosis. In this example, the abnormal cells are larger than adjacent neutrophils located above.

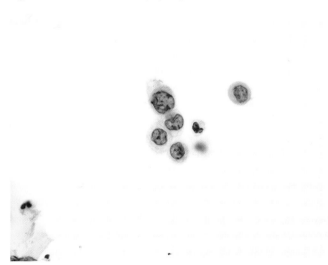

Fig. 2.96 Loosely cohesive sheet of severely dyskaryotic cells with variable chromasia.

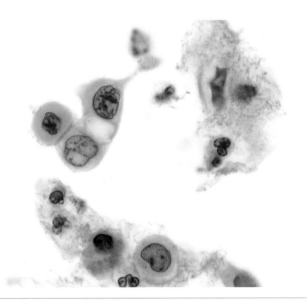

Fig. 2.99 Severely dyskaryotic cells. Note the keratinised severely dyskaryotic cell at the top left.

Fig. 2.100 Severely dyskaryotic cells with keratinisation from a case of keratinising CIN III.

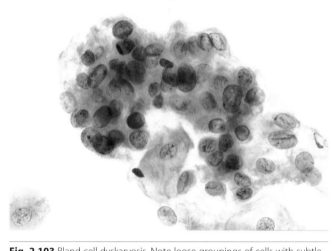

Fig. 2.103 Bland cell dyskaryosis. Note loose groupings of cells with subtle variation in nuclear size and chromatin pattern.

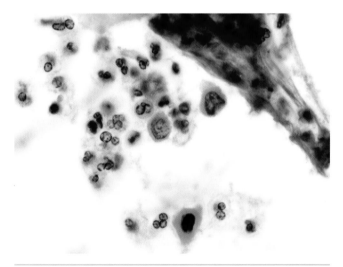

Fig. 2.101 Small severely dyskaryotic cells keratinised in this case, of similar size to surrounding neutrophils.

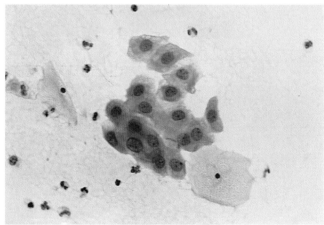

Fig. 2.104† Immature squamous metaplasia, to be distinguished from high-grade (moderate) dyskaryosis. The uniformity of nuclear size and texture, the abundant cytoplasm and pattern of metaplastic cells is characteristic of these normal cells.

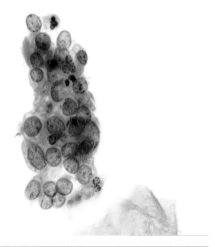

Fig. 2.102 Bland cell dyskaryosis. Chaotic aggregates of cells with a low power glandular arrangement with subtle chromatin abnormalities.

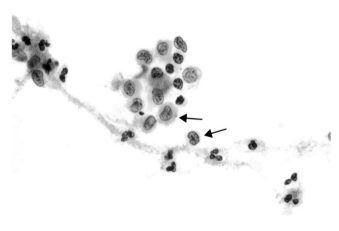

Fig. 2.105 Histiocytes may be mistaken as severely dyskaryotic cells, although notice of reniform nuclei (*arrows*) with delicate cytoplasm should allow correct distinction.

Differential diagnosis (Figs 2.106–2.114)

- Immature squamous metaplastic cells
  - nuclear:cytoplasmic ratio increased but chromatin pattern is normal
- Histiocytes
  - reniform nuclei and delicate cytoplasm distinct from severe dyskaryosis
- Endometrial cells secondary to IUD changes
  - look for three-dimensional clusters of endometrial cells with similar nuclear features. Chromatin, whilst dark, appears 'featureless'
- Follicular cervicitis
  - dispersed lymphocytes may simulate severe dyskaryosis. Coarse lymphocyte chromatin and tingible body macropahges allows correct diagnosis

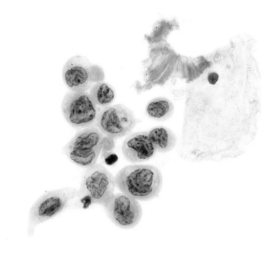

Fig. 2.108 Severely dyskaryotic cells with abnormal nuclei and dense cytoplasm, compared to histiocytes in Fig. 2.109.

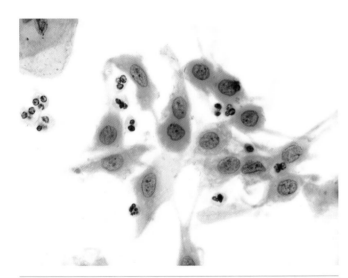

Fig. 2.106 Immature metaplastic cells need to be distinguished from high-grade/moderate dyskaryosis. Uniformity of nuclear size and chromatin texture is reassuring.

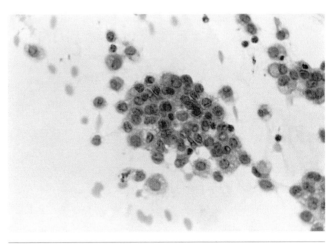

Fig. 2.109† Histiocytes: differential diagnosis of high-grade dyskaryosis. Reniform nuclei, nucleoli, vacuolated cytoplasm and size are features which aid in the identification of histiocytes. These features are seen more clearly in the single cells surrounding the cluster.

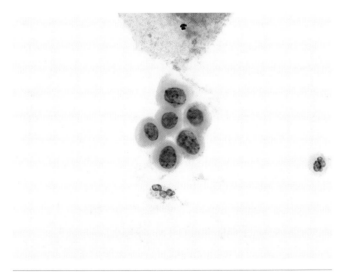

Fig. 2.107 Moderate dyskaryosis. Note irregularity of chromatin pattern and nuclear membranes compared to immature metaplastic population in Fig. 2.106.

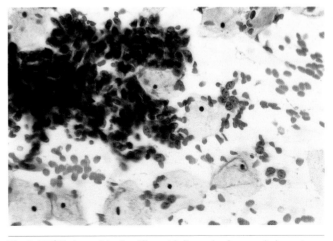

Fig. 2.110† Endometrial cells: differential diagnosis of severe dyskaryosis. Exfoliated endometrial cells tend to form three-dimensional clusters. Distinction of such clusters from fragments of small cell CIN III or invasive carcinoma may require careful scrutiny of the whole sample for additional diagnostic features.

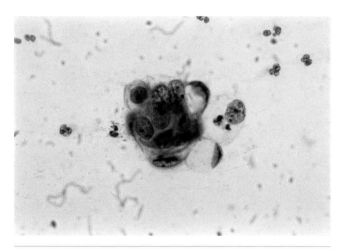

Fig. 2.111[†] Endometrial cells in the sample of an IUD user: differential diagnosis of high-grade dyskaryosis. This small three-dimensional group of endometrial cells with characteristic cytoplasmic vacuolation is easily identified, but see Fig. 2.112.

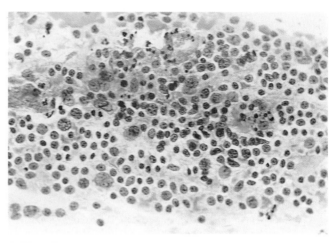

Fig. 2.113[†] Follicular (lymphocytic cervicitis): differential diagnosis of high-grade dyskaryosis. The very coarse chromatin pattern of small lymphocytes and the presence of tingible body macrophages are important features in the identification of these cells.

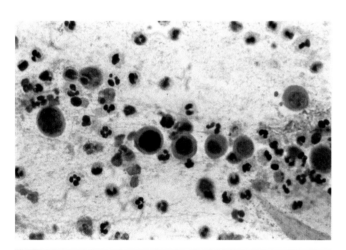

Fig. 2.112[†] Endometrial cells in the smear of an IUD user, same sample as Fig. 2.111. The single cells with high nuclear/cytoplasmic ratios and hyperchromatic nuclei were thought probably to be degenerate endometrial cells, but exclusion of high-grade squamous dyskaryosis was not possible. The patient subsequently underwent a cone biopsy and diagnostic uterine curettage. No neoplastic pathology was demonstrated in either specimen.

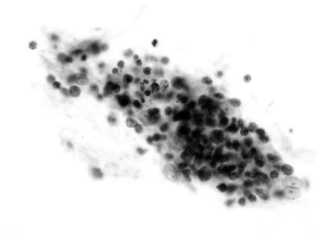

Fig. 2.114[†] Clustered cells in follicular cervicitis in a liquid-based preparation. Note the tingible body macrophages above the centre of the field.

Invasive squamous cell carcinoma of the cervix

- Invasive squamous cell carcinoma develops when neoplastic squamous cells breach the basement membrane and infiltrate into cervical stroma
- Common variants include large cell keratinising and non-keratinising types
- Rarer forms include basaloid and small cell/undifferentiated subtypes and adenosquamous
- FIGO staging is important, as women with 1A1 disease may be treated by cervical cone excision as risk of spread beyond the cervix is very low

Cytological findings (Figs 2.115–2.123)

- Parodoxically, the cytology of high-grade pre-invasive CIN lesions may be easier to diagnose than frank malignancy
- Early invasion arising on a background of CIN III may not be predicted by cytology if only the surface severely dyskaryotic cells are sampled
- In advanced disease, ulceration and necrosis may obscure cytomorphology of diagnostic tumour cells
- Features which suggest invasion include:
  - very large numbers of severely dyskaryotic cells
  - extreme variation in size and shape of severely dyskaryotic cells including small cell types
  - extreme margination of nuclear chromatin producing areas of lucency/clearing between chromatin aggregates ('windowing')
  - large numbers of microbiopsies of abnormal cells
  - large irregular macronucleoli
  - intense keratinisation of cells as well as dense anucleate fragments on a background of severe dyskaryosis
  - bizarrely shaped dyskaryotic cells: 'tadpole' and 'fibre cells'
  - background tumour diathesis in advanced disease reflecting ulceration and necrosis of tumour

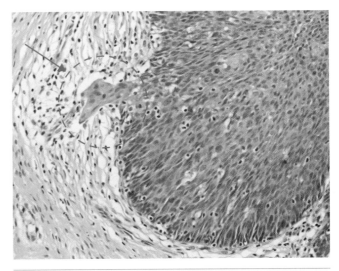

Fig. 2.115 Note the invasive squamous cell carcinoma tumour bud that has just breached the basement membrane of an endocervical crypt containing CIN III (*arrow*).

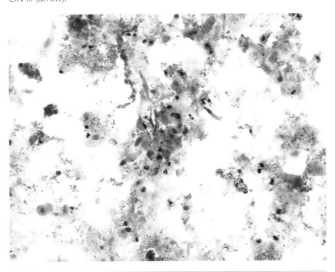

Fig. 2.116 Tumour diathesis. Note the necrotic granular background. In this case, viable tumour cells are not identified, although degenerate forms are present, underscoring the difficulty in cytological diagnosis in advanced cervical cancers.

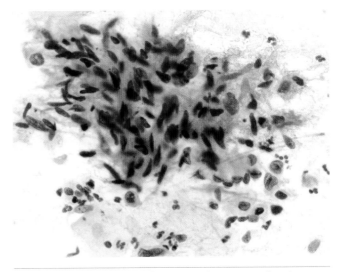

Fig. 2.117 Atypical spindle cells from a case of squamous cell carcinoma.

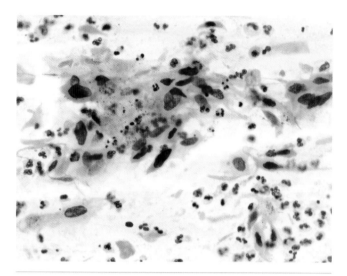

Fig. 2.118 Spindle cells from a case of squamous cell carcinoma of the cervix.

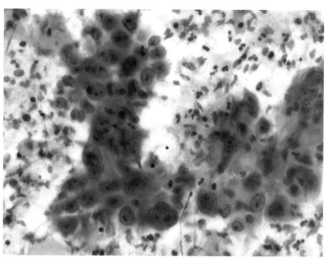

Fig. 2.121 Macronucleoli. Solid sheet of non-keratinising squamous cell carcinoma with macronucleoli.

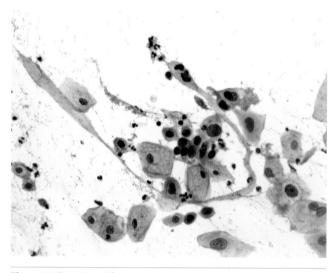

Fig. 2.119 Tadpole cell from a case of invasive squamous cell carcinoma.

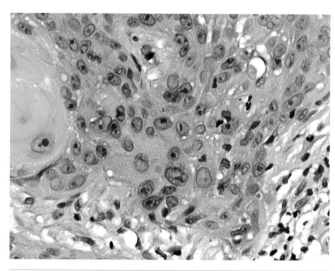

Fig. 2.122 Corresponding histology of invasive squamous cell carcinoma with macronucleoli from the case in Fig. 2.123.

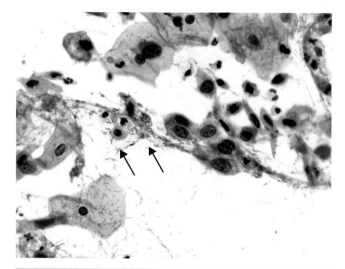

Fig. 2.120 Severely dyskaryotic cells along with scattered tadpole cells (*arrows*) from a case of cervical squamous cell carcinoma.

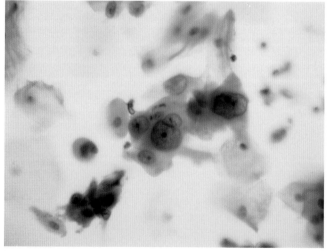

Fig. 2.123[†] Poorly differentiated squamous cell carcinoma. The cells at the centre of the field have non-keratinised cytoplasm but some are of irregular shape. There is focal condensation of chromatin on the nuclear membranes and the nuclei have prominent nucleoli. Such cells should be distinguished from non-neoplastic cells seen in metaplasia or 'repair' change.

Diagnostic pitfalls for cytology of squamous cell carincoma (Figs 2.124–2.127)

Keratinising CIN III

- Characterised by CIN III with surface keratinisation
- Cytology characterised by exfoliation of bizarre severely dyskaryotic cells including tadpole and spindle cell forms
- Coexistent necrotic debris often noted
- May be indistinguishable from well-differentiated squamous cell carcinoma cytologically
- These patients require urgent referral to colposcopy
- On histology, 50% are associated with invasive early squamous cell carcinoma on examination of multiple levels of the cervical cone biopsy samples

Repair and regeneration

- Immature squamous metaplastic cells may appear atypical due to macronucleoli and cellular enlargement
- Always screen for more typical severe dyskaryosis in problematic cases
- Occasionally, cells from non-keratinising squamous cell carcinoma may be misdiagnosed as repair if atypical nuclear features not recognised

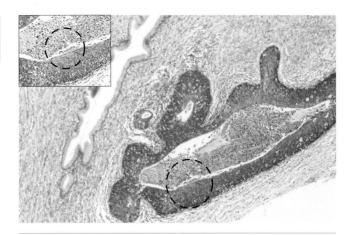

Fig. 2.125 Keratinising CIN III invading endocervical crypt. Circled area shown as inset.

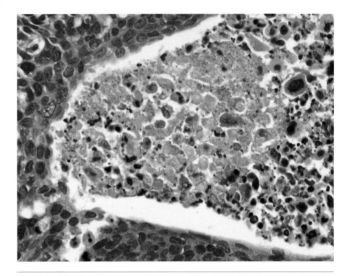

Fig. 2.126 Higher power magnification of Fig. 2.125 showing necrosis and intermingled CIN III cells.

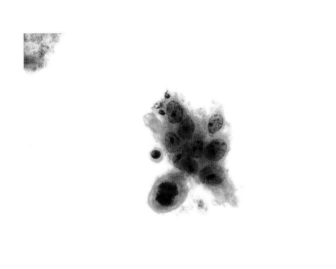

Fig. 2.124 Atypical squamous cells simulating repair changes from a 28-year-old woman with poorly differentiated squamous cell carcinoma.

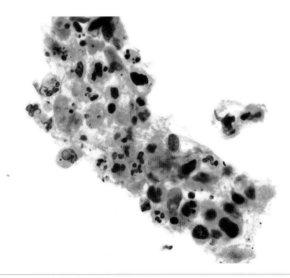

Fig. 2.127 Necrosis and severe dyskaryosis on cytology sample from the same patient as in Figs 2.125 and 2.126.

Borderline nuclear changes in cervical cytology (Figs 2.128–2.136)

'Borderline change' describes morphological cell changes which fall short of unequivocal dyskaryosis.

- It is a poorly reproducible category
- May reflect inflammatory reactive metaplastic or normal processes
- It should be subdivided into borderline (squamous) or borderline (endocervical)
- A small percentage of borderline (squamous) may be associated with underlying ≥ CIN II
- Squamous cells showing borderline changes from a distinct population that are different from surrounding cells
- The cells lack clear-cut evidence of koilocytes (otherwise classified as low-grade dyskaryosis)
- Borderline squamous cells may be binucleate and the nuclei may be enlarged with slightly irregular membranes
- The term 'borderline changes – high-grade dyskaryosis not excluded' (and which is similar to the Bethesda category 'atypical squamous cells suggesting high-grade squamous intraepithelial lesion (ASC-H)' is obsolete following use of high-risk HPV
- Endocervical cells may be reported as 'borderline' if they show some but not all of the features of CGIN, e.g.
  - three-dimensional groups with disorderly cell arrangements
  - coarse grainy chromatin

Management of borderline nuclear changes

- New UK NHSCSP recommendations advise high-risk HPV testing on borderline, including squamous or endocervical (as well as mildly dyskaryotic samples) with colposcopy referral only if positive
- Women with negative HPV testing results can be returned to normal recall

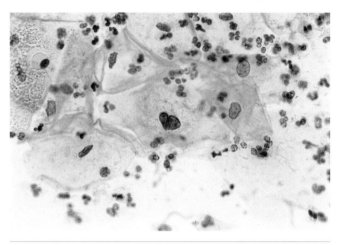

Fig. 2.128[†] Borderline nuclear change. In the centre is a binucleated cell with slight nuclear enlargement and hyperchromasia, but no abnormality of chromatin pattern. Compare with adjacent normal nuclei. The change may be HPV related.

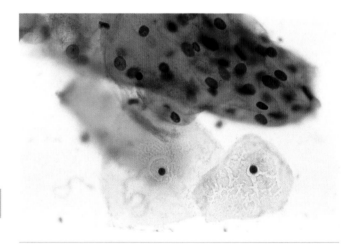

Fig. 2.129[†] Borderline nuclear change. This dyskeratotic cell group shows mild nuclear enlargement and anisonucleosis. Peripheral condensation of chromatin can be seen in some of the nuclei. Compare with adjacent superficial cell nuclei.

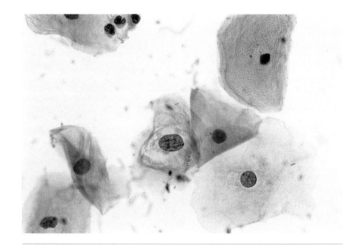

Fig. 2.130[†] HPV-related changes. The cell in the centre is a koilocyte with nuclear enlargement, longitudinal nuclear folding and slight coarsening of the chromatin pattern. The nuclear appearances may be regarded as 'borderline', but because of the presence of koilocytosis this cell would be graded as low-grade dyskaryosis in the BAC/NHSCSP 2013 terminology.

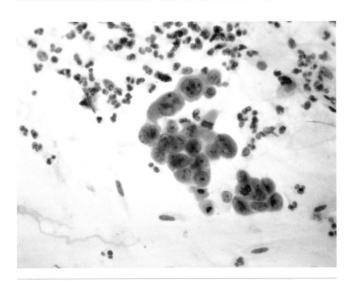

Fig. 2.131 Extreme regenerative atypia, including mitotic activity, in a patient's cervical sample taken 3 days post dilatation and curettage for intermenstrual bleeding. The sample was reported as borderline in immature metaplastic cells. A sample taken 6 months later was normal.

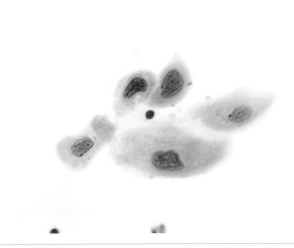

Fig. 2.132 Immature squamous metaplastic cells with subtle changes in chromatin and irregularity of nuclear contour. These were the only atypical cells in the entire sample and were reported as borderline.

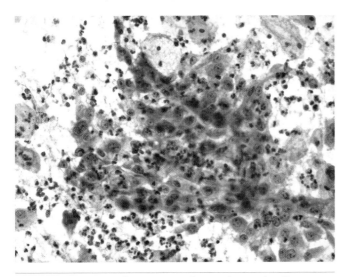

Fig. 2.133 Florid acute inflammation involving endocervical and immature squamous metaplastic cells.

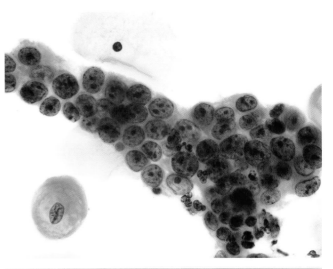

Fig. 2.134 Borderline change in endocervical cells. Note the grainy chromatin and prominent nucleoli without significant associated inflammation.

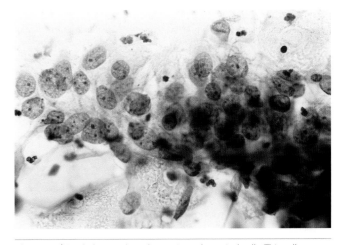

Fig. 2.135[†] Borderline nuclear change in endocervical cells. This cell group is three-dimensional with nuclear crowding. Where individual nuclei can be seen, there is anisonucleosis and mild coarsening of the chromatin.

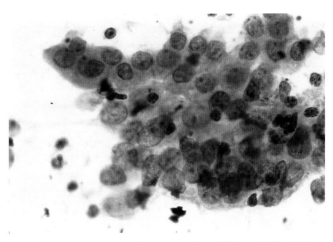

Fig. 2.136[†] Borderline nuclear change in endocervical cells. The endocervical cells in the upper part of the field appear normal but they merge with cells showing disorderly, crowded and enlarged nuclei with coarsening of the chromatin pattern.

Glandular neoplasms in cervical cytology

Primary cervical adenocarcinoma (Figs 2.137–2.144 and Table 2.2)

- Variable incidence worldwide
- Increased rates in UK, Australia and Europe, possibly reflecting increased diagnostic accuracy of screening programmes
- Risk factors include:
  - increased numbers of sexual partners
  - early age of intercourse
  - high-risk HPV 16 and 18 (++)
- Adenocarcinoma preceded by cervical glandular intra-epithelial (CGIN)/adenocarcinoma in situ (AIS)
- CGIN may be subdivided histologically into low and high grade
- Features of low-grade CGIN poorly reproducible and not well described

Cytologic appearances of CGIN

- Abnormal chromatin ranging from fine 'sanded' to coarse aggregated appearance
- Nuclei enlarged and irregular but may be significantly smaller
- Ragged cytoplasmic tags seen at the edge of cells, reflecting forced avulsion of the cell from the basement membrane by the sampling device
- Cells arranged in hyperchromatic crowded groups with chaotic 'supercrowded' honeycomb appearance
- 'Feathering': protruding bare elongated nuclei at different levels ± 'tipped' by wispy cytoplasm
- Pseudostratification: nuclei seen at different levels
- Rosette formation: rounded groups of cells with nuclear palisades at periphery and cytoplasm facing the centre
- Cytological features of CGIN and adenocarcinoma may overlap; features suggestive of invasion include tumour diathesis and abundant single dyskaryotic glandular cells in the background
- Uncommon subtypes of cervical adenocarcinoma may be difficult to categorise via site of origin, i.e. primary or extracervical and will need clinicoradiological correlation

Table 2.2 Comparison of BAC/NHSCSP terminology and the Bethesda System for reporting glandular abnormalities

BAC/NHSCSP terminology	The Bethesda System (TBS) (2001)
Negative	**WNL** Within normal limits Benign atypia
Borderline nuclear changes – endocervical (for endocervical prediction only)	**AGC NOS** (atypical glandular cells – not otherwise specified) (for abnormality from all sites)
?Glandular neoplasia Cervical glandular intraepithelial neoplasia (CGIN) and endocervical adenocarcinoma Non-cervical adenocarcinoma from all non-cervical sites	**AGC favour neoplasia** (from all sites)
	Adenocarcinoma in situ (AIS)
	Adenocarcinoma (from all sites)

BSCC: British Society for Clinical Cytology

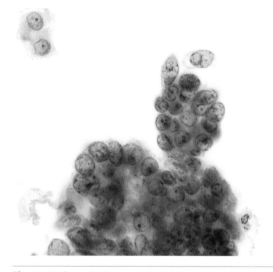

Fig. 2.137 Cervical adenocarcinoma. Enlarged and irregular endocervical nuclei with coarse chromatin.

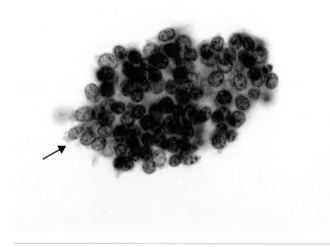

Fig. 2.138 Cervical adenocarcinoma: CGIN. Supercrowded dyskaryotic endocervical cells in which nuclei appear smaller than normal. Note cytoplasmic 'tags' at one end (*arrow*).

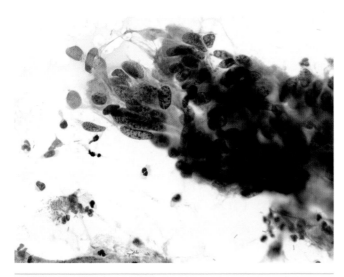

Fig. 2.139 Cervical adenocarcinoma: CGIN. Nuclear elongations and pseudostratification.

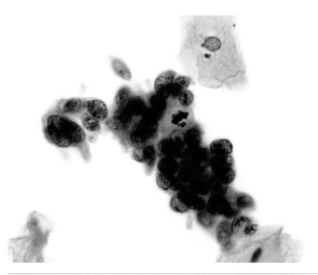

Fig. 2.142 Cervical adenocarcinoma: CGIN. Dyskaryotic endocervical group. Note mitotic figure, nuclear chromatin coarsening and cytoplasmic tags.

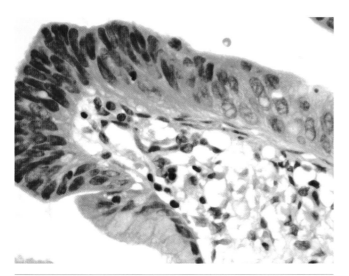

Fig. 2.140 Corresponding histology of high-grade CGIN case illustrated in Fig. 2.139.

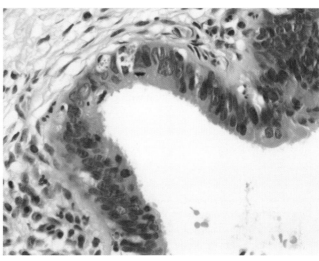

Fig. 2.143 Corresponding histology of high-grade CGIN as in Fig. 2.142. Note mitotic figures and apoptotic debris.

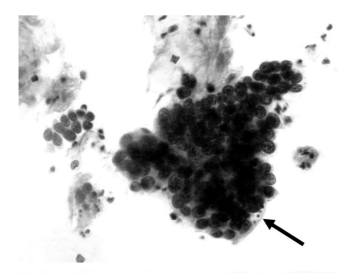

Fig. 2.141 Cervical adenocarcinoma: CGIN. Supercrowded dyskaryotic endocervical group with intermingled apoptotic debris (*arrow*).

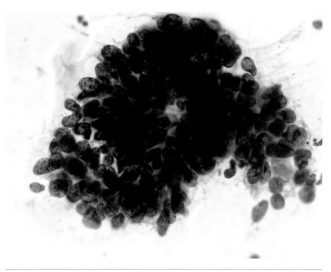

Fig. 2.144 Cervical adenocarcinoma: CGIN. Rosette formation.

Non-cervical adenocarcinoma (Figs 2.145–2.153)

- Endometrial carcinoma is the commonest glandular neoplasm diagnosed on cervical cytology samples
- This reflects incidental 'trapping' of exfoliated malignant cells from the endometrium during cervical sampling. Rarely the tumour may be directly sampled if the tumour has infiltrated the cervix, making distinction from CGIN very difficult
- Primary ovarian and fallopian tube carcinoma as well as extra-genital metastatic tumours are only rarely diagnosed
- The female genital tract is lined by Müllerian-type epithelium which can exhibit a wide range of phenotypes, e.g. endocervical, endometrioid, serous, making site of origin difficult to predict on cytology alone

Cytological appearances of endometrial adenocarcinoma

- Clusters, balls and single atypical glandular cells
- Enlarged and pleomorphic nuclei
- Raised nuclear:cytoplasmic ratios
- Variable chromatin pattern
- Enlarged and irregular nucleoli
- Variable cytoplasmic vacuolation with engulfed neutrophils
- ± mitotic activity
- ± diathesis
- Psammoma bodies with papillary serous differentiation

Further investigations

- Immunocytoclinical panels are helpful in distinguishing cervical from endometrial origin in adenocarcinomas
- Sample adequacy and capricious immunostaining are often limiting factors in cytology compared to histology biopsy material for immunohistochemistry
- Precise identification of site of origin requires clinicoradiological correlation and further histological sampling

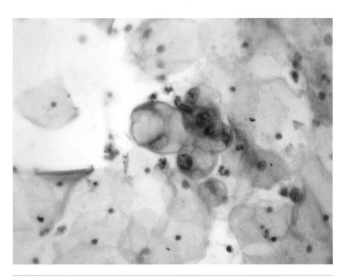

Fig. 2.145 Atypical endometrial cells from endometrial carcinoma.

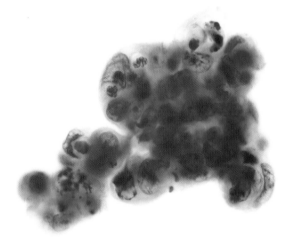

Fig. 2.146 Malignant endometrial cluster. Note engulfed cytoplasmic neutrophils.

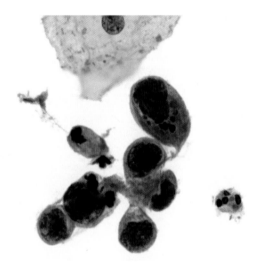

Fig. 2.147 Malignant glandular cells from endometrial adenocarcinoma.

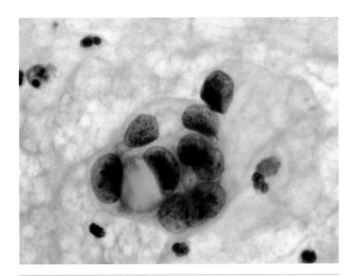

Fig. 2.148 Malignant glandular cluster from papillary serous carcinoma of endometrium.

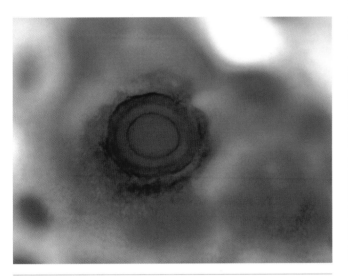

Fig. 2.149 Psammoma body from a case of papillary serous endometrial carcinoma.

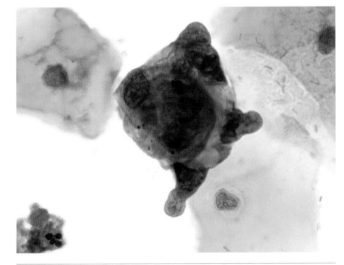

Fig. 2.150 Malignant glandular cluster from clear cell carcinoma of endometrium.

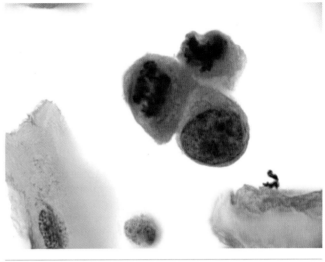

Fig. 2.151 Malignant glandular cluster from clear cell carcinoma of ovary. No discriminating features identified on Papanicolaou cytology to predict exact origin of these neoplastic glandular cells.

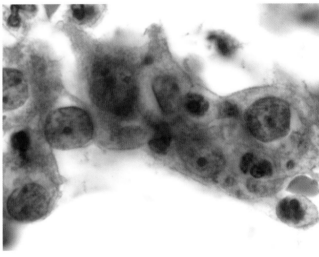

Fig. 2.152 Malignant pleomorphic glandular cells with eosinophilic macronucleoli. Histology was of clear cell carcinoma of endocervical origin.

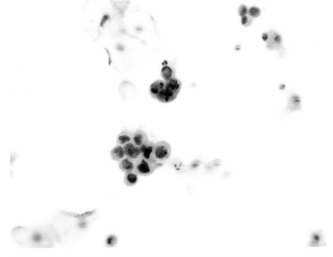

Fig. 2.153† Metastatic lobular carcinoma of the breast in cervical cytology. Clusters of small hyperchromatic cells with marked irregularity in nuclear contour and well-demarcated cytoplasm.

Diagnostic pitfalls of CGIN and adenocarcinoma (Figs 2.154–2.161 and Table 2.3)

- High-grade CIN (Table 2.3)
- Endometrial polyps and hyperplasia: the spectrum of morphology separating normal/atypical and malignant endometrial epithelium cytologically is poorly described. Endometrial cells in post-menopausal women should indicate gynaecological referral to exclude polyps or worse
- Occasionally, direct sampling of an endometrial polyp protruding into the endocervical canal can cause diagnostic difficulty due to the nature of the usual endometrial pseudostratified epithelium masquerading as CGIN. Close attention to the relative monotony of the cells with normal chromatin pattern and kidney-bean-shaped nuclei in at least some cells should aid correct interpretation of endometrial origin
- Endocervical polyps/endocervicitis: inflammatory changes may look worrying but chromatin and architectural features of CGIN are not evident
- Microglandular hyperplasia: cytological features are non-specific. Florid papillary forms may be confused with neoplastic change but chromatin is bland
- Arias–Stella changes: large cells with vacuolated cytoplasm, coarse chromatin and enlarged nucleoli may simulate endometrial neoplasia
- Lower uterine segment: noted more frequently post-conisation due to sampling of artificially shortened endocervical canal. Characterised by dense straight-sided tubular microbiopsies with peripheral palisading and associated delicate tangles of stromal cells
- Tuboendometrioid metaplasia/endometriosis: this is challenging cytologically as crowded and mitotically active groups may be sampled simulating CGIN
- Reserve cell hyperplasia: multinucleated cells with uniform nuclei and typically residual cytoplasmic tufts reflecting forced abrasion of these cells from the basement membrane

Table 2.3 Characteristics of cell clusters in crypt involvement in HG CIN versus CGIN

Crypt involvement	High-grade CIN	CGIN
Group contour	Thick steep-sided microbiopsies	Shallow clusters 2–3 cells deep
Group centre	Crowded, disordered	Residual honeycomb pattern
Group periphery	Haphazard cell arrangement	Palisading or feathering
Nuclear morphology	Variable shape, size, chromasia	Relatively even shape, size, chromasia
Nuclear membrane	Irregular thickness	Irregular thickness
Nuclear outline	Irregular, may be notched	Smooth round/oval
Chromatin	Usually fine granules	Coarse irregular sized granules
	May be maldistributed	Commonly evenly distributed
Nucleoli	Small	Prominent, may be large
Cytoplasm	Dense, smooth edged	Finely vacuolated, wispy edged

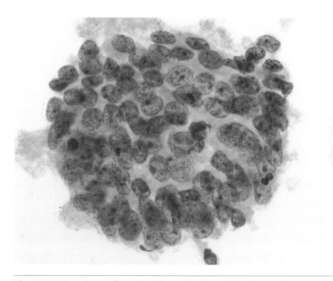

Fig. 2.154 Pseudostratified glandular epithelium originally condensed to reflect possible CGIN but subsequent histology was of a benign endometrial polyp. This is an example of direct sampling of pseudostratified epithelium from a benign endometrial polyp.

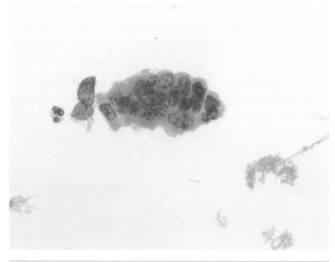

Fig. 2.155 Same case as in Fig. 2.154. Note apparent pseudostratification of glandular epithelium.

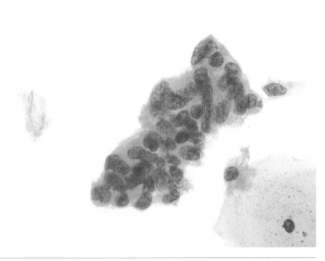

Fig. 2.156 Same case as in Fig. 2.154 and Fig. 2.155.

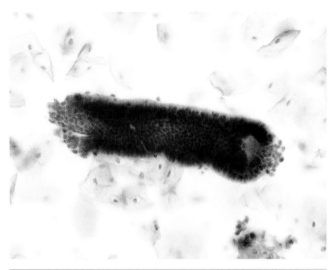

Fig. 2.159[†] Cervical cytology. LUS. Three-dimensional tube of small uniform cuboidal cells with well-demarcated outline and peripheral palisading in association with stromal fragments.

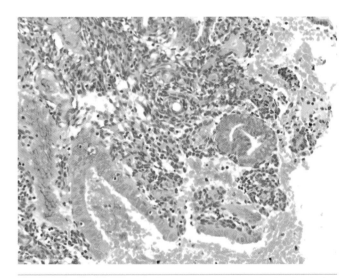

Fig. 2.157 This is the histology of the benign endometrial polyp that had prolapsed down the endocervical canal and had been directly sampled in Figs 2.154–2.156.

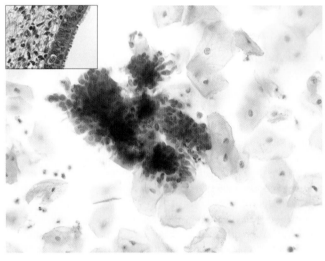

Fig. 2.160[†] Cervical cytology. Tubal metaplasia. Crowded cluster of glandular cells with a well-defined rim of cytoplasm with focal cilia. (Inset) Cervical biopsy. Tubal metaplasia in an endocervical crypt. Although nuclei are enlarged and chromatin pattern vesicular, ciliated cells are numerous.

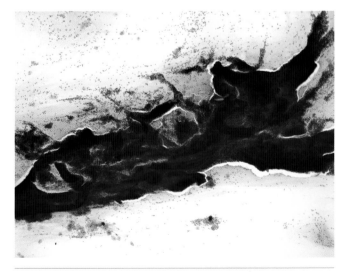

Fig. 2.158 Low-power view of lower uterine segment with well-defined tubular architecture.

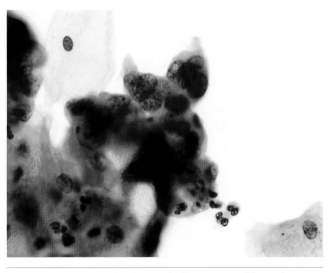

Fig. 2.161 Multinucleated endocervical cells in reserve cell hyperplasia.

Management of women with abnormal cervical cytology

Squamous dyskaryosis

- All women with predicted high-grade (moderate or severe) dyskaryosis (high-grade SIL Bethesda) should be referred for colposcopy
- Referral should be urgent for women with predicted invasive squamous cell carcinoma
- Management for the much more common cytological diagnosis of mild dyskaryosis and borderline changes (low-grade SIL/ASCUS) is less well defined
- High-risk HPV testing offers significant refinement in the management of women with low-grade dyskaryosis
- Only those women with low-grade changes who are high-risk HPV-positive need to be referred
- Women who are high-risk HPV-negative have the same risk of developing cancer in any given screening round as an age-matched woman with negative cytology and can be returned to routine recall

Glandular dyskaryosis

- Women with predicted endocervical dyskaryosis should be urgently referred for colposcopy
- Abnormalities may not always be visualised, as the pathological lesion may be high up the canal and not visualised under colposcopic direct view
- Discussion at the multidisciplinary team meeting should confirm the cytological diagnosis and the patient offered a cone biopsy or large loop excision as a minimum on which to diagnosis and treat CGIN
- Trachelectomy, in which the cervix is amputated with conservation of uterus and adnexa, may be performed to conserve fertility in early glandular and squamous carcinomas of the cervix
- Borderline changes in endocervical cells (AGUS) may be triaged with HR HPV testing analogous to borderline changes in squamous cells

Follow-up after treatment and HPV testing as 'test of cure'

- Women retain an increased risk of recurrent CIN and invasive squamous cell carcinoma after treatment of CIN, and follow-up is essential
- Previous UK guidance advised a 10-year follow-up for all women with treated ≥ CIN II and 2-year follow-up for all women with low-grade abnormalities
- Compliance issues and increased anxiety may occur with such lengthy follow-up

- Additional high-risk HPV testing is a potentially valuable test in this setting
- Current UK guidelines advocate HR HPV testing at 6 months post-treatment for all CIN lesions in women with negative/borderline or mild (low-grade) cytology, therefore so-called 'test of cure'
- If HR HPV testing is negative, the woman may be returned to normal routine recall
- HR HPV testing is NOT indicated following CGIN treatment as lesions may be high up in the canal and/or multifocal and not sampled adequately enough for viral testing
- Figure 2.162 outlines current UK HPV protocol for low-grade abnormalities and 'test of cure'

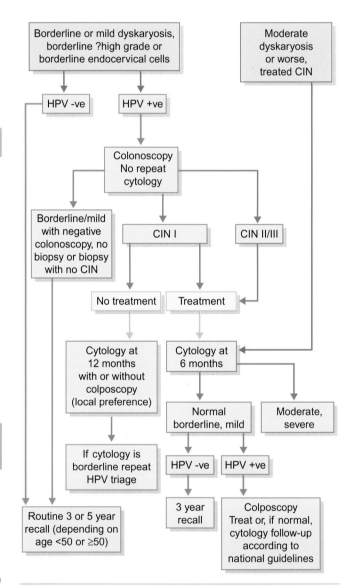

Fig. 2.162 NHSCSP HPV protocol chart.

Cytology of the vulva and vagina

The range of pathology is vast.

- It covers infections, inflammatory conditions, pre-invasive and invasive malignancy
- Women may be referred to dermatologists, gynaecologists or genitourinary physicians
- Cytology is of limited use technically due to scanty and air-dried samples and also because of overlying keratosis that may be scraped, which may not reflect the underlying disease
- Biopsy and histological assessment remains the gold standard

VIN, VAIN and invasive malignancy (Figs 2.163–2.172)

- Occasionally, samples are taken in the diagnosis and follow-up of vulval intraepithelial neoplasia (VIN) and vaginal intraepithelial neoplasia (VAIN) as well as invasive malignancy
- Cytological findings:
  - anucleate squames (non-specific)
  - parakeratotic cells (non-specific)
  - dyskaryotic cells: these are graded identically to those from CIN lesions
  - bizarre cells forms, e.g. tadpole and spindle cells and tumour diathesis can suggest invasive malignancy

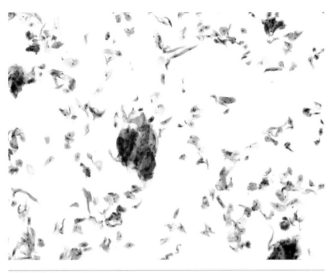

Fig. 2.164 An adequate vulval scrape sample.

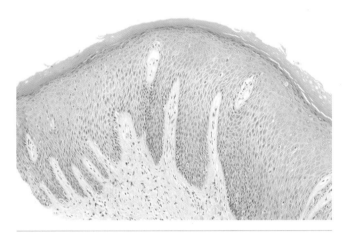

Fig. 2.165 Hyperkeratosis overlying vulval squamous hyperplasia.

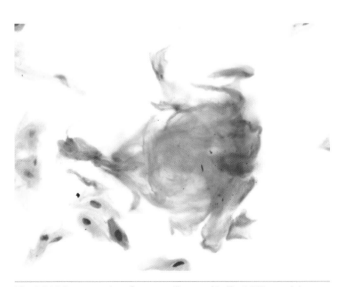

Fig. 2.163 An inadequate vulval scrape sample.

Fig. 2.166 Scrape cytology from case illustrated in Fig. 2.165 containing anucleate squames indicating hyperkeratosis.

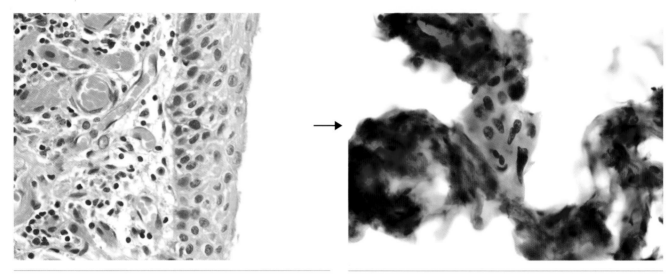

Fig. 2.167 Vulval biopsy with VIN I.

Fig. 2.170 Scrape cytology from case illustrated in Fig. 2.167 showing mild dyskaryosis.

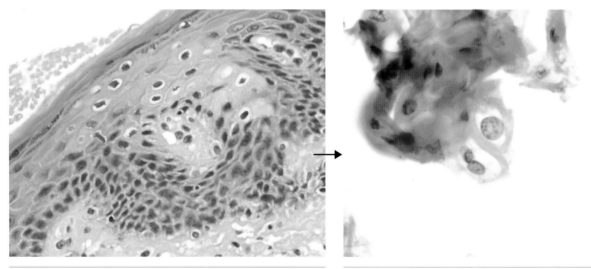

Fig. 2.168 Vulval biopsy showing HPV-related changes with overlying hyperkeratosis.

Fig. 2.171 Scrape cytology from case illustrated in Fig. 2.168 showing mild dyskaryosis and coexistant HPV-related changes.

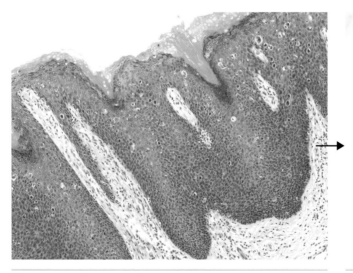

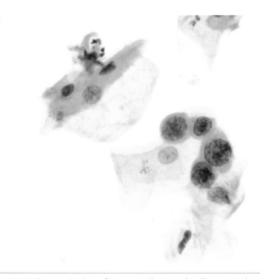

Fig. 2.169 Hyperkeratosis overlying VIN III.

Fig. 2.172 Scrape cytology from case illustrated in Fig. 2.169 showing severe dyskaryosis.

- Rare tumour of vulva and vagina
- Loose clusters of pleomorphic cells
- Nuclei of variable size and shape
- ± intranuclear pseudonuclear inclusions
- ± pigment
- Large cells with pale and indistinct cytoplasm
- Enlarged nuclei and nucleoli

- Histologically Paget's disease is similar to other sites where it occurs in the body
- Unlike breast, only 20–30% of vulval cases associated with underlying tumour
- If untreated may spread to perianal skin, vagina and cervix
- Large cells with pale and indistinct cytoplasm
- Enlarged nuclei and nucleoli

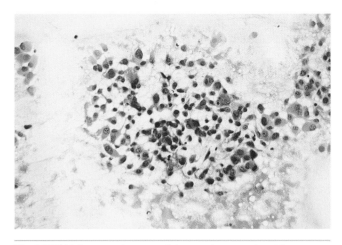

Fig. 2.175[†] Malignant melanoma cells in a touch preparation. A loose cluster of cells with marked pleomorphism. Brown pigment can be seen in some of the cells (PAP).

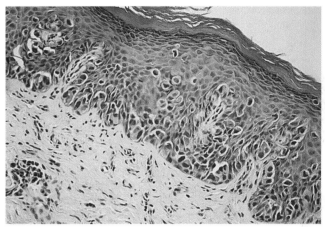

Fig. 2.176[†] A biopsy of Paget's disease of the vulva. The large Paget's cells are present singly and in clusters in the epidermis (H&E).

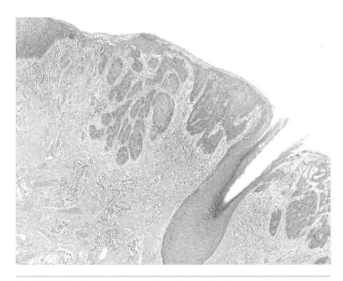

Fig. 2.173 Invasive squamous cell carcinoma of vulva.

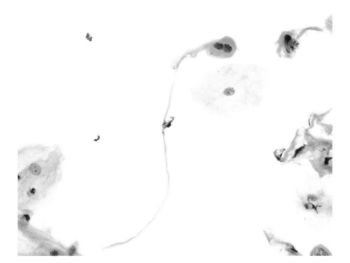

Fig. 2.174 Scrape cytology from case shown in Fig. 2.173 containing a large tadpole cell indicating invasive squamous cell carcinoma.

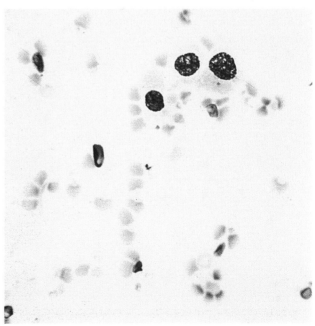

Fig. 2.177[†] A touch preparation from a case of Paget's disease of the vulva. Note the very scanty Paget's cells here in a small cluster. They are clearly adenocarcinoma cells with very abnormal chromatin distribution. The cytoplasm is pale staining and has an indistinct cell boundary (MGG).

Uterine cytology

This section will cover the role of direct sampling cytological methods in the diagnosis of uterine pathology (and is separate to endometrial appearances in cervical cytology samples already described).

Cytology plays a limited role, as biopsy, with histology ± taken under direct vision is the gold standard.

Nevertheless, direct cytological endometrial sampling with brush, suction or lavage techniques may be performed, although often limited by the small amount of tissue retrieved and the 'blind' nature of sampling.

Cytology of normal directly sampled endometrium (Figs 2.178, 2.179)

- Epithelial cell aggregates in tubular or sheet-like arrangements ± cohesion of endometrial stromal cells to the surface
- Small cells with scanty cytoplasm
- Uniform and round nuclei
- Fine granular chromatin with chromocentres
- Stromal clusters, often with nuclear overlapping, irregular outlines and protruding 'bulging' nuclei
- Epithelial and stromal cell appearances can vary with phase of cycle, with more abundant and vacuolated cytoplasm in secretory phase
- Squamous, metaplastic and endocervical cells from the cervix may be intermingled
- Inflammatory cells common
- ± multinucleated histiocytes in post-menopausal samples

Cytology of non-neoplastic conditions

- Usually, a specific diagnosis is not possible
- Biopsy and histology are the mainstay of diagnosis

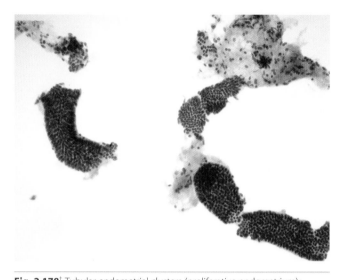

Fig. 2.178[†] Tubular endometrial clusters (proliferative endometrium): endometrial cells show scant cytoplasm and small nuclei. LBC direct endometrial sampling.

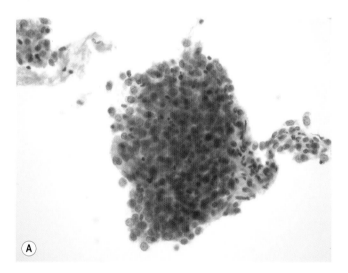

(A)

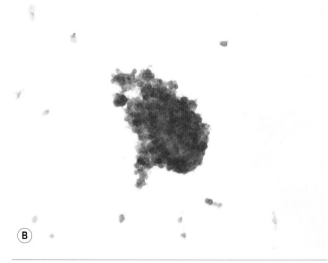

(B)

Fig. 2.179[†] (A) Stromal cluster on progesterone: obvious cytoplasm and isomorphic nuclei showing finely granular chromatin and small chromocentres. (B) CD10-positive immunostaining. LBC direct endometrial sampling.

Endometrial hyperplasia and/or malignancy (Figs 2.180–2.187)

Diagnosis is difficult, with histological assessment the gold standard.

Cytological features that may suggest hyperplasia and/or carcinoma include:

- Architectural
  - loss of polarity
  - papillary cell clusters
  - discohesive cells
- Cellular
  - high nuclear : cytoplasmic ratios
  - anisonucleosis
  - abnormal chromatin pattern
  - macronucleolation
  - irregular nuclear membranes
  - cell cannibalism
- Background
  - paucity of stromal cells
  - necrosis

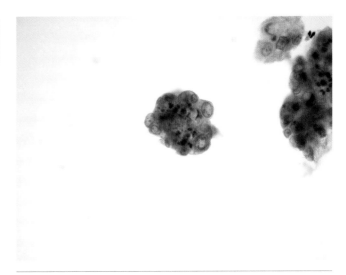

Fig. 2.180[†] Papillary aggregate. LBC direct endometrial sampling.

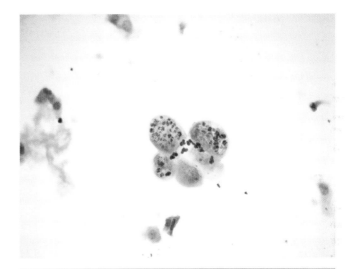

Fig. 2.181[†] Cell cannibalism; polymorphonuclear cells are engulfed in the cytoplasm of the tumour cells (neutrophilic emperipolesis). LBC direct endometrial sampling.

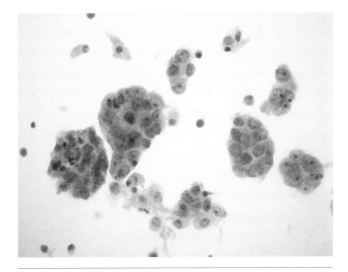

Fig. 2.182[†] Serous carcinoma. Because of the marked exfoliation of this histological subtype, the cytological specimens are rich in neoplastic cells which frequently show a papillary architecture (serous papillary carcinoma). LBC direct endometrial sampling.

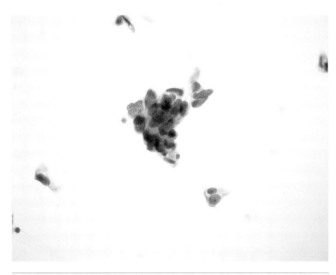

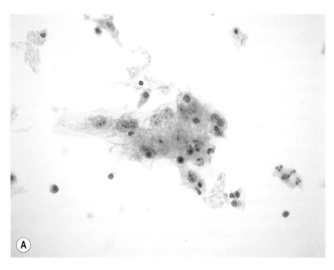

Fig. 2.183[†] Serous carcinoma. A small cluster showing prominent atypia with irregular size and shape of the cells, coarse and marginated chromatin, prominent nucleoli, irregular nuclear contour. LBC direct endometrial sampling.

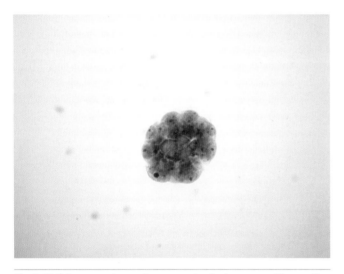

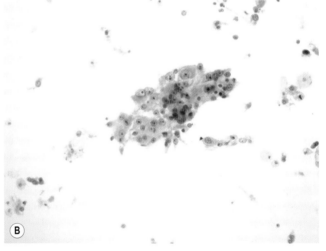

Fig. 2.186[†] Clear cell carcinoma. Neoplastic cells have abundant clear cytoplasm, large nuclei and prominent nucleoli. LBC direct endometrial sampling.

Fig. 2.184[†] Serous carcinoma. Psammoma bodies incorporated in a papilla. LBC direct endometrial sampling.

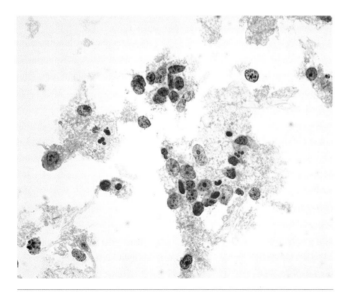

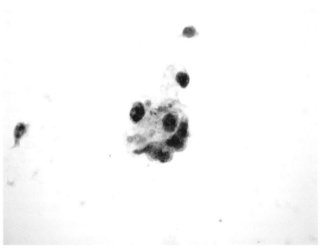

Fig. 2.185[†] Serous carcinoma. Single cells and bare nuclei. LBC direct endometrial sampling.

Fig. 2.187[†] Serous carcinoma. Positive p53 immunostaining. LBC direct endometrial sampling.

Ovarian cytology

Application of ovarian FNA is limited but may be useful in the diagnosis of non-neoplastic ovarian cysts.

Knowledge of aspiration route (transvaginal, transrectal or laparoscopic) is essential to recognise presence of normal-contaminant epithelial cells.

It is difficult to confidently distinguish primary ovarian carcinoma from metastatic to the ovary based solely on cytological findings.

Correlation with the clinicoradiological impression is essential for correct diagnosis ± immunocytochemistry.

Non-neoplastic ovarian cysts (Figs 2.188–2.194)

- Functional cysts
  - include follicular and luteal cysts
  - clear, cloudy or bloody fluid
  - tightly packed and single granulosa cells with longitudinal nuclear grooves and 'pepper-pot' chromatin evident
  - single granulosa cells may resemble macrophages
  - ± mitoses
  - ± pyknotic degenerate cells
  - luteinised cells are large and polygonal with abundant granular/foamy cytoplasm
  - chromatin is grainy with small but distinct nucleoli
- Endometriotic cysts
  - thick, dark brown fluid
  - numerous pigment-laden macrophages
  - background contains abundant debris
  - intact endometrial cells rarely seen
  - distinction from haemorrhagic functional cysts may be difficult in the absence of well-preserved endometrial cells

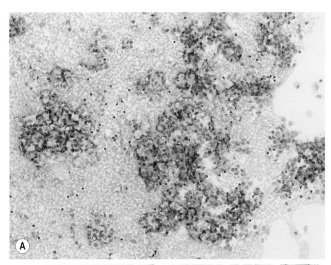

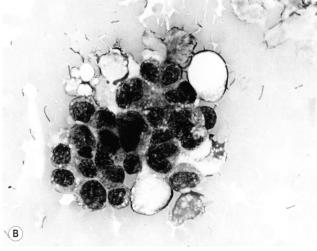

Fig. 2.188 Tightly packed clusters of follicular cells with round to oval nuclei and scanty cytoplasm. FNA of ovary (A, MGG; B, PAP).

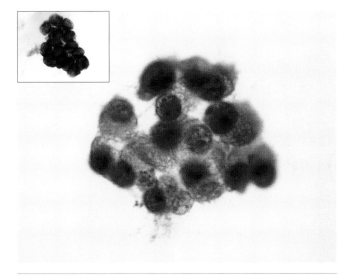

Fig. 2.189[†] Follicular cells with rounded nuclei containing multiple nucleoli and coarse chromatin rendering a pepper-pot appearance. FNA of ovary (PAP). (Inset) Inhibin positivity in functional epithelium.

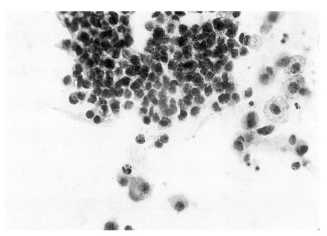

Fig. 2.190[†] Luteinised follicular cyst of ovary. A cluster of granulosa cells with round to oval nuclei and small rim of cytoplasm surrounded by larger luteinised granulosa cells with ample foamy cytoplasm. FNA of ovary (PAP).

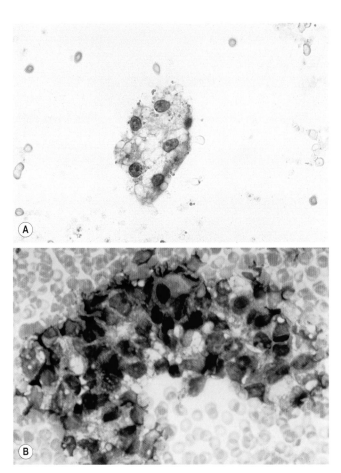

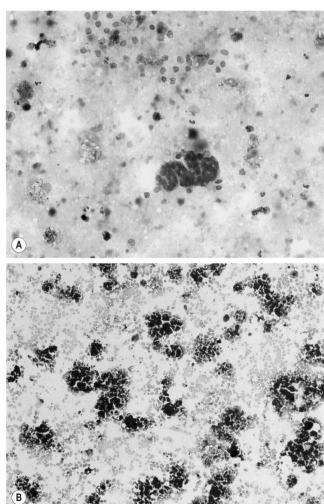

Fig. 2.191[†] Corpus luteum cyst of ovary. A loose cluster of luteinised granulosa cells containing round to oval nuclei with small prominent nucleoli. The cytoplasm is abundant with vacuolisation. FNA of ovary (A, PAP; B, MGG).

Fig. 2.193 Endometriosis of ovary. Degenerate blood in the background with haemosiderin-laden macrophages, indicative of old haemorrhage into cyst, with cytonuclear debris. Other types of cysts may also show old and recent haemorrhage. FNA of ovary (A,[†] MGG; B, PAP).

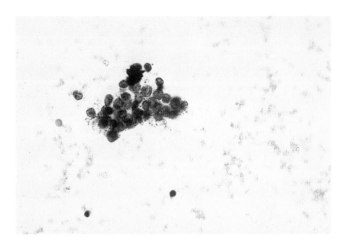

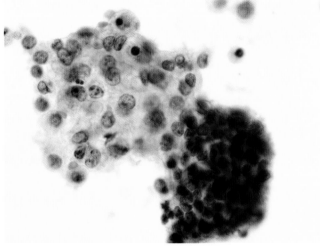

Fig. 2.192[†] Endometriosis of ovary. A tight cluster of small uniform endometrial cells. The background usually shows numerous haemosiderin-laden macrophages as illustrated in Fig. 2.193. FNA of ovary (PAP).

Fig. 2.194 Endometriosis of the ovary. Note tight endometrial cluster in the right hand side.

Simple cysts – including serosal inclusion cysts, paraovarian cysts and regressing follicular cysts

- Clear fluid
- Erythrocytes and debris in the background
- Variable numbers of macrophages
- Degenerate cell groups, ?origin
- Immunocytochemistry can be helpful
- Inhibin positivity supports diagnosis of functional cyst
- BerEP4 and/or Ca 125 indicates epithelial cells (endometriotic or neoplastic)

Ovarian neoplasms (Figs 2.195, 2.196)

- Less commonly aspirated than non-neoplastic cysts
- Epithelium ± atypia in ovarian FNA warrants surgical intervention
- Common benign tumours include:

Serous cystadenoma

- Hypocellular and similar to non-neoplastic cysts
- Macrophages, aggregates and single bland epithelial cells without atypia with cribiform/columnar appearance

Mucinous cystadenoma

- Columnar mucin-secreting cells in honeycomb or picket-fence arrangement without atypia
- ± background mucinous matrix

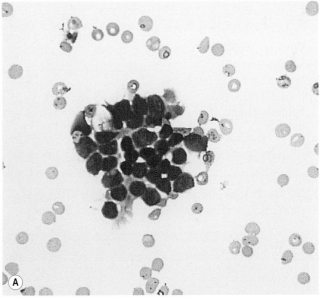

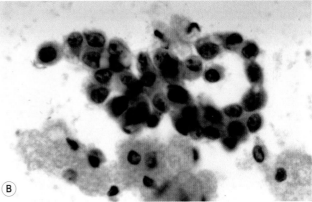

Fig. 2.195 Serous cystadenoma of ovary. A cluster of uniform cuboidal cells with round to oval nuclei and amphophilic cytoplasm, some of which are ciliated. FNA of ovary (A,[†] MGG; B, PAP).

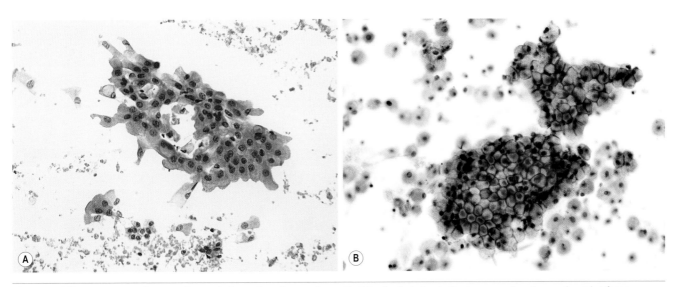

Fig. 2.196 (A)[†] Mucinous cystadenoma of ovary. A sheet of mucin-secreting epithelial cells displaying both a honeycomb pattern and a picket-fence arrangement at the edges. FNA of ovary (MGG). (B) Honeycomb sheet of mucin-secreting cells (PAP).

Borderline epithelial ovarian tumours (Fig. 2.197)

- Often very cellular samples
- Variable atypia
- May be difficult to subclassify
- Presence of invasion cannot be determined; therefore borderline tumours may be indistinguishable from malignant tumours

Malignant ovarian tumours (Figs 2.198–2.203)

- Subclassification may be difficult – particularly if high grade
- Histological examination is mainstay of primary diagnosis

Mature cystic teratoma (Figs 2.204, 2.205)

- Anucleate squames
- Amorphous debris
- Other epithelial and mesenchymal elements, e.g. respiratory, enteric epithelium and adipose
- Knowledge of aspiration procedure important to rule out contamination, e.g. transvaginal squames

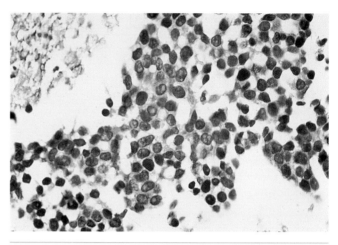

Fig. 2.197[†] Serous tumour of low malignant potential (borderline) of ovary. A loose cluster of cuboidal to columnar cells with irregular arrangement, nuclear hyperchromasia and an irregular chromatin pattern. FNA of ovary (PAP).

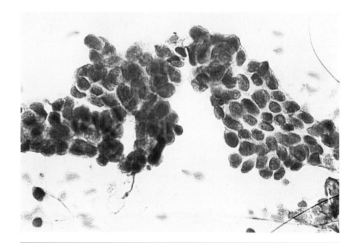

Fig. 2.198[†] Serous cystadenocarcinoma of ovary. Irregular branching group of malignant columnar cells with syncytial and papillary configurations. FNA of ovary (PAP).

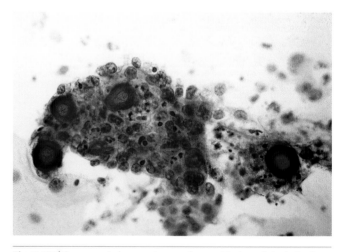

Fig. 2.199[†] Serous cystadenocarcinoma of ovary. Clusters of atypical cells centred around psammoma bodies. FNA of ovary (PAP).

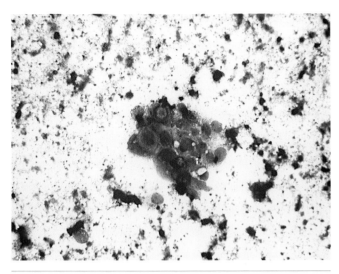

Fig. 2.200† Mucinous cystadenocarcinoma of ovary. Cytologically malignant mucin-secreting cells in a vague picket-fence arrangement. FNA of ovary (MGG).

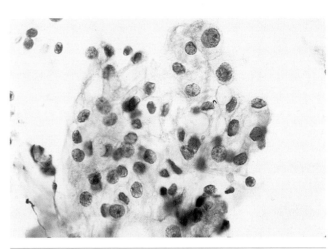

Fig. 2.203† Clear cell carcinoma of ovary. Malignant cells with abundant, granular or vacuolated clear cytoplasm and round nuclei with prominent nucleoli. FNA of ovary (PAP).

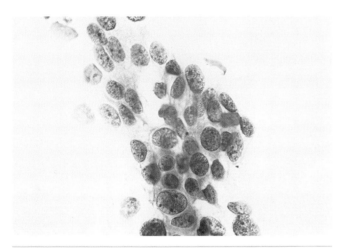

Fig. 2.201† Metastatic colonic adenocarcinoma to ovary. Cytological features show a mucinous adenocarcinoma, indistinguishable from a primary ovarian mucinous adenocarcinoma. Clinical findings were metastatic disease to the ovary. FNA ovary (PAP).

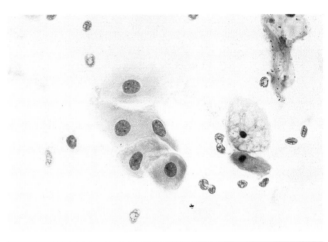

Fig. 2.204† Benign mature cystic teratoma of ovary. Mature superficial squamous cells are present. FNA of ovary (PAP).

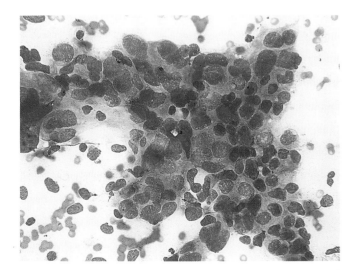

Fig. 2.202† Endometrioid adenocarcinoma of the ovary. Syncytial sheets of malignant cells with moderate amounts of granular cytoplasm and atypical nuclei (MGG).

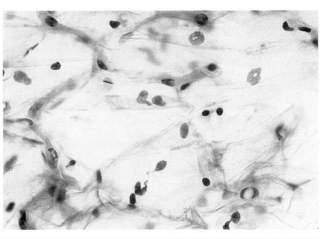

Fig. 2.205† Benign mature cystic teratoma of ovary. Mature adipose tissue. Abundant cellular and keratin debris were also present. FNA of ovary (PAP).

CHAPTER 3

Respiratory

Contents

Introduction	59	Other lung tumours and metastases	79
Normal cytological findings	60	Mesenchymal tumours and lymphomas	81
Reactive changes	62	Mediastinal tumours	84
Common lung tumours	64	Lung infections	88
Carcinoid tumours	77	Other pulmonary conditions	96

Introduction

Historically, sputum was one of the earliest cytological samples used for cancer diagnosis. Lung cancer is now the leading cause of cancer death worldwide, and the incidence is still rising in some countries, largely due to cigarette smoking. Today, fine needle aspiration (FNA) techniques, including endoscopic ultrasound-guided (EBUS-FNA) methods, are frequently used, both for tumour diagnosis and for staging, yielding excellent diagnostic material directly from the lesion. In addition, there are now many immunological markers for tumour identification, for indicators of response to therapy and for prognosis. These may require additional sampling.

Exfoliative samples (sputum, bronchial brushings, washings and bronchoalveolar lavages) from airways (see Figs 3.1 and 3.2) are alcohol-fixed for Papanicolaou staining. FNA specimens are air-dried for Giemsa staining, but some wet-fixed preparations are also made, together with spare slides for ancillary stains where appropriate. Whenever possible, fresh material should also be submitted for microbiological studies to exclude or confirm infection.

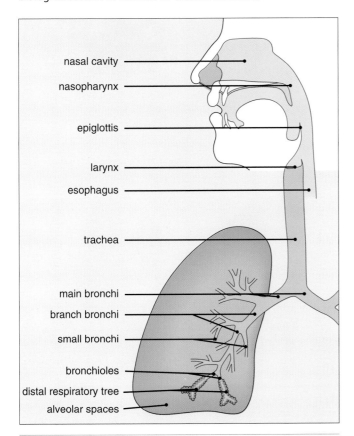

Fig. 3.1 Anatomy of the respiratory tract. (From Stevens A, Lowe J. *Human Histology*, 3rd edn. 2005; Mosby, Philadelphia.)

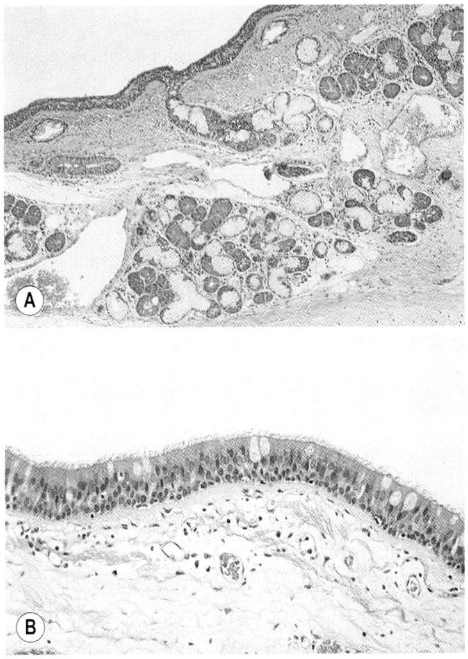

Fig. 3.2[†] (**A**) Bronchial biopsy. Section of brochial lining with surface glandular mucosa and underlying submucosa containging sero-mucinous glands. (**B**) High-power view of columnar epithelium with ciliated border. A few goblet cells also seen.

Normal cytological findings

Cytology varies with type of sample:

- **Sputum:** airways content and exfoliated cells
- **Bronchial brushings and washings:** directly abraded and exfoliated epithelial cells
- **Bronchoalveolar lavage (BAL):** cells from the bronchioles and alveolar spaces
- **FNA samples:** transthoracic or by ultrasound-guided endobronchial (EBUS-FNA): obtain cells directly from a lung mass or carinal lymph nodes

Cytological findings: normal exfoliative sample (Figs 3.3–3.6)

- **Macrophages:** dissociated cells, one or more nuclei, may have ingested material in cytoplasm
- **Macrophages** are used as an indication of a good sample, i.e. are from the airways, not from saliva
- **Mature squamous cells:** from upper airways: abundant cytoplasm, small dark nuclei
- **Mucoid background**
- **Bronchial epithelium:** a few tall columnar cells, some ciliated, occasional goblet cells may be seen but reserve cells are rare
- **Food contamination:** common

Cytological findings: normal aspiration sample (Fig. 3.7)

- **Macrophages:** usually present but are not an indication of a good sample
- **Bronchial epithelium:** often very well-preserved sheets are included
- **Reserve cells:** may be attached to groups of bronchial epithelial cells
- **Mucus and inflammatory cells:** present but not profuse

Differential diagnosis (Figs 3.8–3.11)

- **Inadequate sample:** no/few macrophages, scanty cellularity; important to recognise and repeat sample if necessary
- **Degenerative changes** in normal cells e.g. ciliocytophthoria (Fig. 3.8)
- **Inflammatory/reactive changes** in normal epithelium occur in almost all pathological processes and are non-diagnostic but are a pitfall for overdiagnosis (see p. 62 et seq)
- **Poor sample preparation** due to delays in transit, poor fixation, blood/inflammatory cells. Liquid based cytology (LBC) reduces all of these problems and provides more material for ancillary testing
- **Contaminants:** from sample or processing

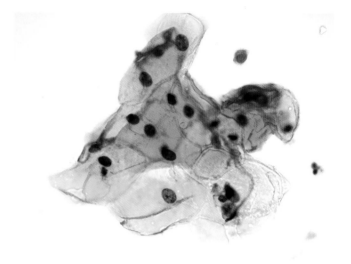

Fig. 3.3[†] Sputum: normal squamous cells with occasional inflammatory cells (LBC).

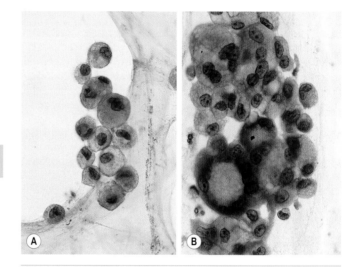

Fig. 3.4[†] (A) Sputum. Macrophages in mucoid background; (B) Sputum. Multinucleated macrophages aggregated with mononuclear forms (PAP).

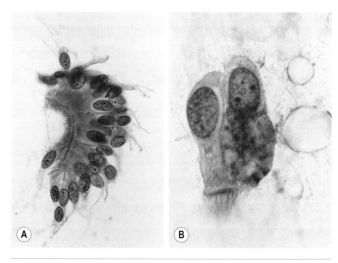

Fig. 3.5[†] (A) Bronchial brushing: epithelial strip of columnar cells with preserved cilia. (B) EBUS-FNA. Normal bronchial epithelium with cilia.

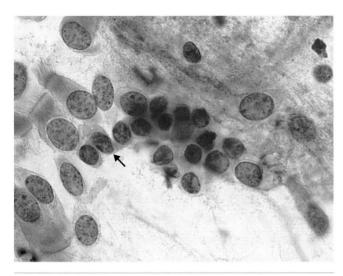

Fig. 3.6[†] Bronchial brushing epithelial cells with a row of small reserve cells at arrow.

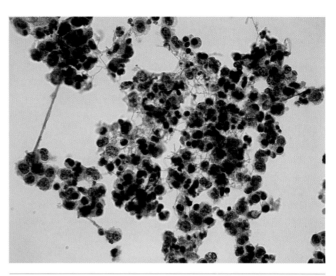

Fig. 3.9[†] Sputum. Unsatisfactory sample with inflammatory cells obscuring other cell detail.

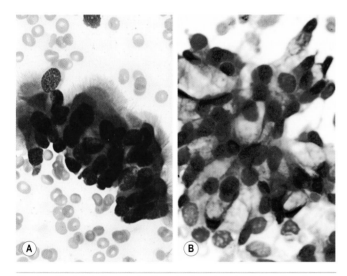

Fig. 3.7 EBUS-FNA. Bronchial cells with cilia in A and goblet cells in B.

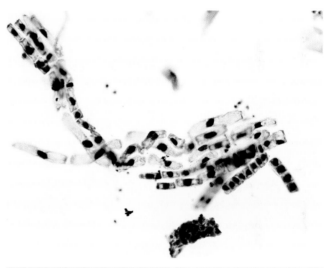

Fig. 3.10 FNA. Contaminant vegetable cells with thick cellulose walls and degenerate nuclei.

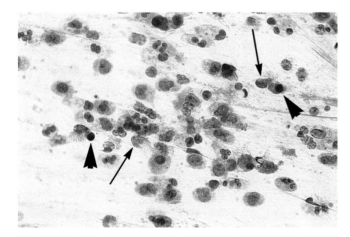

Fig. 3.8[†] Ciliocytophthoria in sputum from a patient with squamous carcinoma. Scattered fragments of cytoplastic remnants present, some ciliated (*arrows*), others with pyknotic nuclei (*arrowheads*).

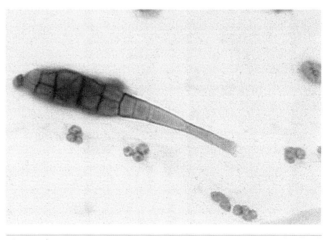

Fig. 3.11[†] Sputum. Aerial or water-borne contaminant (*Alternaria* species).

Reactive changes

- **Reactive changes in bronchial epithelium** are frequently seen in any lung pathology and are especially common after chronic irritation (smoking) or instrumentation, as in post-bronchoscopy samples
- **Clinical details** are essential
- **Squamous metaplasia** is the commonest. This is a change in columnar bronchial epithelial cells which undergo metaplasia to less specialised immature squamous cells. This change is reversible in the early stages
- **Hyperplasia** of bronchial epithelium, or more rarely reserve cells, may be a specific response to toxins or infection. Usually reversible, but the cells' mass may show atypia

Cytological findings: reactive changes (Figs 3.12–3.16)

- **Squamous metaplastic cells:** in the early stages these are partially mature cohesive polygonal cells with variable staining of cytoplasm and dense regular nuclei. Dissociation and keratinisation may be seen in the later stages as the cells become atypical (see p. 3.8)
- **Hyperplastic bronchial/reserve cells:** sheets or clusters of crowded cells, enlarged nuclei with vesicular chromatin and visible nucleoli
- **Degenerative inflammatory changes** are often present in normal-looking epithelial cells as well as in these reactive groups

Differential diagnosis: reactive changes (Figs 3.17–3.19)

- **Atypical squamous metaplasia:** this is a pre-malignant change and shows more dissociation of cells, with greater nuclear abnormality including pleomorphism, increased nuclear cytoplasmic ratio and hyperchromasia (see p. 3.8). Repeat samples may be needed
- **Squamous cell carcinoma:** shows advanced changes of atypical squamous metaplasia (see p. 3.8). Repeat samples may be needed
- **Adenocarcinoma:** a difficult differential diagnosis in some cases of reactive bronchial epithelium. Further sampling or biopsy may be needed to distinguish these. Clinical details are also important (see Case Study on p. 3.5)
- **Specific lung infections;** e.g. herpes simplex and other viruses (see Lung infections)
- **Specific lung disorders;** e.g. fibrosis (see Other conditions)
- **Iatrogenic/therapeutic effects;** see Other conditions (p. 97 et seq) and case study on page 63
- In all cases the clinical details are essential

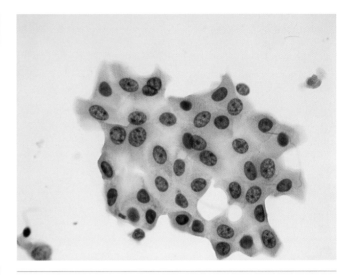

Fig. 3.12[†] Sputum from a smoker: squamous metaplastic cell group with amphophilic cytoplasm and regular nuclei.

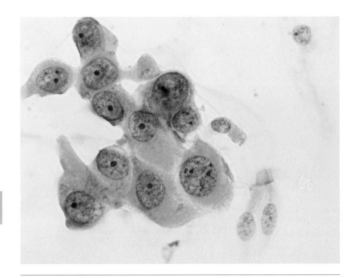

Fig. 3.13 FNA lung. Immature squamous metaplasia with enlarged nuclei but regular contours and even chromatin.

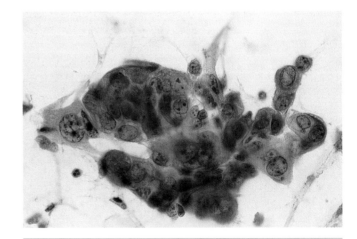

Fig. 3.14[†] Bronchoalveolar lavage. Disorganised irregular clump of pleomorphic hyperplastic bronchial cells, some with prominent nucleoli. Some cells show early metaplasia.

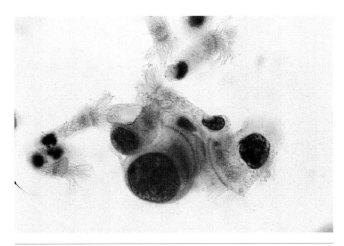

Fig. 3.15† Bronchial brushing. Reactive enlarged bronchial epithelial cells with pleomorphism but regular contours and even chromatin. Some cilia visible.

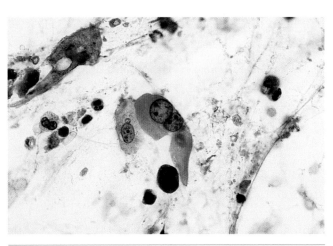

Fig. 3.17† Bronchoalveolar lavage. Patient on cytotoxic treatment; large bizarre degenerate cells probably alveolar lining cells with direct damage.

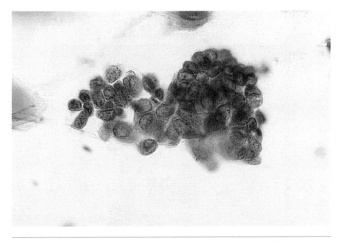

Fig. 3.16† Bronchial brushing. Basal cell hyperplasia in a crowded group of small uniform cells with regular nuclei.

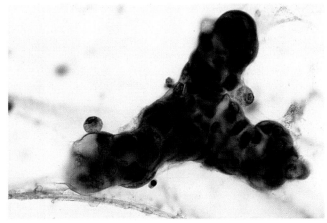

Fig. 3.18† Bronchial brushing. Cluster of hyperplastic bronchial columnar and goblet cells. From a case of ciclosporin toxicity.

Case Study

Reactive atypia due to drug toxicity

A young man with leukaemia treated with cyclophosphamide developed respiratory symptoms and was found to have extensive epithelial atypia with necrosis on BAL (see Fig. 3.19). Cyclophosphamide was discontinued and 3 months later the BAL was normal and the symptoms had disappeared (Fig. 3.20).

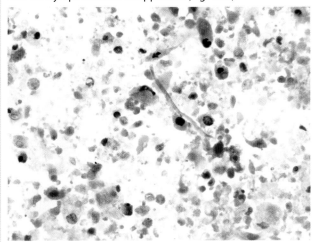

Fig. 3.19 BAL showing widespread necrosis and degenerate atypical epithelial cells with some hyperchromatic nuclei.

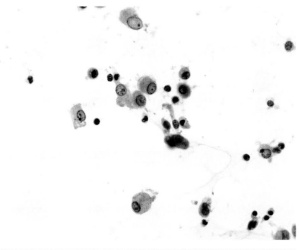

Fig. 3.20 BAL showing well-preserved macrophages and inflammatory cells with occasional columnar cells.

Common lung tumours

- **Most tumours of lung are malignant,** usually bronchogenic carcinomas or other epithelial neoplasms. Heterogeneity within the tumour is common, giving mixed cytological findings
- **Tobacco** is the commonest aetiological agent
- **Neuroendocrine tumours, sarcomas and lymphomas** are much less frequent
- **Metastatic carcinoma** is common in lungs
- See WHO Classification of lung tumours (Table 3.1)

Diagnosis and management of lung tumours

- **Exfoliative methods** of diagnosis are still common but FNA is used increasingly for diagnosis and staging
- **Squamous cell carcinoma, adenocarcinoma and other large cell carcinomas** are treated operatively whenever possible
- **Small cell carcinoma** (oat cell) is often advanced due to early spread, so is usually treated by chemotherapy
- **For the clinician** it is most important to distinguish non-small cell lung cancers from small cell for correct management

Tumour spread

- **Carcinomas spread via lymphatics** to local nodes, which can be sampled by FNA at the time of diagnosis, for tumour type and staging
- **Direct spread** to pleura occurs with peripheral tumours leading to effusions in pleural cavity. These tumours are often not retestable
- **Vascular spread** is late except with sarcomas
- **Central tumours** may obstruct the airways, leading to infection distally and this may be the presenting symptom
- **Haemorrhage (haemophysis)** is common with central tumours

Lung cancer diagnosis by cytology (Figs 3.21–23)

- **Sputum:** 3-5 samples can detect 60–90% of bronchogenic carcinomas but sputum is less effective for peripheral tumours and is not localizing. Used as a preliminary investigation
- **Brushings and washings:** can sample up to 90% of central malignancies, but not effective for diagnosis of peripheral or submucosal tumours
- **Percutaneous** FNA lung: is used for peripheral lesions
- **Endoscopic bronchial ultrasound (EBUS) FNA** probe for sampling tumour or of carinal lymph nodes. FNA provides well-preserved material for ancilliary techniques such as immunocytochemistry and FISH (see Chapter 13)

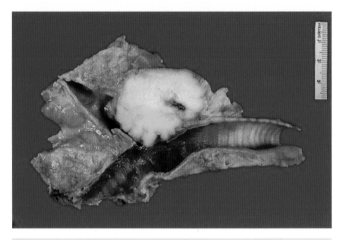

Fig. 3.21 Section of lung with an obstructing necrotic lung tumour in the main bronchus.

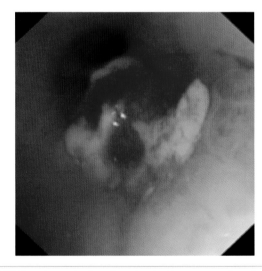

Fig. 3.22 Bronchoscopic view of an ulcerated tumour mass in main bronchus.

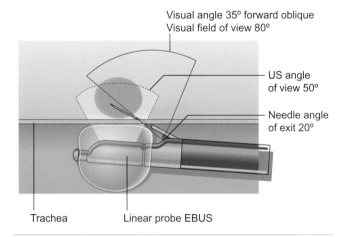

Visual angle 35° forward oblique
Visual field of view 80°

US angle of view 50°

Needle angle of exit 20°

Trachea   Linear probe EBUS

Fig. 3.23 Flexible bronchoscope with integrated ultrasound probe at tip, giving a direct view of needle during FNA (EBUS-TBFNA).

Table 3.1 Pulmonary tumours (adapted from Travis WD, Brambilla E, Muller-Hermelink HK, Harris CC, eds. Pathology and Genetics of Tumors of the Lung, Pleura, Thymus and Heart. 3rd ed. Lyon, France: IARC Press; 2004. World Health Organization Classification of Tumors; vol 10)

CARCINOMA OF THE LUNG

- Squamous cell carcinoma (variants: papillary, clear cell, small cell, basaloid)
- Small cell carcinoma (variants: combined with other forms of carcinoma)
- Adenocarcinoma*
  - Acinar adenocarcinoma
  - Papillary adenocarcinoma
  - Bronchioloalveolar carcinoma (mucinous, non-mucinous or mixed)
  - Solid adenocarcinoma with mucin
  - Other variants: well-differentiated fetal; mucinous, mucinous cystadenocarcinoma; signet ring cell; clear cell
- Large cell carcinoma
  - Large cell neuroendocrine carcinoma
  - Basaloid
  - Lymphoepithelioma-like
  - Clear cell
  - Rhabdoid phenotype
- Carcinomas with pleomorphic, sarcomatoid or sarcomatous elements
  - Spindle or giant cell
  - Carcinosarcoma
  - Pulmonary blastoma

OTHER PRIMARY EPITHELIAL NEOPLASMS

- Carcinoid tumours
  - Typical carcinoid (variants: adenopapillary, clear cell, oncocytic, spindle, melaninogenic)
  - Atypical carcinoid
- Tumours of seromucinous gland/salivary gland type
  - Mucoepidermoid carcinoma
  - Adenoid cystic carcinoma
  - Acinic cell carcinoma
  - Mucous cell adenoma
  - Oncocytic adenoma
  - Pleomorphic adenoma
- Papillary tumours of bronchus/lung
  - Juvenile papillomatosis
  - Squamous cell papilloma and papillary carcinoma
  - Papillary adenoma and adenocarcinoma
- Mucinous cystadenoma
- Alveolar adenoma
- Sclerosing haemangioma/pneumocytoma
- Thymoma
- Malignant melanoma

SECONDARY MALIGNANCIES

Connective tissue neoplasms

- Chondroid hamartoma/chondroma
- Granular cell tumour
- Benign clear cell ('sugar') tumour
- Localised fibrous tumour
- Inflammatory myofibroblastic tumour
- Epithelioid haemangioendothelioma
- Primary pulmonary artery sarcoma
- Leiomyosarcoma
- Malignant fibrous histiocytoma
- Neurogenic sarcoma
- Rhabdomyosarcoma

Germ cell neoplasms

- Teratoma mature/immature

LYMPHOPROLIFERATIVE DISEASE

- Lymphoid interstitial pneumonia
- Nodular lymphoid hyperplasia
- Low-grade marginal zone B-cell lymphoma of the mucosa-associated lymphoid tissue (MALT)
- Lymphomatoid granulomatosis (angiocentric non-Hodgkin lymphoma)
- Other non-Hodgkin lymphomas
- Hodgkin lymphoma
- Plasmacytoma
- Histiocytosis X (Langerhans histiocytosis)

OTHER LOCALISED MASS LESIONS

- Amyloid tumour
- Hyalinising granuloma

*Invasive adenocarcinoma, acinar, lepidic, papillary, solid (Travis WD, Brambilla E, Noguchi M, et al. *J Thorac Oncol.* 2011;6(2):244–85).
Adenocarcinoma in situ, usually nonmucinous lepidic (AIS). Predominantly lepidic (MIA) <5 mm invasion. AIS and MIA were previously bronchioloalveolar carcinoma (BAC)

Squamous cell carcinoma (SqCC)

- **Globally this is the commonest** type of lung cancer today, but in USA adenocarcinoma is commoner in women and is rising in Western countries where smoking is decreasing
- **Usually a central keratinising tumour,** strongly related to smoking, arising from bronchial mucosa following pre-malignant changes (atypia) in squamous metaplasia which takes place over many years
- **Well (keratinising) to poorly (non-keratinising) differentiated**
- **Mixed histological types** can occur (e.g. small cell/squamous cell carcinoma or adeno/squamous cell carcinoma) especially with wide sampling by FNA
- **Spreads to lymph nodes** early and pleural cavity later

Cytological findings (Figs 3.24–3.30)

- **Dissociated abnormal squamous cells** with dense orange (if keratinised) or green cytoplasm (PAP stain), blue cytoplasmic staining with MGG
- **Bizarre angular cell contours,** e.g. tadpole, fibre cells, cell-in-cell arrangement
- **Nuclei dense,** pyknotic or absent if strongly keratinising (ghost cells); pale open chromatin if non-keratinising
- **Nucleoli not seen** unless non-keratinising in type
- **Tumour diathesis present** (necrosis); preserved tumour cells may be scanty, requiring extensive searching and/or further samples
- **FNA samples** may include well-preserved less mature cells in sheets due to deeper sampling than with exfoliative methods which often include material exclusively from the necrotic surface

Differential diagnosis (Figs 3.31–3.38)

- **Atypia/dysplasia/carcinoma in situ sequence** (pre-invasive changes) show lesser nuclear and cytoplasmic changes, no necrosis, less cell dissociation
- **Reactive changes** in bronchial epithelium: full clinical details are essential
- **Other lung tumours,** e.g. adenocarcinoma versus non-keratinising squamous cell carcinoma. This may not be possible in all cases but does not affect management unless a small cell carcinoma is queried
- **Metastatic squamous cell carcinoma** from other sites in lung
- **Metastatic squamous cell carcinoma** from a primary tumour elsewhere. A full history is essential, with comparison of any previous cytology/histology if possible
- **Other metastatic tumours:** immunostaining may be helpful
- **Chemotherapy, radiotherapy changes:** clinical details are essential
- **Bizarre contaminant cells:** note distribution, e.g. only at one edge of slide

Further investigations

- Ensure that full clinical details are available
- Discuss these cases at multidisciplinary team meetings
- Immunocytochemical stains may help
  CK5 and CK7 positive
  p53 positive
  TTF1 negative
- See Fig. 3.50, p. 71 and Table 3.2, p. 79)

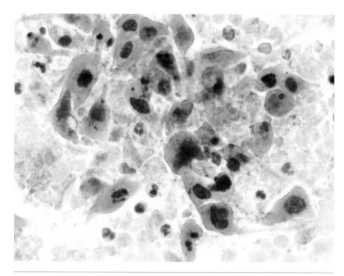

Fig. 3.24[†] Sputum. Squamous cell carcinoma. Densely keratinised dissociated cells with bizarre shapes and pyknotic nuclei; ghost cells also present with faded nuclei.

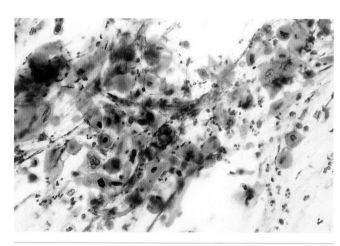

Fig. 3.25[†] Sputum. Squamous cell carcinoma. Non-keratinised malignant squamous cells with open chromatin pattern mixed with keratinised cells and necrosis in the background.

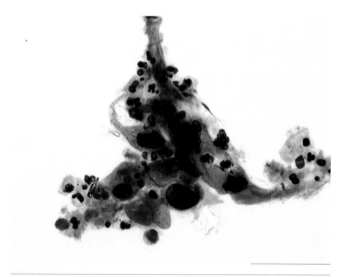

Fig. 3.26 FNA. Well-differentiated squamous cell carcinoma with tadpole cells and inflammatory cells.

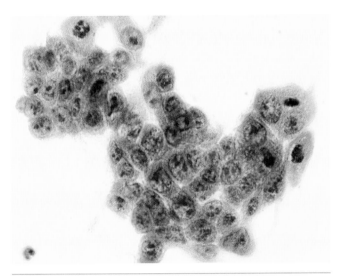

Fig. 3.27 FNA: Poorly differentiated non-keratinising squamous cell carcinoma with scanty cytoplasm and open pale chromatin. Nucleoli visible.

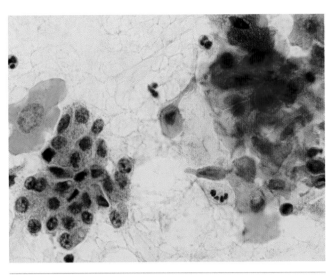

Fig. 3.30 FNA. Separate groups of dyskaryotic squamous cells, keratinised and non-keratinised, more cohesive than in exfoliative samples.

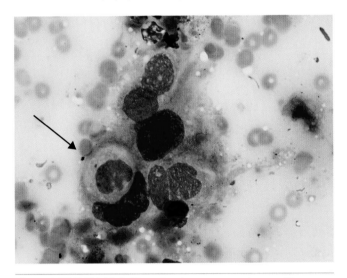

Fig. 3.28 EBUS-FNA. Well-differentiated squamous carcinoma with intensely blue keratinised cytoplasm. Note cell-in-cell at arrow (MGG stain).

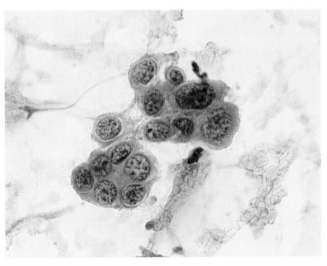

Fig. 3.31 Bronchial brushing. Non-keratinising dysplasia showing cohesive cells with high N/C ratio and abnormal chromatin. Note similarity to Fig. 3.13.

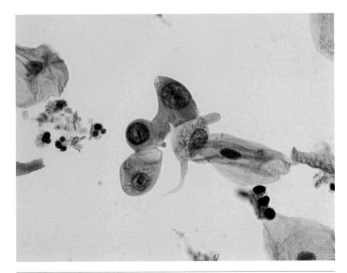

Fig. 3.29 Sputum: Mild atypia in a few metaplastic squamous cells with dyskaryotic nuclei and variable cytoplasm (LBC).

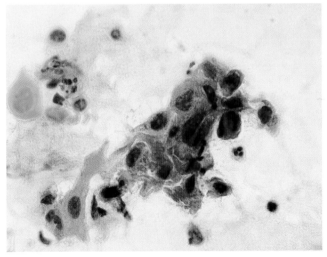

Fig. 3.32 Bronchial brushing. Severe dysplasia/carcinoma in situ with findings indistinguishable from invasive squamous cell carcinoma. In some cases, a biopsy is necessary to establish the presence of stromal invasion.

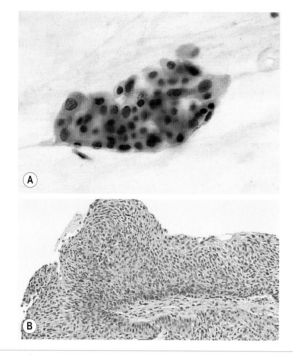

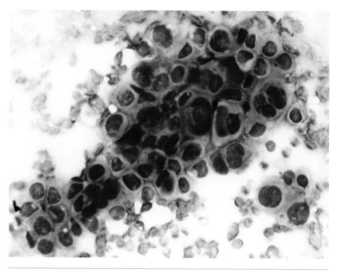

Fig. 3.35 FNA lung (Giemsa stain). Well-differentiated metastatic keratinising squamous cell carcinoma, indistinguishable from a lung primary.

Fig. 3.33† (A) Sputum. Severe dyskoryosis (carcinoma in situ). Note the clean background with no tumour diathesis. (B) Bronchial biopsy histology showing in situ carcinoma with intact basement membrane.

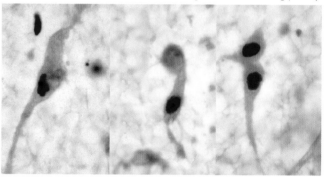

Fig. 3.36† FNA. Metastatic transitional bladder carcinoma cells. Elongated 'cercariform' cells versus non-keratinising tadpole cells.

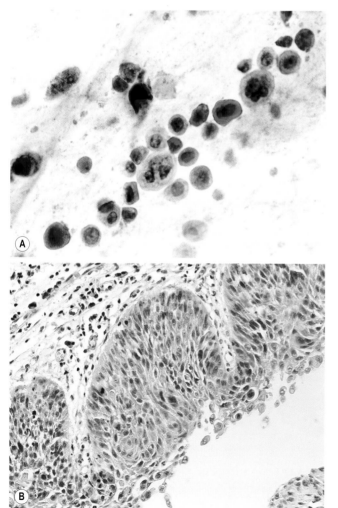

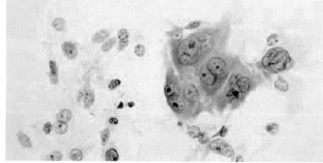

Fig. 3.37† Bronchial brushing. Chemotherapy effect: pleomorphic cells with dense cytoplasm and enlarged pale degenerate nuclei.

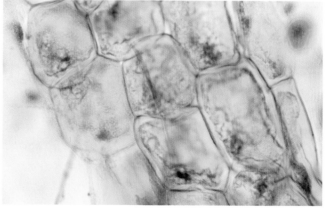

Fig. 3.34 (A) Sputum: severe dyskoryosis in squamous cells. (B) Bronchial biopsy: carcinoma in situ with no invasion below basement membrane.

Fig. 3.38† Sputum. Food contamination: large cells with dense cellulose walls and degenerate nuclei.

Small cell carcinoma

- Accounts for **15–30% of lung tumours**
- Related to **cigarette smoking**
- **Arises from specialised cells** deep in mucosa which have endocrine-like features or neurosecretory granules in their cytoplasm
- **Clinically aggressive,** often central, metastasizes early and widely so usually treated with chemotherapy rather than surgically
- **Mixed with other types** of lung carcinoma in 10% of cases, but still behaves aggressively
- **May present with myaesthenic** or other ectopic hormonal symptoms eg ACTH or ADH secretion

Cytological findings (Figs 3.39–3.43)

- **Cells larger than lymphocytes** but smaller than all other carcinoma cells seen as aggregates of dissociated cells, in elongated streaks in exfoliated samples
- **High N/C ratio** and poorly preserved cytoplasm leads to nuclear moulding which is highly characteristic
- **Hyperchromatic nuclei** with granular chromatin ('salt and pepper' pattern)
- **Other carcinoma cells (e.g. SqCC) may be seen** as well in combined tumours

Differential diagnosis (Figs 3.44–3.47)

- **Lymphocytes:** these are smaller, more uniform and have no moulding
- **Lymphoma:** cells are all dissociated (see Fig. 3.39), may be uniform or pleomorphic depending on lymphoma type. They are often disrupted by the preparation process (smear cells)
- **Degenerate bronchial cells**
- **Metastatic breast/prostatic** carcinoma cells: can be quite small
- **Small cell squamous carcinoma cells:** these have more cytoplasm and do not show moulding
- **Inspissated mucus/debris:** a pitfall in exfoliative material
- **Carcinoids:** these have larger cells, often with distinctive patterns of arrangement (see p. 3.19). No moulding is seen
- **Neuroendocrine carcinoma:** larger cells with more pleomorphism
- **Basal cells,** especially if hyperplastic , no moulding (see Fig. 3.16)

Further investigations

- **Check clinical details** for any evidence of ectopic hormone effects
- **Immunostaining** is usually characteristic
  CD56, TTF1, chromogranin, synaptophysin all positive, cytokeratin dot-like positivity
- See Table 3.2 on p. 79

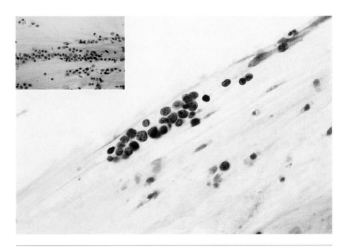

Fig. 3.39[†] Sputum. Small cell carcinoma: streak of small dark cells in line of spread of sample. Note high N/C ratio and poorly preserved cytoplasm. Inset shows sputum from a patient with lymphoma cells, dissociated and with no moulding.

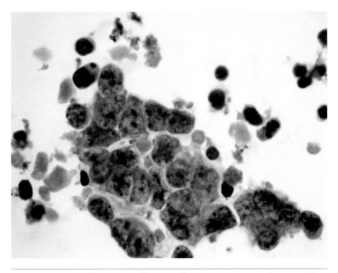

Fig. 3.40 Small cell carcinoma from FNA lung (PAP). Note nuclear moulding and grainy 'salt and pepper chromatin' characteristic of small cell carcinoma.

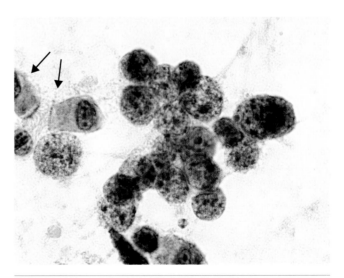

Fig. 3.41 FNA. Cells from small cell carcinoma with stippled chromatin, micro-nucleoli, minimal cytoplasm. Note two normal epithelial cells at left edge (*arrows*).

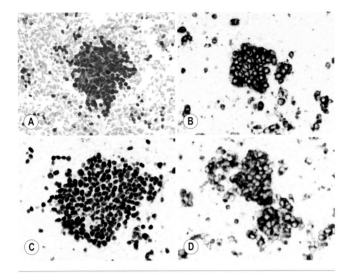

Fig. 3.42 EBUS-FNA, small cell carcinoma. (A) MGG, (B) TTF1, (C) CD56, (D) chromogranin.

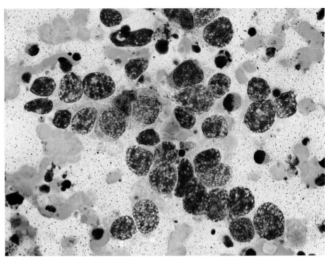

Fig. 3.45 EBUS-FNAC small cell carcinoma. Dissociated cells, difficult to distinguish from non-Hodgkin lymphoma.

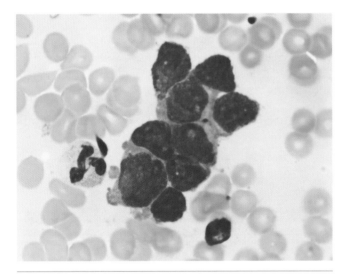

Fig. 3.43 FNA lymph node. Small cell carcinoma MGG stain showing scanty cytoplasm, nuclear moulding and coarse chromatin pattern.

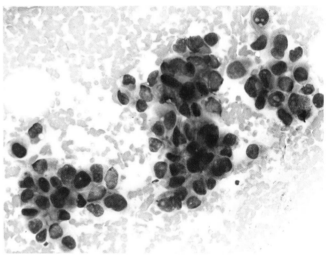

Fig. 3.46 EBUS-FNA. Metastatic breast carcinoma. Clumps of tumour cells with variable cytoplasm

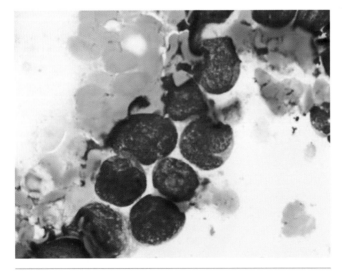

Fig. 3.44 FNA lymph node. Non-Hodgkin lymphoma of lung resembling small cell carcinoma . Cells are all dissociated, polylobated and show no nuclear moulding

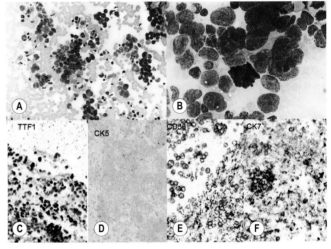

Fig. 3.47 FNA neuroendocrine carcinoma: (A) low power view, (B) high power, cells, larger, some with cytoplasm showing rosetting, (C) TTF1 positive, (D) CK5 negative, (E) CD56 positive, (F) CK7 positive.

Adenocarcinoma

- **Arises from glandular epithelium** of airways and air spaces, with glandular differentiation
- **Now the commonest lung cancer in some countries** e.g. in the USA, particularly for women
- **Many different growth patterns:** acinar, papillary, lepidic, bronchioloalveolar, solid, mucinous or mixed, and all may be well- or poorly differentiated
- **Tend to be situated peripherally** in lung
- **Metastatic adenocarcinoma** is common in lung

Cytological findings (Figs 3.48–3.52)

- **Cell aggregates if well differentiated;** sheets, rosettes, acini, papillary clumps
- **Large eccentric rounded or pleomorphic nuclei,** pale chromatin or hyperchromatic
- **Nuclear membrane** often prominent
- **Prominent nucleoli,** may be large, usually single and round
- **Abundant pale or vacuolated cytoplasm**
- **FNA:** columnar cells, sheets, papillary groups; mucin/ necrosis in background
- **Emperipolesis** (ingestion of polymorphs by malignant cells) may be seen

Differential diagnosis (Figs 3.53–3.56)

- **Reactive bronchial/bronchiolar epithelium,** e.g. post-bronchoscopy, asthma
- **Atypical cells** from alveolar damage
- **Pseudoglandular growth pattern** in squamous cell or large cell carcinoma
- **Metastatic adenocarcinoma:** check clinical details, radiology, immunoprofile

Further investigations

- Immunocytochemistry is helpful: see fig. 3.50 and Table 3.2
- TTF1 and CK7 positive
- CK20 and p63 negative
- Metastatic breast carcinoma: TTF1 negative, ER positive

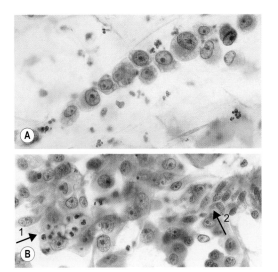

Fig. 3.48[†] Adenocarcinoma. Sputum. (A) Adenocarcinoma. dispersed malignant cells, high N/C ratio, eccentric nuclei, large single, round nucleoli, pale chromatin, prominent nuclear membrane, vacuolated cytoplasm. (B) Brushing: sheets of adenocarcinoma cells, some showing emperipolesis (*arrow 1*) with a clump of normal bronchial cells (*arrow 2*).

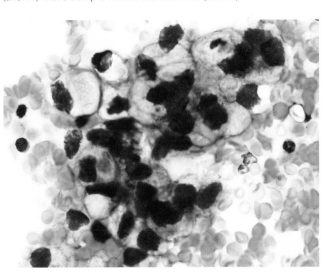

Fig. 3.49 EBUS-FNA. Adenocarcinoma: cohesive pleomorphic cells vacuolated, variable N/C ratio, visible nucleoli.

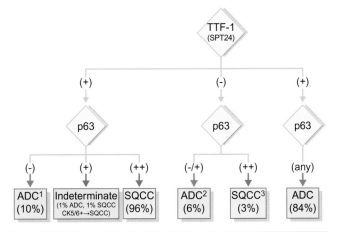

	p63-	p63+	p63++
TTF-1++	ADC	ADC	ADC
TTF-1+	ADC	ADC[2]	SQCC[3]
TTF-1-	ADC[1]	INDET	SQCC

Fig. 3.50 Immunohistochemical algorithm for differentiation of lung adenocarcinoma and squamous cell carcinoma using TTF1 and p63 as a first-line panel and CK5/6 indeterminate cases. (From Rekhtman N et al. Modern Pathology (2011) 24, 1348–1359).

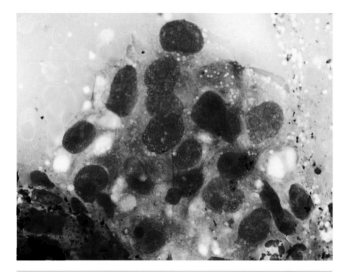

Fig. 3.51 EBUS-FNA. Adenocarcinoma group with vacuolation, high N/C ratio and large prominent nucleoli.

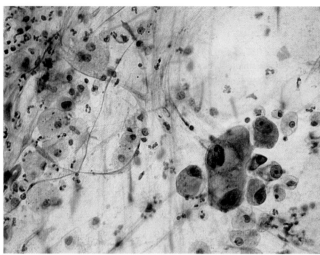

Fig. 3.54[†] Sputum. Adenosquamous carcinoma with malignant glandular (on right) and squamous (left) cells.

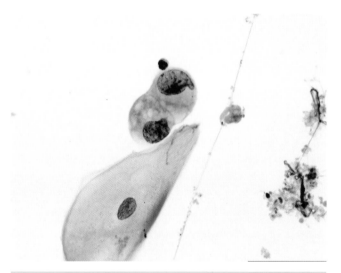

Fig. 3.52 Adenocarcinoma. Pair of cohesive malignant cells with minor vacuolation.

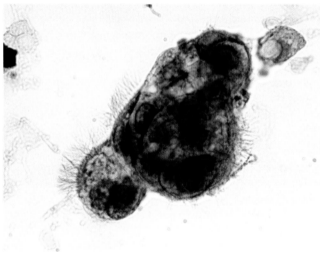

Fig. 3.55[†] Sputum, asthma. Hyperplastic group with ciliated border known as Creola body (asthmatic patient may be misdiagnosed as adenocarcinoma).

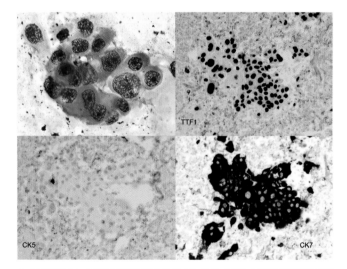

Fig. 3.53 EBUS-FNA adenocarcinoma. Group of cells with no definite glandular features apart from minor vacuolation and eccentric nuclei. Immunostaining: TTF1 and CK7 positive, CK5 negative.

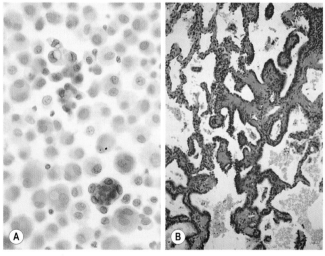

Fig. 3.56[†] Bronchoalveolar lavage. (A) Groups of hyperplastic bronchiolar cells with many macrophages. (B) Histology: fibrosing alveolitis.

Adenocarcinoma – lepidic predominant

- **Previously known as bronchioloalveolar cell carcinoma** (BAC)
- **Usually non-mucinous,** but has a mucinous variant
- **Usually peripheral,** may be a solitary lesion or diffusely spreading (lepidic spread), hence may exfoliate easily into alveolar spaces
- **May be non-invasive** (adenocarcinoma in situ, AIS) or minimally invasive (MIA) on resection specimens
- **Requires close clinicopathological correlation** for accurate diagnosis; radiological findings may be characteristic
- **Good prognosis** if fully resected
- **Easier to diagnose on FNA** material than in exfoliative samples

Cytological findings (Figs 3.57–3.62)

- **Many small cohesive glandular/ papillary clusters**
- **Regular small rounded cells** with dense or vacuolated, non-phagocytic cytoplasm with mucin content in mucinous variant
- **N/C ratio slightly raised,** some irregular shaped nuclei and hyperchromasia
- May have **prominent nucleoli**
- **Intranuclear cytoplasmic inclusions** seen (on FNA)
- **Clean or mucoid background**
- Rare cases show **psammoma bodies** (concretions) on FNA

Differential diagnosis (Figs 3.63–3.65)

- **Reactive bronchial/bronchioloalveolar cell groups** are sometimes present post- infection, trauma, asthma, artificial respiration. The groups are often still ciliated
- **Fibrosing lung diseases** with alveolar cell hyperplasia, e.g. adult respiratory distress syndrome (ARDS): difficult to distinguish radiologically, need full clinical details
- **Metastatic carcinoma** especially breast, prostate and pancreas have a tendency to spread along alveolar walls: history and ancillary tests help
- **Mesothelioma** (epithelial type): clinico-pathological correlation

Further investigations

- **Full clinical details** are needed, including the radiological findings
- Discussion at multidisciplinary meetings is important
- Immunoprofile:
  Nonmucinous: TTF1 positive
  Mucinous: CK7 and CK20 positive
- See Table 3.2 on p. 79

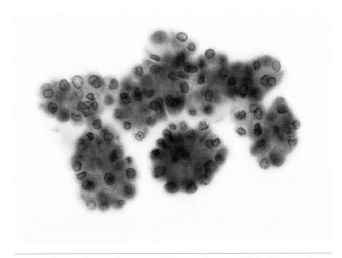

Fig. 3.57[†] Bronchoalveolar lavage. Adenocarcinoma with lepidic growth pattern. Papillary clusters of crowded cells with mild nuclear variation and hyperchromasia.

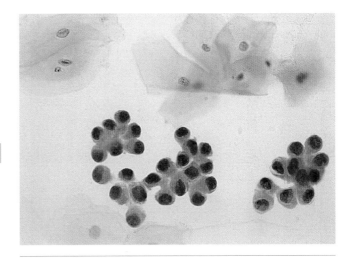

Fig. 3.58[†] Sputum. Adenocarcinoma with lepidic growth pattern. Tumour cell clusters in clean background.

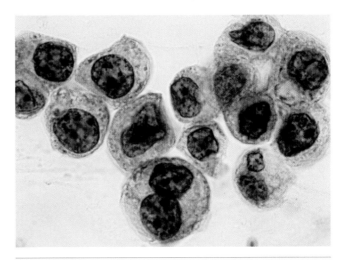

Fig. 3.59[†] Sputum. Adenocarcinoma with lepidic growth pattern showing lacy vacuolated cytoplasm and pleomorphic hyperchromatic nuclei.

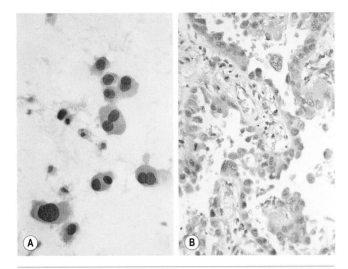

Fig. 3.60† (A) Adenocarcinoma with lepidic growth pattern. Dispersed pleomorphic cells with dense cytoplasm. (B) Biopsy: lepidic spread of tumour cells

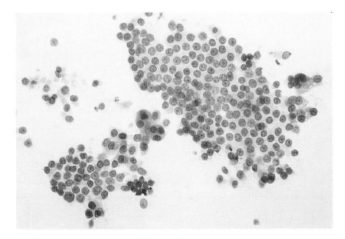

Fig. 3.61† FNA. Adenocarcinoma with lepidic growth pattern. Sheets of regular bronchiolar cells; some have intranuclear cytoplasmic inclusions.

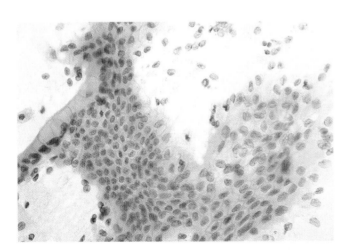

Fig. 3.62† FNA. Mucinous adenocarcinoma: monolayered sheet of regular cells with abundant apical mucin.

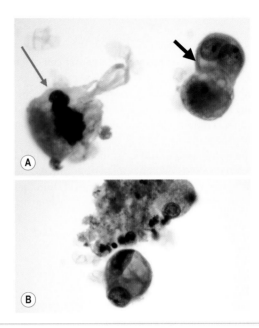

Fig. 3.63 Mucinous BAC cells. (A) Red arrow identifies normal bronchial epithelial cells and the black arrow identifies malignant glandular cells. (B) Two malignant glandular cells with an obvious mucinous vacuole indenting the nucleus of one cell.

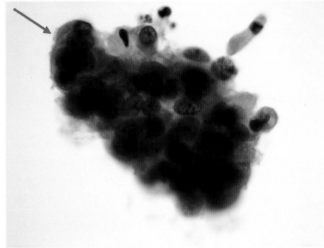

Fig. 3.64 Brushing, post-bronchoscopy. Cluster of reactive bronchiolar epithelial cells. Note the ciliated border of one cell (arrowed).

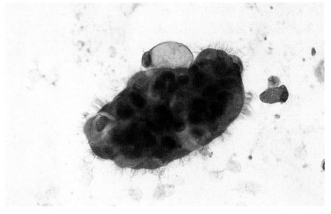

Fig. 3.65† Bronchial lavage. Fibrosing alveolitis, papillary grouping of regular cells with cilia.

Large cell carcinoma

- **A heterogeneous group** of non-small cell tumours without evidence of squamous or glandular differentiation
- **Usually poorly differentiated** with a relatively poor prognosis
- **May be difficult to diagnose** definitively in cytological specimens or small biopsies due to limited areas of sampling
- **Immunomarkers** may help in identification

Cytological findings (Figs 3.66–3.70)

- **Large clearly malignant cells**
- **Disorganised groups** and pleomorphic single cells, sometimes with ingested polymorphs or debris from nucleus
- **High N/C ratio,** irregular nuclei, multinucleation are all frequently seen
- **Dense or open chromatin pattern,** often with visible nucleoli
- **Necrotic background** frequently present
- **Spindle cell forms** sometimes seen

Differential diagnosis (Figs 3.71–3.73)

- **Cell aggregates** suggesting adenocarcinoma due to pseudo-glandular differentiation
- **Poor staining** may resemble keratinisation, suggesting squamous carcinoma
- **Metastatic tumour,** e.g. melanoma with no visible pigment, sarcoma (see Case Study Fig. 3.73)
- **Drug and chemotherapy effects**
- **Radiation changes**
- **Repair changes,** e.g. post-bronchoscopy
- **Viral degenerative effects** as seen in sputum

Further investigations

- Obtain **full clinical details**
- **Immunoprofiles:** positive for a range of epithelial markers, including CK7, CK5/6 and TTF1 negative for specific tissue markers such as melanoma
- See Table 3.2 on p. 79

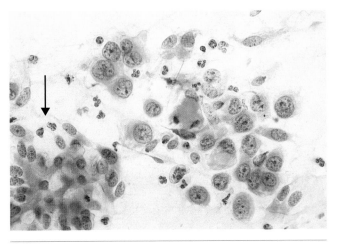

Fig. 3.66[†] Bronchial brushing. Poorly differentiated large cell carcinoma: dissociated pleomorphic cells. Normal bronchial cells lower-left corner (arrow) and two normal columnar cells in lower right corner.

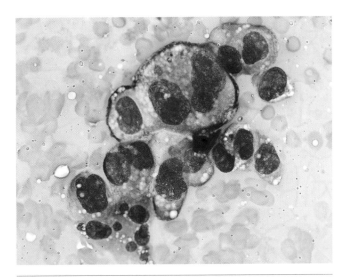

Fig. 3.67 FNA. Large cell carcinoma: pleomorphic malignant cells, some multinucleated. Note huge nucleoli and non-mucinous vacolated cytoplasm.

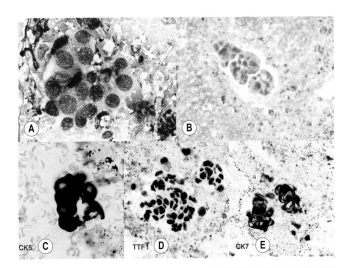

Fig. 3.68 FNA. Large cell carcinoma: (A) MGG, (B) H&E cell block, (C) CK5 positive, (D) TTF1 poitive, (E) CK7 positive.

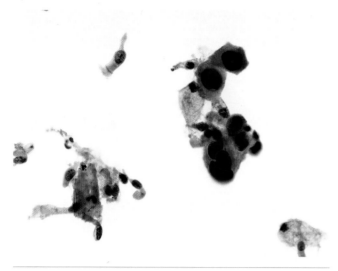

Fig. 3.69 FNA. Large cell carcinoma: obviously malignant cells with no differentiation. A few normal bronchial cells present.

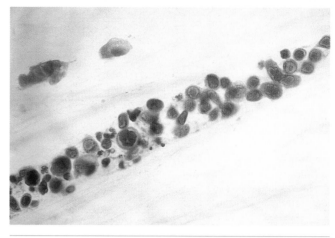

Fig. 3.71† Sputum. Herpes simplex virus degenerative changes resembling large cell carcinoma on low-power view.

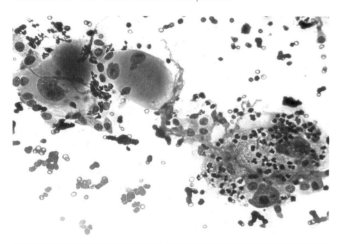

Fig. 3.70† FNA. Pure giant call carcinoma: very large multinucleated cells with ingested polymorphs, necrosis.

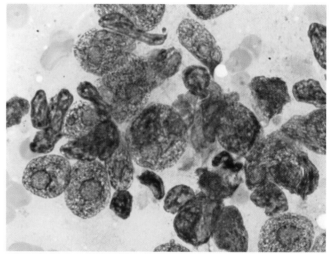

Fig. 3.72 FNA. Lung metastasis of malignant melanoma. Note the large nucleoli, granular chromatin and pale blue cytoplasm.

Case Study (Fig 3.73)

Large cell tumour

Multiple rounded lung masses were found on chest X-ray in a middle-aged man on follow-up after resection of a malignant fibrous histiocytoma of thigh 5 years previously. There was no evidence of tumour spread at the time of his surgery.

FNA of one of the nodules was performed (A and B). No clinical or past history details were given on the request form.

Initial impressions were of a poorly differentiated large cell tumour of lung but laboratory records revealed the past history. Comparison with histology section (C) gave a correct diagnosis: metastatic sarcoma.

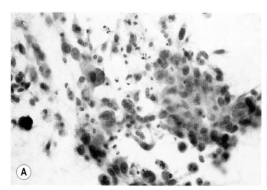
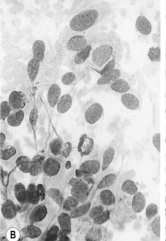
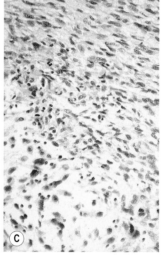

Fig. 3.73† (A) and (B): FNA lung nodule (PAP and MGG stains), (C) Original histology section.

Carcinoid tumours

- **A group forming 1% of lung tumours,** all showing evidence of neuroendocrine differentiation
- **Typical (classic) carcinoids** are usually central and submucosal, with a good prognosis. Atypical carcinoids often peripheral, especially the spindle cell variant
- **Occur in younger age group** (40–50 years) than bronchogenic carcinoma and are not related to smoking
- **Neuroendocrine features** confirmed by immunostains (e.g. chromogranin, synaptophysin)

Cytological findings (Figs 3.74–3.77)

- **Best seen in brushings and FNAs** due to their submucosal origin; rare in sputum
- **Uniform small cells,** rounded/oval nuclei, eccentric, finely stippled chromatin
- **Marked cell dissociation,** some palisades, trabeculae
- **Bare nuclei** are common but necrosis is rare
- **FNA: plexiform vascular fragments** seen
- **FNA spindle cell carcinoid:** elongated cells with delicate cytoplasm, occasional cytoplasmic granules

Differential diagnosis (Figs 3.78–3.82)

- **Small cell carcinoma:** atypical carcinoid cells have more uniform nuclei, not moulded or smeared, no background debris
- **AIS/MIA:** cells are larger, often in sheets with more cytoplasm and no vascular component
- **Lymphoma:** dissociated, more polymorphous cells
- **Mesenchymal tumours:** pleomorphic cells, variable cytoplasm

Further investigations

- Check history and clinical details for ectopic hormone effects
- **Immunoprofile**
- Strongly positive with chromogranin and synaptophysin
- See Table 3.2 on p. 79

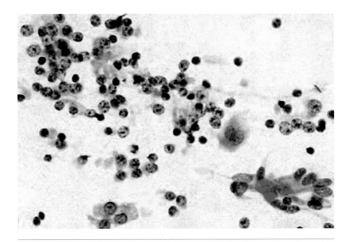

Fig. 3.74[†] Bronchial brushing. Typical carcinoid: dispersed cells, small, regular, preserved nuclei with coarse chromatin, no moulding. Cytoplasmic granules may be seen.

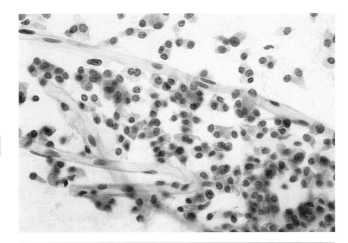

Fig. 3.75[†] Bronchial brushing. Typical carcinoid: dispersed regular cells with 'neuroendocrine' round eccentric nuclei with stippled chromatin. Plexiform capillaries in background.

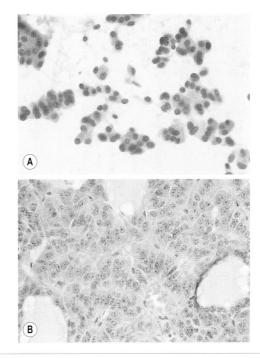

Fig. 3.76[†] Typical carcinoid. (A) FNA: clumps, cords, trabeculae of uniform tumour cells in clean background. (B) Histology.

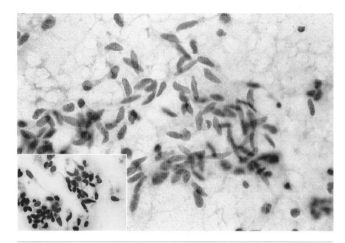

Fig. 3.77[†] Imprint from spindle cell carcinoid: elongated cells with spindle-shaped nuclei, coarse chromatin (inset).

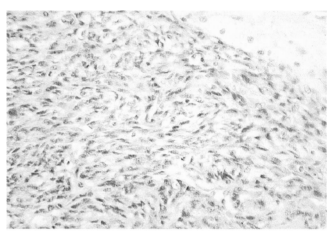

Fig. 3.80[†] FNA lung. Spindle cell thymoma (cf. Fig. 3.77 spindle cell carcinoid).

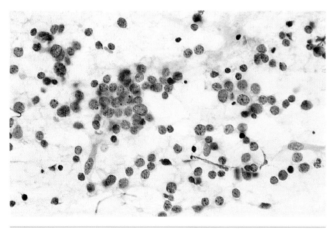

Fig. 3.78[†] Brushing. Small cell carcinoma: dispersed pleomophic small cells with some nuclear moulding.

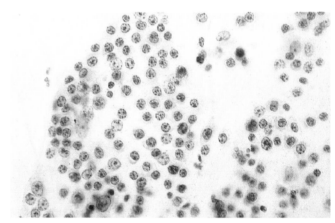

Fig. 3.81[†] Sputum. Non-Hodgkin lymphoma: dissociated cells, some nuclear variation, open chromatin, visible nucleoli.

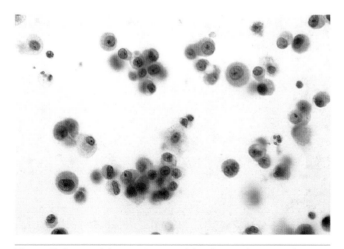

Fig. 3.79[†] Sputum. Adenocarcinoma with lepidic growth pattern showing pleomorphic cells with dense cytoplasm, some vacuolation.

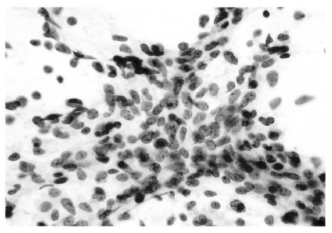

Fig. 3.82[†] FNA lung. Primitive neuroectodermal tumour (PNET): rare lung tumour with spindle cells, diagnosed with immunocytochemistry antibodies for C-myc antigen.

Other lung tumours and metastases

- **Adenoid cystic carcinoma:** primary tumour in main bronchus or peripheral metastasis from a distant primary site
- **Mucoepidermoid carcinoma:** low-grade bronchial tumour of mixed glandular and squamous cell type
- **Metastatic carcinoma:** 15–20% of FNA lung lesions in some series, e.g. breast, prostate, GIT, renal, bladder, melanoma, etc.
- **Benign bronchial papilloma** of epithelial origin
- **Juvenile papillomatosis:** arises in upper airways, may be due to human papillomavirus

Cytological findings (Figs 3.83–3.87)

- **Adenoid cystic carcinoma:** FNA: small epithelial cells with eosinophilic spheres of basement membrane material (Figs 3.83, 3.84)
- **Mucoepidermoid carcinoma:** squamous and mucinous cells with some intermediate forms
- **Metastatic tumours:** may show similar features to the primary for comparison. Immunostaining may help (Figs 3.85–3.87)
- **Papillomas:** benign-looking squames and/or glandular cells. Need clinical details for diagnosis

Differential diagnosis

- **Adenoid cystic carcinoma:** resembles small cell tumours if no spheres present
- **Mucoepidermoid carcinoma:** resembles squamous or adenocarcinoma if the FNA is not representative
- **Metastases:** remember that it could be a second primary tumour of the same histological type
- **Papillomas:** exclude well-differentiated malignancy of same histological type on clinical grounds and/or biopsy

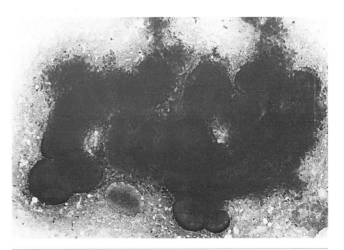

Fig. 3.83[†] FNA. Adenoid cystic carcinoma: globules of basement membrane material with sheets of small tumour cells.

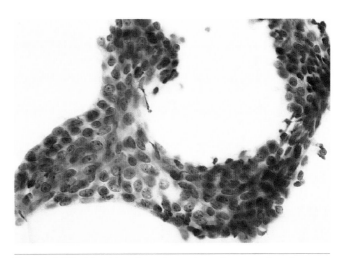

Fig. 3.84[†] FNA. Adenoid cystic carcinoma: intact fragment of poorly differentiated basaloid cells with no basement membrane spheres.

Table 3.2 Immunocytochemical markers for primary and metastatic lung carcinomas

	CK5/6	CK7	CK20	TTF1	CD56	chromogr	synapto	p63	ERP
Squamous carcinoma	+	+	–	–	–	–	–	+	–
Small cell carcinoma	–	±	–	+	+	+	+	–	–
Adenocarcinoma NOS	–	+	–	+	–	–	–	–	–
Bronchioloalveolar	–	+	±	±	–	–	–	–	–
Large cell NOS	±	+	–	±	–	–	–	±	±
Carcinoid tumour	–	–	–	±	–	+	+	–	–
Metastatic breast	±	±	–	–	–	–	–	±	+

CK, cytokeratin series; TTF, thyroid transcription factor; CD, lymphocyte marker series; Chromogr, chromogranin; Synapto, synaptophysin; ERP, oestrogen receptor protein.

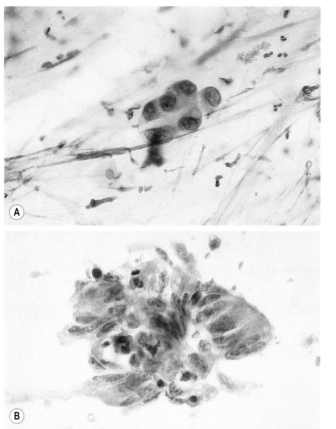

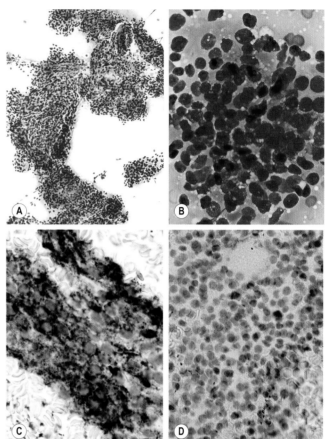

Fig. 3.85[†] (A) Sputum. Metastatic breast carcinoma cells. (B) Metastatic colonic carcinoma cells.

Fig. 3.86 EBUS-FNA. Metastatic prostatic carcinoma: (A) MGG low-power view; (B) high-power view shows an undifferentiated aggregate of tumour cells; (C) PSA positive; (D) TTF1 negative.

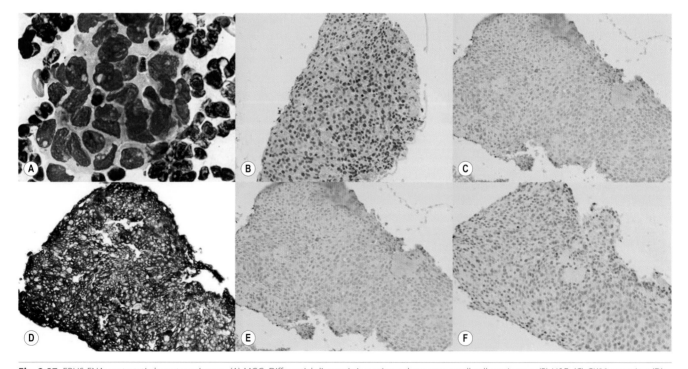

Fig. 3.87 EBUS-FNA: metastatic breast carcinoma. (A) MGG. Differential diagnosis is a primary lung non-small cell carcinoma; (B) H&E; (C) CK20 negative; (D) CK7 positive; (E) ER negative; (F) TTF1 negative. Immunocytochemistry performed on the cell block favours metastasis from a breast carcinoma.

Mesenchymal tumours and lymphomas

- **Chondroid hamartoma:** peripheral round mass (Figs 3.88 and 3.89)
- **Sclerosing haemangioma:** (pneumocytoma) mainly in women (Fig. 3.90)
- **Granular cell tumour:** bronchial Schwann cell origin (Fig. 3.91)
- **Inflammatory myofibroblastic tumour:** fibroblasts, inflammatory cells including plasma cells (Fig. 3.92)
- **Solitary fibrous tumour** of lung or pleura (Fig. 3.93)
- **Primitive neuroectodermal tumour (PNET):** mixed neural and endocrine differentiation (Fig. 3.94)
- **Pulmonary blastoma:** rare, aggressive sarcoma
- **Carcinosarcoma:** rare, aggressive, may present as an endobronchial pedunculated mass, dual malignant cell types

Cytological findings (Figs 3.88–3.96)

- **Chondroid hamartoma:** cartilage, myxoid tissue, epithelial cells, fat, macrophages
- **Sclerosing haemangioma** (pneumocytoma): epithelial cells, intranuclear inclusions
- **Granular cell tumour:** abundant granular cytoplasm, small regular nuclei
- **Solitary fibrous tumour:** spindle cells
- **Sarcomas: FNA:** metastatic or primary, discohesive spindle cells, fragile cytoplasm
- **Primitive neuroectodermal tumour:** small rounded cells in loose sheets, patchy glycogen-laden cells

Differential diagnosis

- Some of these tumours have characteristic cytology, e.g. myxoid tissue in chondroid hamartoma, granular cytoplasm in granular cell tumours, others have no specific findings
- Reactive mass: e.g. plasma cell granuloma (see Fig. 3.92)
- Sarcomas may have a characteristic biphasic picture or striations; usually clearly malignant. Distinguish from carcinomas with epithelial features, mucin production

Further investigations

- **Clinical details** are vital, e.g. location, duration, gender, past history
- **Immunoprofile**
- Variable epithelial and connective tissue positive staining according to the histological type (see other sections on carcinoma, lymphoma and metastases)

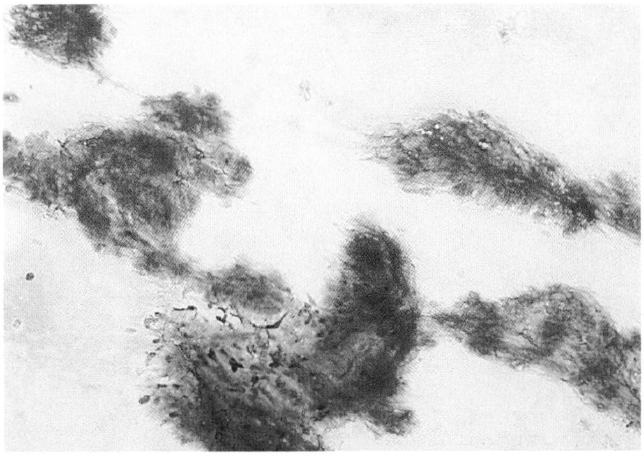

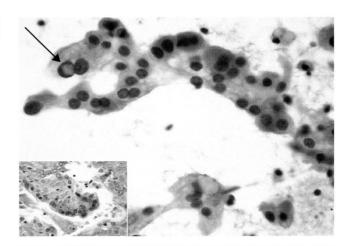

Fig. 3.88† Chondroid hamartoma. FNA: magenta-stained chondromyxoid tissue.

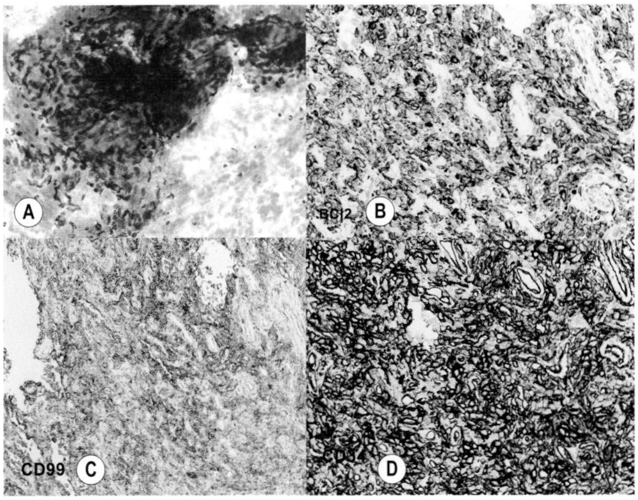

Fig. 3.89 EBUS-FNA. Solitary fibrous tumour. (A) MGG shows bundles of spindle cells; (B) Bcl 2 positive; (C) CD99 weakly positive; (D) CD34 positive.

Fig. 3.90† Pneumocytoma (sclerosing haemangioma). Group of mildly pleomorphic bronchiolar type cells with intranuclear cytoplasmic inclusions (arrow). Inset: Biopsy of pneumocytoma.

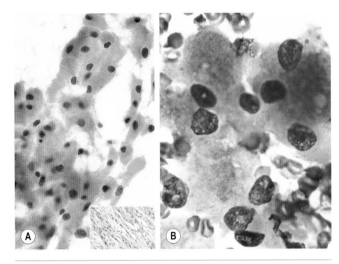

Fig. 3.91 Granular cell tumour FNA. (A)[†] Loose aggregates of cells (PAP). Inset[†]: Cords of granular cells on biopspy specimen; (B) MGG: granular cytoplasm, round eccentric nuclei.

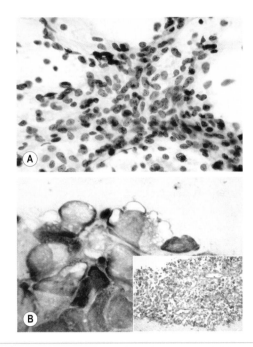

Fig. 3.94[†] FNA: primitive neuroectodermal tumour (PNET). (A) Loose sheet of small round cells (PAP); (B) Glycogen laden cells. Inset: histology shows CD99++.

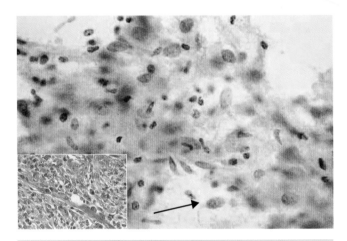

Fig. 3.92[†] Inflammatory myofibroblastic tumour. FNA: mixed spindle and inflammatory cells including plasma cells (arrow), also in inset showing biopsy with mixed cellularity.

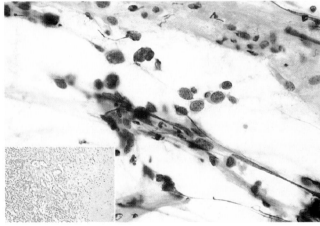

Fig. 3.95[†] Bronchial brushing, pulmonary blastoma: pleomorphic small celled tumour. Inset: original histology section of tumour.

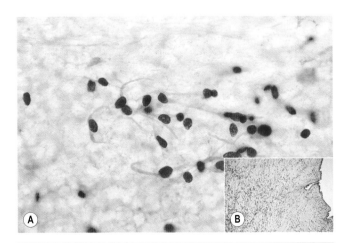

Fig. 3.93[†] (A) Solitary fibrous tumour of pleura. FNA: spindle cells with mild nuclear pleomorphism. (B) Inset: Biopsydense fibrous tissue, variable cellularity.

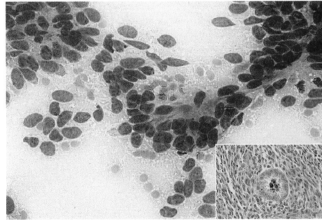

Fig. 3.96[†] Pulmonary blastoma FNA. Groups include spindle cells and suggestion of biphasic pattern as seen in histology (inset).

Pulmonary lymphomas, leukaemia

- **Primary lymphoproliferative disorders of lung** are uncommon but lung is often involved at some stage in non-Hodgkin lymphomas
- **Low-grade B-cell MALT lymphoma** in adults is the commonest primary lymphoma of lungs. High-grade B cell lymphoma is also seen
- **Angiocentric pattern** of infiltration is common
- **Hodgkin lymphoma** rarely occurs as a primary lung tumour

Cytological findings: lymphoma (Figs 3.97–3.99)

- **Lavage or FNA** are better diagnostic material than sputum
- **Large cell lymphomas** are easier to diagnose than small or mixed cell types
- **Discohesive cells,** intact cytoplasm
- **Hodgkin lymphoma:** mixed cellularity with a few Hodgkin and Reed–Sternberg cells

Differential diagnosis: lymphoma

- **Reactive lymphocytic infiltrate:** mixed population of lymphocytes, plasma cells, macrophages
- **Small cell carcinoma:** nuclear moulding is absent in lymphoma, but crush artefact of bare nuclei is seen (see Figs 3.43 and 3.44)
- **Hodgkin lymphoma** versus anaplastic or giant cell carcinoma (see Fig. 3.118 and see Fig. 3.70)

Further investigations

Immunocytochemistry
- **Reactive proliferation:** mixed immunostaining with lymphoid markers, no clonality
- **Small cell versus low-grade lymphoma:** CD56, keratin (dot-like), chromogranin all positive; CD20 and other lymphoid markers positive according to type
- **Hodgkin and Reed–Sternberg cells** are CD20 and often CD15 positive, carcinoma markers negative
- See Table 3.2 of lung carcinoma markers (see page 79)

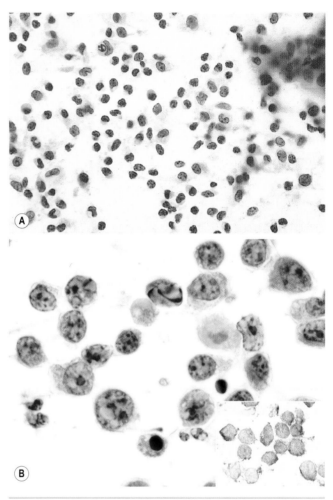

Fig. 3.98 (A)[†] Non-Hodgkin lymphoma T-cell type (FNA). (B) Dissociated mildly pleomorphic lymphoid cells. Inset CD20 immunomarker uniformly positive, confirming B cell type lymphoma.

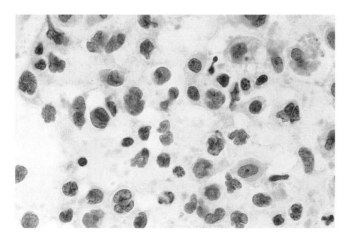

Fig. 3.97 Lung/mediastinal mass (FNA). Dispersed cells with unequivocal nuclear features of malignancy and suggesting hyperlobated malignant lymphoma cells. The diagnosis was confirmed by biopsy (H&E).

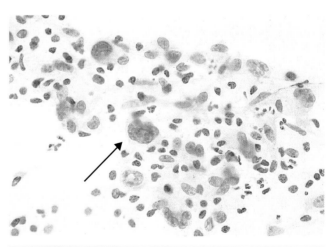

Fig. 3.99 Hodgkin lymphoma FNA. Reed–Sternberg cells (arrow) with lymphoid cells and atypical mononuclear cells.

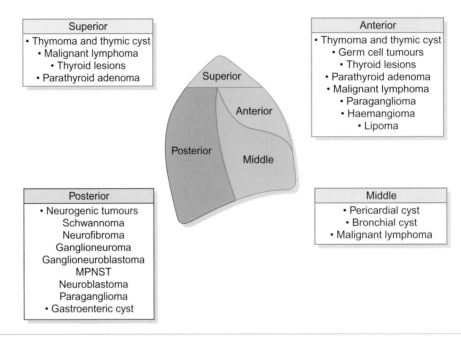

Superior
- Thymoma and thymic cyst
- Malignant lymphoma
- Thyroid lesions
- Parathyroid adenoma

Anterior
- Thymoma and thymic cyst
- Germ cell tumours
- Thyroid lesions
- Parathyroid adenoma
- Malignant lymphoma
- Paraganglioma
- Haemangioma
- Lipoma

Posterior
- Neurogenic tumours
  Schwannoma
  Neurofibroma
  Ganglioneuroma
  Ganglioneuroblastoma
  MPNST
  Neuroblastoma
  Paraganglioma
- Gastroenteric cyst

Middle
- Pericardial cyst
- Bronchial cyst
- Malignant lymphoma

Fig. 3.100† Location of the most common tumours and cysts of the mediastinum. MPNST: Malignant peripheral nerve sheath tumour.

Mediastinal tumours

Thymoma (Figs 3.100–3.104)
- **Commonest tumour** in anterior mediastinum in adults
- **Classified** as: type A epithelial, type B epithelial atypia, with or without a lymphocytic component
- **Many variants:** spindle cell, lymphocyte rich, mixed A&B, encapsulated tumours, minimally invasive
- **Cytology:** cohesive pale epithelial cells, regular nuclei, variable numbers of lymphocytes
- **Differential diagnosis:** NHL or Hodgkin lymphoma, soft tissue tumours if spindle cell type of thymoma

Thymic carcinoma (Figs 3.105–3.106)
- **A spectrum** from atypical thymoma to a frankly invasive metastasising tumour
- **Cytology:** dispersed or aggregated clearly malignant cells, or frankly epithelial, e.g. squamous carcinoma of thymus
- **Origin** from thymus must be established by excluding other primary sites, e.g. lung cancer
- **Immunoprofile:** panel for benign and malignant thymomas CK7 and TTF1 negative (adenocarcinoma lung CK7 positive), CD5, CD99 positive
- **Exclude neuroendocrine carcinoma** with immunocytochemistry (see Fig. 3.47)

Thymic/mediastinal lymphomas
- **Anterior/superior mediastinum** or separate from thymus, arising in lymph nodes (Figs 3.107, 3.113 and 3.116)
- **Cytology:** dissociated cells of lymphoid type, mono-morphic or pleomorphic. Hodgkin lymphoma also seen
- **Immunocytochemistry** required for firm diagnosis (see Chapter 7)

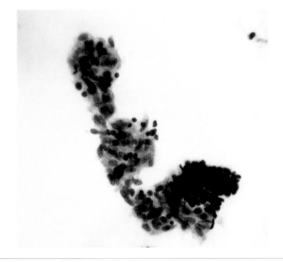

Fig. 3.101† Benign thymoma FNA. Bland spindle cells with many lymphoid cells.

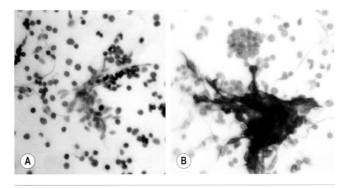

Fig. 3.102† FNA. Thymoma: thin prep sample from Fig. 3.101. (A) lymphocyte marker positive for T lymphocytes (CD3), (B) epithelial marker positive (AE1-AE3).

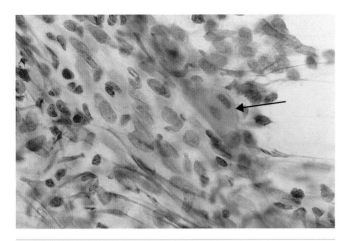

Fig. 3.103† Lymphoepithelial thymoma metastasis to lung: oval pale epithelial cells, few lymphocytes, Hassall's corpuscle (*arrow*).

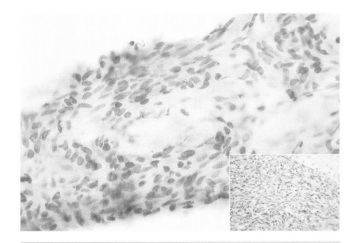

Fig. 3.104† Spindle cell thymoma FNA. Cohesive fragment of spindle cells, mildly pleomorphic as in histology (inset).

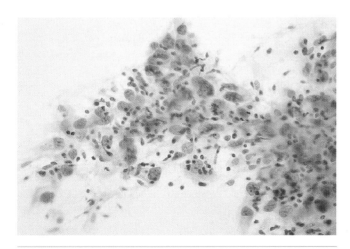

Fig. 3.105† Thymic carcinoma FNA. Disorganised aggregate of large cohesive (? epithelial) malignant cells, few lymphocytes.

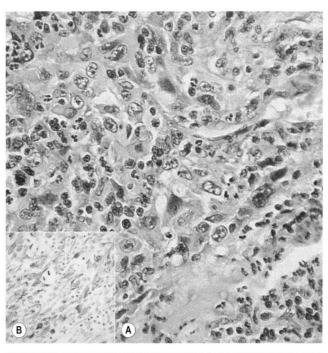

Fig. 3.106† (A) Histological section of tumour in Fig. 3.104 showing epithelial malignancy with scattered lymphocytes. (B) Positive staining with CK7 (AE1-AE3).

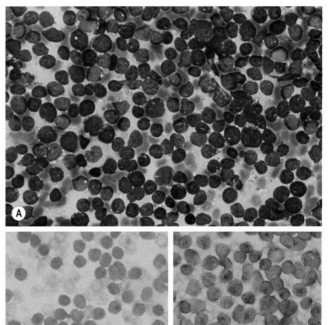

Fig. 3.107† Lymphoblastic lymphoma of thymus FNA. (A) Small to medium sized blast cells, all dissociated. (B) B-cell marker negative. (C) T-cell marker positive.

Mediastinal germ cell tumours (GCTs)

- **25% of childhood mediastinal tumours** (15% in adults, mainly males) are of this type
- **Occur as seminomas, non-seminomatous germ cell tumours and teratomas**
- **GCTs** may be associated with acute leukaemia
- **Seminomas** are usually solid, teratomas cystic, non-seminomatous GCTs heterogeneous
- **Most GCTs develop adjacent to the thymus** or in the posterior mediastinum; and may invade lung

Cytological findings (Figs 3.108–3.116)

- **Seminoma**: dispersed fragile cells with 'tigroid' background
  - Pleomorphic nuclei, prominent nucleoli
  - Macrophages and inflammatory cells in cystic lesions
- **Mature teratoma**: anucleate squames, keratin, columnar cells, mucus, macrophages
- **Malignant teratoma**: malignant epithelial and connective tissue groups, necrosis
- **Embryonal carcinoma:** primitive cells CD30 positive

Differential diagnosis

- **Metastatic tumours** (e.g. Fig. 3.116): clinical details, include immunostaining for carcinoma, melanoma, etc.
- **Metastatic GCT** from primary testicular tumour: identical cytologically
- **Other cystic lesions:** thymic tumours, NHL, Hodgkin disease (Figs 3.113 and 3.116). Use lymphoma markers

Further investigations

- Clinical details essential
- PLAP, CD117 both positive in seminoma
- CD30 positive in embryonal carcinoma
- α fetoprotein positive in yolk sac tumour
- β-HCG positive in choriocarcinoma
- CD15 negative in all GCTs
- Lymphoma markers (see Chapter 7)

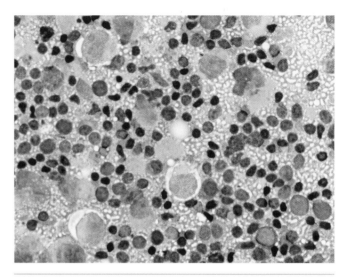

Fig. 3.108[†] Mediastinal seminoma FNA. Dissociated cells with poorly defined cytoplasm, large eccentric nuclei and prominent nucleoli, note 'tigroid' background, a few lymphocytes.

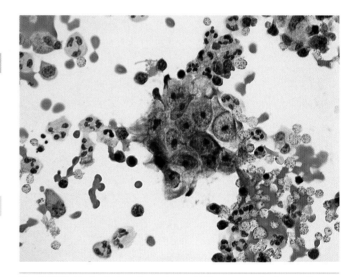

Fig. 3.109[†] Mediastinal cystic seminoma FNA, young male. Group of malignant cells with large nucleoli, inflammatory cells, blood (see Fig. 3.110).

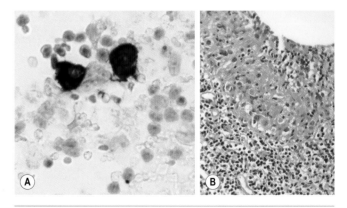

Fig. 3.110[†] (A) Pan cytokeratin stain on case in Fig. 3.109 showing seminoma cells with lymphocytes. (B) Histology.

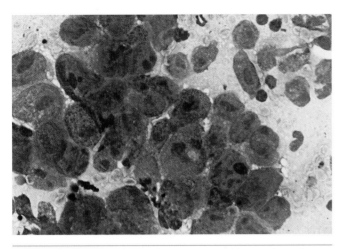

Fig. 3.111† Mediastinal embryonal carcinoma FNA. Pleomorphic malignant cells with high N/C ratio, prominent nucleoli.

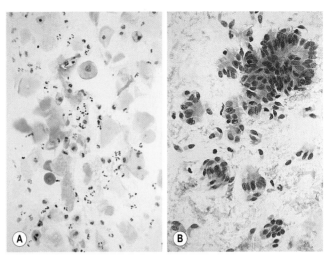

Fig. 3.114† Mediastinal mature cystic teratoma FNA. Squames, keratin, inflammatory cells on left, ciliated columnar cells on right.

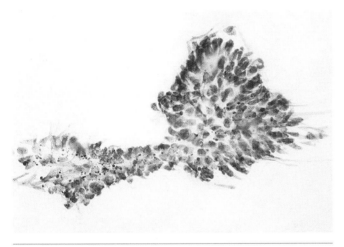

Fig. 3.112† Lung and mediastinal malignant teratoma FNA: cohesive epithelial cells with apoptotic nuclei (see Fig. 3.115).

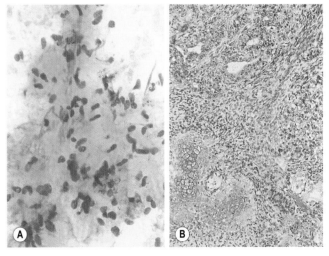

Fig. 3.115† Same case as Fig. 3.112. (A) Fibromyxoid mesenchymal fragment. (B) Histology, mixed malignant tissue.

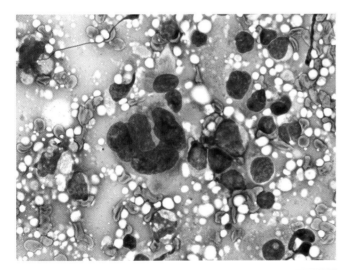

Fig. 3.113† Mediastinal lymphoma, young man, touch prep. Pleomorphic malignant cells from high-grade B-cell non-Hodgkin lymphoma.

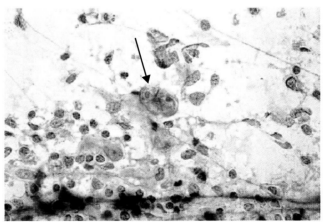

Fig. 3.116† FNA mediastinal mass. Hodgkin lymphoma; Reed–Sternberg cell (arrow) in a background of lymphoid cells and atypical mononuclear cells. Cytological findings suggesting Hodgkin lymphoma, confirmed on formal biopsy (PAP).

Lung infections

- **Cytological findings** are often non-specific, diagnosis usually made by culture of organism
- **Viral infections** may show cytopathic diagnostic features in exfoliated samples e.g. lavage fluid containing well-preserved cells
- **Fungal and parasitic infections** can sometimes be identified directly in certain samples e.g. lavage with well-preserved fungi/parasites
- **Immunosuppression** may be an underlying factor in unusual infections (see Table 3.3 on p. 91)

Bacterial infections

Acute bacterial infections (Figs 3.117–3.119)

- **Lobar or bronchopneumonia** may be present with purulent/bloodstained sputum
- **Polymorphonuclear exudate debris and degenerate cells** may obscure sample, a robust screen for malignant cells as tumour may be the underlying cause
- **Gram stains** do not definitively identify organisms: culture of sample is necessary for diagnosis

Chronic bacterial infections (Figs 3.120–3.125)

- **Pulmonary tuberculosis** (TB) is increasing in frequency worldwide due to bacterial resistance and immunosuppression (see below)
- **Early acute inflammatory changes** are replaced by chronic inflammation with granulomata and caseation necrosis (an immune response)
- **Atypical mycobacteria:** are seen with immunosuppression
- **Other organisms** may induce granulomata, e.g. fungi

Bacterial infections: differential diagnosis

- **Epithelia atypia may be present:** need clinical details and a 'wait and see' policy to exclude an underlying tumour
- **Overgrowth of organisms** from mouth (Fig. 3.119): recognised by absence of inflammatory cells
- **Obstructing tumour** may present with pneumonia; screen slides fully for malignant cells
- **Other causes** of granulomatous inflammation (see Other pulmonary conditions on p. 97)

Pulmonary TB: cytological findings (Figs 3.120–3.125)

- **Chronic inflammatory cells:** mainly lymphocytes, macrophages, plasma cells
- **EBUS-FNA:** epithelioid histiocytes, caseous necrosis and Langhans giant cells with arc of eccentric nuclei
- **Ziehl–Neelsen stain positive** for acid fast bacilli, including atypical types

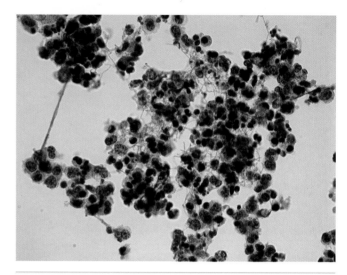

Fig. 3.117[†] Bronchial lavage fluid from transplant patient. Polymorph exudate obscuring cells. Organisms visible (see Fig. 3.118).

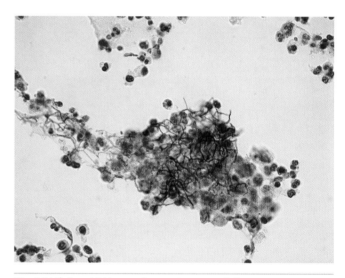

Fig. 3.118[†] Bronchial lavage. Gram stain on sample from Fig. 3.117 showing Gram-positive bacilli consistent with *Nocardia asteroides* confirmed on microbiology culture (opportunistic).

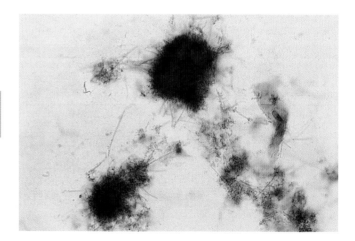

Fig. 3.119[†] Actinomycotic bacteria in sputum, forming balls of organisms with no inflammation, probably oral contaminant.

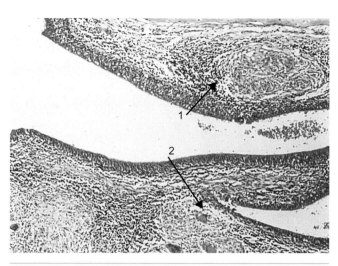

Fig. 3.120[†] Bronchial wall histology. TB with submucosal granulomas (*arrow 1*) and chronic inflammation. Giant cells visible (*arrow 2*).

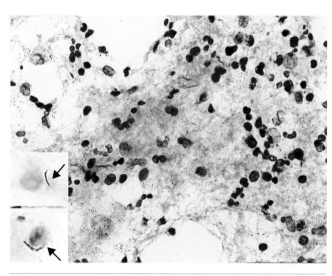

Fig. 3.123 Acid-fast bacilli in bronchial washing with ZN stain. Insets: organisms on high power (arrows). Note bended shapes, beaded staining.

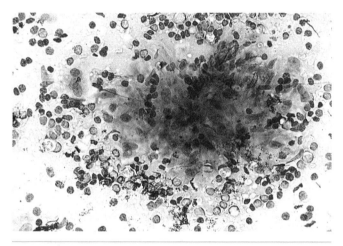

Fig. 3.121[†] TB granuloma in FNA, with chronic inflammatory cells, pale-stained epithelioid histiocytes and central necrosis.

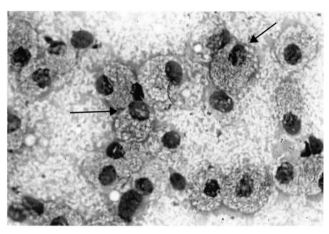

Fig. 3.124[†] *Mycobacterium avium-intracellulare* in lymph node FNA. Swollen foamy macrophages with negative images of bacilli (arrows) (see Fig. 3.125).

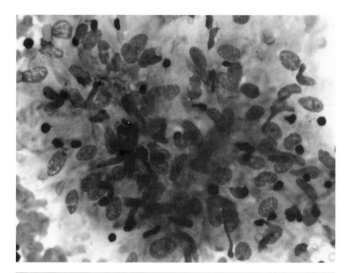

Fig. 3.122 EBUS-FNA. Granuloma with chronic inflammatory cells and pale-stained epithelioid histiocytes.

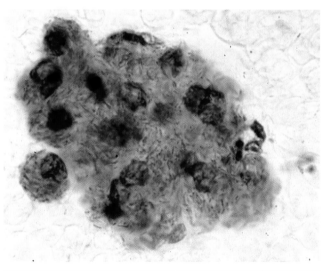

Fig. 3.125[†] Ziehl–Neelsen stain on material from Fig. 3.124. Immunosuppressed patient with numerous acid-fast bacilli.

Viral infections

- Viral infections may cause characteristic cytopathic effects in epithelial cells and alveolar macrophages although the virus is within the nucleus
- Non-specific inflammatory and reactive changes also seen in the same sample
- Changes seen best in sputum and bronchial secretions, using PAP staining
- Immunosuppression is a common factor (see Table 3.3 on p. 91)

Cytological findings: non-specific viral effects

- Non-specific inflammation and debris
- Necrosis
- Ciliocytophthoria (see Fig. 3.8): fragmented cells with separate nuclei and cilia
- Bronchial and alveolar cell hyperplasia
- Swollen degenerate epithelial cells with loss of nuclear structure

Cytological findings: specific changes (Figs 3.126–3.132)

- Intranuclear inclusion bodies (herpes (HSV), cytomegalovirus (CMV), adenovirus)
- Loss of chromatin pattern (all viruses)
- Multinucleation (herpes, measles, respiratory syncytial virus (RSV))
- Nuclear moulding (herpes, varicella)
- Cytoplasmic inclusion bodies (herpes, cytomegalovirus)

Differential diagnosis: viral infections

- Need to exclude malignancy in cases with marked bronchial hyperplasia especially if cells are atypical
- Specific cytological viral changes may overlap with other viral type changes
- Mixed viral infection may be present

Further investigations

- Detailed screening of sample for specific features of viral infection or definitive changes of underlying malignancy
- Submit material for microbiological culture
- Request further samples if in doubt
- Check all clinical information
- Immunomarkers may identify viral type accuracy e.g. HSV, CMV (see Fig. 3.131)

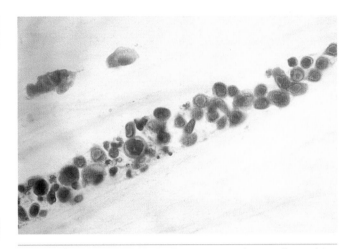

Fig. 3.126[†] Sputum. HSV changes, degenerate cytoplasm, swollen nuclei, loss of chromatin pattern (cf. malignant cells look-alike).

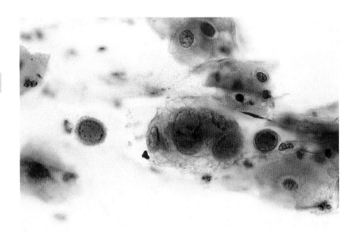

Fig. 3.127[†] HSV changes in sputum (immunosuppressed patient). Swollen bronchial cells, ground-glass chromatin, moulding.

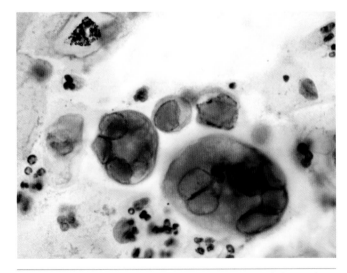

Fig. 3.128 HSV changes in sputum showing swollen ground-glass nuclei with inclusions.

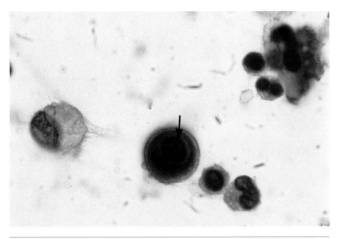

Fig. 3.129† Bronchoalveolar lavage. CMV inclusion bodies in lavage fluid from a transplant patient.

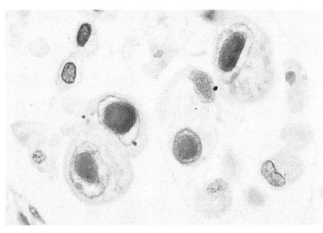

Fig. 3.131† Immunoperoxidase stain with anti-CMV antibody on same sample as Fig. 3.130, confirming diagnosis of CMV.

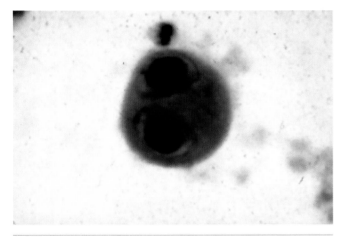

Fig. 3.130† Bronchoalveolar lavagae. High-power view of CMV inclusions giving an 'owl's eye' appearance.

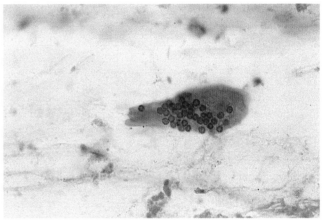

Fig. 3.132† Sputum. Measles virus pneumonia; multinucleated macrophage (giant cell). Note loss of chromatin pattern.

Table 3.3 Principal causes of pulmonary dysfunction in the immunosuppressed

INFECTION	NEOPLASIA
• Bacterial	• Lymphoproliferative disorders
– *Staph. aureus*	• Leukaemia
– *Strep. pneumoniae*	• Hodgkin's lymphoma
– *H. influenzae*	• Myeloma
– *P. aeruginosa*	• Kaposi's sarcoma
– *L. pneumophila*	• Bronchial carcinoma
– *M. tuberculosis*	• Secondary carcinoma
– *M. avium-intracellulare*	**IATROGENIC PROCESSES**
• Viral	• Irradiation
– Cytomegalovirus	• Drug toxicity
– Herpes simplex	• Oxygen toxicity
– Adenovirus	• Graft-versus-host disease
• Fungal	• Rejection of lung allograft
– *P. jiroveci*	**IDIOPATHIC AND MISCELLANEOUS PROCESSES**
– *Candida* spp.	• Lipoproteinosis
– *Aspergillus* spp.	• Alveolar haemorrhage
– *C. neoformans*	• Lymphocytic interstitial pneumonia
– *H. capsulatum*	• Non-specific interstitial pneumonia
– *C. immitis*	
• Parasitic	
– *T. gondii*	
– *S. stercoralis*	

Fungal infections

- Fungi: septate or non-septate branching hyphae with chains of spores if aerobic (fruiting head)
- May be dimorphic with hyphae and yeast forms
- May be true pathogen or opportunistic infection in lung, or saprophytic in diseased tissue
- Remember that contaminants from mouth/slide/stain are common
- Allergic reaction to the fungus may occur

Aspergillus spp.: clinical settings in lung

- **Saprophytic colonisation** of airways, e.g. mucosal damage, bronchiectasis
- **Allergic bronchopulmonary aspergillosis,** e.g. in asthma, causes severe mucoid plugging
- **Aspergilloma:** a fungal colony formed in a cavity within the lung
- **Invasive aspergillosis:** occurs in immunosuppression

Cytological findings: *Aspergillus* spp. (Figs 3.133–3.135)

- Septate hyphae 3–4 μ in width
- Dichotomous branching at 45° angle
- Fruiting heads form in aerobic conditions, e.g. in lung cavities
- Oxalate crystals form within colonies due to degenerative changes
- May be a contaminant but should be reported

Differential diagnosis: *Aspergillus* spp.

- Degenerative changes may alter fungal structure making recognition difficult
- Fungal hyphae may be contaminants (see above)
- Other infections, e.g. viral, bacterial may also be present if patient is immunosuppressed

Further investigations

- Clinical details and radiology findings are essential to assess the significance of the findings
- Culture for confirmation is necessary but results take time
- Ensure that the sample is from the airways (if exfoliative), not from the mouth – macrophages help if present
- Ensure that specimens for cytology are prepared without delay to avoid overgrowth of fungi

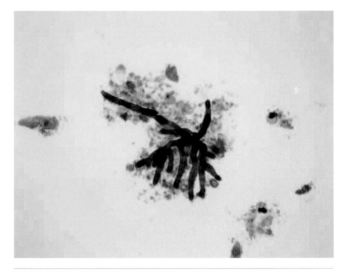

Fig. 3.133[†] BAL from patient with lymphoma. *Aspergillus* spp. hyphae in radiating 'sunburst' pattern.

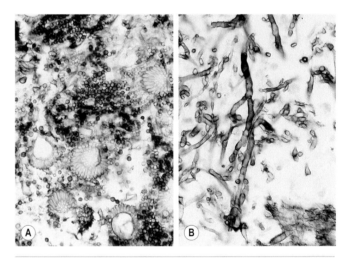

Fig. 3.134[†] (A) Cavitated lung carcinoma with mycetoma: septate hyphae, fruiting heads, spores. (B) Septate branching hyphae.

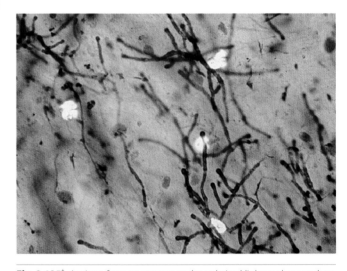

Fig. 3.135[†] Aspirate from mycetoma under polarised light to show oxalate crystals among the hyphae.

Pneumocystis jirovecii (previously *P. carinii*)

- An opportunistic fungus, present in soil and atmosphere, previously thought to be a protozoon
- Causes pneumonia in untreated AIDS cases with breathlessness, cough and fever due to a foamy proteinaceous exudate in alveolar spaces
- May cause lung infections with other immunosuppressive conditions but this is less common
- Organisms (trophozoites) attach to type 1 pneumocytes then form cysts containing merozoites which are released as trophozoites, completing the life cycle

Cytological findings (Figs 3.136–3.138)

- Amphophilic alveolar casts with honeycomb appearance due to unstained cysts (PAP)
- Grocott silver stain shows cysts 5–8 μ diameter
- Free trophozoites not easily seen but may be visible using MGG stain
- Empty cup-shaped cysts often seen
- BAL fluid or induced sputum are the best samples for diagnosis

Differential diagnosis

- Other fungi, e.g. *Histoplasma*, *Candida*, *Cryptococcus* spp. may resemble *P. jirovecii*
- Alveolar casts occur in other conditions, e.g. pulmonary alveolar proteinosis, amyloidosis
- Artefacts, e.g. degenerate blood cells and air trapped under the slide
- Missed diagnosis: too few cysts present if already treated

Further investigations

- PAP and Grocott stains mainly used but others, e.g. Toluidine blue, fluorescent microscopy with monoclonal antibodies, immunocytochemistry may be used
- Polymerase chain reaction has high diagnostic sensitivity with DNA amplification
- All preparations must be fully screened to avoid missing mixed infections

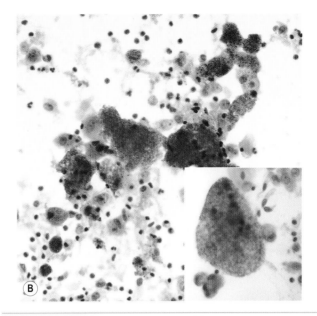

Fig. 3.136[†] (B) BAL from HIV-positive haemophiliac patient. Note amphophilic alveolar casts with honeycomb pattern. Inset: high-power view of the alveolar casts.

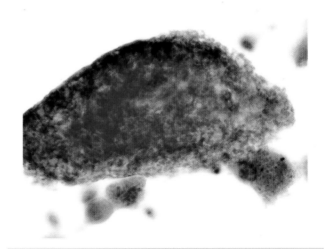

Fig. 3.137[†] Alveolar cast from HIV-positive patient. Note alveolar three-dimensional shape, amphophilia and honeycomb appearance.

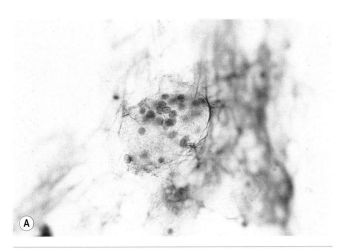

Fig. 3.136[†] (A) *Pneumocystis jiroveci* in a plaque stained with modified toluidine blue method, a more rapid technique than the traditional Grocott stain. Bronchoalveolar lavage.

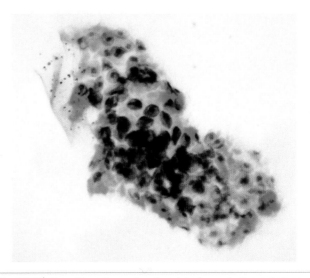

Fig. 3.138[†] Grocott's methenamine silver stain demonstrating cysts in an alveolar plaque.

Other fungal infections (Figs 3.139–3.144)

- **Candida** spp.: budding yeast or hyphae
- Zygomycetes (e.g. *Mucor* species): hyphae
- **Cryptococcus neoformans:** yeast with mucoid capsule, narrow-necked single budding
- **Histoplasma capsulatum:** intracellular yeast
- **Paracoccidiomycosis:** cyst-forming yeast (mainly in the Americas)
- **Blastomycetes:** budding yeast forms

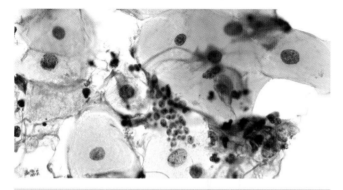

Fig. 3.139† Sputum. Contaminant spores and hyphae in salivary specimen, no inflammation.

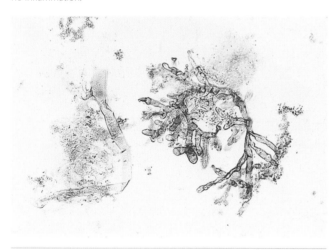

Fig. 3.140† Bronchial washing (diabetic patient). *Mucor* sp. Broad non-septate hyphae, irregular branching.

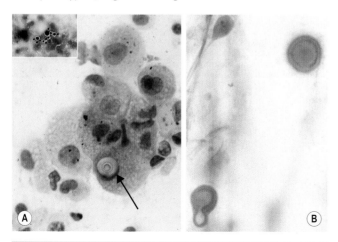

Fig. 3.141 Sputum. (A) *Cryptococcus neoformans*: at arrow. Inset: Grocott stain shows translucent capsule. (B)† Mucicarmine stain showing dense capsule and budding.

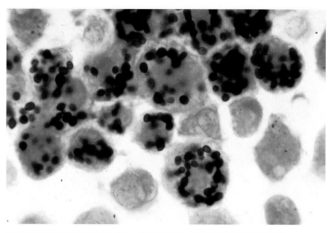

Fig. 3.142† BAL from immunosuppressed patient. Alveolar macrophages containing *Histoplasma* yeasts (Gomori stain).

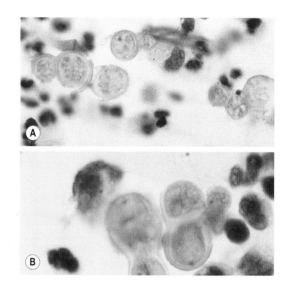

Fig. 3.143† BAL *Blastomyces dermatiditis*. Large yeasts, refractile cell wall, single broad-based budding in A and B.

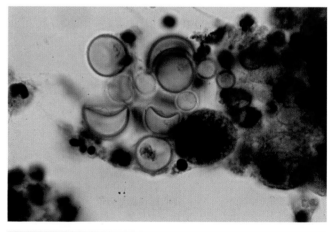

Fig. 3.144 Paracoccidioidomycosis. Cystic bodies including some empty cup-shaped forms. (Bronchoalveolar lavage)

Parasitic infections

- These are rare as a primary lung infection unless the patient is immunosuppressed
- Protozoa, nematodes, trematodes, cestodes, arthropods and leeches have been recorded clinically, but may not be sampled cytologically
- Protozoa include *Entamoeba gingivalis* and *E. histolytica*, *Giardia lamblia*, *Trichomonas* spp.
- Worms: *Strongyloides stercoralis*

Cytological findings (Figs 3.145–3.148)

- **Entamoebae:** amoeboid 10–40 μ; *E. gingivali*s – ingested polymorphs, *E. histolytica* – ingested red blood cells
- **Strongyloides:** worm-like larva, 400–500 μ in length, expanded at one end, notch at tail
- Most protozoa and other parasites infecting lung have not yet been described in cytology samples

Differential diagnosis

- Firm identification may be possible from sputum sample or washing but appearances within species often overlap
- Could be oral contaminants (e.g. *E. gingivalis* if dental hygiene is poor) or may be due to atmospheric contamination during collection of sample or processing
- Awareness of immune status important

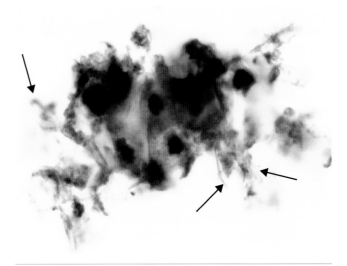

Fig. 3.146 *Entamoeba* gingivitis associated with food (*arrows*). (Sputum)

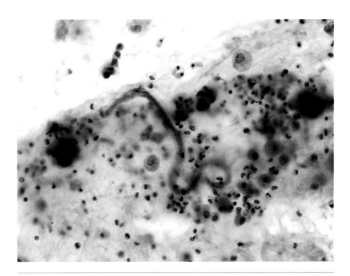

Fig. 3.147[†] BAL from immunosuppressed patient. *Strongyloides* with inflammatory debris.

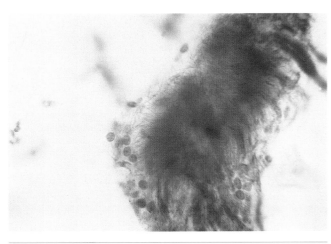

Fig. 3.145[†] Sputum. *Entamoeba gingivalis* organisms adherent to *Actinomyces* spp. colony, probably saprophytic from mouth.

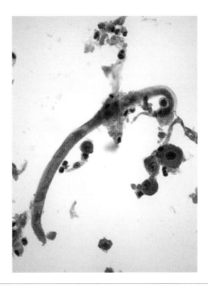

Fig. 3.148[†] BAL from HTLV-1-positive patient. *Strongyloides* larvum (notch not visible).

Other pulmonary conditions

Chronic obstructive pulmonary disease (COPD)

- Spectrum of chronic bronchitis and emphysema
- Hypertrophied bronchial glands, excess sputum
- Recurrent chest infections
- Strong association with smoking and lung cancer
- Less common today than in the past (less atmospheric pollution)

Cytological findings (Figs 3.149, 3.150)

- Groups of hyperplastic bronchial cells
- Goblet cells, reserve cell hyperplasia
- Degenerative changes, ciliocytophthoria
- Squamous metaplasia with increasing atypia
- Curschmann's spirals

Differential diagnosis

- All of the above findings are non-specific: need good clinical details
- Hyperplasia can mimic adenocarcinoma: look for uneven chromatin, macronucleoli
- Atypical metaplasia versus squamous carcinoma: difficult since they may coexist

Bronchiectasis (Fig. 3.151)

- Less common now due to antibiotic use
- Permanently dilated damaged bronchi, foul sputum, recurrent infections and risk of carcinoma developing in wall of a bronchiectatic cavity

Cytological findings

- Purulent, mucoid or bloody sputum
- Many polymorphs, lymphocytes, cell debris present
- Hyperplastic epithelium or squamous metaplasia with or without atypia

Further investigations

- Clinical details are important since there is often a long history
- May require examination of further samples to exclude malignancy

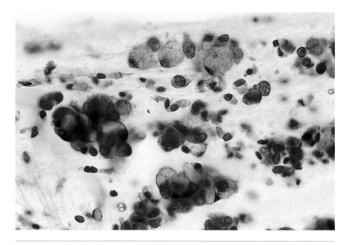

Fig. 3.149† Bronchial washing, COPD. Clusters of swollen bronchial cells, a few goblet cells, inflammatory cells.

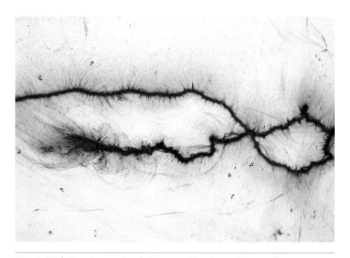

Fig. 3.150† Curschmann's spiral, a cast of inspissated mucus from a bronchiole. (Sputum, COPD)

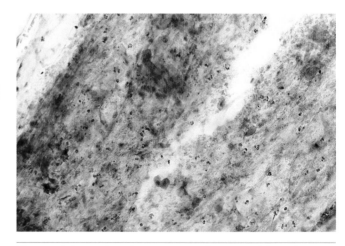

Fig. 3.151† Sputum bronchiectatic cavity. Inflammatory debris with degenerate keratinised cells, no obvious atypia.

Allergic bronchopulmonary disease

- **Bronchial asthma** is the commonest type; allergic bronchopulmonary aspergillosis, eosinophilic pneumonia and extrinsic allergic alveolitis are uncommon types
- **Acute asthma** causes outpouring of fluid with mucus and shedding of cells and eosinophils
- **Aspergillus spp.** induces type III allergic reaction with asthmatic symptoms (see p. 3.34)

Cytological findings (Figs 3.152–3.155)

- Mucus plugs (lavage fluid)
- Ciliated hyperplastic epithelial cell clumps (Creola bodies)
- Eosinophils, Charcot–Leyden (C–L) crystals form degenerate eosinophil granules
- Curschmann's spirals: inspissated casts from small airways
- Inflammatory debris ± fungal hyphae may be seen

Differential diagnosis

- Hyperplastic bronchial epithelial groups have been mistaken for adenocarcinoma cells: Creola bodies were an early example of this, diagnosed as adenocarcinoma in a young woman
- Eosinophils may be due to eosinophilic pneumonia, tumour or parasites, with symptoms of asthma
- Degenerate fungi may be missed, leading to inappropriate treatment

Further investigations

- A full clinical history usually confirms the diagnosis

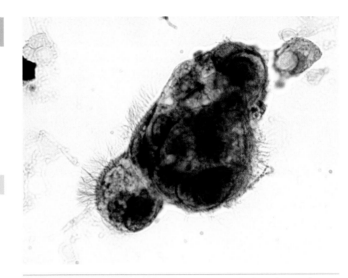

Fig. 3.153[†] Sputum from asthmatic patient. Creola body with typical curved (embryo-like) shape, visible mucus in cytoplasm, prominent ciliated borders.

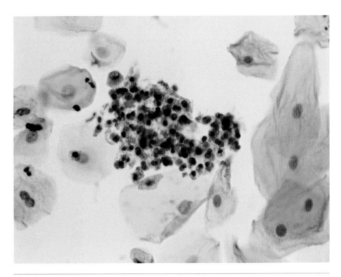

Fig. 3.154 Sputum from asthmatic child. Many eosinophils with bi- and single-lobed nuclei.

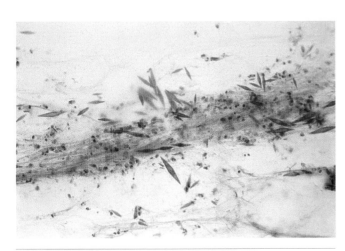

Fig. 3.152[†] Sputum, asthma. Charcot–Leyden crystals bright orange with acicular octahedral shape.

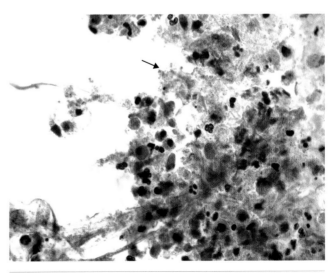

Fig. 3.155[†] Washings from patient with allergic bronchopulmonary aspergillosis: debris with eosinophils, C-L crystals, few hyphae (*arrow*).

Sarcoidosis (Figs 3.156, 3.157)

- Commonest of non-infective granulomas, 90% of cases of sarcoidosis involve the respiratory tract
- Cell-mediated immunity depressed
- Cytology: epithelioid histiocytes, variable giant cells, many lymphocytes (T-helper cells)
- Inclusions: Schaumann bodies, asteroids
- No necrosis
- See Table 3.4 for sources of granulomas

Table 3.4 Conditions associated with pulmonary granulomata

INFECTIONS

Bacterial
- *Mycobacterium tuberculosis* and other mycobacteria
- *Nocardia asteroides*

Fungi
- *Aspergillus fumigatus, niger, flavus*
- *Blastomyces dermatitidis*
- *Candida albicans*
- *Coccidioides immitis*
- *Cryptococcus neoformans*
- *Histoplasma capsulatum, duboisii*
- *Paracoccidioides brasiliensis*
- *Rhinosporidium seeberi*
- *Sporothrix schenkii*
- *Torulopsis glabrata*
- *Trichosporon capitatum*
- *Zygomycetes*

Parasites
- Arthropods
- Cestodes
- Nematodes
- Protozoa
- Trematodes

OCCUPATIONAL EXPOSURE

- Asbestosis
- Silicosis
- Heavy metals
- Aluminium
- Beryllium
- Organic dusts (extrinsic allergic alveolitis)

IDIOPATHIC LUNG DISEASES

- Sarcoidosis
- Rheumatoid disease
- Wegener's granulomatosis
- Allergic angiitis and granulomatosis
- Necrotising sarcoid granulomatosis
- Lymphomatoid granulomatosis
- Bronchocentric granulomatosis
- Granulomatous disease of childhood

IATROGENIC CAUSES

- Drug toxicity
- Radiation exposure
- Oxygen therapy

OTHER CONDITIONS

- Foreign body reaction
- Tumour-related granulomas

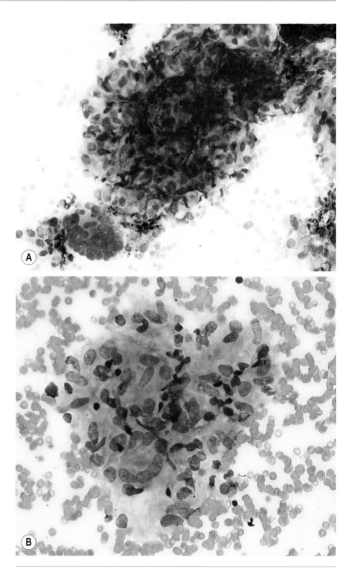

Fig. 3.156 (A) EBUS-FNA. Sarcoidosis: intact granuloma with many epithelioid histiocytes. (B) Tissue imprint. Fibrosing alveolitis: macrophages, inflammatory cells, carbon particles. Also see Figs 3.54 and 3.64.

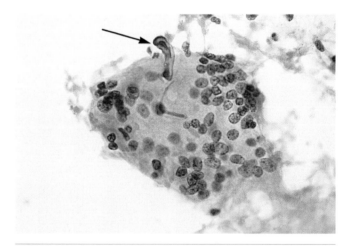

Fig. 3.157 Multinucleated giant cell in a bronchial brushing sample from a patient with sarcoidosis. The cytoplasm contains a partly dislodged Schaumann body, seen at the upper border of the cell *(arrow)* (PAP). (Courtesy of Professor B. Naylor, Michigan.)

Diffuse parenchymal lung disease (Fig. 3.158)

- Many causes of lung damage (see Tables 3.5 and 3.6) but all end in pulmonary fibrosis
- Problems can be assessed sequentially by BAL on the balance of inflammatory cell types
- Epithelial cell and type II pneumocyte hyperplasia and atypia develop over time
- Clinical details important to avoid mistaking for malignancy

Occupational lung diseases (Figs 3.159 and 3.160)

- Many causes (see Table 3.5), ultimately fibrosing the lung parenchyma especially if carcinogenic
- Mineral pneumoconioses common: asbestos fibres identifiable on cytology as pointed long fibres coated with iron, thicker at ends (dumbbell-shaped)
- Small numbers of asbestos bodies in sample are significant (litigation)

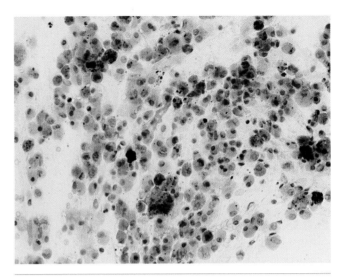

Fig. 3.158 Tissue imprint of fibrosing alveolitis showing many macrophages, some inflammatory cells and patchy carbon deposition

Table 3.5 Conditions associated with pulmonary fibrosis

INDUSTRIAL DISEASES

- Silicosis
- Coal worker's pneumoconiosis (massive pulmonary fibrosis)
- Asbestosis
- Heavy metal exposure
- Organic dusts exposure

IMMUNE DISORDERS

- Rheumatoid disease
- Systemic sclerosis
- Dermatomyositis
- Sjögren's syndrome
- Coeliac disease

END-STAGE GRANULOMATOUS DISEASE

- Sarcoidosis
- Fungal infections
- Mycobacterial infections
- Viral infections
- *Mycoplasma* pneumonia

IATROGENIC CAUSES

- Cytotoxic antibiotics
- Alkylating agents
- Antimetabolites
- Antirheumatic drugs
- Radiation therapy
- Oxygen toxicity

DIRECT LUNG INJURY

- Adult respiratory distress syndrome
- Paraquat poisoning

IDIOPATHIC CONDITIONS

- Fibrosing alveolitis
- Bronchiolitis obliterans
- Organising pneumonia
- Pulmonary haemosiderosis
- Histiocytosis X
- Alveolar proteinosis

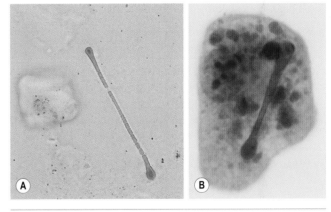

Fig. 3.159[†] (A) Beaded dumbbell-shaped asbestos body coated with iron. (B) Asbestos body ingested by an iron-laden macrophage.

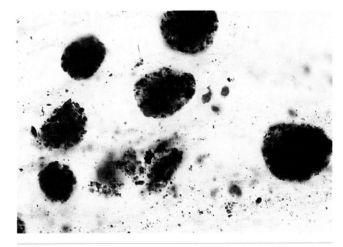

Fig. 3.160[†] Carbon pigment-laden macrophages (coal miner's sputum).

Iron pigment deposition (Fig. 3.161)

- Usually due to microscopic haemorrhages into the lung parenchyma
- **Congestive cardiac** failure is the commonest cause
- **Goodpasture's syndrome** causes haemorrhages due to vasculitis
- **Pulmonary infarction:** many causes
- **Idiopathic pulmonary hemosiderosis:** childhood condition
- **Haemorrphagic diathesis:** a generalised bleeding tendency
- Mineral pneumoconiosis (industrial exposure)

Cytological findings (Fig. 3.161)

- PAP stain shows grey/black pigment-laden macrophages, often with red blood cells present
- Perl's stain for iron shows deep blue stain

Further investigations

- Clinical history is important
- **Patient's age is significant:** childhood vs adult vs old age
- The presence of iron pigment (confirmed by special staining) does not provide a firm diagnosis

Lipoid pneumonitis (Fig 3.162)

- **Exogenous** due to e.g. inhaled oil
- **Endogenous** e.g. distal to bronchial obstruction or due to drug reaction (Amiodorone)
- **Cytology:** finely vacuolated swollen macrophages, multinucleated giant cells with a mixed inflammatory background
- A few small fat droplets are not significant

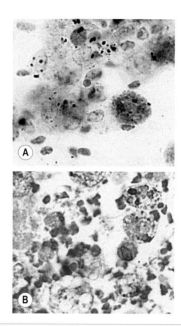

Fig. 3.161[†] (A) Sputum CCF: iron-laden macrophages (Perl's stain). (B) BAL Goodpasture's syndrome: blood and iron in macrophages.

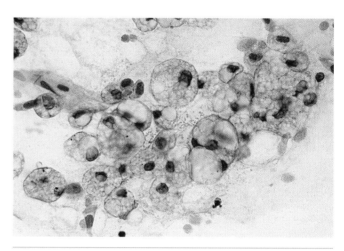

Fig. 3.162[†] Lipoid pneumonitis. Finely vacuolated macrophages with lipid content. (Alveolar lavage)

Table 3.6 Some drugs associated with pulmonary toxicity

Non-cytotoxic drugs	Cytotoxic drugs
Antibacterial agents	**Cytotoxic antibiotics**
Nitrofurantoin	Bleomycin
Sulphalazine	Mitomycin
Analgesics	Ciclosporin A
Aspirin	**Nitrosoureas**
Anticonvulsants	Carmustine
Antiarrhythmic agents	**Alkylating agents**
Amiodarone	Busulphan
Antirheumatic drugs	Cyclophosphamide
Penicillamine	Chlorambucil
Gold salts	Melphalan
Colchicine	**Antimetabolites**
Diuretics	Methotrexate
Opiates	Azathioprine
Sympathomimetics	Cytosine arabinoside
Tranquillisers	**Other cytotoxic drugs**
	Procarbazine
	Vinca alkaloids

Pulmonary alveolar proteinosis (Fig. 3.163)

- Associated with dust exposure originally, also now with immunosuppression
- Lavage fluid milky, opaque
- Rounded amphophilic plaques of surfactant and debris in alveolar spaces
- Pneumocystis lookalike: foamy plaques with cysts on silver stains are the distinguishing feature

Amyloidosis (Fig. 3.164)

- Amyloidosis deposits may be diffuse or localised as a tumour mass
- Can be tracheobronchial or parenchymal
- May be detected in brushings (usually tracheobronchial) or on FNA
- Consist of fibrillary protein forming irregular plaques with amphophilic staining on PAP stain
- The diagnosis is confirmed by Congo red positive staining

Talc granuloma (Fig. 3.165)

- Typical reaction to many foreign materials
- May follow intravenous infection of substances mixed with talc
- Diffuse or focal lung nodules which may be subjected to FNA
- Granulomatous reaction with refractile material, often birefringent

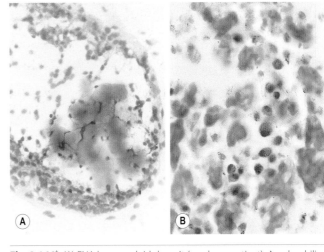

Fig. 3.164[†] (A) FNA lung amyloid deposit (myeloma patient). Amphophilic plaque. (B) Congo red positive.

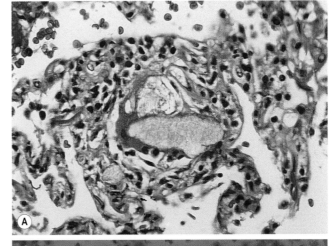

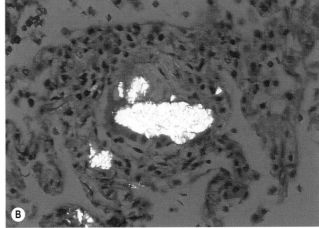

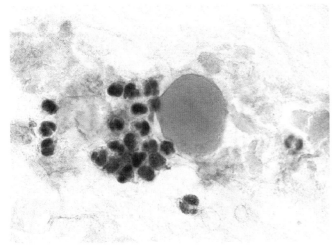

Fig. 3.163[†] BAL alveolar proteinosis. Plaque of amphophilic material from alveolus, surrounded by debris and inflammation.

Fig. 3.165 (A) Refractile talc particles in cell block of FNA lung, with surrounding macrophage reaction. The patient was thought to be an intravenous drug user. Birefringence is apparent with polarised light (B) (H&E). (Courtesy of Professor B. Naylor, Michigan.)

CHAPTER 4

Serous effusions

Contents

Introduction   103

Cytology of normal and reactive mesothelial cells   105

Other benign findings in reactive effusions   108

Benign reactive effusions with specific features   110

General diagnostic approach to malignant effusions   112

Mesothelioma   123

Diagnostic approach: mesothelioma morphology   127

Diagnostic approach: immunocytochemistry   128

Introduction

The term serous effusion refers to an excess of fluid in any of the three main body cavities – pleural, pericardial or peritoneal (Fig. 4.1). It is always pathological and examination of the cellular content of the fluid may reveal the underlying cause.

Normally, the cavities contain a film of clear serous fluid, allowing smooth movement of the internal viscera. The fluid is produced by a single-layered sheet of mesothelial cells lining the parietal (outer) and visceral (inner) surfaces of each cavity. Serous fluid is reabsorbed from the cavities via gaps (windows) between mesothelial cells containing fine microvilli projecting from each mesothelial cell (Fig. 4.2).

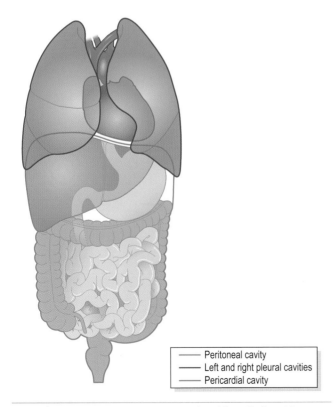

- Peritoneal cavity
- Left and right pleural cavities
- Pericardial cavity

Fig. 4.1[†] Four major serous cavities. (Reproduced from Shidham VB, Atkinson BF. Cytopathologic Diagnosis of Serous Fluids. 1st ed. London: Elsevier; 2007.)

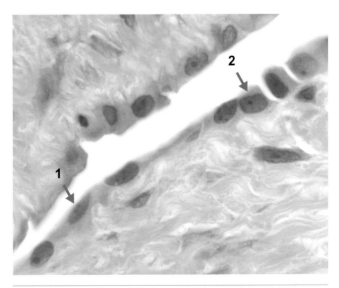

Fig. 4.2[†] Histology of serous lining (inguinal hernia sac). The flat mesothelial cells (*arrow 1*) line the fibrous tissue. They assume a focal cuboidal contour (*arrow 2*) as they undergo reactive changes.

Clinicopathological significance of serous effusions (Table 4.1)

- Fluid accumulates due either to pressure or permeability changes within the body affecting all cavities, or due to local disease producing fluid within one cavity
- All effusions are pathological, most being reactive, with a mixture of mesothelial cells and non-specific inflammatory cells
- An effusion containing malignant cells may be the presenting sign of malignancy or may develop in a patient with a known history of cancer. However, note that effusions in patients with known cancer may just be reactive, with no tumour cells
- Recognition of a second population of 'foreign cells' differing from a reactive population of mesothelial cells highlights cells that are suspicious for malignancy
- Clinical details, gross appearance of fluid and careful processing are critical; ancillary techniques including histochemical stains, immunocytochemistry, and flow cytometry are also often necessary for diagnosis (see Chapter 12)
- A bloodstained effusion is not necessarily indicative of malignancy (see Fig. 4.3)

Table 4.1 Types of effusions

	Transudate	Exudate	Chylous
Biochemical features	Accumulation of fluid as an ultra-filtrate of plasma a. Total protein, 3.0 g/dL (30 g/L) b. Specific gravity, 1.015 c. Ratio of fluid lactic dehydrogenase to serum lactic dehydrogenase, 0.6 d. Does not coagulate	Associated with increased permeability of the capillaries leading to exudation of protein-rich fluid a. Total protein, 3.0 g/dL (30 g/L) b. Specific gravity, 1.015 c. Ratio of fluid lactic dehydrogenase to serum lactic dehydrogenase, 0.6 d. May coagulate on standing	Leakage of lymphatic fluid secondary to trauma or the obstructed thoracic duct or cisterna chyli, caused by malignant neoplasms including lymphomas and carcinomas a. Milky white fluid b. Wet preparations usually show small free fat droplets
Cytological features	Hypocellular smears. Mostly mesothelial cells	Hypercellular smears. Predominantly inflammatory cells with reactive mesothelial cells with or without malignant cells	The smears are rich in lymphocytes and some lipid-laden macrophages
Causes	Cardiovascular conditions, e.g. heart failure Chronic renal disease Liver disease, e.g. cirrhosis Collapsed lung Meig's syndrome Vena caval obstruction/hypertension	Malignant neoplasms Infections, e.g. pneumonia, peritonitis Collagen diseases, e.g. SLE, rheumatoid arthritis Pulmonary embolism Abdominal diseases, e.g. pancreatitis, liver abscess Post-myocardial infarction, cardiac rupture	Metastatic cancer Trauma, blunt or operative Retroperitoneal cancer Lymphoma Tuberculosis Congenital lymphatic anomalies

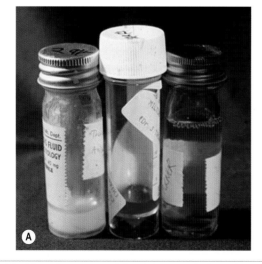
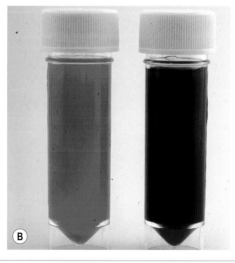

Fig. 4.3 (A) Pleural fluid from three patients: left – chylous sample due to blocked lymphatic duct; centre – bloodstained fluid due to metastatic tumour deposits; right – clear fluid due to cardiac failure. (B) Gross appearance of effusions must be recorded, and history is essential. The bloodstained fluid on the left contained malignant cells, the right-hand one with altered blood staining was benign (due to endometriosis).

Cytology of normal and reactive mesothelial cells

Mesothelial cells

- In fluid, single mesothelial cells round up or form aggregates, with a spectrum of reactive changes
- Although mesodermal in origin, the cells have some features of epithelial cells or may have macrophage-like features, imbibing fluid by pinocytosis
- Flat sheets of mesothelial cells may be present, e.g. in peritoneal washings, with windows between cells containing microvillous projections of mesothelial cytoplasm

Cytological findings (Figs 4.4–4.12)

- **Mesothelial cells** are the hallmark of a serous effusion, varying in number
- Rounded cells with marked variation in size, usually 15–30 μm, but can be much larger
- Cells arranged singly, in pairs and small groups; over time, they may form larger clusters
- Nuclei large, round, dark, usually central but irregular if highly reactive. Separated from the cell border by cytoplasm. Multinucleation seen frequently
- Cytoplasm often voluminous with two-zone staining, darker around nucleus
- Normal cells merge with reactive ones
- Microvilli are seen as blebs or a fringe of fine vacuolation at the cell membrane
- PAP-stained mesothelial cells are smaller with dense cytoplasm but show more nuclear detail than in air-dried MGG-stained preparations
- Over time, mesothelial cells imbibe fluid (pinocytosis) giving a macrophage-like appearance with vacuolation of cytoplasm
- Mitotic figures are often seen (normal forms)
- Degenerative changes are common, e.g. vacuolated cytoplasm, condensed nuclei (pyknosis, apoptotic bodies)

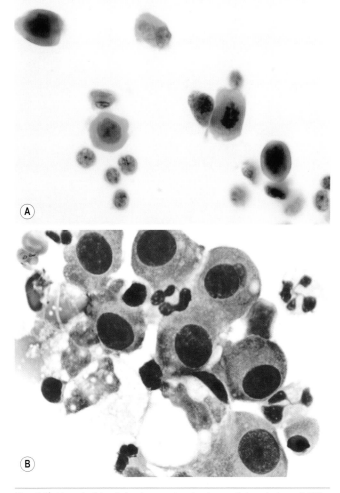

Fig. 4.5† Mesothelial cells in clusters showing intercellular windows (MGG stain LBC).

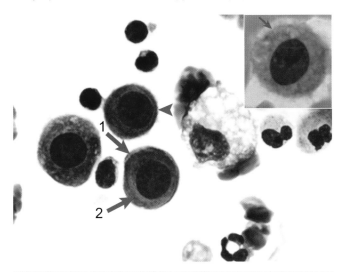

Fig. 4.4† Rounded mesothelial cells (1) with central round nuclei (2), paler outer cytoplasm. Microvilli at arrowhead. Degenerate inflammatory cells and macrophage in background. Inset: blebs (*arrow*).

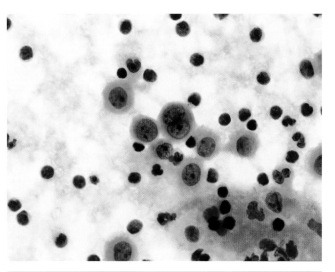

Fig. 4.6 Mesothelial cells stained by PAP showing central rounded nuclei, including binucleation. Background lymphocytes present.

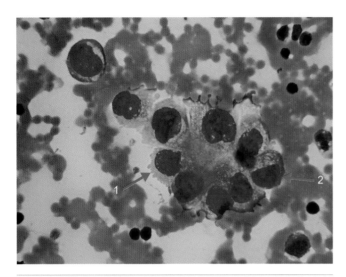

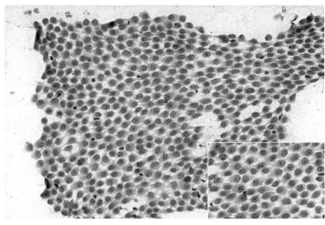

Fig. 4.10 Peritoneal washing: flat sheet of mesothelial cells with visible intercellular windows. Inset: microvilli visible between cells.

Fig. 4.7† Reactive mesothelial cell group with knobbly contours (1), pleomorphic nuclei, vacuolation of cytoplasm, eccentric nuclei (2).

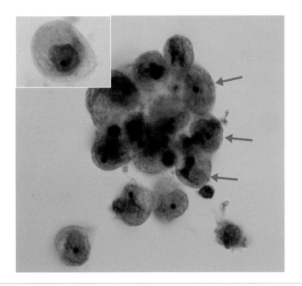

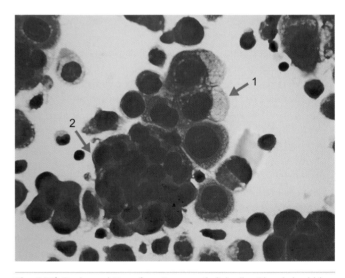

Fig. 4.11† Dual population of reactive mesothelial cells with pale knobbly outer contours (*arrow 1*) and carcinoma cell group with smooth contour (*arrow 2*).

Fig. 4.8† Peritoneal fluid: PAP stain cf. Fig. 4.7: reactive and degenerative changes. Arrows and inset: cytoplasmic borders.

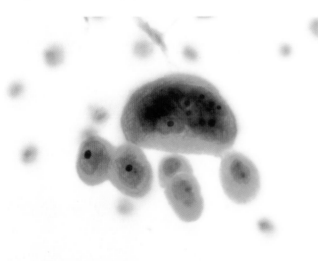

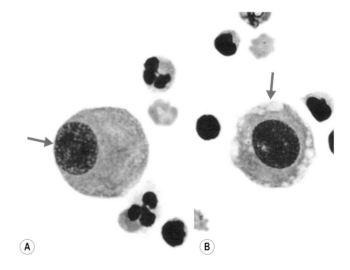

Fig. 4.9† Peritoneal dialysis fluid: mesothelial cells with bi- and multinucleation.

Fig. 4.12† Pleural fluid. (A) Adenocarcinoma cell with no two-zone staining and nucleus abutting on the cell membrane. (B) Mesothelial cell with central nucleus and pale periphery with blebbing.

Diagnostic pitfalls: non-specific reactive mesothelial cells (Figs 4.13–4.15)

- Due to the wide morphological spectrum of mesothelial cell morphology, overdiagnosis of malignancy is the commonest problem in serous effusion cytology
- Underdiagnosis of malignancy will usually lead to repeat sampling or other investigation, such as biopsy, to obtain a diagnosis. Effusions usually recur if malignant
- The dual cell approach to malignancy diagnosis is discussed more fully on page 128

Conditions causing non-specific effusions

1. **Congestive cardiac failure/organ ischaemia**
   - Effusions in heart failure usually involve all cavities to a variable extent
   - Hepatomegaly leads to shedding of mesothelial sheets
   - Haemosiderin and/or red blood cells may be present
2. **Trauma to organs**
   - Spleen, liver and lung
3. **Large retroperitoneal masses**
   - Hyperplasia of mesothelium due to stretching of peritoneum
4. **The washings procedure**
   - Common source of large sheets of mesothelial cells, especially in pelvic or peritoneal washings (see Figs 4.10 and 4.14)

'Atypical' mesothelial cells (Fig. 4.15)

- Marked changes (atypia) in mesothelial cells may occur in the above conditions, simulating malignancy
- The absence of a recognisable second 'foreign cell' population raises the possibility of a mesothelioma (see Fig. 4.15B), especially if the cells form large balls
- Awareness of the clinical details and past history is essential for correct evaluation of 'atypical' mesothelial cells

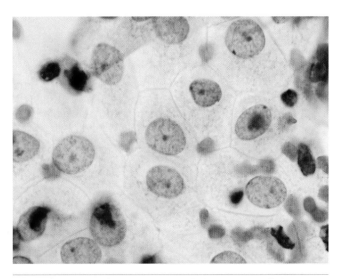

Fig 4.14[†] Flat sheet of mesothelial cells dislodged mechanically by peritoneal washing procedure. Note the active nuclei and nucleoli. (PAP stain).

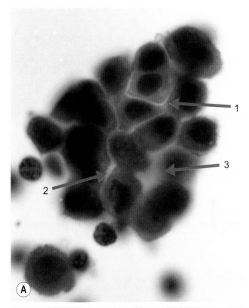

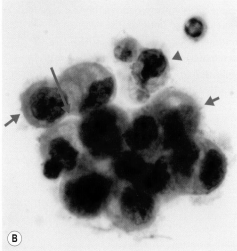

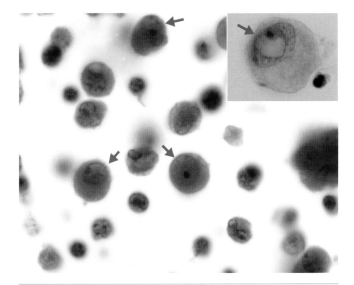

Fig 4.13[†] Benign reactive effusion; pleomorphic mesothelial cells with large nuclei. Note the cytoplasmic rim between the nucleus and the cell membrane, characteristic of mesothelial cells (*arrows*).

Fig 4.15[†] (A) Flat group of reactive mesothelial cells in a benign effusion (windows at arrows). (B) Mesothelioma group (window at long arrow, microvilli at short arrows).

Other benign findings in reactive effusions

- A mixture of cell types with many macrophages can be seen in most effusions, usually having no diagnostic significance (unless they can be identified as malignant cells)
- Their importance lies in recognising that they are not a malignant cell population, but sometimes the cell types are characteristic of benign pathology, e.g. pus cells
- The ability of mesothelial cells to act as facultative macrophages blurs the dividing line between these two cell types, but the distinction is rarely important

Macrophages

- Macrophages are common in longer standing effusions
- Some are derived from mesothelial cells which act as facultative macrophages

Cytological findings: macrophages (Figs 4.16–4.17)

- Pale cells, variable in size but usually large (similar in range to mesothelial cells)
- Irregular cytoplasmic contours with poorly visualised cell borders
- Random coarse vacuolation which may distort or overlap with the nucleus
- Nuclei often eccentric, sometimes indented (cf. histiocytes), often degenerate
- Cytoplasmic content may be significant, e.g. iron pigment, mucin

Cytology of other cells/entities (Figs 4.18–4.23)

- Blood may be present without any clinical significance (see Fig. 4.3)
- Inflammatory/haematological cells: RBCs, lymphocytes and neutrophils usually present in small numbers, others rare
- Psammoma bodies occur in benign or, more often, in malignant effusions: round lamellated dark concretions (see Fig. 4.20)
- Collagen balls: benign mesothelial cells covering a collagen core may be seen in peritoneal washings (Fig. 4.21)
- Detached ciliary tufts: seen in peritoneal washings, arising from the pouch of Douglas (Fig. 4.22)
- Cell fragments, e.g. endometriosis (Fig. 4.23)
- Contamination from other samples (Fig. 4.18)
- Squames due to skin contamination at collection, or due to fistula formation (see Fig. 4.19)

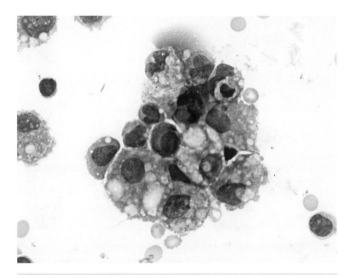

Fig. 4.16 Reactive effusion: macrophages and mesothelial cells, some of which show macrophage-like features.

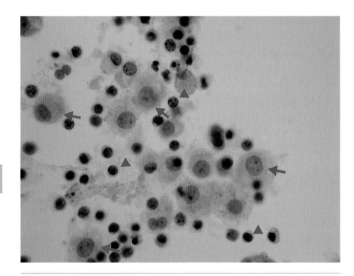

Fig. 4.17[†] Reactive effusion: many mesothelial cells and macrophages (*arrows*). Also inflammatory cells with degenerative changes (*arrowheads*) and air-drying artefact.

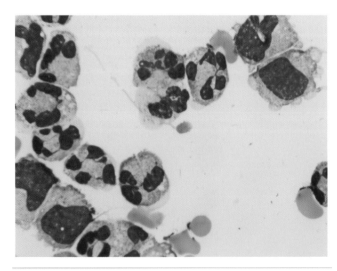

Fig. 4.18[†] Ascitic fluid with inflammatory cells, mainly polymorphs, a few lymphocytes and occasional red blood cells.

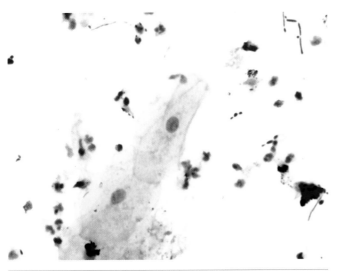

Fig. 4.19 Pleural fluid with squamous cells, inflammatory cells and debris due to bronchopleural fistula.

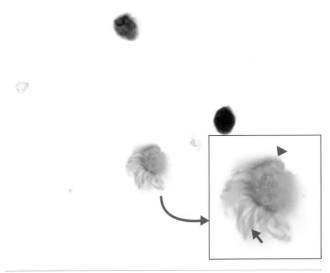

Fig. 4.22[†] Peritoneal washing: detached ciliary tuft. Anucleate cell fragment with cilia at arrows, cytoplasm at arrowhead.

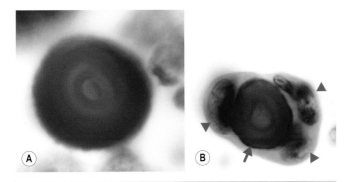

Fig. 4.20[†] (A) Psammoma body. A solitary psammoma body and carcinoma cells elsewhere. (B) Psammoma body: round, acellular, calcific structures with concentric lamellation in association with abnormal tumour cells (*arrowheads*).

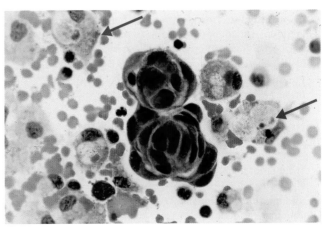

Fig. 4.23 Pleural effusion from patient with endometriosis involving the pleural cavity. Note scattered macrophages (some with iron particles (*arrows*) from recurrent haemorrhages). Central cohesive group of rounded-up endometrial cells from pleura (see Fig. 4.3B).

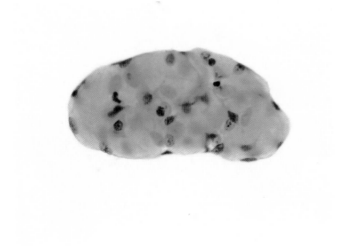

Fig. 4.21 Collagen ball. A ball of mesothelial cells covering a collagen core, as seen in 4–29% of peritoneal washings.

Benign reactive effusions with specific features

- There are numerous causes of benign effusions, including the presence of an underlying malignancy causing lymphatic obstruction but with no malignant cell component in the fluid
- Most of these effusions have no specific features, cytology contributing by helping to exclude malignancy
- There is a risk of false-positive diagnosis, especially if the mesothelial cells show marked reactive changes overlapping with adenocarcinoma cells ('atypical' mesothelial cells) or if there is a history of previous malignancy, with risk of over-interpretation

Cytological findings: specific features (Figs 4.24–4.32)

- **Acute infection:** numerous polymorphs, cells often too degenerate for interpretation (Fig. 4.24)
- **Chronic infection:** e.g. tuberculosis: usually a non-specific lymphocytosis; granulomas rarely seen; culture is essential for diagnosis (Fig. 4.25)
- **Cirrhosis of liver:** markedly reactive mesothelial cells, singly, in groups, pseudopapillary forms or acinar groups; large dark nuclei, multinucleation, large nucleoli, mitoses. Uraemia and acute pancreatitis have similar findings (Figs 4.26–4.28)
- **Pulmonary embolism/infarction:** markedly reactive mesothelial cells resembling adenocarcinoma
- **Systemic lupus erythematosus:** usually a pleural or pericardial fluid; many inflammatory cells, with LE cells formed from polymorphs or macrophages filled with homogeneous basophilic nuclear material. Characteristic of SLE but not pathognomonic as can be due to drug toxicity (Figs 4.29, 4.30)
- **Rheumatoid effusions:** not common; occur with or after joint manifestations, mainly in men. Necrotic debris, degenerate cells, spindle cells, few or no mesothelial cells. Pitfall: spindle cells may resemble squamous carcinoma cells or other malignancy (Fig. 4.31)
- **Other causes:** asbestos, talc, fistula, endometriosis, parasites (eosinophils ++), amoebiasis, hydatids, etc. (Fig. 4.32)

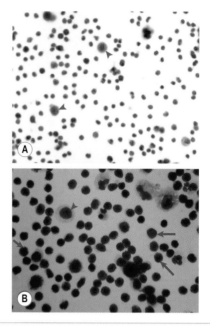

Fig. 4.25[†] (A) PAP. (B) MGG. Reactive effusion as seen in cirrhosis, etc. (*arrowheads*, mesothelial cells; *arrows*, lymphocytes).

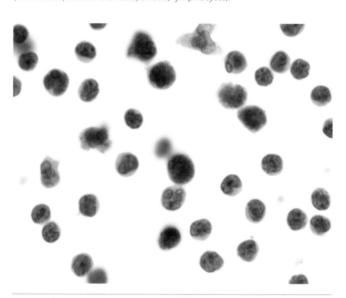

Fig. 4.26[†] Pleural fluid: lymphocytosis; distinguish TB from low-grade lymphoma using immunocytochemistry and culture.

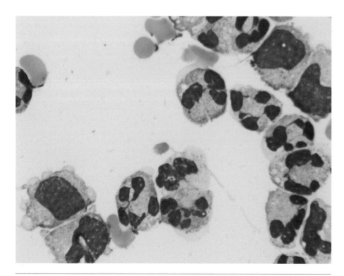

Fig. 4.24[†] Ascitic fluid: many neutrophil polymorphs with a few lymphocytes, and red blood cells.

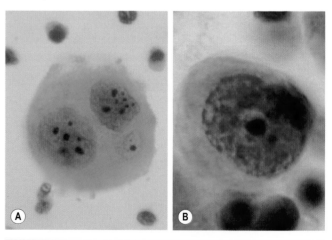

Fig. 4.27[†] Reactive mesothelial cells from a patient with active cirrhosis. Note the nuclear degenerative changes in (B).

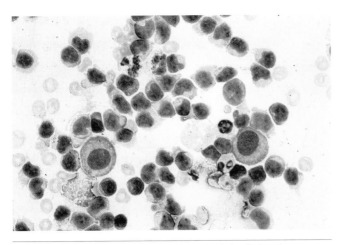

Fig. 4.28 Uraemia: non-specific reactive mesothelial cells, lymphocytes, degenerate macrophages, few polymorphs.

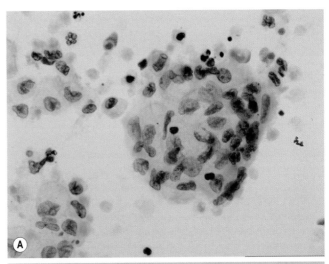

(A)

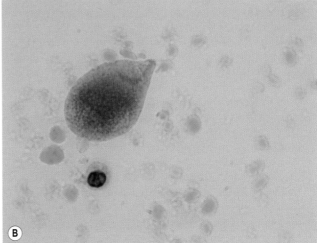

(B)

Fig. 4.31 Rheumatoid arthritis. (A) Serous fluid with granuloma and inflammatory debris. (B)[†] Atypical mesothelial cell showing multinucleation and a squamoid shape, with potential for over-diagnosis.

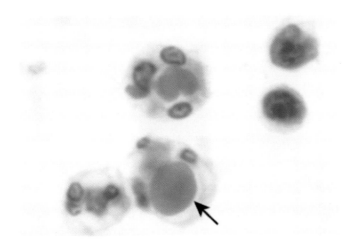

Fig. 4.29[†] Pleural fluid showing large haematoxyphil body (*arrow*) displacing polymorph nuclei (LE cell) (Diff-Quik stain).

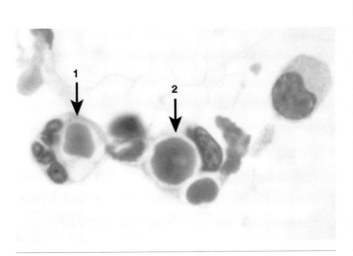

Fig. 4.30[†] Same case as Fig. 4.29. Several LE cells, in polymorph (*arrow 1*) and macrophage (*arrow 2*) (PAP stain).

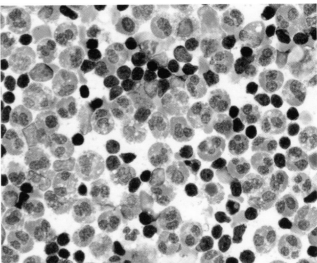

Fig. 4.32 Eosinophilic effusion with many eosinophils, a few lymphocytes and polymorphs. Causes: drugs, autoimmune diseases, parasites, idiopathic.

General diagnostic approach to malignant effusions

Cytological identification of a malignant cell population in serous fluid presents unique problems for cytologists because of the complex and variable cellular findings:

- Metastatic malignant cells in serous fluid may be epithelial (carcinoma) or, less often, non-epithelial in origin (melanoma, sarcoma, haematolymphoid); rarely, the primary is a mesothelioma arising within the cavity

- Typically, cancer cells mingle with reactive mesothelial cells, both having overlapping features

- Identifying malignant cells usually depends on recognition of a second population of cells foreign to the spectrum of mesothelial cells – this is the '**dual population approach**' to diagnosis of malignancy (Fig. 4.33)

- Most carcinomas, melanomas and sarcomas present as a mixed pattern of single cells and cell groups or loose cellular aggregates (see Figs 4.33A and B). Diagnosis of malignancy may be achieved using routine stains but tumour type may not be certain

- A population composed entirely of single malignant cells is seen, especially in haematolymphoid malignancies (see Fig. 4.33C), and also in certain metastatic carcinomas such as breast, risking a false-negative diagnosis because the dual population approach cannot be used

- With high-grade tumours, nuclear changes of malignancy may be obvious, especially with PAP stains; these include frequent mitoses, atypical mitotic figures and apoptotic bodies

- Mesothelioma effusions usually have no evidence of a dual cell population, and the tumour cells may lack overt malignant features

- Haematological malignancy may be difficult to distinguish from background inflammatory cells

- Confirmation of a foreign cell population and firm classification of tumour type may not be possible without the use of ancillary techniques such as histochemical stains and immunocytochemistry, which can be conclusive

- A definitive diagnosis of malignancy may be possible without a conclusive diagnosis of the primary site

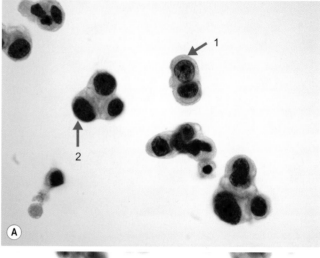

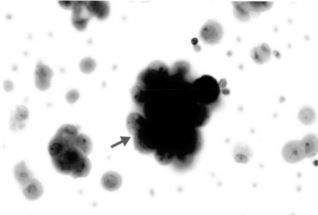

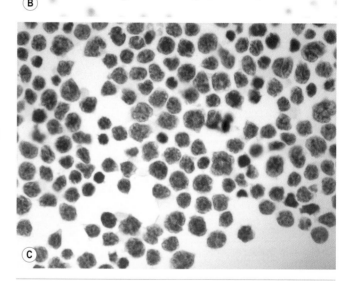

Fig. 4.33[†] (A) Metastatic adenocarcinoma: single cells and small groups at arrow 2 (cf. mesothelial cells at arrow 1). (B) Metastatic breast carcinoma with proliferation sphere (*arrow*). (C) Malignant lymphoma: a monotonous population of non-cohesive cells.

Metastatic carcinoma cells in serous effusions

- Metastatic carcinoma is the commonest cause of a malignant effusion
- Primary tumour often already known but cells in effusion may differ from the primary due to effects of fluid
- Breast cancer is the commonest source of malignancy in women, then ovarian, GI tract, lung. Lung cancer is the commonest primary site in men
- Carcinoma cells in fluid tend to have overlapping morphology, usually preventing firm identification of the likely primary site without the use of ancillary stains

Cytological findings: metastatic carcinoma cells (Figs 4.34–4.41)

General features:

- Cells are often similar in size to mesothelial cells, with some cytoplasmic and nuclear features in common
- The 'dual population approach' can help identify carcinoma cells as distinct from mesothelial cells
- Mesothelial cells show a continuum of subtle morphological change, differing from the range of carcinoma cells which form a 'foreign' cell population, better seen in MGG stains than PAP as the cells are larger
- Many carcinoma cells show nuclei touching the nuclear membrane, mesothelial cells having a rim of finely vacuolated cytoplasm separating nucleus from cell border (see Figs 4.34 and 4.12)
- Other features of carcinoma, e.g. mucous vacuoles, must be distinguished from degenerative vacuolation (Table 4.2, p. 119)
- Classification of carcinomas in fluid can be established with immunostains in many cases, combined with the clinical details

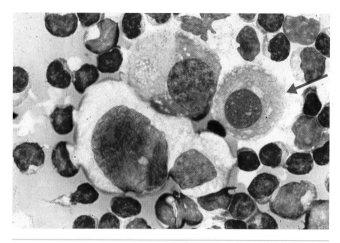

Fig. 4.34 Pleural fluid: with dual population of metastatic breast carcinoma cells and mesothelial cells. Note two different cell types, malignant nuclei touching the cell border, and the smaller mesothelial cell (*arrow*) has a rim of cytoplasm between with fine peripheral vacuolation.

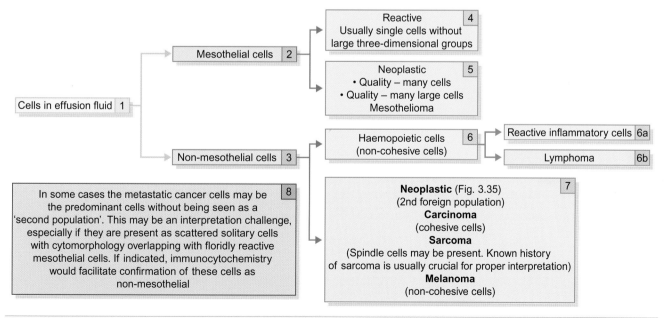

Fig. 4.35[†] Algorithm for evaluation of a 'second foreign population'. (From Shidham VB, Atkinson BF. Cytopathologic Diagnosis of Serous Fluids. 1st ed. London: Elsevier; 2007).

Cell arrangements in carcinomatous effusions

- Retained intercellular cohesion leads to formation of cell clusters, later to large proliferation spheres
- Glandular structures, acini and papillary patterns are seen in some metastatic well-differentiated adenocarcinomas
- Single scattered cells, with few or no mesothelial cells, are seen in small cell carcinomas, often with no obvious dual cell population (risk of false-negative reporting)

Cytoplasmic features in carcinomatous effusions

- Malignant cell cytoplasm lacks the two-zone pattern of mesothelial cells as seen with MGG stains
- Mucous vacuolation is PASD and mucicarmine positive and may indent the nucleus (signet ring cell); glycogenic fine vacuolation is PASD negative
- Keratinisation (squamous carcinoma) best seen in MGG stains. Psammoma bodies within papillary clusters or isolated are seen mainly in thyroid and ovarian carcinoma metastases

Nuclear features in carcinomatous cells

- Standard criteria, i.e. enlarged irregular nuclei, hyperchromasia with prominent nucleoli, are often present, seen best in PAP stained preparations
- Adenocarcinoma nuclei tend to abut on the nuclear membrane (cf. mesothelial cells with cytoplasm between). Mitoses are common, often atypical
- Apoptotic bodies may be seen (nuclear disintegration) (see Fig. 4.43)

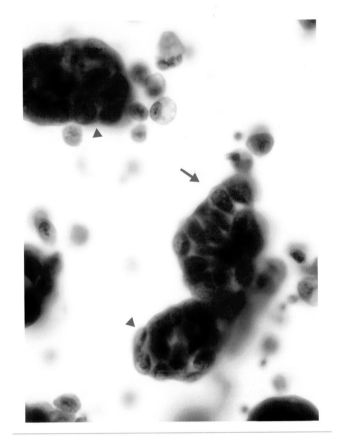

Fig. 4.37[†] Ascites; papillary and glandular structures with psammoma bodies (ovarian seous papillary carcinoma). Note anatomical border (*arrow*) and papillary formation (*arrowheads*).

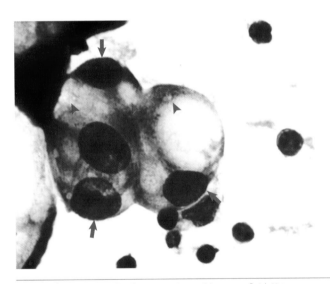

Fig. 4.36[†] Mucin vacuoles (breast carcinoma) in serous fluid. Note hard-edged vacuoles (*arrowheads*) and nuclei touching cell walls (*arrows*).

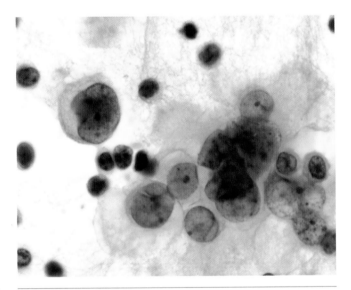

Fig. 4.38[†] Poorly differentiated carcinoma cells showing obvious nuclear features of malignancy (PAP stain, lung carcinoma).

Differential diagnosis of carcinoma cells in serous effusions

- **Carcinoma versus reactive mesothelial cells:** no two-zone pattern in cytoplasm of malignant cells
- **Carcinoma versus mesothelioma:** malignant cells merge with normal mesothelial cells, no dual population
- **Carcinoma of unknown primary:** cell arrangement and cellular morphology may give clues, e.g. lobular breast carcinoma with a single-cell pattern (but lung, gastric, etc. can also show this), papillary ovarian carcinoma (but thyroid carcinoma is similar)
- **Non-epithelial tumour versus carcinoma:** melanoma is a look-alike for adenocarcinoma; low-grade lymphoma with a single-cell monotonous population resembles small cell carcinomas with this pattern
- **Therapeutic effects:** degenerative changes due to radiotherapy or chemotherapy can lead to false-negative or false-positive diagnosis
- **Benign reactive effusions** with atypical cells, e.g. rheumatoid effusion (see Fig. 4.31B)

Further investigation

- **Full clinical details** are needed including previous cytology findings and histology of primary tumour if the primary is known (N.B. serous fluid alters cell morphology so original primary site FNA findings may not be fully comparable)
- **Histochemical stains** for cytoplasmic content:
  - mucin: mucicarmine and PASD positive
  - glycogen: PASD negative
  - lipid: oil red O positive
  - thyroid: colloid present
  - pigment: Masson–Fontana for melanin, Perl's stain for iron
  - immunoglobulin: in plasma cells
- **Immunocytochemistry:** this is one of the most useful techniques and often gives definite confirmation of the likely primary tumour. See section on diagnostic approach for details on p. 112 and Chapter 13 for technical details
- **Further samples** of fluid may be needed and are usually obtainable as malignant effusions generally reaccumulate
- Establishing the primary site of carcinomatous cells in an effusion or the cell morphology alone is usually only tentative. Examples of some of the commonest findings are given on the following pages (see Figs 4.42–4.63). Note the similarity in many of the patterns
- See Table 4.3 on p. 122 for several features of carcinoma cells and other neoplastic cells

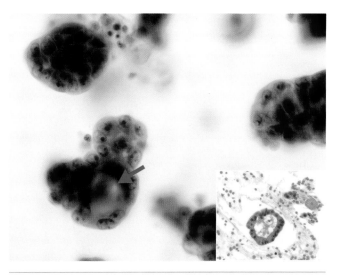

Fig. 4.39[†] Proliferation sphere in pleural fluid with central clearing (*arrow*). Inset shows hollow core in section from cell block (breast carcinoma).

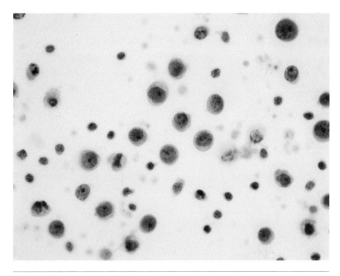

Fig. 4.40[†] Ascites with discohesive malignant cell population, a few lymphocytes and no mesothelial cells (gastric carcinoma).

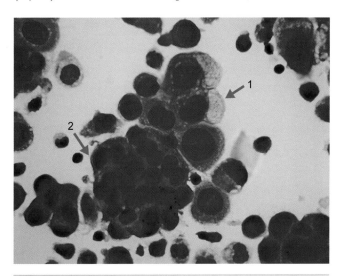

Fig. 4.41[†] Dual cell population in metastatic breast carcinoma. (*Arrow 1*) Mesothelial cell group. (*Arrow 2*) Malignant cells with nucleus touching cell border.

Examples of metastatic carcinoma effusions from breast (Figs 4.42–4.44)

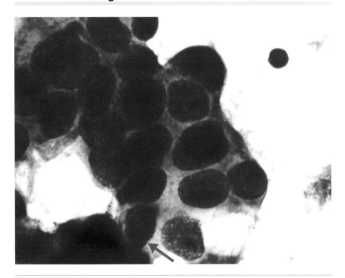

Fig. 4.42† Adenocarcinoma cells from breast metastasis. Note acinus at arrow and adjacent vacuolated cell. Nuclei touch cell borders.

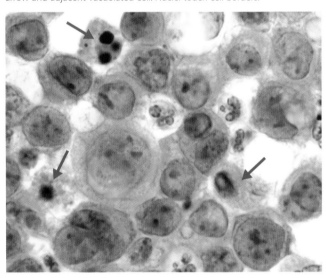

Fig. 4.43† Metastatic poorly differentiated breast carcinoma in ascitic fluid. Note obvious malignant nuclear features and suggestion of a glandular pattern. Apoptotic bodies present at arrows. (PAP stain).

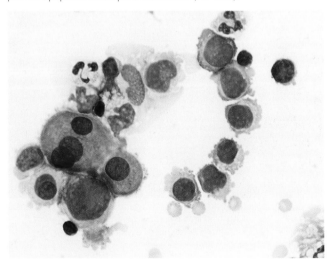

Fig. 4.44 Metastatic lobular carcinoma of breast in pleural fluid. Tendency to single-cell pattern with 'Indian file' arrangement.

Examples of metastatic carcinoma effusions from lung (Figs 4.45–4.47)

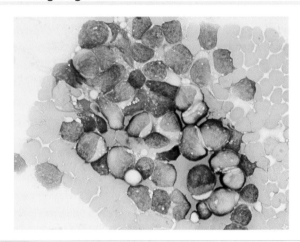

Fig. 4.45 Metastatic small cell carcinoma of lung showing nuclear moulding and scanty cytoplasm (cf. other small cell tumours in Figs 4.44, 4.53, 4.56 and 4.68).

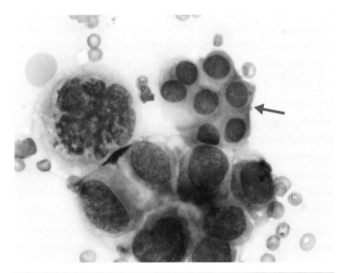

Fig. 4.46 Metastatic carcinoma cells (lung). Cells are clearly malignant but have no distinguishing features. Group of mesothelial cells is seen above the malignant group for comparison (*arrow*).

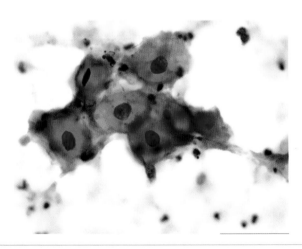

Fig. 4.47 Malignant squamous cells showing keratinisation.

Examples of metastatic effusions from female genital tract carcinomas (Figs 4.48–4.53)

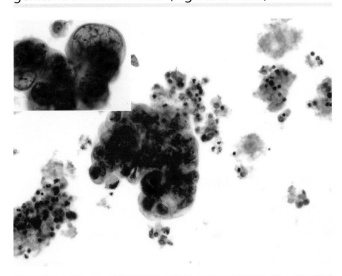

Fig. 4.48† Peritoneal fluid: ovarian papillary carcinoma showing papillary frond; obviously malignant nuclei (*inset*).

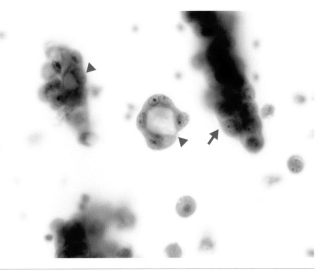

Fig. 4.51† Metastatic mucinous papillary cystadenocarcinoma of the ovary (ascitic fluid). Cohesive clusters may show ill-defined papillary structures (*arrow*) without peripheral palisading. Some cells show cytoplasmic vacuoles (*arrowheads*). Psammona bodies were absent.

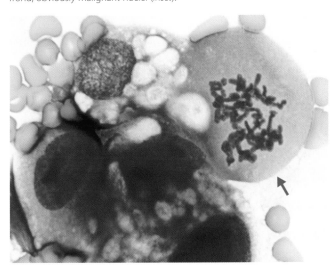

Fig. 4.49† Abnormal mitotic figure in a group of carcinoma cells found to be ovarian in origin.

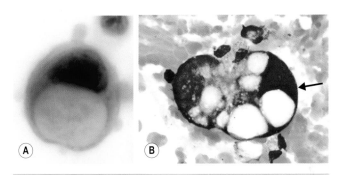

Fig. 4.52† Secretory vacuoles in adenocarcinoma cells from ovarian cancer metastasis. Note: vacuoles indent nuclei (*arrow*) and have sharp margins.

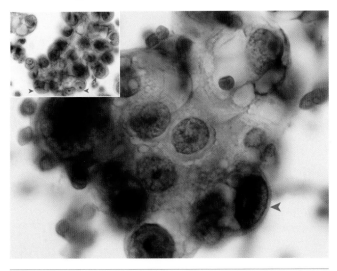

Fig. 4.50† Cohesive carcinomatous cells (ovarian origin). Note nuclei touch the cell borders (*arrowheads*). (Inset) Mesothelial cell group with rim of cytoplasm at cell border (*arrowheads*).

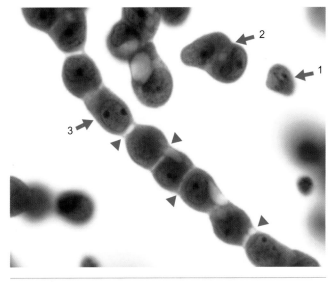

Fig. 4.53† Ascites metastatic ovarian carcinoma with solitary (1), groups (2) and single cell file (3). Nuclei abut on cell border (*arrow*). Narrow spaces between some cells (*arrowheads*).

Examples of metastatic carcinoma effusions: gastrointestinal tract (Figs 4.54–4.59)

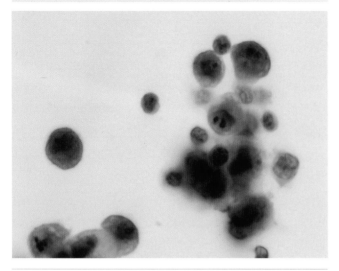

Fig. 4.54† Malignant cell groups and single cells with no differentiating features (gastric carcinoma).

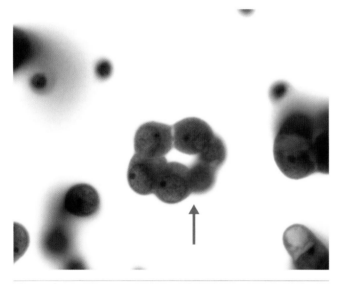

Fig. 4.55† Acinus formation (*arrow*) in ascitic fluid from metastatic duodenal carcinoma.

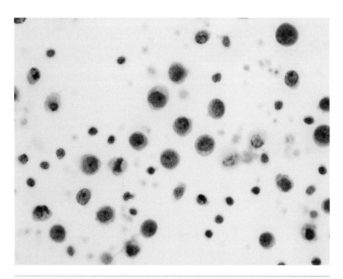

Fig. 4.56† Single cell variant of gastric adenocarcinoma resembling small discohesive malignant cells from lung, breast or lymphoma.

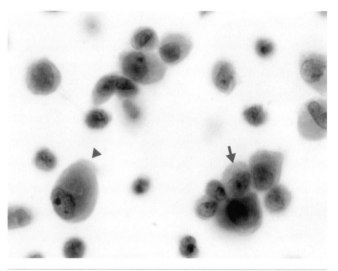

Fig. 4.57† Adenocarcinoma cells varying in size (*arrow and arrowhead*). This is a duodenal carcinoma but other adenocarcinomas can look similar.

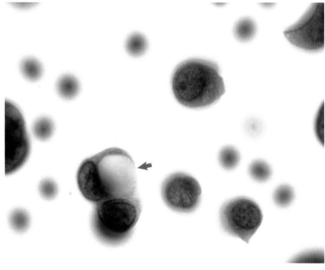

Fig. 4.58† Signet ring cell: (gastric primary) firm-edged vacuole pushing and indenting nucleus to one side (*arrow*). Remember this is not a specific finding for metastatic gastric carcinoma.

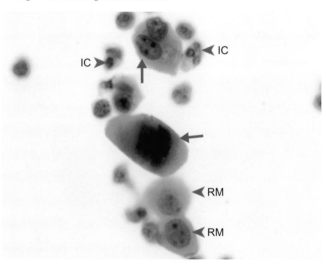

Fig. 4.59† Pleomorphic carcinoma cells (*arrows*), inflammatory cells (IC), reactive mesothelials (RM) (pancreatic carcinoma).

Other metastatic carcinoma examples in effusions (Figs 4.60–4.63, Table 4.2)

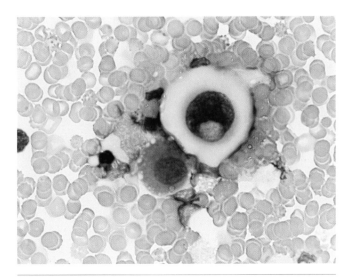

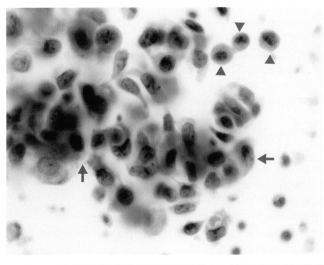

Fig. 4.60 Large well-formed malignant cell with finely vacuolated cytoplasm due to lipid content, consistent with renal carcinoma metastasis but not specific without immunocytochemistry for confirmation.

Fig. 4.62† Malignant cells in loosely cohesive clusters (*arrows*) with some spindle-shaped or cercariform, as seen in some urothelial tumours (bladder carcinoma). Note a few mesothelial cells (*arrowheads*).

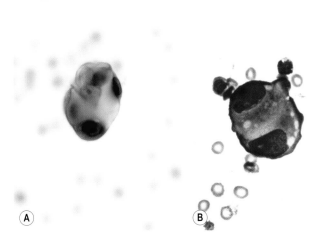

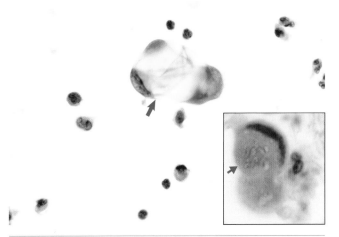

Fig. 4.61† Small clusters of carcinoma cells with markedly eccentric nuclei and finely vacuolated cytoplasm. No specific features (prostatic primary adenocarcinoma (ascites)).

Fig. 4.63† Vacuolated cluster of malignant cells compressing the nuclei (*arrow*). (Inset) Mucicarmine stain confirms mucous content of vacuole (cholangiocarcinoma).

Table 4.2 Comparison of degenerative intracytoplasmic vacuoles versus secretory vacuoles

Degenerative intracytoplasmic vacuoles	Secretory intracytoplasmic vacuoles
Do not occupy the entire cytoplasm of a cell and do not show ballooning	Secretory vacuoles with mucin and other material such as colloid in the vacuoles, usually balloon the entire cell and occupy most of the cytoplasm
Borders of vacuoles: usually ill-defined	Borders of vacuoles: well-defined
Do not show secretion in the lumen	May show secretion in the lumen (targetoid vacuole)
PAS stain after diastase digestion, and mucicarmine stain: negative	PAS stain after diastase digestion and mucicarmine stain: may show positive secretion
May show other associated degenerative features such as nuclei with hyperchromatic smudgy chromatin	Hyperchromatic nuclei show features of malignancy with clumped crisp chromatin

Haematolymphoid malignancies in effusions (Figs 4.64–4.69)

- Third commonest cause of malignant effusions in pleural cavity (after breast and lung in adults) and in peritoneal fluid after ovary and breast. Malignant childhood effusions are usually haemopoietic in origin
- Fluid may look milky (chylous) due to lymphocytosis and triglycerides if obstructive (chylothorax)
- Effusions in Hodgkin lymphoma are usually reactive, not malignant, due to obstruction by enlarged glands

Cytological findings: haemopoietic malignancy

- Discohesive cell pattern almost always present
- Low-grade lymphoma/lymphocytic leukaemia cells resemble reactive lymphocytes
- High-grade lymphoma cells may be monotonous or pleomorphic. Reactive lymphocytes are also present
- Leukaemic effusions: mixed leukaemic and reactive cell population present

Differential diagnosis

- Reactive effusion: usually mixed cells but can be monomorphic, e.g. TB
- Remember that there is a risk of concomitant infections in patients with haematological malignancy
- Epithelial malignancy with cell dissociation resembles high-grade lymphoma or low-grade if small cell type, e.g. breast, lung, etc.
- Melanoma metastases may have a dissociated cell pattern resembling lymphoma

Further investigations (Table 4.3)

- Full clinical details are necessary
- Immunocytochemistry is essential to confirm cell type, light chain restriction, etc. In known cases, immunomarkers may be needed to exclude second malignancy or transformation to a high-grade type (see Chapter 7 for full details)
- Flow cytometry is needed sometimes for diagnosis
- Special stains for non-haematological malignancy may be needed, e.g. pigment for melanoma
- See Table 4.3 on p. 122 for cytological features of malignant cells of different types including lymphomas

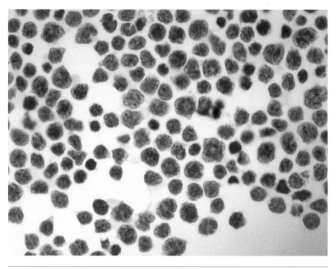

Fig. 4.64[†] Malignant lymphoma single-cell pattern with some irregular contours, nuclear pleomorphism, hyperchromasia.

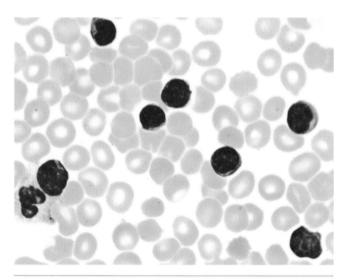

Fig. 4.65[†] Chronic lymphocytic leukaemia/low-grade lymphocytic lymphoma: coarse chromatin, no nucleoli seen, little cytoplasm.

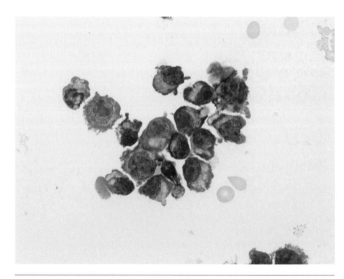

Fig. 4.66 Multiple myelomatosis: plasmacytoid cells with eccentric nuclei and degenerate cytoplasm.

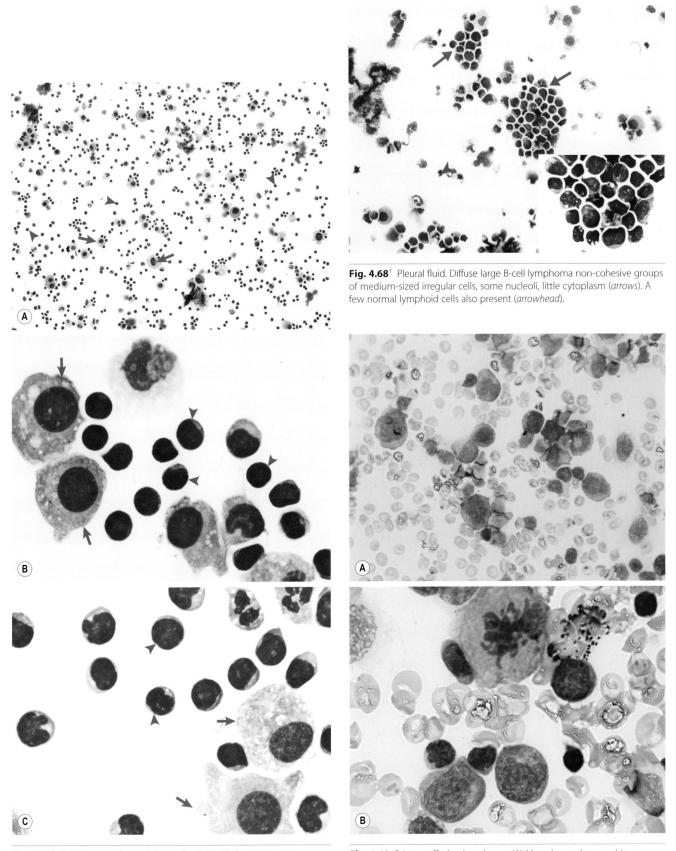

Fig. 4.68† Pleural fluid. Diffuse large B-cell lymphoma non-cohesive groups of medium-sized irregular cells, some nucleoli, little cytoplasm (*arrows*). A few normal lymphoid cells also present (*arrowhead*).

Fig. 4.67† Follicular lymphoma (pleural fluid). (A–C) Flow cytometry demonstrated a distinct population of light chain-restricted B cells with an immunophenotype consistent with follicular lymphoma (reactive mesothelial cells, *arrows*; lymphoma cells, *arrowheads*) (Wright–Giemsa stain cytospin, courtesy of Horatiu Olteanu, MD, PhD).

Fig. 4.69† Primary effusion lymphoma. (A) Many large pleomorphic malignant cells of lymphoid type with scattered small lymphocytes in the background. (B) High-power view of abnormal lymphoid cells with bizarre mitotic figures (pleural fluid).

Table 4.3 Cytomorphological features suggestive of different primary sites in metastatic effusions

Cytomorphology	Possible primary carcinoma	Cytomorphology	Possible primary carcinoma
ARCHITECTURE-BASED FEATURES		**INDIVIDUAL CELLULAR FEATURES**	
Predominantly scattered isolated malignant cells	Gastric adenocarcinoma Non-cohesive variant of lung adenocarcinoma Breast lobular carcinoma Adrenocortical carcinoma Also lymphoma, melanoma and sarcoma)	Extensive cytoplasmic vacuolation	Renal cell carcinoma (glycogen, fat) Adrenocortical carcinoma (fat) Benign mesothelial cells Pancreatic adenocarcinoma (mucin) Ovarian adenocarcinoma (mucin) Lung adenocarcinoma Clear cell carcinoma endometrium
Three-dimensional round cell groups – proliferation spheres or 'cannonballs'	Breast adenocarcinoma Ovarian adenocarcinoma Mesothelioma of epithelioid type Reactive mesothelial proliferations	Targetoid intracytoplasmic vacuole containing secretion	Breast adenocarcinoma (especially lobular) Thyroid carcinoma (colloid) Ovarian carcinoma Pancreatic carcinoma
Acini/glands	Adenocarcinoma of breast, lung, colorectum, stomach, ovary, endometrium, etc. Mesothelioma of epithelioid type	Prominent nucleoli	Hepatocellular carcinoma Renal cell carcinoma Prostatic adenocarcinoma
Three-dimensional groups in papillary configurations	Bronchioloalveolar carcinoma Colonic adenocarcinoma Endometrial adenocarcinoma Breast adenocarcinoma	Signet ring cells	Gastric adenocarcinoma Colorectal adenocarcinoma
Three-dimensional papillary groups containing psammoma bodies	Ovarian carcinoma – serous papillary Thyroid papillary carcinoma Pancreatic papillary carcinoma	Cytoplasmic pigment	Hepatocellular carcinoma (bile pigment) Melanoma (melanin)
Carcinoma cells in chains and rows ('Indian file' pattern)	Breast – lobular and ductal carcinoma Poorly differentiated small cell carcinoma Gastric adenocarcinoma Ovarian adenocarcinoma	Small cells	Small cell carcinoma of lung Carcinoma of breast (lobular) Non-Hodgkin lymphoma (low grade)
Pseudomyxoma peritonei	Mucinous neoplasms of ovary and appendix Carcinoma of pancreas, endocervix and breast	Giant tumour cells	Lung large cell carcinoma (giant cell type) Pancreatic adenocarcinoma Thyroid anaplastic carcinoma Squamous cell carcinoma Melanoma and pleomorphic sarcoma
Cell groups of tall columnar cells with a picket fence pattern	Colonic adenocarcinoma Pancreato-biliary carcinoma	Cellular pleomorphism	Poorly differentiated carcinomas of lung, pancreas, ovary, thyroid, urothelium
		Sharp angulated cell borders with keratinisation	Keratinising squamous cell carcinoma
		Squamous cells	Squamous cell carcinomas
		Spindle cells	Sarcomas Spindle cell carcinoma Melanoma Mesothelioma
		Large polyhedral cells	Hepatocellular carcinoma Transitional cell carcinoma Large cell type squamous cell carcinoma

(Modified from Shidham VB, Metastatic carcinoma in effusions. In: Shidham VB, Atkinson BE, editors. Cytopathologic Diagnosis. New York: Igaku-Shoin; 1994)

Mesothelioma

The tumour arising from mesothelial cells, a mesothelioma, can develop in any of the body cavities but around 90% occur in the pleural cavity (Fig. 4.70), followed by the peritoneum and the pericardial sac (6–10%). Almost all mesotheliomas are malignant, although localised mesothelial tumours exist with variable behaviour (Table 4.4).

Clinical details

- Aetiologically, the vast majority of malignant mesotheliomas are associated with exposure to asbestos, a natural mineral fibre mined from rock
- Long interval (20 years +) between exposure and development of a mesothelioma
- Today, individuals with mesothelioma and a history of industrial exposure are entitled to compensation in many countries, making accurate early diagnosis important
- With control of asbestos use globally, the incidence of mesothelioma should start to fall over the next decades but some natural exposure will still occur
- Serous effusion, pain in the chest, breathlessness are common presentations
- Spread to other cavities and distant metastases often occur within a year
- Histologically, most mesotheliomas are either epithelial or mixed in type
- Sarcomatoid type is rare, especially as a cause of effusion
- In situ mesothelioma is occasionally seen, involving the surface of the cavity only

N.B. Mesothelioma cells must be distinguished from reactive mesothelial cells but also from metastatic carcinoma cells, both of which it resembles.

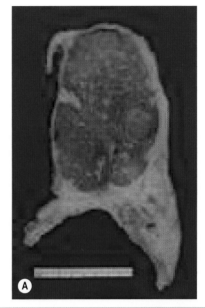

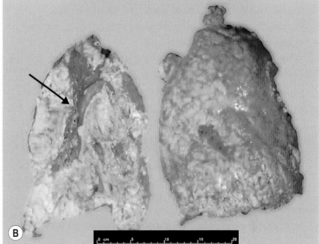

Table 4.4 Working classification of mesothelial-related neoplasms

Malignant mesothelioma	Epithelial Biphasic Sarcomatous
Unusual or rare variants	Clear cell, decimoid, lymphohistiocytoid, signet ring and small cell type
Other neoplasms of mesothelial origin or differentiation	Well-differentiated papillary mesothelioma of peritoneum Cystic mesothelioma Adenomatoid tumour of male and female genital tract
Neoplasms likely to be of subserosal origin	Benign fibrous tumour of pleura (so-called localised fibrous mesothelioma, benign pleural fibroma) Localised malignant fibrous tumours of pleura

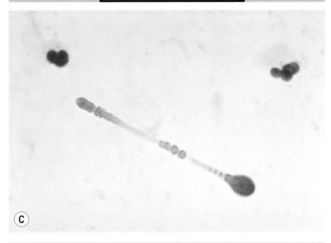

Fig. 4.70 (A) Pleural mesothelioma showing dense tumour tissue encasing the lung. (B) Mesothelioma from left pleural cavity removed intact and bisected revealing a central compressed streak of lung tissue (*arrow*) (PM specimen). (C) Asbestos body showing beaded fibre due to iron coating.

Clues to cytological diagnosis (Tables 4.5, 4.6, p. 127)

- Fluid may be viscous due to hyaluronic acid content
- Quantitative features: smears usually hypercellular with many single mesothelial-type cells and cell groups
- Qualitative features: large knobbly groups and cell balls, exaggerated mesothelial cell features
- No foreign cell population: cell pattern important
- MGG stain: cytoplasmic features, PAP: nuclear details

Cytological findings (Figs 4.71–4.82)

- Hypercellular fluid
- Enlarged single cells have mesothelial cytoplasmic features: metachromasia, vacuoles, blebs
- Groups vary in size, with scalloped contours, sometimes papillary with stromal cores
- Wide intercellular windows may be seen with cytoplasmic microvilli
- Nuclei usually central, often enlarged, usually regular
- Multinucleation often present, giant cells occasionally seen
- Visible nucleoli, may be enlarged
- Mitotic figures may be seen, normal or atypical
- Cell-in-cell arrangements are not uncommon
- Frankly malignant nuclear changes are not commonly seen
- Nuclear pyknosis, apoptosis sometimes present

Differential diagnosis (Figs 4.83–4.85)

- Reactive mesothelial cells (Table 4.5): mesothelioma shows a spectrum of mesothelial cell changes but more cells have exaggerated mesothelial cell features in effusions due to mesothelioma
- Adenocarcinoma cells (Table 4.6): equally cellular with groups that have smooth contours, may show acinar formation or contain mucin; nuclear malignancy changes may be marked in effusions due to metastatic carcinoma
- Variants of mesothelioma are hard to diagnose by cytology alone: immunostains are needed to exclude other tumour types

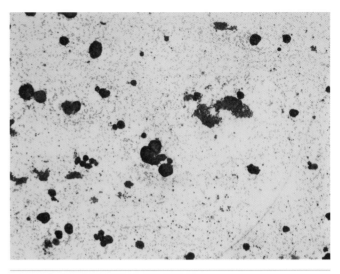

Fig. 4.71[†] Pleural mesothelioma: cellular smear with single cells and variably sized goups. Note pinkish background of hyaluronic acid.

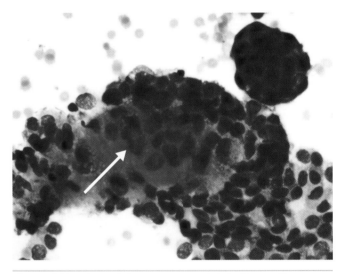

Fig. 4.72[†] Pleural mesothelioma: many mesothelial cells, a papillary group and a metachromatic stromal core at arrow.

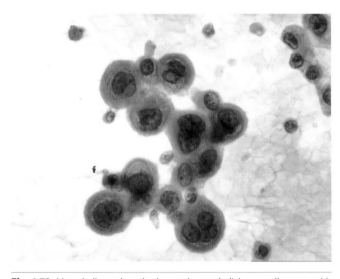

Fig. 4.73 Mesothelioma: loosely clustered mesothelial-type cells, some with nuclear atypia, multinucleation (PAP stain).

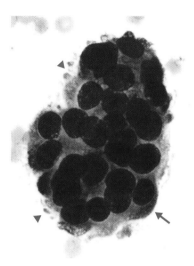

Fig. 4.74† Pleural mesothelioma: large crowded group of mesothelial cells with peripheral blebs (*arrowheads*) and cytoplasmic scalloped border (*arrow*) (MGG stain).

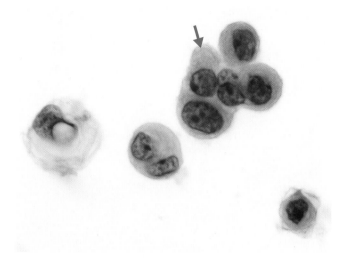

Fig. 4.77† Individual and grouped mesothelioma cells: note similarity to reactive mesothelial cells, no definite features of malignancy. Note the peripheral vacuolation (*arrow*).

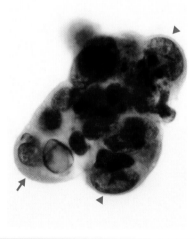

Fig. 4.75† Same case as Fig. 4.74: PAP stain showing malignant nuclear features, inconspicuous rim at arrowheads and microvilli at arrow.

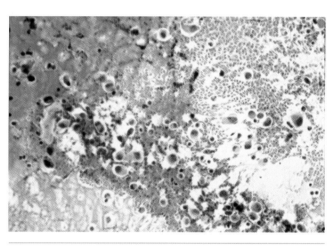

Fig. 4.78† Peritoneal deciduoid mesothelioma: single atypical enlarged mesothelial cells. See also Fig. 4.75, same case.

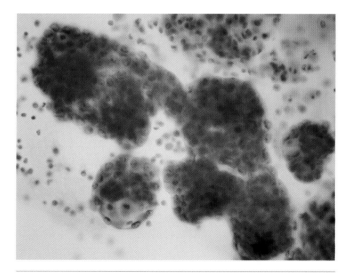

Fig. 4.76† Pleural mesothelioma: numerous large cell balls in three-dimensional papillary groups. See also Fig. 4.77, same case.

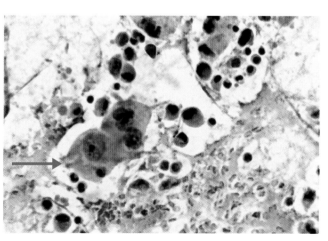

Fig. 4.79† Deciduoid mesothelioma with large bizarre cells, glassy cytoplasm and multinucleation (*arrow*). Note the malignant nuclear features (cf. Fig. 4.78) (PAP stain).

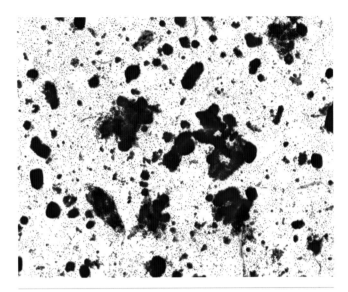

Fig. 4.80† Mesothelioma: hypercellular with crowded cells in large papillary groups, smaller groups and single cells.

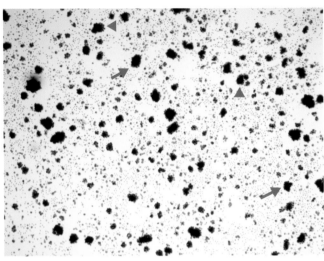

Fig. 4.83† Metastatic breast carcinoma in pleural fluid: many small- to medium-sized cell groups (*arrows*), some suggesting papillary forms (*arrowheads*) (cf. Figs 4.84 and 4.85).

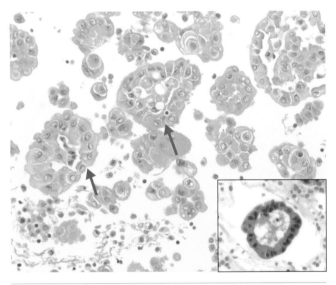

Fig. 4.81† Cell block from mesothelioma (Fig. 4.80), with solid groups, and some stromal cores (*arrows*). (Inset) Breast metastasis hollow sphere.

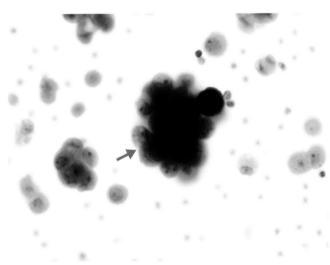

Fig. 4.84† Detail of Fig. 4.83: note dual cell population with normal mesothelial cells and epithelial-type malignant cells (*arrow*).

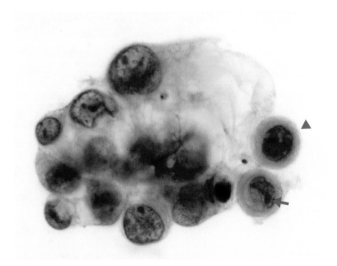

Fig. 4.82† Mesothelioma: three-dimensional group of cells with nuclear pleomorphism, obvious nucleoli (*arrow*), cytoplasmic rim preserved (*arrowhead*).

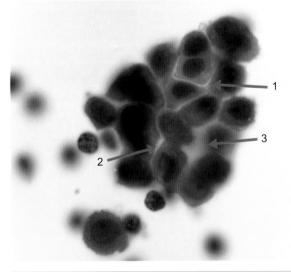

Fig. 4.85† Flat group of reactive mesothelial cells with large active nuclei (cf. Fig. 4.74) and windows increasing in width in arrows 1–3.

Diagnostic approach: mesothelioma morphology (Tables 4.5, 4.6)

Table 4.5 Comparison of reactive mesothelial cells and mesothelioma in effusions

	Feature	Reactive mesothelial cells	Mesothelioma
QUANTITATIVE FEATURES			
1	Specimen cellularity	Moderate to low	Hypercellular
2	Size of cell groups	Relatively smaller	Relatively larger
3	Number of cells in each group	Usually few	Usually more
QUALITATIVE FEATURES			
1	Morphology of cell groups	Mainly mono-layered with knobbly outlines	Two- and three-dimensional cell groups with knobbly outlines
2	Cell size variability	Mild variation	Greater variation
3	Giant mesothelial cells and multinucleate cells	Usually absent	May be present
4	Peripheral cytoplasmic blebs and microvilli	Present, but not very prominent	Usually prominent
5	Nuclear features of malignancy – pleomorphic enlarged nuclei, prominent nucleoli, atypical mitoses	Not a feature	May be present

Table 4.6 Comparative cytomorphology of mesothelioma versus adenocarcinoma in effusions

Feature	Mesothelioma	Adenocarcinoma
Specimen cellularity	Hypercellular	Hypercellular
Cell groups	Two- and three-dimensional	Two- and three-dimensional
Outlines to groups	Knobbly	Smooth ('community borders')
Acinar formations	Usually absent	Usually present
Cellular variability	Present	Usually present
Abnormal cells	Giant mesothelial cells present	Bizarre malignant cells present
Overt features of malignancy – pleomorphic enlarged nuclei, prominent nucleoli, and atypical mitoses	Present, but usually subtle	Usually present
Two-zone cytoplasmic appearance	Present	Absent
Intercellular windows	Present: large windows may resemble acini	Absent: narrow acini may resemble windows
Cytoplasmic blebs with microvilli	Present	Absent
Distinct 'foreign' second population	Absent	Present

Diagnostic approach: immunocytochemistry (Fig. 4.86 and Tables 4.7, 4.8)

- There are many overlapping features in the cytological findings in effusion cytology using routine stains such as MGG (Diff-Quik) and PAP. Histochemical stains for secretory products, e.g. glycogen (PAS), mucin: (PASD after diastase to remove glycogen, or mucicarmine stain) may be conclusive if positive for mucin but cannot distinguish one adenocarcinoma primary site from others
- Mesothelial cells have no diagnostic staining properties but can be identified in some cases by their negative staining reactions for mucin (PASD negative)
- Benign reactive lymphoid effusions may not be distinguishable from low-grade lymphoma on morphology alone, and high-grade lymphomas can closely resemble some metastatic carcinomas in fluids, as the cells tend to round up
- An ever-increasing range of markers for cytoplasmic and nuclear proteins can be used on cells from effusions but usually a more limited selection can be used as a panel, determined by the routine morphology of the cells in question. (See Chapter 13 for technical details)

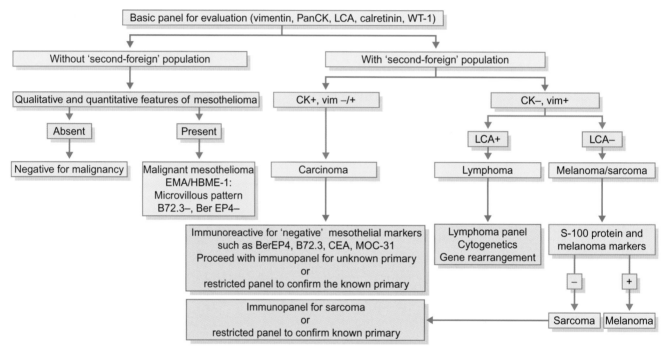

Effusions containing numerous lymphocytes and suspicious for lymphoma (even if lymphoid population is polymorphic) should be immunophenotyped by flow cytometry (or by immunocytochemistry on cell block sections). In high-grade large cell lymphoma the atypical cells seen as 'second-foreign' population will be LCA (CD45) immunoreactive at the initial SCIP approach.

Fig. 4.86[†] Algorithm for immunocytochemial evaluation of effusions.

Table 4.7 Recommended immunocytochemistry markers for routine diagnosis

Mesothelial cell markers	Non-mesothelial cell markers
Calretinin	Ber-EP4
Cytokeratin 5/6	mCEA
D2–40 (podoplanin)	MOC-31
WT-1	BG-8
Thrombomodulin	B72.3
LESS SENSITIVE OR SPECIFIC	**LESS SENSITIVE, FAIRLY SPECIFIC**
Mesothelin, HBME-1, N-cadherin, OV632, CD44S	TTF-1, prostate-specific antigen (PSA), calcitonin, ER, CDX2

Table 4.8 Immunomarkers (in alphabetical order) for immunocytochemical evaluation of effusions

Immunomarker	Pattern	Immunoreactivity in	Remarks
Anti-mesothelial cell antibody	Cytoplasmic	Mesothelioma	Not evaluated and reported by a study other than Donna et al. 1992
B72.3	Membranous	AdCa	Good general immunomarker for adenocarcinoma. Slightly weaker than BerEP4
BerEP4	Membranous	AdCa	Good general immunomarker for adenocarcinoma. Relatively better than B72.3
CA19–9	Cytoplasmic; luminal	AdCa	Most pancreatic, gastric, colonic and gall bladder adenocarcinomas 50% of ovarian carcinomas and 35% of mucoepidermoid carcinomas of salivary gland
E-Cadherin (HECD-1)	Membranous; cytoplasmic	AdCa and reactive/neoplastic meso in some cases	Not a significantly useful immunomarker in effusion immunocytochemistry
N-Cadherin	Membranous; cytoplasmic	AdCa and reactive/neoplastic meso in some cases	Not a significantly useful immunomarker in effusion immunocytochemistry
Calretinin	Nuclear (with or without cytoplasmic)	Mesothelioma; mesothelial cells	Relatively specific mesothelial immunomarker in effusion immunocytochemistry
CD15 (LeuM1)	Membranous; cytoplasmic	AdCa; haemopoietic cells	Weaker immunomarker for adenocarcinoma. Overlaps with mesothelioma. Less useful immunomarker for effusion immunocytochemistry
CD44S (CD44H)	Membranous	Mesothelial cells; AdCa	Not a useful immunomarker in effusion immunocytochemistry
CD45 (LCA)	Cytoplasmic	Inflammatory cells and lymphoma cells	Useful immunomarker in effusion immunocytochemistry. Distinguishes the inflammatory cells from mesothelial cells and metastatic carcinoma
CD68 (preferably PGM1, not KP1)	Cytoplasmic	Inflammatory cells and lymphoma cells	Useful immunomarker in effusion immunocytochemistry. Distinguishes the inflammatory cells from mesothelial cells and metastatic carcinoma
CDX2	Nuclear	Colon (and gastric) AdCa	Useful immunomarker for differential diagnosis of specific primary site
mCEA (monoclonal CEA)	Cytoplasmic	AdCa	Good immunomarker for adenocarcinoma, but less sensitive than BerEP4
CRxA-01	Membranous	Breast Ca	Useful immunomarker in the differential diagnosis of specific primary site. Slightly more non-specific than Mammaglobin
Cytokeratin	Cytoplasmic	Carcinoma; mesothelioma (with concentric pattern)	Useful immunomarker for differential diagnosis from non-mesothelial/non-carcinoma neoplasms
Cytokeratin 5/6	Cytoplasmic	Carcinoma (rare); mesothelial cells	Useful immunomarker to distinguish mesothelial cells from carcinoma cells. Less effective than calretinin and D2–40, but popular with some groups
Cytokeratin 7	Cytoplasmic	Carcinoma (some); mesothelial cells	Useful immunomarker to distinguish mesothelial cells from some carcinoma cells
Cytokeratin 19	Cytoplasmic	Carcinoma; mesothelial cells (rarely)	Useful immunomarker to distinguish lung carcinoma cells from mesothelial cells
Cytokeratin 20	Cytoplasmic	Carcinoma (some)	Useful immunomarker to distinguish some carcinoma cells from mesothelial cells
D2–40 (Podoplanin)	Membranous (microvillous)	Mesothelioma; lymphatic endothelium; testicular germ cell tumours	Specific mesothelial immunomarker in effusion setting. Approaches that for calretinin
EMA (epithelial membrane antigen)	Membranous (microvillous); cytoplasmic	Mesothelioma; AdCa, large cell anaplastic lymphoma	Not a useful immunomarker in effusion immunocytochemistry
HBME-1	Membranous (thick microvillous)	Epithelioid mesothelioma; thyroid Ca; sarcoma; lymphoma	Not a useful immunomarker in effusion immunocytochemistry (but popular with some groups)
HMFG-2 (human milk fat globule)	Cytoplasmic	AdCa; some mesothelioma	Not useful immunomarker in effusion immunocytochemistry
Mammaglobin	Cytoplasmic	Breast Ca	Useful immunomarker for differential diagnosis of specific primary site.
Mesothelin	Membranous	Mesothelioma; many AdCa	Not useful immunomarker in effusion immunocytochemistry
MOC-31	Cytoplasmic	AdCa	Good immunomarker for adenocarcinoma, but is less sensitive and specific than BerEP4
OV632		Ovarian ca; mesothelioma	May be useful immunomarker for differential diagnosis of specific primary site
Thrombomodulin	Membranous	Mesothelial cells; AdCa	Not useful immunomarker in effusion immunocytochemistry
TTF-1	Nuclear	AdCa; lung and thyroid	Useful immunomarker for differential diagnosis of specific primary site
Vimentin	Cytoplasmic	Mesothelioma; sarcoma; lymphoma	Useful immunomarker in effusion immunocytochemistry. Distinguishes most metastatic carcinomas by negative immunostaining
WT-1	Nuclear (with or without cytoplasmic)	Mesothelioma; ovarian Ca; DSRCT	May be specific mesothelial immunomarker in pleural and pericardial effusion setting, but less useful than calretinin and D2–40

(Modified from Shidham VB, Appendix II: Immunocytochemistry of effusions – processing and commonly used immunomarkers. In: Shidham VB, Atkinson BE, editors. Cytopathologic Diagnosis of Serous Fluids. 1st ed. Elsevier; 2007)
AdCa, adenocarcinoma; Ca, carcinoma; DSRCT, desmoplastic small round cell tumour; EMA, epithelial membrane antigen; meso, mesothelial cells; TTF-1, thyroid transcription factor-1; WT-1, Wilms' tumour-1.

Immunomarker examples: malignant cell types (Figs 4.87–4.100)

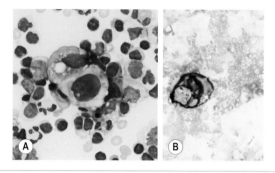

Fig. 4.88 Metastatic adenocarcinoma. (A) Malignant cells with no distinctive features. (B) BerEP4 positive, confirming adenocarcinoma.

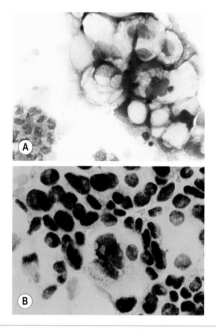

Fig. 4.89 Serous adenocarcinoma of ovary. (A) Vacuolated malignant cells. (B) WT-1 positive for serous (not mucinous) ovarian carcinoma.

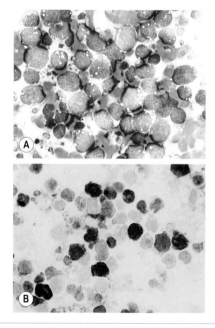

Fig. 4.90 Burkitt's lymphoma. (A) Many atypical lymphoid cells. (B) KI67 positive (proliferation marker).

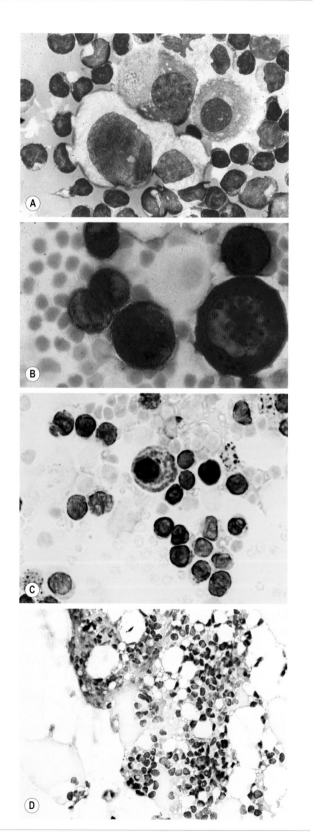

Fig. 4.87 Metastatic breast carcinoma in pleural fluid. (A) Tumour cells, MGG stain. (B) Ber EP4 positive. (C) CK7 positive. (D) Cell block: ER (oestrogen receptor) positive.

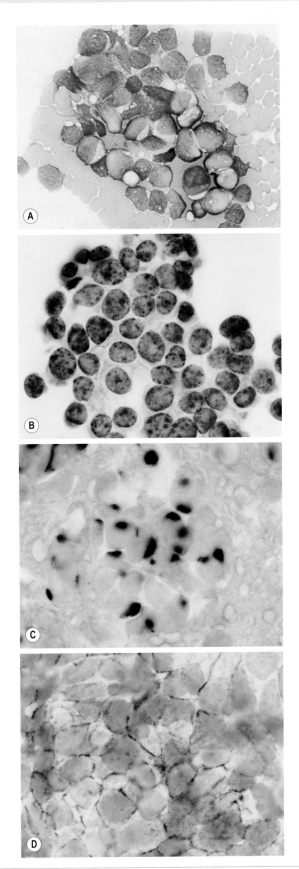

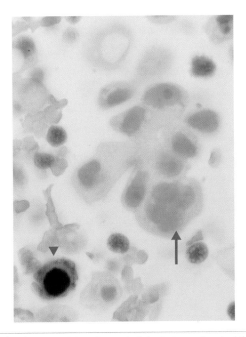

Fig. 4.92[†] Calretinin staining of mesothelial cell at arrowhead, while carcinoma cells at arrow are negative.

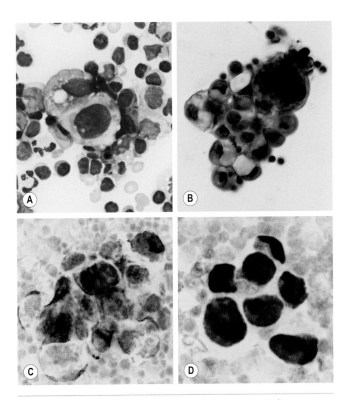

Fig. 4.91 Small cell carcinoma of lung. (A & B) MGG and PAP stains showing typical features. (C) CAM 5.2 dot positivity in tumour cells. (D) CD56 cytoplasmic membrane staining in tumour cells.

Fig. 4.93 Carcinoma of colon. (A & B) MGG and PAP stains with adenocarcinoma cells. (C & D) CK20 positive, CDX2 positive confirming colonic primary site.

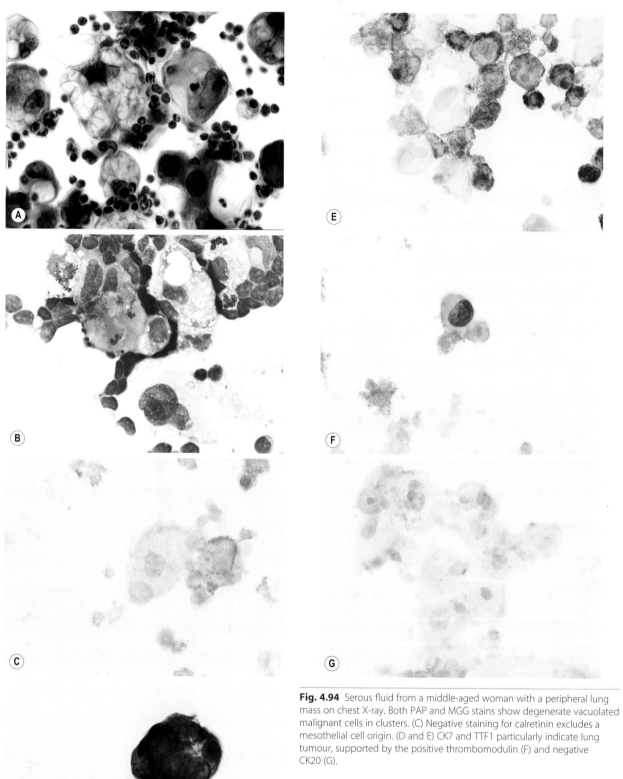

Fig. 4.94 Serous fluid from a middle-aged woman with a peripheral lung mass on chest X-ray. Both PAP and MGG stains show degenerate vacuolated malignant cells in clusters. (C) Negative staining for calretinin excludes a mesothelial cell origin. (D and E) CK7 and TTF1 particularly indicate lung tumour, supported by the positive thrombomodulin (F) and negative CK20 (G).

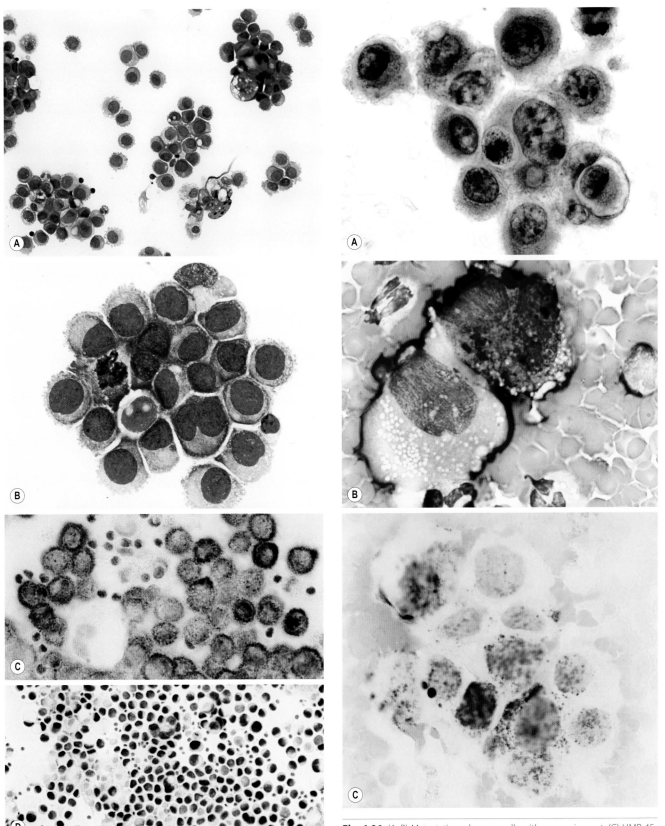

Fig. 4.95 Linitis plastica gastric carcinoma. (A & B) Dissociated small malignant cells. (C & D) BerEP4 and CDX2, both positive, confirming GIT primary.

Fig. 4.96 (A, B) Metastatic melanoma cells with some pigment. (C) HMB 45 positive staining confirming melanoma.

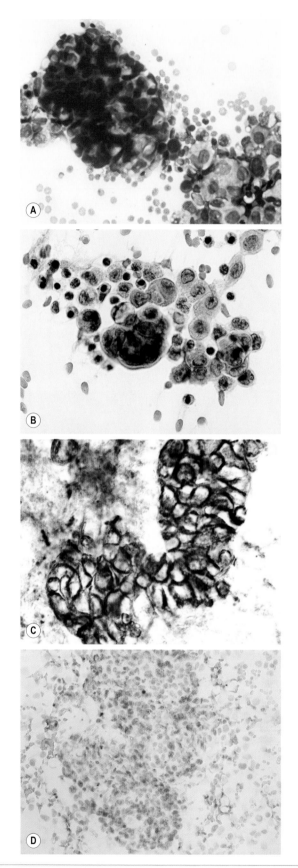

(A)

(B)

(C)

(D)

Fig. 4.97 Primary peritoneal carcinoma (rarity). (A & B) MGG and PAP: ? adenocarcinoma or mesothelioma. (C & D) BerEP4 positive confirms an epithelial origin, calretinin negative indicating tumour is not a mesothelioma. No primary site outside the peritoneum was found.

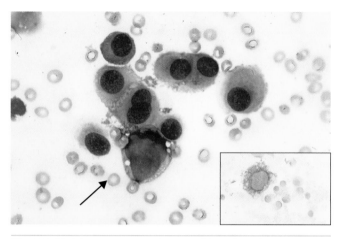

Fig. 4.98 Rhabdomyosarcoma: malignant cell (*arrow*), no diagnostic features. (Inset) Desmin positive cell confirming sarcoma.

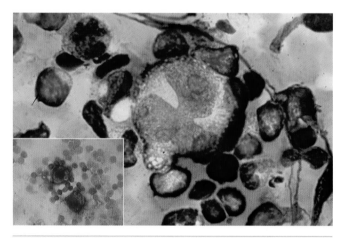

Fig. 4.99 Hodgkin lymphoma: Reed–Sternberg cell in pleural fluid. (Inset)[†] CD30 confirms the presence of Hodgkin cells.

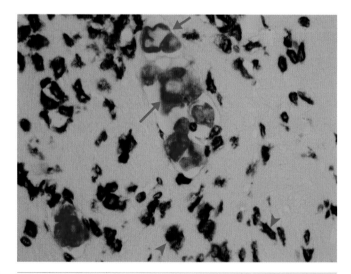

Fig. 4.100[†] Dual immunostaining. Metastatic breast carcinoma in pleural fluid: cytokeratin CK7 positive red staining of cytoplasm of malignant cells (*arrow*) but negative for vimentin (brown staining), which is only present in inflammatory cells (*arrowheads*). Mesothelial cells in other fields stained with both CK7 and vimentin.

CHAPTER 5

Urine cytology

Contents

Introduction   135

Specimen type and appearances   135

Malignancy in urine cytology   139

Differential diagnosis in urothelial malignancy   143

Instrumentation effects   144

Introduction

- The interpretation of urinary tract cytology is used for the diagnosis of urothelial malignancy
- Urine specimens provide a critical role in the evaluation of patient symptoms of painless haematuria and/or other symptoms that may reflect urinary tract pathology
- Urine cytology is used as a screening tool after bladder carcinogen exposure and in surveillance of patients with previous urinary malignancy
- Processing of urine samples may be by centrifugation, monolayer techniques, filtration or cell block preparation

Specimen types and appearances (Figs 5.1–5.9)

Voided urine sample:
- Must be fresh for optimal cellular preservation
- Variable cellularity – often relatively cell-poor
- Bland urothelial cells
- Squamous cells – may be from trigone or urethra, or of vulvovaginal origin
- Cells of prostatic origin in men including seminal vesicle cells
- ± very occasional red blood cells, sperms, and corpora amylacea
- ± casts – red cell casts may suggest a renal cause of blood loss
- Rarities include endometrial contamination in women – although endometriosis should be considered
- VIN and VAIN changes in contaminant exfoliated cells from vulva and vagina (see later)

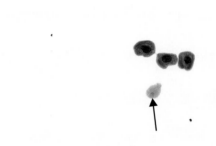

Fig. 5.1 Normal voided urine with occasional bland urothelial cells and a degenerate form (*arrow*).

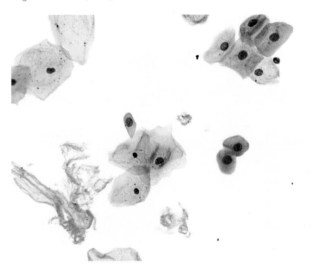

Fig. 5.2 Normal squamous and urothelial cells.

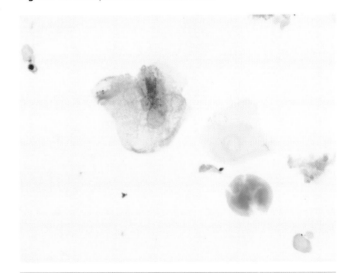

Fig. 5.3 Corpus amylaceum in normal voided urine.

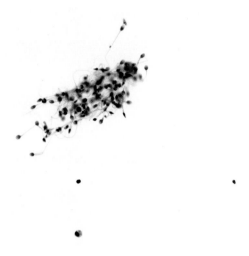

Fig. 5.4 Spermatozoa in normal voided urine.

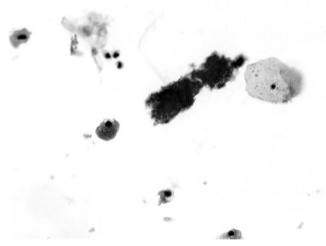

Fig. 5.7 Red blood cell cast.

Fig. 5.5 Red blood cells and seminal vesicle cells. Note spermatozoa within and around cytoplasm of cells.

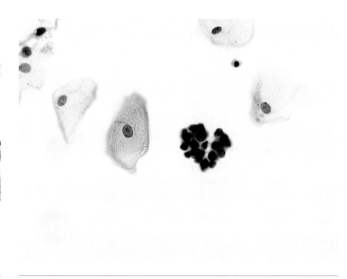

Fig. 5.8 Normal morphology endometrial cluster in voided urine typically indicating menstrual contamination.

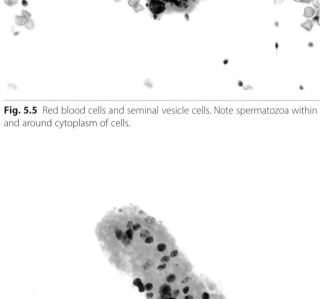

Fig. 5.6 A tubular cast.

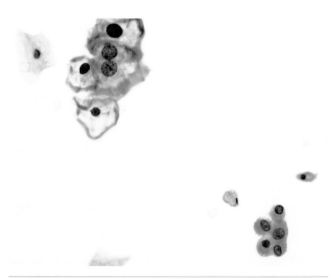

Fig. 5.9 Mild dyskaryosis in vulvovaginal squamous cells. Normal urothelial cells bottom right of picture.

Instrumented samples (Figs 5.10–5.15)

These samples are generated from cystoscopy, bladder/renal pelvis wash-outs, catheterization and direct brush sampling.

- Extremely cellular
- Cells present from superficial and deeper layers – the latter may have a columnar configuration
- Catheter samples may have a significant associated acute inflammatory cell reaction

Ileal conduit samples (Figs 5.16–5.18)

These samples need to be screened to exclude recurrent/other urinary tract malignancy.

Rarely adenocarcinoma may arise, reflecting the adenoma/carcinoma sequence as a consequence of altered bacterial population as a result of the diverted urinary flow.

- Initially very cellular, reflecting the increased surface area of small bowel with enteric cell exfoliation
- Over time, the small bowel villi atrophy and the cell number dwindles
- The exfoliated intestinal cells typically show marked degenerative changes secondary to 'bathing' in the urinary environment

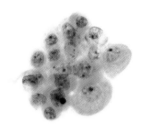

Fig. 5.10 Superficial and deeper urothelial cells in an instrumented sample.

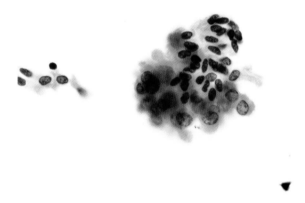

Fig. 5.11 Instrumented samples with columnar-shaped urothelial cells.

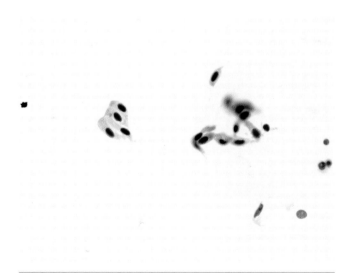

Fig. 5.12 Columnar-appearing urothelial cells in a cystoscopy urine sample.

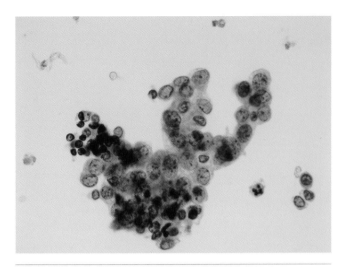

Fig. 5.13[†] A large staghorn cluster of urothelial cells infiltrated by a few acute and chronic inflammatory cells. The urothelial cell nuclei are round to oval and contain thickened nuclear rims, although the chromatin pattern is hypochromatic. A small red nucleolus is present in most of the nuclei. The urothelial cell cytoplasm is finely granular and not homogeneous (catheter sample).

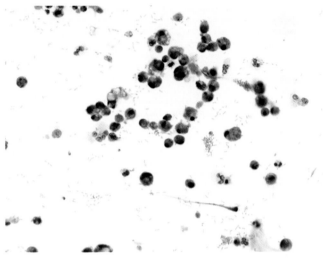

Fig. 5.16 Ileal conduit sample 3 months after surgery.

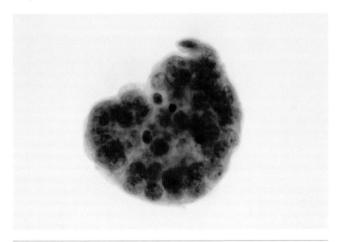

Fig. 5.14[†] A three-dimensional group of urothelial cells show round nuclei with evenly distributed granular nuclear chromatin. Although the nuclei show overlapping, other characteristics of neoplasia are lacking (catheter sample).

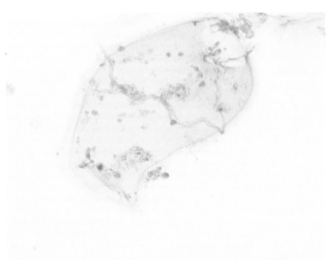

Fig. 5.17 Same patient as Fig. 5.16. Ileal conduit 12 months after surgery. Sample is virtually acellular.

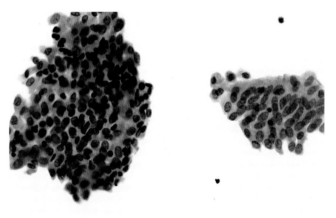

Fig. 5.15 Large normal urothelial cell fragments in a urine sample taken at cystoscopy.

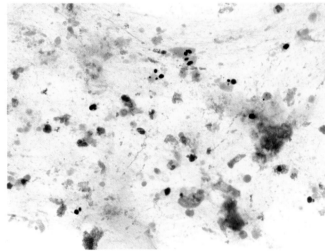

Fig. 5.18 Extreme degeneration of exfoliated intestinal epithelial cells in ileal conduit sample.

Malignancy in urine cytology (Figs 5.19–5.27)

- Urothelial carcinoma is the most common cancer detected by urine cytology
- The most common site of origin is the bladder
- Typically 90% of bladder cancers are urothelial in origin, 5% squamous and 5% mixed urothelial/squamous
- Primary adenocarcinoma of the bladder is rare and the cytomorphology not well described – reflecting their typical non-specific high-grade morphology
- 75% of patients present with painless haematuria
- Other symptoms include urinary frequency, dysuria and urgency
- Sensitivity of voided urine for diagnosis of high-grade urothelial carcinoma (in situ and/or invasive) is >90%
- Low-grade urothelial malignancy is very difficult to diagnose on urinary cytology samples reflecting the blandness of epithelium. The reported sensitivity ranges from 0% to 73%

Cytological findings of high-grade urothelial carcinoma/carcinoma in situ

- No discriminating features between high-grade transitional cell carcinoma (grade 2/3) and carcinoma in situ
- Typically increased cellularity sample
- Malignant cells have enlarged nuclei with abnormal chromatin distribution – including dense hyperchromasia, raised nuclear:cytoplasmic ratios
- The cells are arranged in loosely cohesive groups, sheets and singly
- Necrosis and/or red blood cells are evident in the background

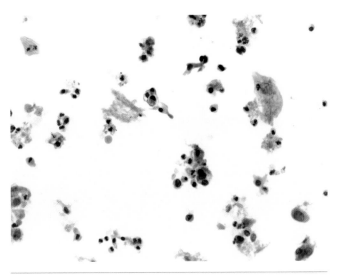

Fig. 5.19 Low-power view of transitional cell carcinoma.

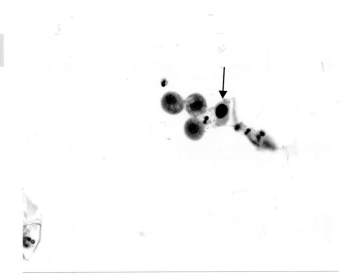

Fig. 5.20 A single malignant urothelial cell (*arrow*) with adjacent normal urothelial cells with degenerative changes for the normal urothelial cells.

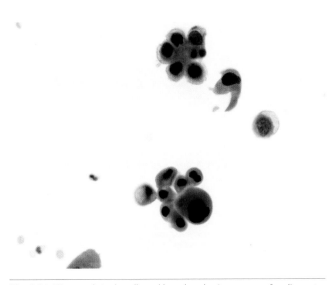

Fig. 5.21 Dispersed single cells and loosely cohesive groups of malignant urothelial cells from high-grade transitional cell carcinoma.

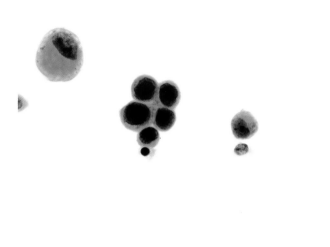

Fig. 5.22 Dense hyperchromasia in malignant urothelial cells.

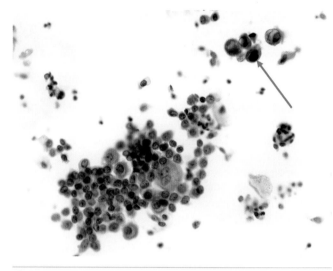

Fig. 5.25 Ureteric brush sample with instrumentation changes and scattered atypical urothelial cells (*arrow*).

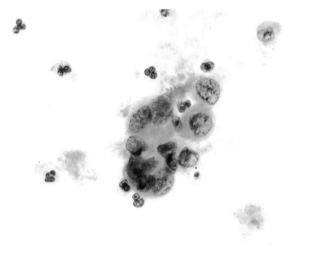

Fig. 5.23 Malignant urothelial cells with abnormal chromatin pattern (but not dense hyperchromasia).

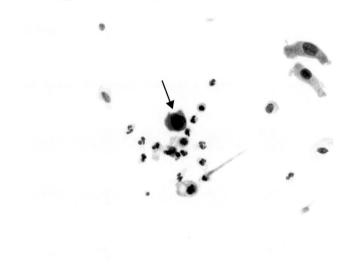

Fig. 5.26 Same patient as Fig. 5.25. Single unequivocal malignant urothelial cell (*arrow*).

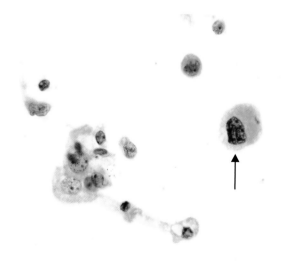

Fig. 5.24 A single malignant urothelial cell with enlarged, hyperchromatic and irregular nucleus (*arrow*).

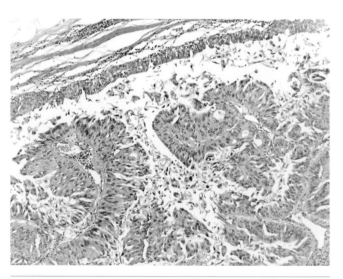

Fig. 5.27 Same patient as Figs 5.25 and 5.26. Low-power view of left ureter showing grade II papillary transitional cell carcinoma.

Cytological findings of low-grade transitional cell carcinoma (Figs 5.28–5.29)

- True papillae with fibrovascular cores rarely identified, but the sample may be extremely cellular with papillaroid structures and dispersed single cells
- Subtle cytological features may suggest atypia/underlying neoplasia including:
  - mild increase in nuclear:cytoplasmic ratios
  - increased density/homogenisation of urothelial cytoplasm

Cytological findings of other urological malignancies (Figs 5.30–5.36)

- **Squamous cell carcinoma**
  - malignant squames evident
  - it is more likely to reflect squamous differentiation in a TCC than primary squamous cell carcinoma *per se*
  - metastatic squamous cell carcinoma should be excluded with clinicoradiological correlation
- **Adenocarcinoma**
  - primary adenocarcinomas are rare and when glandular differentiation evident more likely to represent spread from an extra-urinary site such as prostate, colorectum and female genital tract
  - rarer metastatic tumours include stomach and breast
  - microscopic features show obvious glandular differentiation
  - colorectal tumours have a necrotic background. The component cells appear analogous to CGIN in cervical cytology samples
  - prostatic adenocarcinoma characterised by small cells with prominent orangeophilic nucleoli. Distinction from TCC/CIS may be difficult and require biopsy

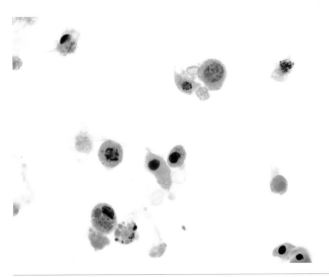

Fig. 5.28 Mild atypia in urothelial cell from a case of grade I transitional cell carcinoma.

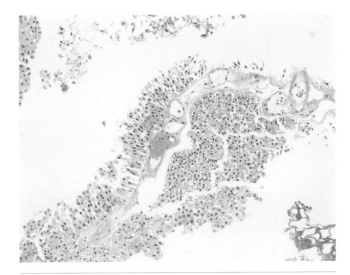

Fig. 5.29 Subsequent histology of grade I transitional cell carcinoma from same patient as in Fig. 5.28.

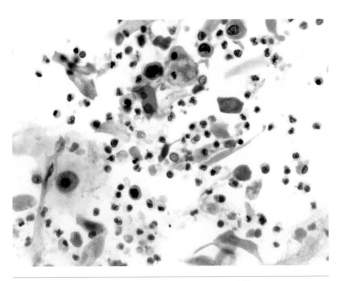

Fig. 5.30 Transitional cell carcinoma with squamous differentiation.

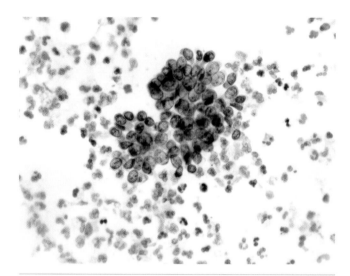

Fig. 5.31 Malignant glandular cluster from a colorectal adenocarcinoma. Note purulent background.

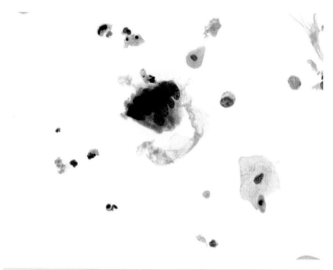

Fig. 5.34 Pseudostratified malignant glandular cluster from colorectal adenocarcinoma.

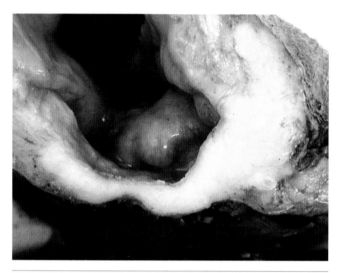

Fig. 5.32 Cross-section of gastrectomy specimen in which wall diffusely thickened secondary to signet cell carcinoma.

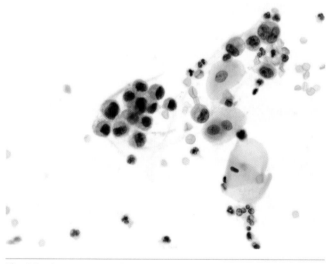

Fig. 5.35 Same patient as Fig. 5.32. Developed haematuria 6 months after gastrectomy. Malignant signet cells seen in urine.

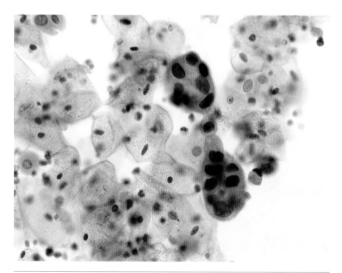

Fig. 5.33 Metastatic ductal carcinoma of breast.

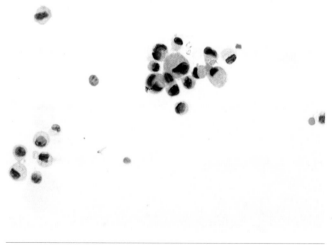

Fig. 5.36 Prostatic carcinoma cells in urine.

Differential diagnosis in urothelial malignancy

Degenerative changes (Figs 5.37–5.39)

- Dark, hyperchromatic nuclei
- Normal nuclear:cytoplasmic ratios which may reduce as the nucleus becomes pyknotic and degenerate
- Degenerate cytoplasmic features include ragged borders, orangeophilic cytoplasmic blebs and vacuolation

BK/human polyomavirus

- Usually seen in immunosuppressed patients; a full clinical history is essential
- When identified, indicates reactivation rather than a primary infection *per se*
- May be associated with haematuria

Characterised by:

- Inclusional 'decoy' cells with dense homogenised and uniformly enlarged nuclei due to a single large inclusion body virtually filling the nucleus
- Post-inclusional cells with 'chinese character'/spireme nuclei
- Often both cell types coexist
- The decoy cells may masquerade as malignant cells. Careful attention to the nuclear features should allow the diagnosis

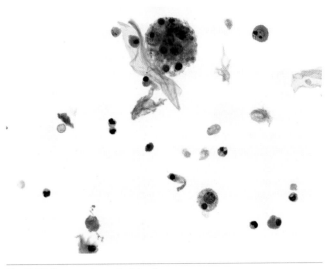

Fig. 5.37 Degenerate urothelial cells.

Fig. 5.38 Papovavirus. Inclusional stage – this is a 'decoy' cell containing a single large inclusion body.

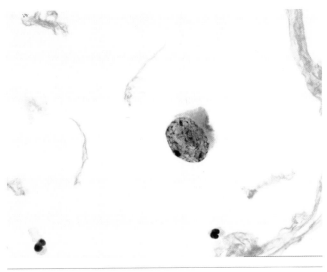

Fig. 5.39 Papovavirus. Post-inclusional stage.

Instrumentation effects (Figs 5.40–5.47)

- Although increased cellularity there is no significant atypia
- Always screen to exclude coexistent tumour

Papillaroid groups

- May be found in low-grade TCC but also instrumentation, exfoliated renal tubular cells, normal voided urines and lithiasis
- May require follow-up/further investigation if the component cells show atypia

Lithiasis/calculus formation

- A voided urine sample may be extremely cellular with inflammatory atypia mimicking low-grade malignancy
- Lack of cytological atypia and clinical history are important

Other reactive conditions

- Chemotherapy and radiotherapy effects may induce urothelial cells with enlarged, hyperchromatic nuclei but normal nuclear:cytoplasmic ratios
- BCG treatment may result in exfoliated granulomata and inflammatory changes. Always screen to exclude recurrent malignancy

Other infections

- Human papillomavirus changes may reflect origin from vulvovaginal contamination in cases of VIN/VAIN or urethral infection. High-grade dyskaryotic cells which may be indistinguishable from high-grade TCC
- Cytomegalovirus infection: infects renal tubular cells in immunosuppressed patients. In urine samples, the infected cells are often degenerate and simulate high-grade TCC/CIS if inclusions not identified

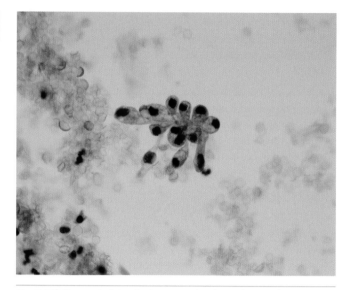

Fig. 5.40 The urothelial cells show vacuolated cytoplasm and degenerative features. The nuclei are hyperchromatic, but small and not larger than the accompanying red cells. The cytoplasm of these reactive cells is often known as 'bubbly'.

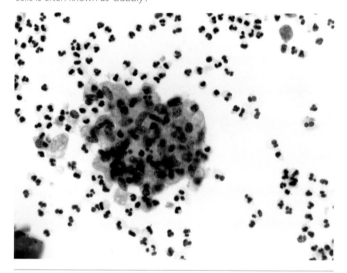

Fig. 5.41 Epithelial granuloma in urine following BCG treatment.

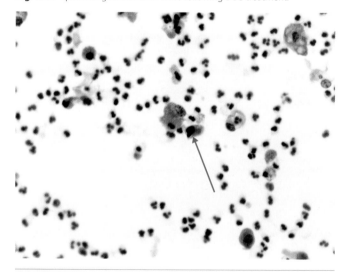

Fig. 5.42 Same as patient as Fig. 5.41. Sample contains an occasional atypical urothelial cell, indicating recurrent transitional cell carcinoma (*arrow*).

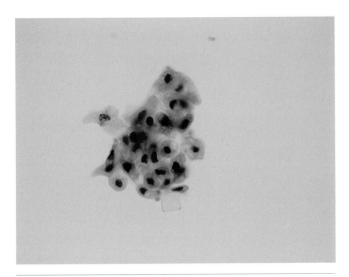

Fig. 5.43† The urothelial cells show vacuolated cytoplasm and low nuclear:cytoplasmic ratios, although nuclear hyperchromasia and nuclear membrane irregularities are present. The patient has a history of lithiasis.

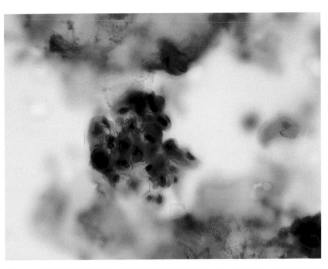

Fig. 5.46† A cluster of squamous cells showing slightly enlarged, hyperchromatic nuclei is seen. The large, eosinophilic structure at the top of the microscope field is a stone fragment. The parakeratotic cell group is representative of reactive change. The patient is 35 years old.

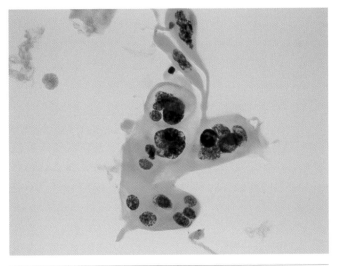

Fig. 5.44† Human papillomavirus findings in bladder are similar to those seen in the cervix or vagina. In this specimen, the infected cells show multinucleation, nuclear hyperchromasia, and perinuclear cytoplasmic halos.

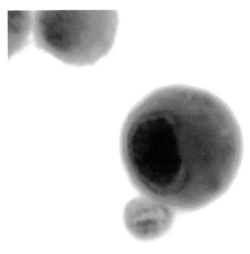

Fig. 5.47† A cytomegalic infected cell shows a very large nuclear inclusion.

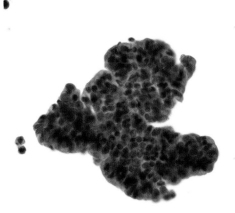

Fig. 5.45† Large groups of benign urothelial cells often are dislodged with instrumentation. In this group, superficial urothelial cells overlie numerous intermediate urothelial cells. The urothelial cells are crowded but do not exhibit significant atypia.

CHAPTER 6

Thyroid gland

Contents

Introduction   147

Benign thyroid nodules   148

Thyroid hyperplasia/hyperthyroidism   156

Follicular lesions   158

Thyroid neoplasms   160

FNA thyroid reporting categories and their management implications   170

Introduction (Figs 6.1–6.3)

The thyroid is currently the organ most frequently sampled by means of fine needle aspiration (FNA) cytology, the main purpose of which is the diagnostic triage of palpable and impalpable nodules into those that require surgery and those that do not. Surgery (total or hemi-thyroidectomy) is currently the recommended treatment for thyroid neoplasms, both benign and malignant. Since the overwhelming majority of thyroid nodules are non-neoplastic colloid nodules, FNA helps reduce the rate of surgery for benign disease. Results of thyroid FNA have to be correlated with other clinical, biochemical, isotope and imaging findings, preferably at the regular multidisciplinary team (MDT) meetings.

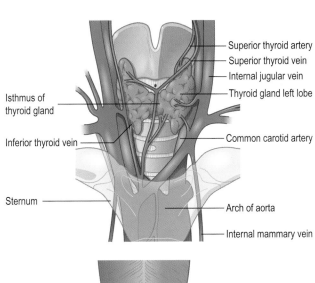

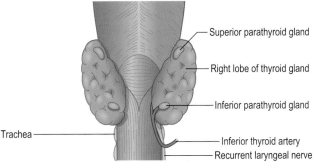

Fig. 6.1 The thyroid is situated on either side of the trachea and oesophagus, joined anteriorly by an isthmus. The gland produces thyroxine under the control of thyroid stimulating hormone (TSH) secreted by the pituitary. It also contains neuroendocrine parafollicular cells, which produce calcitonin.

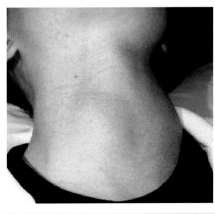

Fig. 6.2 A prominent, soft and fluctuating swelling of the right lobe of the thyroid in a 20-year-old patient from which 10 mL of clear fluid was obtained by FNA. The microscopic finding was of a benign thyroid cyst.

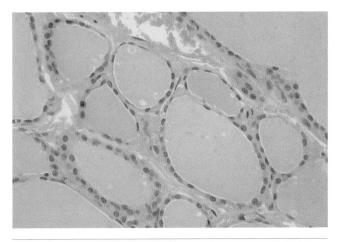

Fig. 6.3 Normal thyroid tissue. Histologically, thyroid consists of numerous follicles lined by a row of cuboidal cells surrounding the lakes of colloid.

Benign thyroid nodules

Benign thyroid nodules include:

- colloid nodular disease such as:
  - nodular goitre
  - hyperplastic/adenomatoid nodule
  - macrofollicular adenoma
- thyroiditis (see p. 153)

The risk of malignancy is low (<3%).

A dominant nodule in the context of a multinodular goitre is the most frequent indication for FNA, and correct diagnosis of a colloid nodule or cyst with the exclusion of malignancy allows the avoidance of surgery in most cases.

Cytological findings: colloid goitre (Figs 6.4–6.12)

- Abundant thin colloid
- Relatively sparse follicular cells
- Follicular cells usually arranged in sheets
- Occasional microfollicles may be present
- Follicular cells have round nuclei and fine granular chromatin pattern
- Cytoplasm is ill defined and may contain granules
- Mild anisonucleosis is not uncommon
- Macrophages

Types of goitre – diffuse enlargement of the thyroid

- Simple non-toxic goitre
  - physiological (including endemic, due to dietary iodine deficiency)
  - dietary goitrogens, goitrogenic drugs and chemicals
  - dyshormonogenetic: inborn errors of thyroxine synthesis
- Multinodular goitre
  - syn: colloid goitre, nodular goitre, adenomatous goitre
- Toxic goitre
- Thyroiditis

Further investigations

- Thyroid function tests
- Ultrasound examination
- Isotope scan (optional)

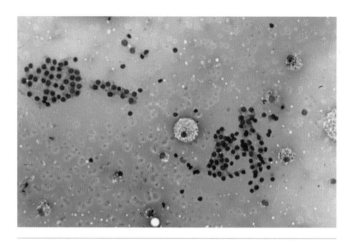

Fig. 6.4 Colloid nodule. Densely blue background representing thin colloid with sheets of thyroid epithelium and a macrophage.

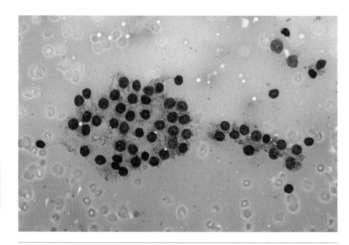

Fig. 6.5 Colloid nodule. High-power view of Fig. 6.4 reveals bland, regularly spaced epithelial cells arranged randomly or in flat sheets.

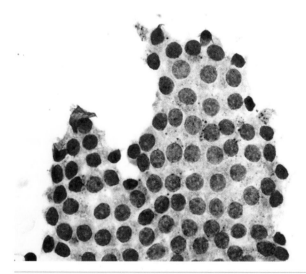

Fig. 6.6 Colloid goitre. Follicular epithelium with bland nuclear features and ill-defined cytoplasm containing granules, sometimes placed within cytoplasmic vacuoles.

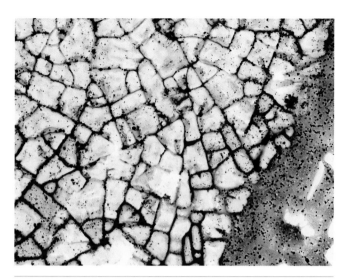

Fig. 6.7 Colloid goitre. Colloid can sometimes assume the appearance of 'crazy paving'.

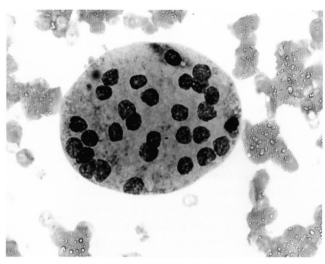

Fig. 6.10 Colloid nodule. Thyroid epithelium can present as microfollicles with a well-defined border.

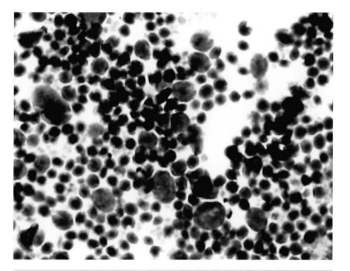

Fig. 6.8 Benign colloid goitre. Colloid appearing as dense proteinaceous globules.

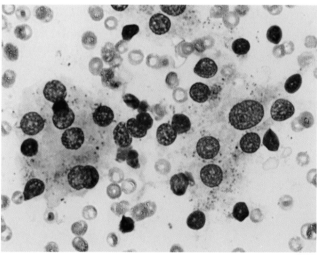

Fig. 6.11 Colloid goitre. Follicular epithelium can show mild anisonucleosis. Note paravacuolar granulations similar to Fig. 6.6.

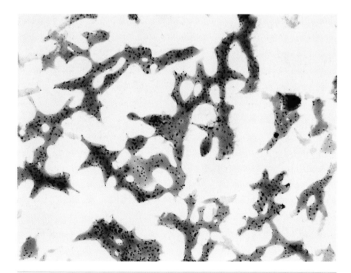

Fig. 6.9 Colloid nodule. Colloid in the shape of 'Chinese letters'.

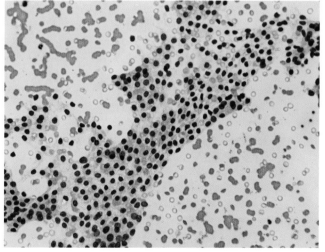

Fig. 6.12 Colloid goitre. Follicular epithelium of thyroid in flat sheet of uniformly sized nuclei and pale, ill-defined cytoplasm.

Thyroid cysts

Multinodular goitre presents clinically as a mass in the neck, which may cause tracheal or oesophageal compression, often predated by a haemorrhage into a colloid nodule forming a thyroid cyst.

The sudden and painful appearance or enlargement of a mass in the neck is frequently an indication for FNA.

Cytological findings (Figs 6.13–6.21)

- Macrophages
- Contain haemosiderin and lipofuscin
- Colloid
- Degenerate follicular cells, vary from being few in number to numerous
- Occasionally atypical cells from the wall of a cyst

Differential diagnosis

- Papillary cystic carcinoma
- Other cystic lesions of the neck

It is important to consider the epithelial component of cystic lesions, particularly if they are haemorrhagic. If epithelium is absent, FNA procedure may need to be repeated.

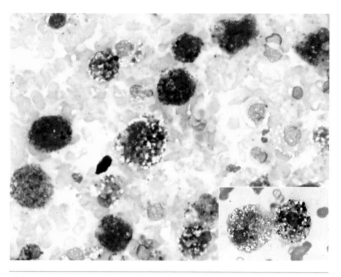

Fig. 6.14 Thyroid cyst. Most of the macrophages are laden with haemosiderin as evidence of haemorrhage into the cyst (*inset*).

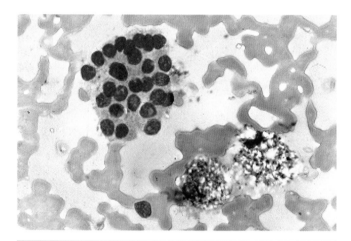

Fig. 6.15 Thyroid cyst. Relatively sparse and degenerate follicular cells are seen.

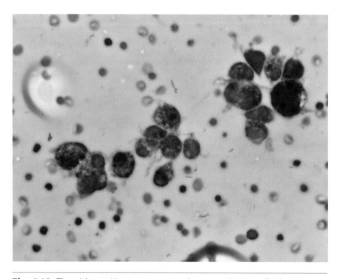

Fig. 6.13 Thyroid cyst. Numerous macrophages against a colloid background.

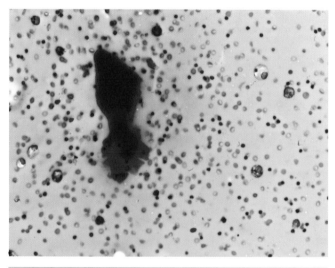

Fig. 6.16 Thyroid cyst. Thin and thick colloid, blood and macrophages.

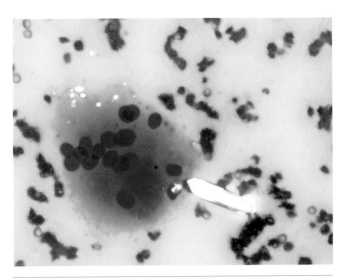

Fig. 6.17 Thyroid cyst. Colloid may contain oxalate crystals which can be polarised. Crystals seen next to multinucleate giant cell.

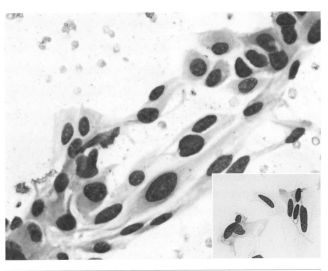

Fig. 6.19 Thyroid cyst. Epithelium from the wall of the cyst may show spindle cell features (*inset*).

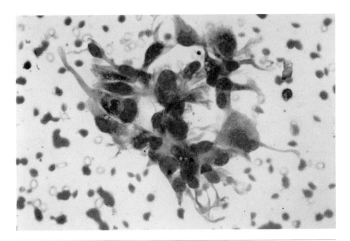

Fig. 6.18 Thyroid cyst. Epithelium from the cyst wall may show bizarre cytoplasmic features. Note cytoplasmic haemosiderin (MGG).

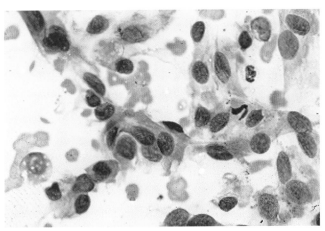

Fig. 6.20 Thyroid cyst. Thyroid epithelium shows degenerative changes and may contain haemosiderin.

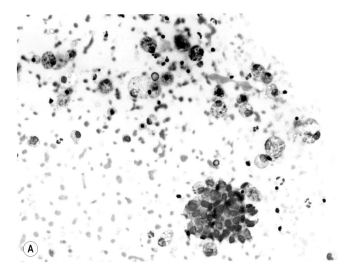

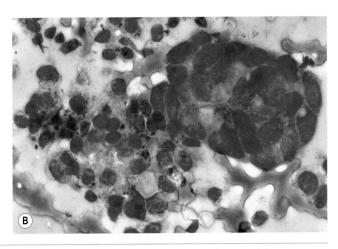

Fig. 6.21 Papillary carcinoma. (A) Metastasis in the neck. Papillary carcinoma, either primary or metastatic, may present as a cystic lesion and show very sparse or no epithelium in the FNA sample. (B) Same case, FNA thyroid also shows prominent cystic change. Malignancy can be overlooked.

Thyroglossal cyst

Clinical presentation

- Midline swelling
- Immediately below the hyoid bone
- Typically occurs in children or young adults
- History of a painless mass of long duration

Cytological findings (Figs 6.22–6.24)

- Degenerate foamy macrophages
- Cholesterol crystals
- Inflammatory cells in infected cysts
- Occasionally, respiratory or squamous cells
- Rarely, thyroid follicular cells or colloid

Differential diagnosis

- Colloid cyst in multinodular goitre
- Cystic papillary carcinoma
- Other neck cysts such as branchial cleft cyst

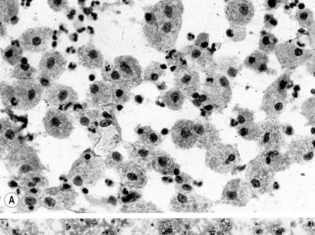

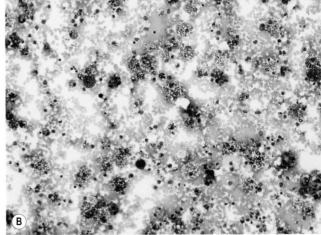

Fig. 6.23 Thyroglossal cyst. Colloid and haemosiderin-laden macrophages are indistinguishable from a colloid cyst (A: PAP, B: MGG).

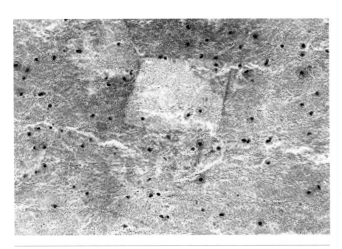

Fig. 6.22 Thyroglossal cyst. Backround of macrophages with inflammatory cells and cholesterol crystals.

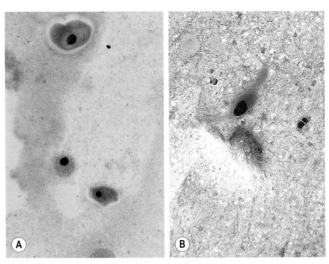

Fig. 6.24 Thyroglossal cyst. Occasional squamous cells may be seen (A: PAP, B: MGG). However, this is exceedingly rare. The presence of squamous cells in a cystic neck lesion is a significant finding. A metastatic squamous cell carcinoma has to be excluded.

Thyroiditis

Inflammation of the thyroid can be subdivided into the following conditions listed in the order of frequency:

- Lymphocytic and autoimmune (Hashimoto's) thyroiditis
- Subacute (de Quervain's) thyroiditis
- Riedel's thyroiditis
- Acute bacterial thyroiditis

Cytological findings: lymphocytic and autoimmune thyroiditis (Figs 6.25–6.29)

- Reactive lymphoid cells including follicle centre cells and plasma cells
- Oncocytic (Hürthle) cells
- Multinucleate and epithelioid histiocytes
- Usually little colloid

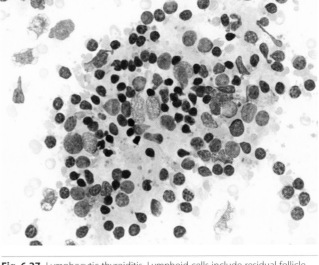

Fig. 6.27 Lymphocytic thyroiditis. Lymphoid cells include residual follicle centre fragments with follicular dendritic cells, centroblasts, centrocytes and plasma cells.

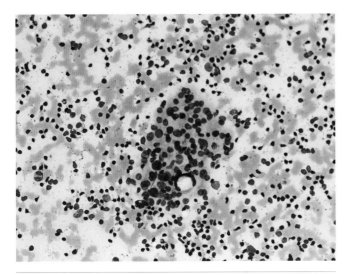

Fig. 6.25 Lymphocytic thyroiditis. Islands of oncocytic epithelium surrounded by lymphoid cells.

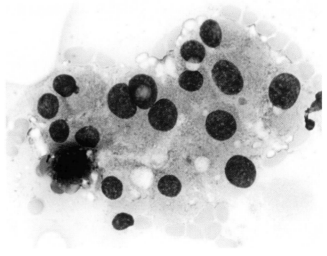

Fig. 6.28 Diagnostic pitfall. Lymphocytic thyroiditis. Oncocytic epithelium may show anisonucleosis and intranuclear clearing mimicking papillary carcinoma. However, lymphocytic thyroiditis may be associated with a coexisting papillary carcinoma. When in doubt, repeat FNA is advised.

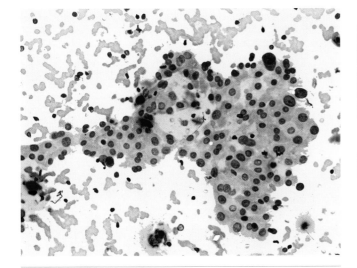

Fig. 6.26 Lymphocytic thyroiditis. Oncocytic epithelium has central round nuclei and dense, well-defined cytoplasm.

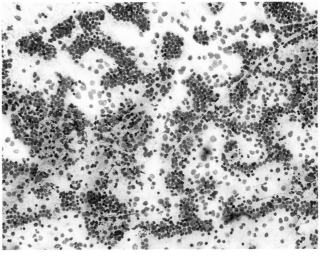

Fig. 6.29 Lymphocytic thyroiditis. Lymphoid cells may dominate and mimic non-Hodgkin lymphoma. Residual follicle centre fragments may be helpful in the differential diagnosis (see Fig. 6.27).

Subacute thyroiditis (de Quervain's) (Figs 6.30–6.34)

- A self-limiting condition of unknown, probably viral, origin
- Patients present with a history of thyroid pain, typically radiating to the ears
- Pain and symptoms subside after a short course of aspirin

Cytological findings

- Numerous multinucleate histiocytes
- Mixed lymphocytes and epithelioid granulomata
- Degenerative changes in follicular cells, cell debris and colloid

Differential diagnosis

- Lymphocytic (Hashimotos's) thyroiditis
- Other systemic granulomatous conditions
- Granulomatous reaction to metastatic tumours

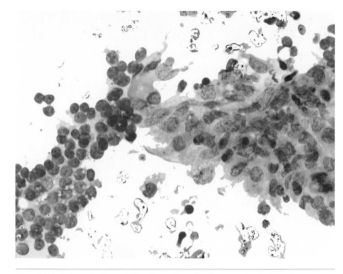

Fig. 6.32 Subacute thyroiditis. Thyroid epithelium on the left and epithelioid cells on the right.

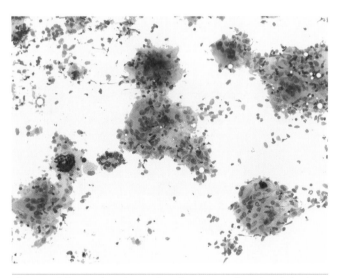

Fig. 6.30 Subacute thyroiditis. Multinucleate giant cells and epithelioid granulomata dominate. Thyroid epithelium is sparse.

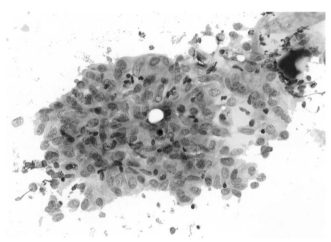

Fig. 6.33 Subacute thyroiditis. Epithelioid granulomata resemble a shoal of fish. Colloid is usually sparse.

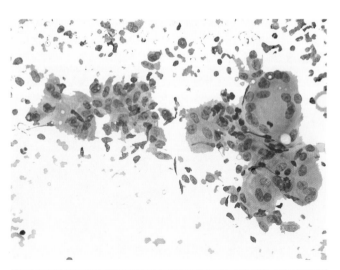

Fig. 6.31 Higher-power view shows giant cells and epithelioid cells found in subacute thyroiditis.

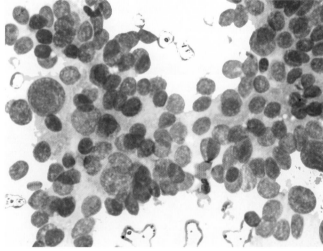

Fig. 6.34 Subacute thyroiditis. Epithelium may show marked anisonucleosis.

Riedel's thyroidtis (Riedel's struma) (Figs 6.35–6.38)

- A rare condition, previously considered as the end stage of thyroiditis
- Currently considered an IgG disease
- Important since clinically and radiologically often mimics anaplastic carcinoma

Cytological findings

- Usually of low cellularity with fragments of fibrous tissue
- Fibroblasts and myofibroblasts
- Occasional lymphocytes, plasma cells and polymorphs
- Absence of necrosis, germinal centre cells, oncocytic cells
- Multinucleate and epithelioid histiocytes

Differential diagnosis

- Anaplastic thyroid carcinoma
- Sarcoma
- Fibromatosis colli
- Fibrosing type of Hashimoto's thyroiditis

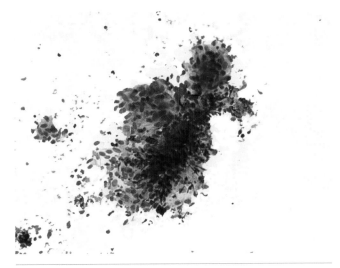

Fig. 6.36 Riedel's thyroiditis. Clusters are often tightly cohesive and hyperchromatic, only the outlying cells showing their spindle shape.

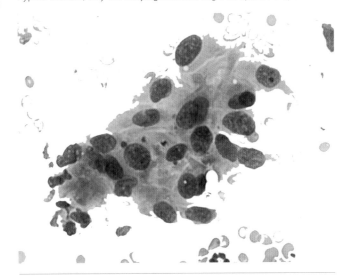

Fig. 6.37 Riedel's thyroiditis. Individual cells have an oval nucleus and relatively plentiful cytoplasm, giving them almost an epithelial appearance. Note metachromatic stroma.

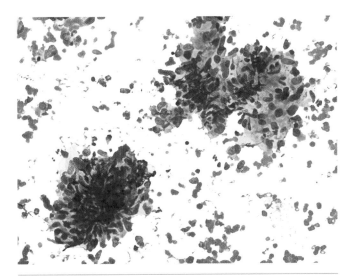

Fig. 6.35 Riedel's thyroiditis. Sparse, tightly cohesive clusters of spindle-shaped cells associated with metachromatic stroma.

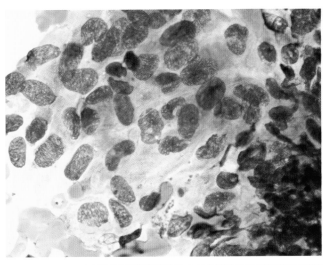

Fig. 6.38 Diagnostic pitfall. This is a case of Riedels' thyroiditis in which some of the cells show overlapping, crowding and irregular chromatin and may be mistaken for anaplastic carcinoma.

Thyroid hyperplasia/hyperthyroidism

- Subtle morphological changes reflect endocrine function of the thyroid
- These changes may be mistaken for neoplasms

Cytological findings (Figs 6.39–6.48)

- Blood-stained aspirates
- Thin, often barely visible colloid
- Moderate cellularity, with low cell:colloid ratio
- Dispersed follicular cells with an enlarged round nucleus and single nucleolus
- Mild anisonucleosis
- Cytoplasmic marginal vacuolation ('fire flares')
- Intracytoplasmic lipofuscin granules

Differential diagnosis

- Differentiation between thyroid hyperplasia and follicular neoplasia may be difficult
- Features favouring hyperplasia are usually a low cell:colloid ratio
- If the sample is both cellular and contains colloid, the presence of flat sheets (not forming microfollicles with central lumina) favours hyperplasia
- Findings need to be correlated with thyroid function tests

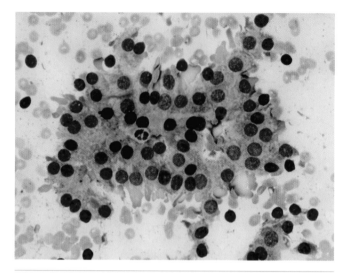

Fig. 6.40 Thyroid hyperplasia. Cytoplasm may show pink soap bubble, colloid suds, flame or 'fire flare' appearances. Although seen more frequently in hyperplasia, these features are non-specific.

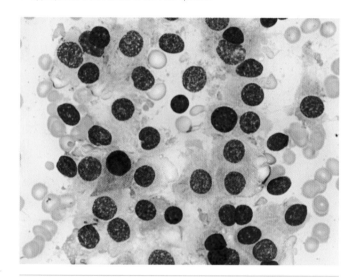

Fig. 6.41 Thyroid hyperplasia. Nuclei are regular and round. Chromatin is finely granular. Nucleoli are usually not prominent.

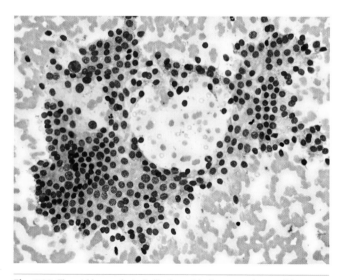

Fig. 6.39 Thyroid hyperplasia. Follicular epithelium may show mild to moderate anisonucleosis.

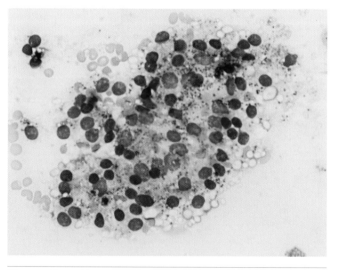

Fig. 6.42 Thyroid hyperplasia. Note cytoplasmic paravacuolar granules and peripheral soap bubbles. Both features are non-specific.

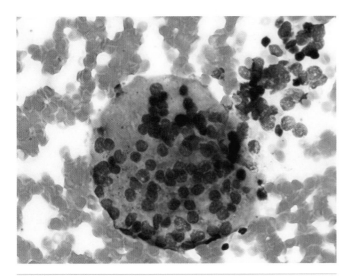

Fig. 6.43 Thyroid hyperplasia. Complete three-dimensional microfollicles can be seen in hyperplastic nodules. This one burst upon being smeared (see Fig. 6.10).

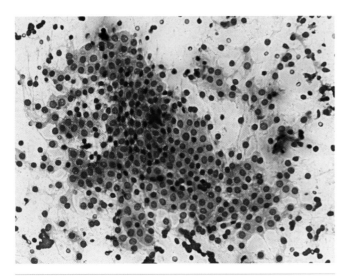

Fig. 6.44 Thyroid hyperplasia. Sheets of follicular cells show regular arrangement and background colloid. Cytoplasm is ill defined.

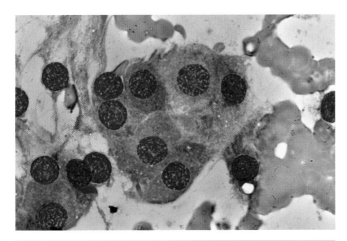

Fig. 6.45 Thyroid hyperplasia. Oncocytic change may be seen in Graves' disease. Papillary carcinoma is not usually associated with Graves' disease but exceptions are possible.

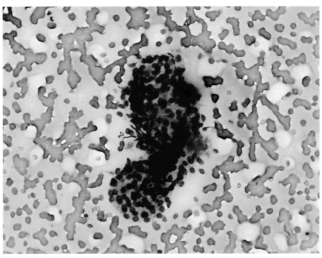

Fig. 6.46 Thyroid hyperplasia. Occasional follicular and papillary structures may be seen. They should be viewed in context of the rest of the sample.

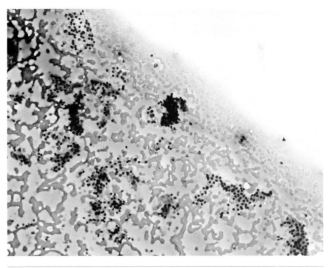

Fig. 6.47 Thyroid hyperplasia. Focally increased cellularity, particularly at the edge of the smear, may be a preparation artefact. Colloid in the background. No follicular arrangement. High cellularity may make distinction from a 'follicular lesion' (see Figs 6.49–6.56).

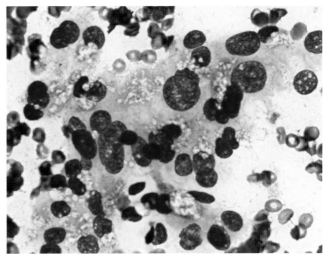

Fig. 6.48 Diagnostic pitfall. Thyroid hyperplasia. The drugs which interfere with thyroid hormone biosynthesis can cause marked nuclear atypia, as can the previous use of ablative radioactive iodine. This can lead to confusion with anaplastic or even papillary carcinoma.

Follicular lesions

'Follicular lesions' is a term which encompasses several pathological entities that have some common morphological characteristics and are often indistinguishable on morphology alone.

Cytological features (Figs 6.49–6.56)

- High cellularity and/or high cell:colloid ratio
- Sparse colloid, usually thick
- Follicular cell arrangement with central colloid
- Bland cell features except in atypical adenoma

Differential diagnosis

- Follicular adenoma
- Follicular carcinoma (follicular adenoma and follicular carcinoma cannot be distinguished on cytomorphology alone)
- Hyperplastic change/thyrotoxicosis
- Follicular variant of papillary carcinoma (FVPC)

The classification and management of follicular lesions is outlined on p. 170, Table 6.2 and p. 171, Fig. 6.103.

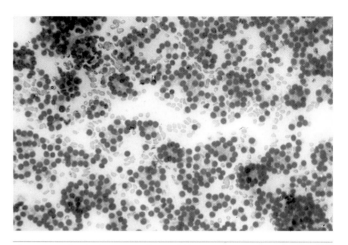

Fig. 6.50 Follicular lesion. FNA from a follicular neoplasm including microfollicular aggregates. FNA diagnosis: follicular lesion. Histology: follicular adenoma.

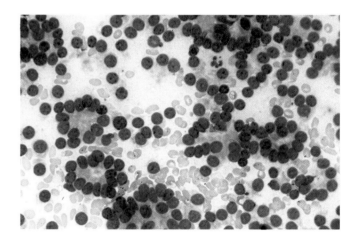

Fig. 6.51 Follicular lesion. High-power view of Fig. 6.50. Note monotonous cell appearance and follicular structures.

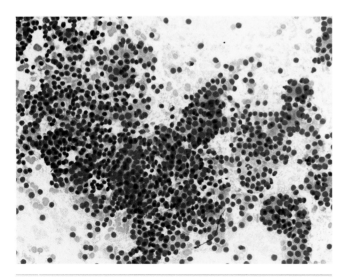

Fig. 6.49 Follicular lesions show increased cellularity and background colloid. Epithelium in flat sheets with follicular arrangement. FNA diagnosis: follicular lesion. Histology: hyperplastic nodule.

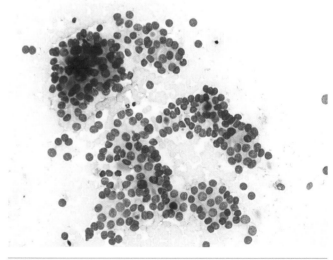

Fig. 6.52 Follicular lesion. Microfollicular aggregates show bland nuclei and ill-defined cytoplasm. Nuclear overlapping is present. FNA diagnosis: follicular lesion. Histology: minimally invasive follicular carcinoma.

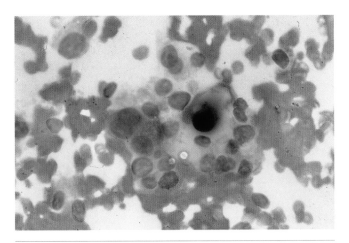

Fig. 6.53 Follicular lesion. Follicular epithelium shows thick colloid centred on the follicles, almost always a sign of a neoplasm. Histology: follicular adenoma.

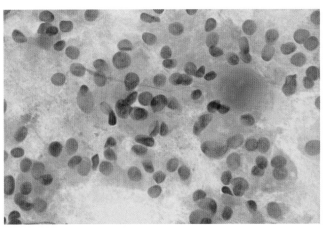

Fig. 6.54 Aspirate from a follicular neoplasm including an inspissated globule of colloid.

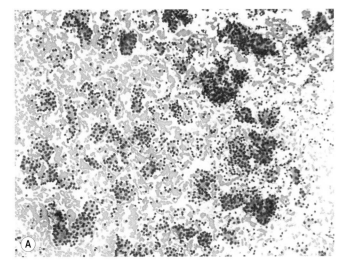

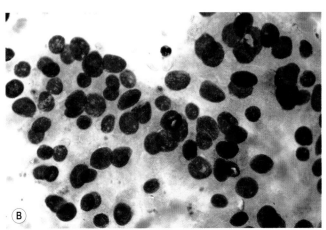

Fig. 6.55 Follicular lesion. (A) Low-power view shows a cellular FNA with numerous follicular aggregates and blood in the background. Scanty colloid centred on the follicles. (B) High-power view shows crowding in cell groups, increased nuclear size, overlapping and crowding. Histology: minimally invasive follicular carcinoma (see p. 160 for follicular neoplasms).

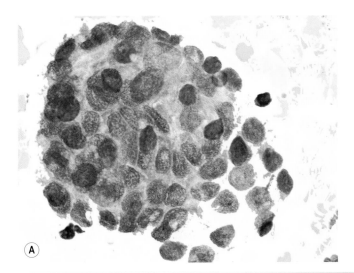

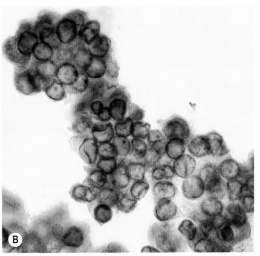

Fig. 6.56 Follicular lesion. Follicular arrangement is sometimes seen together with nuclear features of papillary carcinoma, in particular, intranuclear inclusions (A, MGG) and nuclear grooves (B, PAP). This was a follicular variant of papillary carcinoma, correctly reported as 'follicular lesion'. For further details see pp. 162–165 (papillary carcinoma).

Thyroid neoplasms

Follicular and oncocytic (Hürthle cell) neoplasms

Primary neoplasms*

- Benign
  - Adenoma
  - Atypical adenoma
- Malignant
  - Angioinvasive follicular carcinoma
  - Follicular carcinoma
  - Papillary carcinoma
  - Mixed follicular and medullary carcinoma
  - Medullary carcinoma
  - Anaplastic carcinoma
  - Lymphoma
  - Sarcomas

Secondary neoplasms

Follicular adenoma and carcinoma often cannot be fully characterised and distinguished from other 'follicular lesions' (see previous page) on FNA. However, it is often possible to give a probable diagnosis of a neoplasm. This is helpful for further management (see p. 170, Table 6.2 and p. 171, Fig. 6.103).

Oncocytic (Hürthle cell) neoplasms, cannot be defined on FNA alone as benign and malignant. According to US Bethesda classification, they are considered a separate diagnostic category (class IV). UK terminology considers them part of 'follicular lesions' and are managed accordingly (see p. 170, Table 6.2).

Cytological findings (Figs 6.57–6.65)

- Follicular neoplasms (see p. 170, Table 6.2 and p. 171, Fig. 6.103)
- High cellularity and/or high cell:colloid ratio
- Sparse colloid, usually thick
- Follicular cell arrangement with central colloid
- Bland cell features except in atypical adenoma (see p. 158–159)
- Oncocytic (Hürthle cell) neoplasms: abundance of oncocytic cells, in aggregates and singly
  - abundant dense well-defined cytoplasm
  - prominent nuceloli
- Little or no colloid

*World Health Organization Classification of Tumours. Pathology and Genetics of Tumours of Endocrine Organs, IARC Press, Lyon, 2004, 49–134.

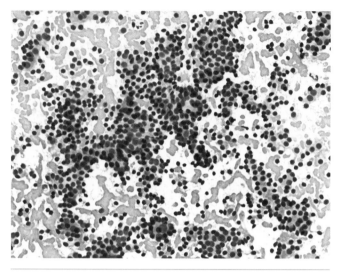

Fig. 6.57 Follicular lesion. Cellular aspirate with little or no colloid in the background is suggestive of a neoplasm. Cytomorphology alone cannot distinguish between follicular adenoma and follicular carcinoma.

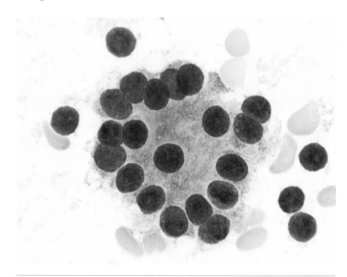

Fig. 6.58 Follicular arrangement with round, relatively evenly sized nuclei, bland chromatin pattern and ill-defined cytoplasm. Histology: follicular adenoma.

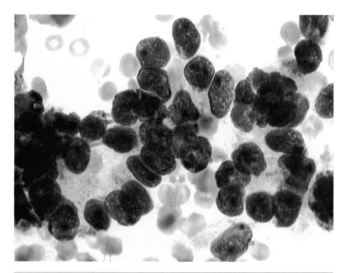

Fig. 6.59 Follicular adenoma may exhibit a marked cytological atypia, as well as overlapping and crowding. This case was diagnosed cytologically as follicular carcinoma. Histology: follicular adenoma.

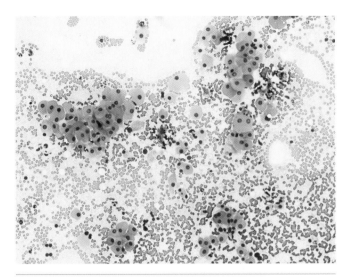

Fig. 6.60 Oncocytic tumour shows large polygonal or oval cells with a well-defined grey-blue dense cytoplasm. Histology: oncocytic adenoma.

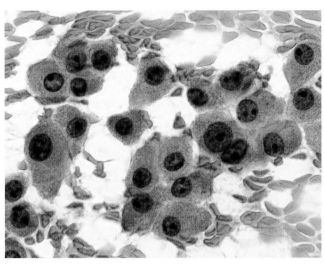

Fig. 6.63 The characteristic nuclear enlargement and pleomorphism of oncocytic cells is seen with prominent nucleoli. Binucleation is common. Intranuclear inclusions may be present though Hürthle cell tumours with nuclear features of papillary carcinoma may actually be oncocytic.

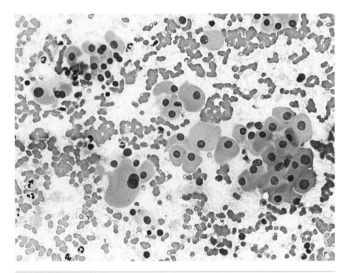

Fig. 6.61 Low-power view of oncocytic tumour showing aggregates of oncocytic cells. Histology: oncocytic adenoma.

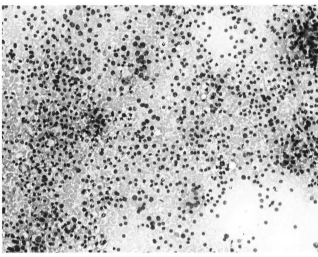

Fig. 6.64 Cellular sample composed of dispersed oncocytic cells reported on FNA as oncocytic tumour. Histology: oncocytic carcinoma.

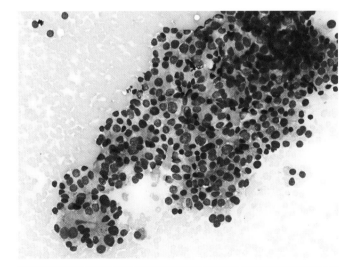

Fig. 6.62 Follicular lesion. FNA shows follicular aggregates with some anisonucleosis. Colloid centred on the follicles. FNA diagnosis: follicular lesion. Histological diagnosis: follicular carcinoma.

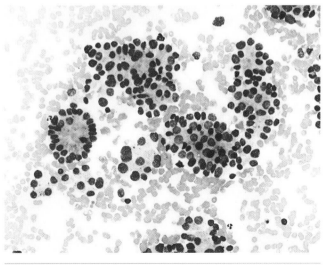

Fig. 6.65 Follicular lesion diagnosed on cytology was excised. Histology: follicular carcinoma. Note bland nuclear features. Mild anisonucleosis.

Papillary carcinoma

- The most common malignancy of the thyroid
- Constitutes 70% of the clinically apparent carcinomas
- Female predominance of approximately 3:1
- Most commonly found in the 30–50 age range
- Exposure to irradiation during childhood, either therapeutically or due to radioactive fall-out, is a risk factor

Cytological findings (Figs 6.66–6.74)

- Cellular aspirate with little colloid usually, but can contain abundant colloid
- Papillary fronds and sheets of cells
- Dense blue-grey cytoplasm with well-defined cell boundaries
- Intranuclear inclusions
- Nuclear grooves
- Psammoma bodies
- Multinucleate histiocytes, particularly where there is cystic degeneration
- 'Chewing-gum' colloid

Differential diagnosis

In practice, the papillary architecture, nuclear inclusions, abundant nuclear grooves, the quality and definition of the cytoplasm are found to be of most use in diagnosis.

Intranuclear inclusions and nuclear grooves can be seen in other lesions including:
- Multinodular goitre
- Hashimoto's thyroiditis
- Hyalinising trabecular adenoma
- Hürthle cell tumours
- Follicular tumours
- Insular carcinoma
- Medullary carcinoma

Psammoma bodies are a very valuable finding but are seen rarely. They can also be seen in:
- Thyroid hyperplasia
- Multinodular goitre
- Hashimoto's thyroiditis
- Hyalinising trabecular adenoma
- Can be confused with inspissated colloid

Papillae are valuable but may be absent if a predominantly follicular area of the tumour is sampled and can also occur in:
- Thyroid hyperplasia
- Multinodular goitre

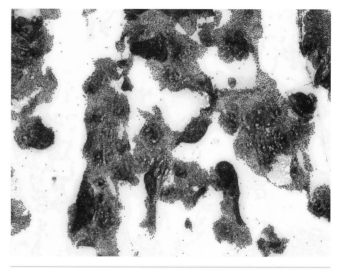

Fig. 6.66 Papillary carcinoma. Low-power view of FNA sample from a papillary carcinoma shows high cellularity and papillary arrangement.

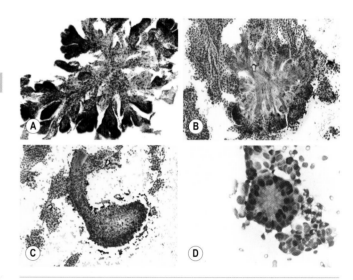

Fig. 6.67 Papillary carcinoma. (A) Low-power view of FNA of papillary carcinoma in PAP stain showing numerous well-defined papillae with central vascular cores. (B, C, D) MGG stain shows papillary fragments with well-defined borders.

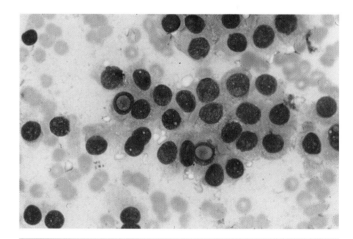

Fig. 6.68 Papillary carcinoma. Intranuclear inclusions are cytoplasmic invaginations in the nucleus. They have sharp borders and cytoplasmic staining.

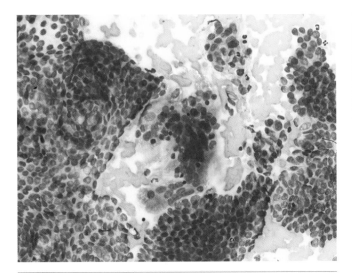

Fig. 6.69 Papillary carcinoma. Well-defined border of papillary clusters. Multinuclear giant cells are a frequent finding.

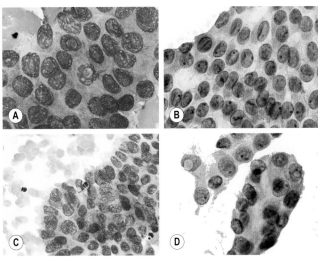

Fig. 6.72 Papillary carcinoma. Intranuclear inclusions and grooves as shown in MGG (A and C) and PAP stains (B and D) are characteristic of papillary carcinoma.

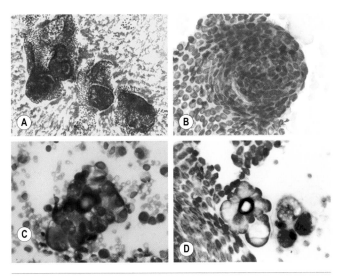

Fig. 6.70 Papillary carcinoma. (A, B) Cell whorls. (C) Psammoma bodies in the centre of the papillae. (D) Psammoma body refracts light.

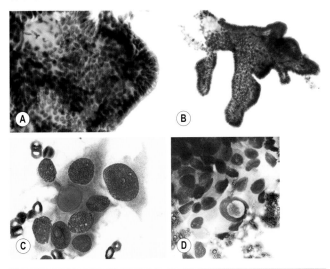

Fig. 6.73 Papillary carcinoma. The combination of papillary structures (A and B), psammoma bodies (C) and intranuclear inclusions (D) is diagnostic of papillary carcinoma.

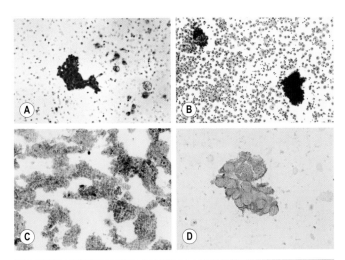

Fig. 6.71 Papillary carcinoma. (A, B) Presence of colloid is variable in papillary carcinoma. Occasionally, much colloid and only a minor epithelial component is seen, such as in the cystic neck metastases of papillary carcinoma. (C) CK19 positive. (D) Thyroglobulin positive.

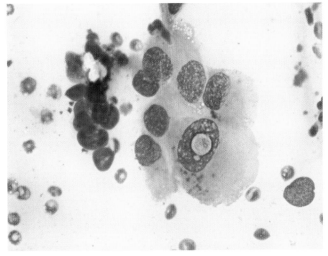

Fig. 6.74 Diagnostic pitfall. Intranuclear inclusions can be seen in other conditions including multinodular goitre, as shown here.

Papillary carcinoma: special types

- Follicular variant of papillary carcinoma
- Diffuse sclerosing
- Tall cell
- Columnar cell
- Oncocytic (Hürthle cell)
- Clear cell
- Warthin-like tumour
- Papillary carcinoma with a nodular fasciitis-like stroma

Cytological findings (Figs 6.75–6.83)

- **Follicular variant**: cell arrangement predominantly follicular with nuclear features of classic type
- **Columnar cell variant**: elongated cells with hyperchromatic and ovoid nuclei in the absence of intranuclear inclusions and nuclear grooves
- **Tall cell variant**: elongated cells with dense cytoplasm and typical nuclear features of papillary carcinoma
- **Diffuse sclerosing variant**: chronic inflammatory element, abundant psammoma bodies and squamous metaplasia
- **Warthin-like** papillary carcinoma: prominent lymphoid cell component
- **Papillary carcinoma with NF-like stroma**: stromal cells have had myofibroblastic features
- **Cribriform-morular variant**: contains numerous hyaline globules and mimics adenoid cystic carcinoma

Differential diagnosis

- **Follicular arrangement**: follicular variant of papillary carcinoma (FVPC) poses most diagnostic difficulties and is often reported as 'suggestive' of papillary carcinoma or as a 'follicular lesion'. Nuclear grooves and intranuclear inclusions are helpful for diagnosis (see p. 171, Fig. 6.103)
- **Lymphoid infiltrate** may be seen in papillary carcinoma as part of pre-existing Hashimoto's but also in Warthin's-type PC and diffuse sclerosing variant
- **Psammoma bodies** and hyaline globules are seen in hyalinising trabecular adenoma, diffuse sclerosing and cribriform morular variants

A diagnosis of papillary carcinoma subtype is often not possible on cytology but the awareness of various types is necessary to avoid pitfalls.

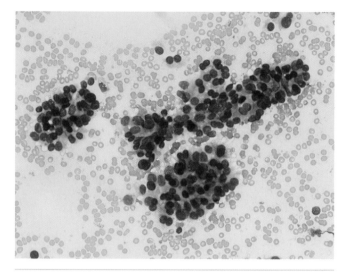

Fig. 6.75 Follicular variant of papillary carcinoma. Confluent follicular structures in a cellular sample indicate follicular lesion (see pp. 158 and 159).

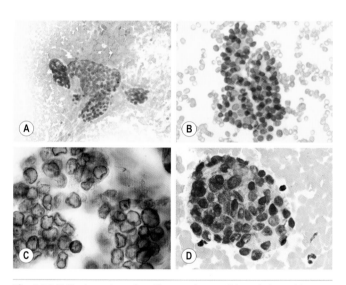

Fig. 6.76 Follicular variant of papillary carcinoma. Although the architecture is follicular, cell details including grooves and intranuclear inclusions are diagnostic of papillary carcinoma.

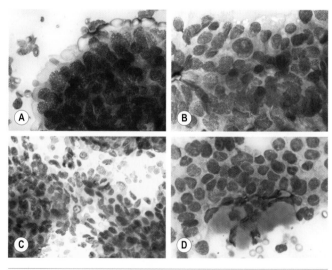

Fig. 6.77 Tall cell variant of papillary carcinoma. Apart from elongated cells, appearances are those of classic papillary carcinoma.

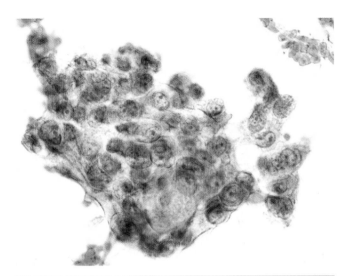

Fig. 6.78 Diagnostic pitfall. Hyalinising trabecular adenoma can be a diagnostic pitfall since it can have intranuclear inclusions.

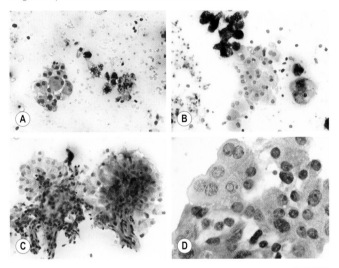

Fig. 6.79 Diagnositc pitfall. (A–D) Predominantly cystic papillary carcinoma, such as in this case, may be mistaken for a colloid cyst. Note abundant colloid, papillary vascular cores and well-defined cytoplasm of epithelial cells. Intranuclear inclusions may be rare or absent.

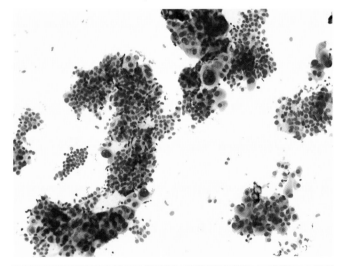

Fig. 6.80 Oncocytic variant of papillary carcinoma should not be mistaken for lymphocytic thyroiditis with focal oncocytic change..

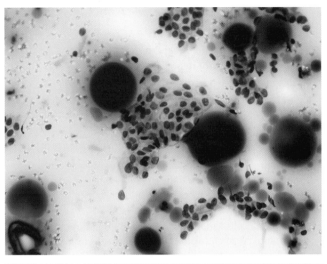

Fig. 6.81 Diagnostic pitfall. Globules of colloid may be seen in nodular goitre, hyalinising trabecular adenoma as well as in diffuse sclerosing variant and cribriform morular variant of papillary carcinoma (see Fig. 6.82).

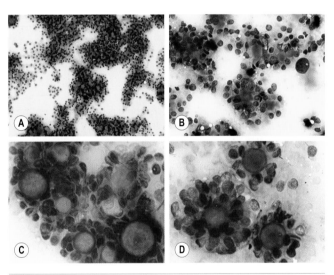

Fig. 6.82 Cribriform morular variant of papillary carcinoma. (A–D) Note hyaline globules reminiscent of adenoid cystic carcinoma (laminin positive) and intranuclear inclusions.

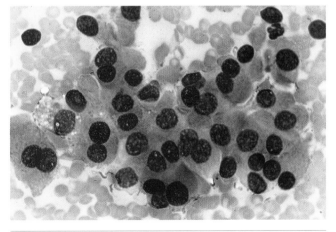

Fig. 6.83 Diagnostic pitfall. Oncocytic variant of papillary carcinoma may be mistaken for oncocytic adenoma. All oncocytic lesions should be reported according to the current guidelines (see p. 170, Table 6.2 and p. 171, Fig. 6.103) and discussed at the MDT meetings.

Medullary carcinoma

- Parafollicular cell differentiation
- Constitutes 5–10% of thyroid carcinomas
- Most commonly sporadic
- Part of multiple endocrine neoplasia syndromes (MEN)
- Amyloid deposition occurring in 80%
- Cells contain neurosecretory granules
- Immunocytochemically, 80% stain positively for calcitonin
- A rare group of tumours, which show features of both medullary and follicular differentiation with immunocytochemical positivity for both calcitonin and thyroglobulin
- Carcinoma cells variable, usually polyhedral but may show spindling, be small ovoid carcinoid-like cells or may mimic small cell carcinoma
- Giant cell, clear cell, melanotic, mucinous and oncocytic forms rarely

Cytological findings (Figs 6.84–6.93)

- Dispersed cellular aspirate
- Variable cell size and shape
- Cytoplasmic granularity
- Amyloid
- Calcitonin positivity

It is of essence that a medullary carcinoma is not missed on the initial FNA examination and is diagnosed correctly prior to any surgery. Once diagnosed, it attracts a different management protocol from the conventional carcinomas. Given that it is relatively rare and morphologically variable, it should be considered in the differential diagnosis of all 'unusual' appearances of the FNA samples. Both serum and FNA calcitonin should be performed (see Fig. 6.93).

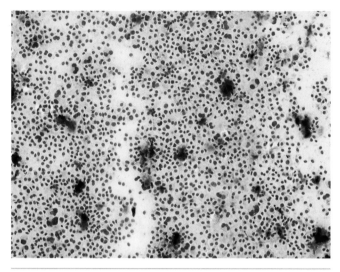

Fig. 6.85 Medullary carcinoma. Dispersed cell pattern showing cells of variable shape and size.

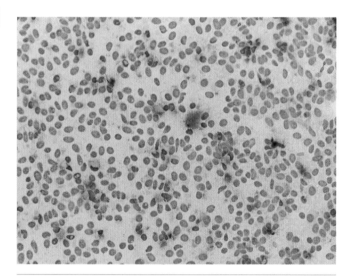

Fig. 6.86 Diagnostic pitfall. Medullary carcinoma. Amyloid deposits amidst monotonous cells may be mistaken for colloid.

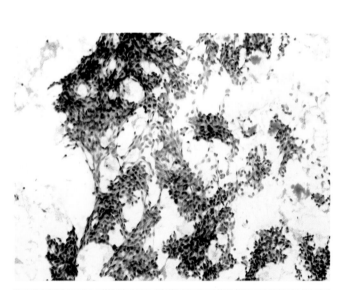

Fig. 6.84 Medullary carcinoma. PAP stain shows a cellular sample composed of monotonous small cells in clusters and single.

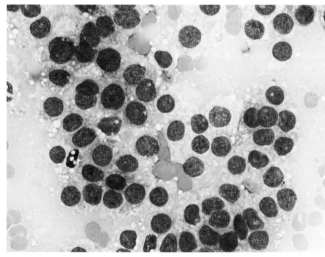

Fig. 6.87 Medullary carcinoma. Neck metastasis shows monotonous round cells with finely vacuolated cytoplasm.

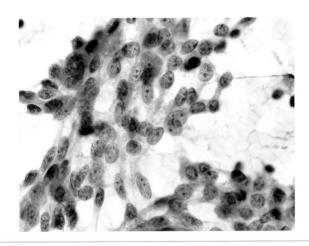

Fig. 6.88 Medullary carcinoma. PAP stain shows mainly single cells with eccentric nuclei.

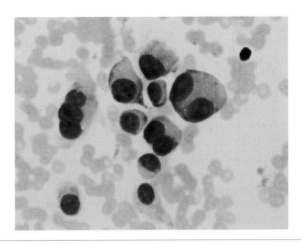

Fig. 6.91 Medullary carcinoma. Eccentric nuclei and plasmacytoid appearance are seen in some cases.

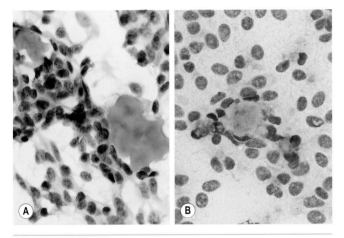

Fig. 6.89 Medullary carcinoma. Different cases showing amyloid in both alcohol fixed (A) and air-dried preparations (B). Note spindle cell pattern in the PAP stain (A).

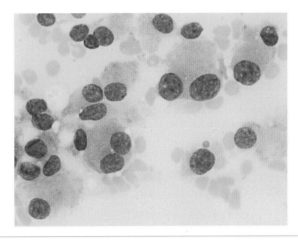

Fig. 6.92 Medullary carcinoma. Binucleation and multinucleation in the cells with eccentric nuclei. Nucleoli may be prominent.

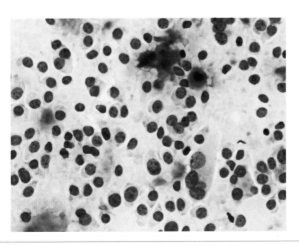

Fig. 6.90 Medullary carcinoma. Amyloid may be well defined or randomly distributed within the sample.

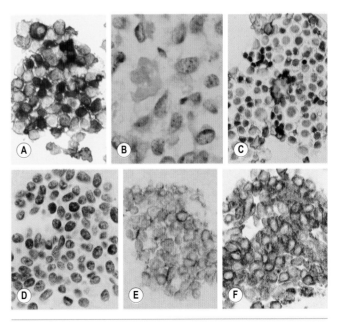

Fig. 6.93 Immunocytochemistry of medullary carcinoma: (A) calcitonin (positive), (B) Congo red (positive), (C) thyroglobin (negative), (D) TTF1 (positive), (E) CD56 (positive), (F) AE1/3 (positive).

Anaplastic carcinoma

- A highly aggressive tumour
- Presenting as a rapidly advancing hard mass in the thyroid
- Often hoarseness, stridor and dysphagia
- Most cases inoperable at presentation
- Radiotherapy and chemotherapy are generally ineffective
- Survival limited to a few months
- FNA confirms malignancy without the need for needle core biopsy or surgery – this enables appropriate management
- FNA allows the distinction from treatable thyroid lymphomas, which may present in an identical fashion to anaplastic carcinoma

Cytological findings (Figs 6.94–6.96)

- Elderly patients with a rapidly advancing hard mass in the neck
- Bizarre giant, squamoid or spindle cells with clear features of malignancy
- Necrosis may be present

Differential diagnosis

- Immunocytochemistry is often useful to distinguish between anaplastic carcinoma, lymphoma and metastatic carcinoma (Table 6.1)
- Morphologically: metastatic carcinoma (Figs 6.97–6.99)
- Clinically: other thyroid tumours including lymphoma (Figs 6.100–6.102)

Table 6.1 Anaplastic carcinoma of the thyroid (undifferentiated carcinoma)

Immunocytochemistry	
Cytokeratin	50%
EMA	33–55%
Vimentin	50–100%
Thyroglobulin	Almost always negative (0/4[2])
CEA	Squamous component may be positive

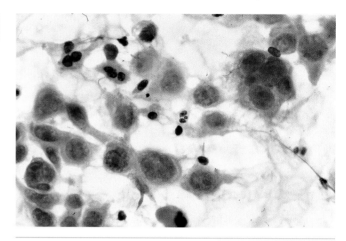

Fig. 6.94 Anaplastic carcinoma. Spindle-shaped malignant cells with central nuclei, coarse chromatin pattern and prominent nucleoli.

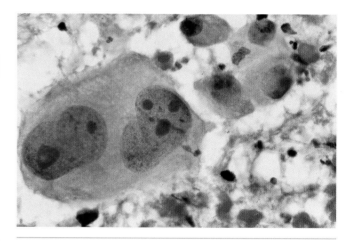

Fig. 6.95 Anaplastic carcinoma. Same case as Fig. 6.94. Malignant cells may show squamous metaplasia.

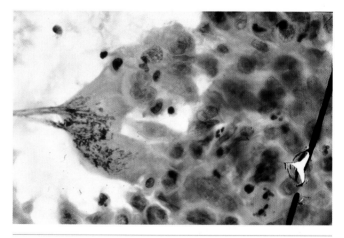

Fig. 6.96 Anaplastic carcinoma. Mitotic figures are common. Overlapping, crowding, coarse chromatin and prominent multiple nucleoli.

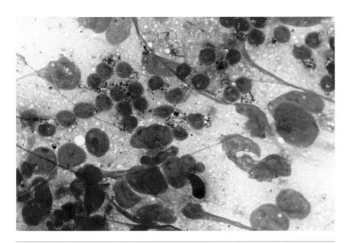

Fig. 6.97 Metastatic carcinoma thyroid. Thyroid epithelium with cytoplasmic granules is infiltrated by large bizarrely shaped cells.

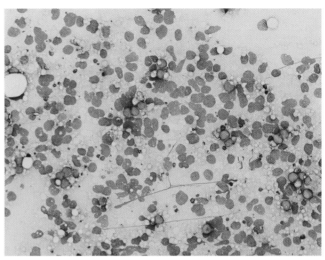

Fig. 6.100 Non-Hodgkin lymphoma, high grade. Dissociated large blastic lymphoid cells usually with the typical background of pale-blue fragments of cytoplasm. Immunostaining for leucocyte common antigen and the absence of cytokeratin staining is usual for confirmation.

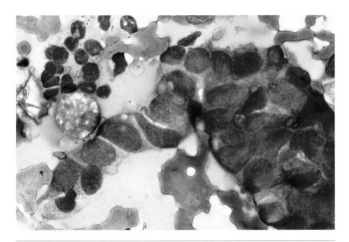

Fig. 6.98 Metastatic carcinoma thyroid. Thyroid epithelium (*top left*) is uniform, round and regular. Malignant cells are large, overlapping, crowding. Primary carcinoma was in the breast.

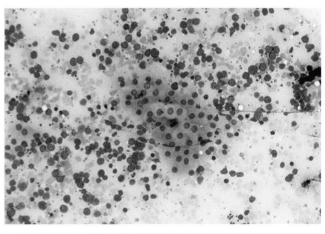

Fig. 6.101 The low-grade lymphomas are more difficult to diagnose, particularly if the aspirates also harvest cells from the surrounding autoimmune thyroiditis. A mixed cell population of reactive and neoplastic lymphoid cells, together with oncocytic cells, may be seen.

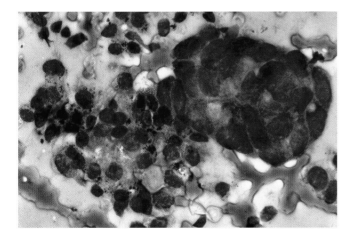

Fig. 6.99 Metastatic carcinoma. Thyroid epithelium is well preserved and in close proximity to metastatic malignant cells. FNAs from primary thyroid tumours usually do not contain normal thyroid epithelium.

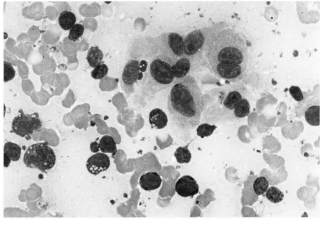

Fig. 6.102 Non-Hodgkin lymphoma. An infiltrate of lymphoid blasts from a high-grade non-Hodgkin lymphoma and residual isolated oncocytic (Hürthle) cells. More commonly, lymphoma infiltrates the whole gland with no residual thyroid epithelium (see Fig. 6.100).

FNA thyroid reporting categories and their management implications

Currently, the most widely used reporting systems are the Bethesda System for Reporting of Thyroid Cytology (TBSRTC) and the five-tier UK Royal College of Pathologists (UK RCPath) thyroid FNA classification (Table 6.2).

To ensure effective use of thyroid cytology, pathologists should agree with local surgeons, endocrinologists, radiologists and oncologists on the use of any particular terminology, and ideally meet regularly on the clinical site to discuss individual cases. The various terminologies share a common goal: clarity of clinical management by predicting the probable outcome, in particular the risk of malignancy (see Table 6.3).

Whilst the TBSRTC is more prescriptive in its management recommendations associated with particular categories, the UK RCPath terminology recommends that all atypical, suspicious and malignant cases be discussed at the multidisciplinary meetings prior to definitive management (Table 6.3).

Table 6.2 Comparison table of the UK Royal College of Pathologists' Thyroid FNA reporting Classification and The Bethesda System for Reporting Thyroid Cytopathology

RCPath*	Bethesda system for reporting Thyroid Cytopathology**	
Non-diagnostic for cytological diagnosis (Thy1)	I.	Non-diagnostic or unsatisfactory Virtually acellular specimen Other (obscuring blood, clotting artifact, etc.)
Non-diagnostic for cytological diagnosis – cystic lesion (Thy1c)		Cyst fluid only
Non-neoplastic (Thy2)	II.	Benign Consistent with a benign follicular nodule (includes adenomatoid nodule, colloid nodule, etc.) Consistent with lymphocytic (Hashimoto's) thyroiditis in the proper clinical context Consistent with granulomatous (subacute) thyroiditis Other
Non-neoplastic – cystic lesion (Thy2c) Neoplasm possible – atypia/non-diagnostic (Thy3a)	III.	Atypia of undetermined significance or follicular lesion of undetermined significance
Neoplasm possible, suggesting follicular neoplasm (Thy3f)	IV.	Follicular neoplasm or suspicious for a follicular neoplasm Specify if Hürthle cell (oncocytic) type
Suspicious of malignancy (Thy4)	V.	Suspicious for malignancy Suspicious for papillary carcinoma Suspicious for medullary carcinoma Suspicious for metastatic carcinoma Suspicious for lymphoma Other
Malignant (Thy5)	VI.	Malignant Papillary thyroid carcinoma Medullary thyroid carcinoma Undifferentiated (anaplastic) carcinoma Squamous cell carcinoma Carcinoma with mixed features (specify) Metastatic carcinoma Non-Hodgkin lymphoma Other

Helpful websites: *http://www.rcpath.org/Resources/RCPath/Migrated%20Resources/Documents/G/g089guidanceonthereportingofthyroidcytologyfinal.pdf.
**http://www.papsociety.org./atlas.html.

Table 6.3 The Bethesda system for reporting thyroid cytopathology with RCPath equivalents and the implied risk of malignancy (positive predictive value)

Diagnostic category	Risk of malignancy (%)
Non-diagnostic or unsatisfactory/Thy1/Thy1c	0–10
Benign/Thy2/Thy2c	0–3
Atypia of undetermined significance or follicular lesion of undetermined significance/Thy3a	5–15
Follicular neoplasm or suspicious for a follicular neoplasm/Thy3f	15–30
Suspicious for malignancy/Thy4	60–75
Malignant/Thy5	97–99

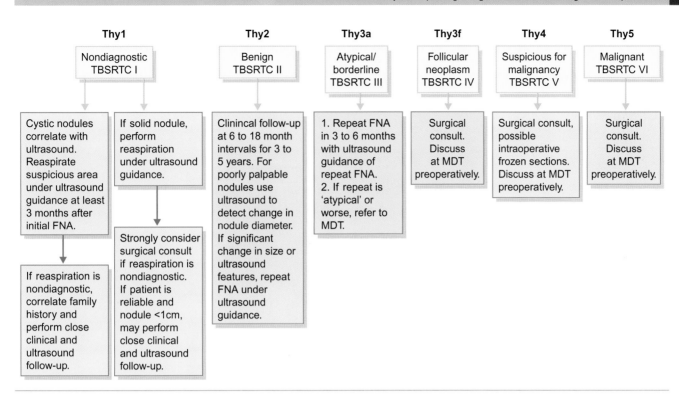

Fig. 6.103 Clinical management implications following from the six main categories of thyroid cytology reporting as described by The Bethesda System for Reporting Thyroid Cytology and compared with the UK Royal College of Pathologists' terminology. Adapted from Kocjan G., Chandra A., Cross P. A., et al. The interobserver reproducibility of thyroid fine-needle aspiration using the UK Royal College of Pathologists' classification system. Am J Clin Pathol 2011;135: 852–859.

CHAPTER 7

Haemopoietic

Contents

Introduction   173

Normal lymph node   176

Reactive lymphadenopathy   178

Neoplastic lesions of lymph node   182

Myeloid neoplasms   209

Myelodysplastic/myeloproliferative neoplasms (MDS/MPN)   217

Introduction

Enlarged lymph node (LN) is a perfect model for the patient, the clinician/primary practitioner and the cytologist to see how a sample obtained by cytological fine-needle aspiration (FNA) can serve to differentiate a non-malignant from a malignant process with certainty, using both cytomorphology and adjuvant technologies. Besides blood cell count (red blood cells, leukocytes and platelets), a haematologic patient's condition is monitored by morphological analysis of peripheral blood (PB) smear, i.e. differential blood count. The next step in the diagnosis of haematologic conditions and diseases is bone marrow (BM) analysis. When performed by an experienced professional, the procedure is very simple, easily done in an outpatient setting, and the patient can immediately resume his/her daily activities.

Fine needle aspiration of the lymph node

- All lymph nodes are accessible to FNA
- FNA in superficial, palpable LN is performed as an outpatient procedure, without anaesthesia, by means of thin needles (0.5–0.7 mm in diameter, 25 or 22 gauge)
- FNA of deep-seated lymph nodes (abdominal or mediastinal) with ultrasound (US), computerised tomography (CT), magnetic resonance (MR), or endoscopic instruments guidance, requires one-day hospitalisation (intrathoracic and retroperitoneal nodes in particular)
- In cases of enlarged mesentheric nodes or nodes located more superficially in the abdomen, FNA can be performed as a day procedure where the patient stays for several hours afterwards for observation
- FNA procedures are done under US, CT or MR guidance, mostly also without local or general anaesthesia, with the use of longer and very thin, CHIBA needles (0.7 mm in diameter, 22 gauge)
- Fine needle aspiration of superficial lymph nodes (Fig. 7.1) should preferably be performed with a 23-gauge (0.6 mm) needle
- The smear should be thin to ensure instant fixation, which will allow an optimal evaluation of cytological detail
- Thin smears should be prepared without using too much pressure
- Lymphoid cells are fragile and readily lose their cytoplasm
- Fragmented cytoplasm will appear as small pale grey structures with Romanowsky stains, and these are often called 'lymphoglandular bodies'
- Whenever possible, both air-dried and alcohol-fixed smears should be prepared for May–Grünwald–Giemsa (MGG) and Papanicolaou (PAP) staining
- If mycobacterial or fungal infections are suspected, extra material should be sent for PCR and/bacteriology

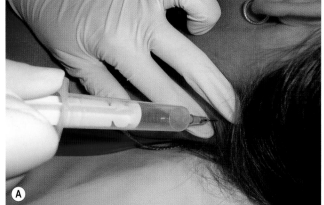

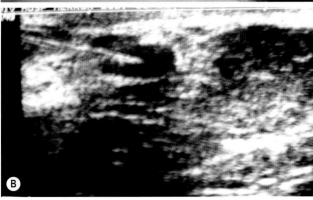

Fig. 7.1 (A) A palpation-guided fine needle aspiration of superficial lymph node. (B) Ultrasound-guided fine needle aspiration of deep-seated lymph node.

Bone marrow aspiration

- FNA is performed in the region of the sternum, spina cristae anterior or posterior or in the tibial area (in children)
- The aspiration of marrow is painful but it only takes a moment
- Complications are extremely rare:
  - haemorrhage at the puncture site may occur in case of inappropriate compression or in the case of haemorrhagic disorder
  - infection due to non-sterile manipulation or premature removal of sterile needle cover
  - rare complications are fractures (sternum in particular) in cases of extensive osteolytic lesions due to metastatic bone lesions or multiple myeloma
- The person performing FNA should be familiar with the indication and should have the clinical history available

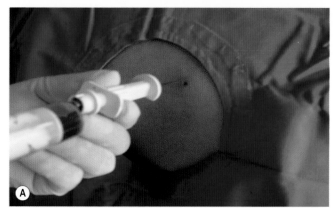

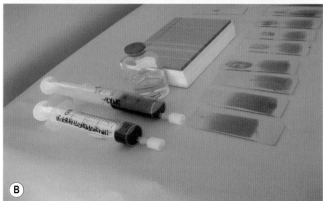

Fig. 7.2 (A) Bone marrow aspiration. (B) Smears of bone marrow on the slides, samples of bone marrow in syringes for ancillary analyses and tiny sample (core) of bone marrow in bottle.

The role of FNA in management of lymphadenopathy

The majority of enlarged lymph nodes need not be excised and can be diagnosed by morphology and various ancillary techniques. In cases of reactive lymphadenopathy, excision is necessary only if the lymphadenopathy persists long term without a known cause and microbiology tests are negative. Flow cytometry and polymerase chain reaction (PCR) for assessment of clonality, may be useful. In cases of metastatic carcinoma, there is no need for excision; special immunocytochemistry markers such as oestrogen receptor (ER), progesterone receptor (PR), thyroglobulin (Tg), thyroid transcription factor 1 (TTF1) and prostate specific antigen (PSA), may narrow the search or specifically indicate the site of the primary tumour. In cases of lymphoma, FNA cytology can give a diagnosis and classify the lymphoma with the help of PCR, cytogenetics, immunocytochemistry and flow cytometry. In some centres, primary diagnosis of lymphoma will require a histological diagnosis. A recurrence of a known lymphoma may be diagnosed on FNA alone, thus avoiding excision biopsy. The following algorithm shows a cascade of the diagnostic role of FNA in the management of patients with lymphadenopathy.

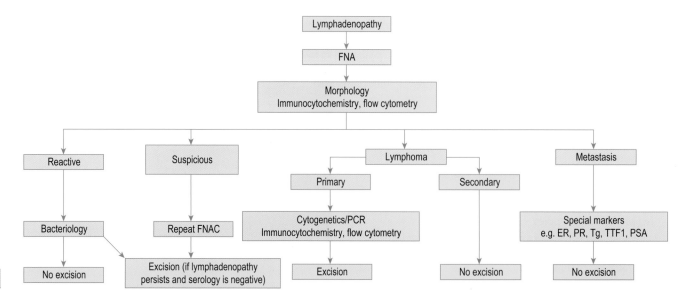

Ancillary technologies and the tumour bank

- The following ancillary techniques may be helpful in diagnosing LN and BM conditions:
  - flow cytometry and immunocytochemistry
  - polymerase chain reaction (PCR)
  - conventional cytogenetics and/or fluorescent in situ hybridisation (FISH)
  - kinetic methods (Ki 67, DNA cytometry etc.)
  - tumour bank

Cytospin preparations

- After using parts of the aspirates for smear making, the remainder should be suspended in a buffered balanced salt (BBS) solution at pH 7.4 for cytospin preparations
- The number of suspended cells should be calculated and the concentration adjusted to $1–2 \times 10^6$ cells/mL
- Cell-rich suspensions can be diluted to optimal concentration by adding BBS solution
- If the cell concentration is low, the cells can be concentrated by centrifugation at 700 rpm for 3–5 min. The resulting pellet is then gently resuspended in a reduced volume of BBS solution
- To prepare the cytospin slides, the cell suspension is spun in a cytocentrifuge at 700 rpm for 3 min
- Each cytospin should contain $1–2 \times 10^5$ nucleated cells
- One of the cytospins should always be stained with MGG and compared with the smears
- If the suspension contains a rich admixture of red blood cells, it is possible to purify the lymphoid cells by density gradient centrifugation

Flow cytometry

- Aspirated cells can also be immunologically characterised by flow cytometry (FC)
- One part of the aspirate should be used for smear making
- The second part should be suspended in BBS solution at pH 7.4
- A cell concentration of approximately 1 million cells per mL buffer will be sufficient for a complete characterisation of reactive lesions as well as most B- and T-cell lymphomas
- At the moment, four-colour FC is standard procedure in immunophenotyping of lymphomas

Important: Results of FC need to be correlated to cytomorphology on routinely stained smears.

- A close cooperation between the FC laboratory and the cytopathologist is strongly recommended

Molecular techniques

- Aspirated cells also perform well in PCR rearrangement analysis (see Ch. 13)
- Aspirated cells suspended in BBS at pH 7.4 should be pelleted immediately, snap frozen and stored at −70°C until used for rearrangement analysis
- Cytospin preparations can also be used for FISH analysis of specific translocations to aid subtyping of reactive lymph node conditions

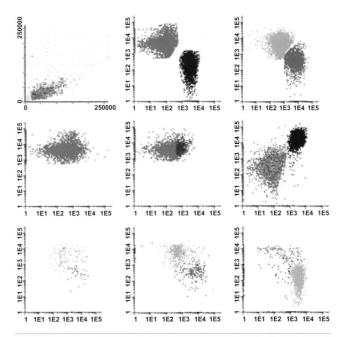

Colour flow cytometry analysis of fine needle aspirate from a lymph node with reactive follicular hyperplasia. Upper row: Left: forward scatter/side scatter plot shows that most cells were in the lymphocyte area. Dead cells (*yellow*) are excluded from analysis. Middle: CD19 versus CD3 plot shows 47% B cells (*red*) and 43% T cells (*blue*). Right: Kappa (*orange*)/lambda (*green*) analysis in CD19/SSC gated B cells shows normal kappa/lambda ratio 1.3. Middle row: Left: CD19 versus CD5 plot within CD19/SSC gate shows a small population of CD5 − B cells that correspond to mantle zone B cells (5% of B cells). Middle: CD19 versus CD10 plot within CD19/SSC gate shows a somewhat larger population of CD10 − B cells that correspond to germinal centre cells (20% of B cells). Right: CD3 versus CD5 plot shows that most T cells were positive for both markers (*blue*). Lower row: Left: Kappa/lambda analysis of CD5 − B cells shows normal kappa/lambda ratio (1.2). Middle: Kappa/lambda analysis of CD10 − B cells shows normal kappa/lambda ratio (1.5). Right: CD4 and CD8 expression in CD3-gated T-cell population. CD4/CD8 ratio was increased to 8.5 (Courtesy Professor A. Porwit, Hematopathology Division, Department of Pathology and Cytology, Karolinska University Hospital Solna, Stockholm, Sweden).[†]

Normal lymph node

Normal lymph node contains a variety of cells which can be present in various ratios depending on the antigenic stimulus causing lymphadenopathy.

Cytological findings (Fig. 7.3)

- Mature lymphocytes
  - of either B or T phenotype, measure around 8 μ
  - dense nucleus with coarse chromatin
  - pale-blue rim of cytoplasm
- Plasma cells
  - eccentrically placed nucleus
  - chromatin arranged in a cartwheel-like pattern
  - abundant cytoplasm often shows a less intense basophilic staining in the paranuclear area
- Centrocytes
  - B cells measuring around 10 μ
  - usually irregular in shape and may be cleaved
  - sparse, weakly stained basophilic cytoplasm
  - fine chromatin pattern
- Centroblasts
  - larger than centrocytes
  - charcteristic round nucleus, usually with several marginal nucleoli
  - cytoplasm sparse and may contain vacuoles
- Immunoblasts
  - of either B or T phenotype
  - the largest of the lymphoid cells (20–30 μ)
  - round nucleus, often eccentrically placed
  - 1–3 large, strongly basophilic nucleoli
  - cytoplasm intensely basophilic
- Macrophages
  - round to oval nucleus
  - evenly distributed chromatin
  - inconspicuous nucleolus
  - poorly defined cytoplasm varies markedly in size
  - may contain phagocytosed cellular debris referred to as 'tingible bodies'

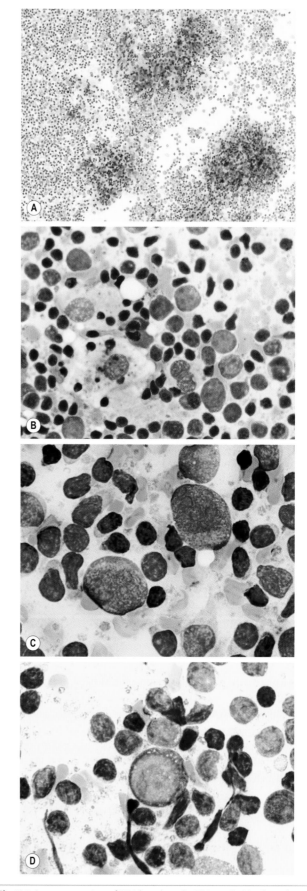

Fig. 7.3 Low-power view of FNA lymph node. (A) Lymphoid cells and residual follicle centre fragments. Normal lymph node cells: centroblasts, centrocytes, plasma cells, tingible body macrophages. (B) Immunoblasts. (C) Centroblasts. (D) Follicular dendritic cells and tingible body macrophages.

Non-specific lymph node hyperplasia (Fig. 7.4)

Cytological pattern depends on the proportion of follicular and interfollicular cells in the aspirate.

- Large follicles with active germinal centres
  - containing many centroblasts and centrocytes
  - may mimic follicular NHL
- Predominance of interfollicular cells
  - smears rich in plasma cells, immunoblasts
  - may mimic low-grade NHL

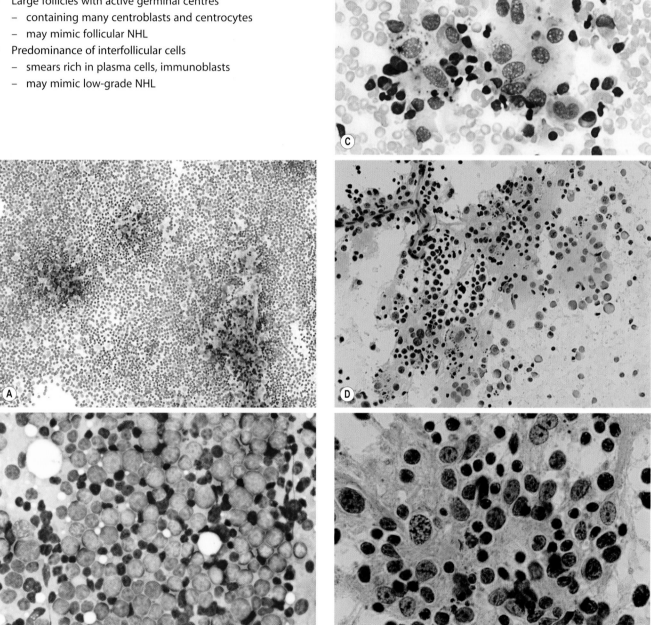

Fig. 7.4 Smears from lymph nodes showing non-specific hyperplasia. (A) Low-power view showing a cellular sample with aggregates representing residual follicle centre fragments. (B) High-power view shows numerous centrocytes and centroblasts. Patient had HIV but similar appearances may be seen in EBV and other non-specific infections. (C) Residual follicle centre in a hypocellular node showing follicular dendritic cells (FDC). (D) Residual follicle centre fragment in alcohol-fixed preparation (PAP stain). (E) High-power view showing FDCs and other follicle centre cells.

Reactive lymphadenopathy

Sinus histiocytosis – Rosai–Dorfmann disease (Fig. 7.5)

Rosai–Dorfman disease: sinus histiocytosis with massive lymphadenopathy. Most patients are in good health and develop massive bilateral non-tender enlargement of the cervical lymph nodes followed by fever.

- Characteristic dilatation of subcapsular and trabecular sinuses, which are partially or completely filled with histiocytes/macrophages
- Dominated by small lymphocytes, some blasts and numerous, sometimes multinucleated macrophages with abundant foamy cytoplasm and round, oval or kidney-shaped nuclei
- The histiocytes often have well-preserved lymphocytes in the cytoplasm, which is referred to as lymphophagocytosis or emperipolesis

Granulomatous lymphadenopathy

The most common cause of granulomatous lymphadenopathy in developed countries is sarcoidosis.

- Infections are a particularly important group:
    - tuberculosis is the commonest
    - leprosy
    - cat-scratch disease
    - paracoccidioidomycosis
    - histoplasmosis
    - leishmaniasis
    - lymphogranuloma venereum
    - brucellosis
    - tularaemia
- Non-infectious causes include:
    - foreign bodies such as talc or silica
    - malignant lymphoma
    - nodes draining a carcinoma

Tuberculous lymphadenitis (Figs 7.6, 7.7)

Tuberculous lymphadenitis shows three major cell patterns.

- Epithelioid granulomas without necrosis
    - small clusters of epithelioid histiocytes and single forms
    - reactive lymphocytes
    - Langhans giant cells are not often seen
- Epithelioid granulomas with necrosis
- Necrosis without epithelioid granuloma

For definitive diagnosis, acid-fast bacilli can be identified using the Ziehl–Neelsen (ZN) stain or other stains for acid-fast bacilli. These stains have a relatively low sensitivity and are nowadays mostly replaced by PCR techniques to identify the mycobacteria.

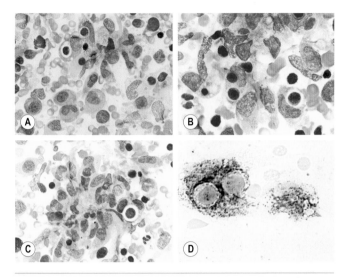

Fig. 7.5 Sinus histyocytosis (Rosai–Dorfman) disease. (A–C) Macrophages showing lymphophagocytosis (emperipolesis). (D) CD68 positivity in macrophages.

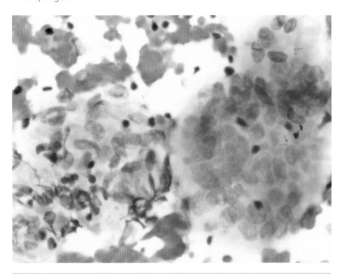

Fig. 7.6 Granulomatous lymphadenitis. Langhans giant cell (*right*) and an aggregate of epithelioid cells (*left*).

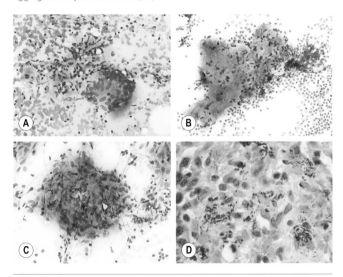

Fig. 7.7 Granulomatous lymphadenitis. (A) Multinucleate giant cell and epithelioid granuloma, (B) necrosis, (C) epithelioid histiocytes forming a granuloma, (D) ZN-positive acid-fast bacilli confirming a mycobacterial infection/tuberculosis, in this case *Mycobacterium avium-intracellulare* (bacilli in the macrophages in large numbers). Patient was immunosuppressed.

Sarcoidosis (Fig. 7.8)

This systemic disorder of young adults is characterised histologically by the presence of non-caseating granulomata and tends to affect lungs and lymph nodes mainly, but most organs can be involved.

Cytological findings

- Cohesive clusters of epithelioid cells and numerous small mature lymphocytes
- In most cases multinucleated giant cells are present
- The background is free from necrosis

Differential diagnosis

If Langhans-type giant cells are absent, the differential diagnosis should include Hodgkin disease and low-grade T-cell lymphoma. Techniques such as PCR and special stains for organisms such as mycobacteria and fungi, as well as immunocytochemistry to characterise the lymphoid cells, are of value in reducing the number of diagnostic alternatives. In sarcoidosis, the lymphoid population is dominated by T cells, while the B cells are polyclonal.

Kikuchi–Fujimoto disease – histiocytic necrotising lymphadenitis (Fig. 7.9)

A benign, self-limiting disorder of unknown aetiology, prevalent in Asian people, presenting with acute tender, cervical lymphadenopathy, predominantly in the posterior cervical region.

Cytological findings

- Numerous foamy macrophages as well as tingible body macrophages containing karyorrhectic debris
- Background of necrotic material
- Small lymphocytes, as well as activated lymphocytes (plasmacytoid monocytes)
- No neutrophils, epithelioid cells and a few plasma cells

Cat-scratch disease (Fig. 7.10)

Granulomatous lymphadenopathy caused by *Bartonella henselae*, the most common cause of chronic lymphadenopathy among children and adolescents. Neoplasia may initially be suspected clinically in 38% of the cases.

Cytological findings

- Confluent epithelioid cells
- Central scattering of neutrophils
- Background of polymorphic inflammatory cells
- Medium-sized to large lymphoid cells (monocytoid B lymphocytes)

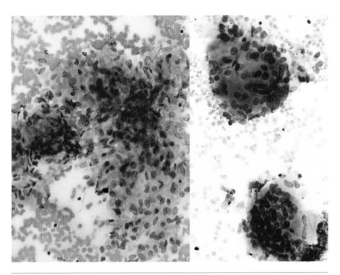

Fig. 7.8 Non-caseating granulomas composed of epithelioid cells (*left*). Multinucleate giant cells (*right*). No necrosis.

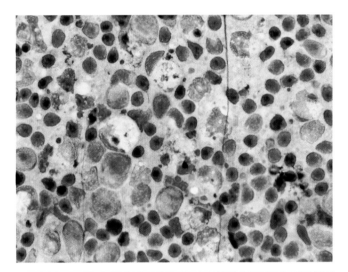

Fig. 7.9 Kikuchi–Fujimoto disease is recognised by the karyorrhectic debris, crescentic macrophages, plasmacytoid monocytes and absence of neutrophils.

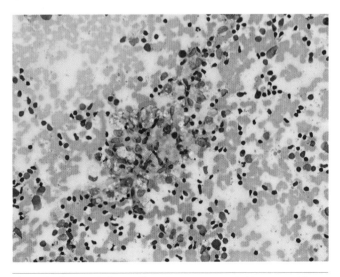

Fig. 7.10 Cat-scratch disease. Necrotic areas surrounded by neutrophils, epithelioid cells and lymphoid cells.

Kimura's disease (Fig. 7.11)

- Chronic inflammatory disorder with a benign course
- Primarily seen in young Asian males
- Warthin–Finkeldey-type giant cells
- Background of a mixed population includes lymphocytes and eosinophils

Differential diagnosis

- Malignant lymphoma
- Langerhans cell histiocytosis (Fig. 7.12)
- Angiolymphoid hyperplasia with eosinophilia
- Other reactive lymphadenopathies
- Foreign body granulomas
- Talc, silicone or beryllium can induce massive lymphadenopathy which is impossible to differentiate clinically from metastatic lymph node disease
- Surgical sutures can induce a granulomatous reaction that can be difficult to distinguish from malignancy (Fig. 7.13)

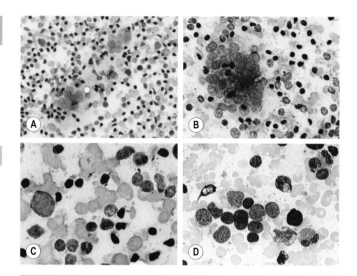

Fig. 7.11 Kimura's disease. (A) Giant cells and a mixed lymphoid cell population, (B) Warthin–Finkeldey giant cell, (C,D) mixed lymphoid cells and eosinophils.

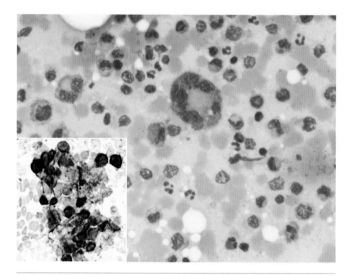

Fig. 7.12 Langerhans cell histiocytosis. Multinucleate giant cell, numerous histiocytes with central grooves, eosinophils. (Inset) CD1-positive histiocytes.

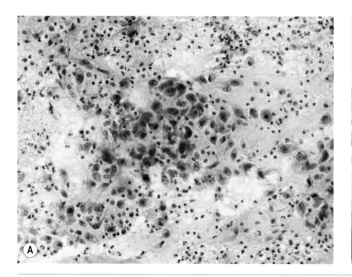

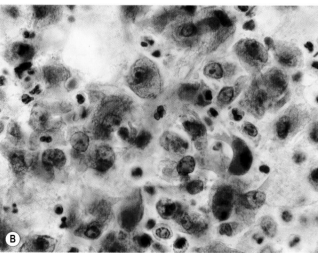

Fig. 7.13[†] Suture granuloma. (A,B) The granulation tissue cells and histiocytes may produce an exuberant reaction which can sometimes be mistaken for malignancy, particularly if there is a clinical history of a lump at the site of tumour surgery.

Castleman's disease (giant or angiofollicular lymph node hyperplasia, lymphoid hamartoma)

- An uncommon lymphoproliferative disorder that can involve single lymph node stations or can be systemic
- Three histological variants (hyaline-vascular, plasma-cell, and mixed) and two clinical types (unicentric and multicentric)

Cytological findings (Fig. 7.14)

- Fine needle aspiration cytology shows non-specific findings
- Lymphoid cells of follicle centre with piercing, fine capillary vessels
- Background with polymorphous lymphocytes with a predominance of B lymphocytes
- Focal hyaline deposits, characteristic of hyaline–vascular type

Further investigations

- CD21 positive
- CD20 negative
- CD3 negative
- CD15 negative
- CD30 negative

Despite some of the features described and the immunocytochemistry that may suggest Castleman's disease, the cytological appearances of this condition are non-specific and may require biopsy if lymphadenopathy persists.

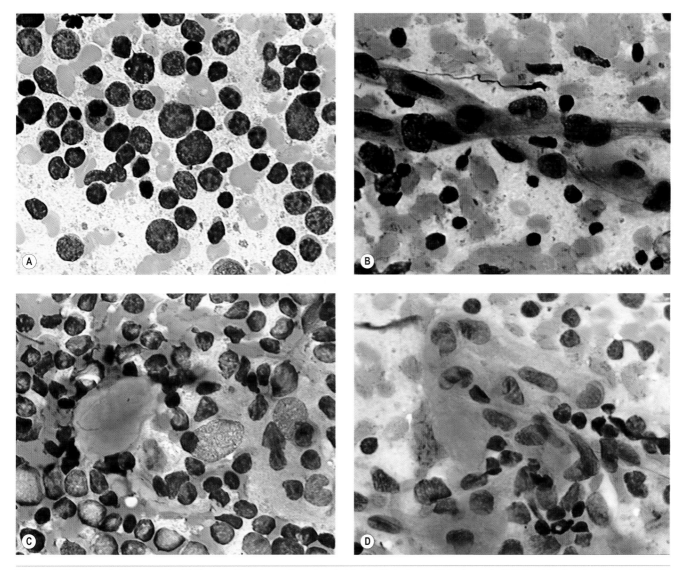

Fig. 7.14 FNA of cervical lymph node. (A) Non-specific polymorphous lymphoid cells. (B) A cluster of blood vessels. (C,D) Focal hyaline deposits and cells of vascular origin. Cytological findings of Castleman's disease are non-specific.

Neoplastic lesions of lymph node

Malignant lymphomas (Hodgkin and non-Hodgkin) are primary tumours of lymph node.

Secondary (metastatic) tumours represent lymphatic involvement from primary tumours of different origin, such as epithelial (metastatic carcinoma), mesenchymal (metastatic sarcoma), germinal (metastatic germ tumour), etc.

Lymphoid neoplasms

The World Health Organization (WHO) classification of lymphoid neoplasms is based on the recognition of distinct diseases, using a multidisciplinary approach comprising morphology, immunophenotype, genetic or molecular and clinical features (Table 7.1).

Table 7.1 WHO classification of lymphoproliferative disorders

Precursor lymphoid neoplasms	B-lymphoblastic leukaemia/lymphoma
	B-lymphoblastic leukaemia/lymphoma with recurrent genetic abnormalities
	T-lymphoblastic leukaemia/lymphoma
Mature B-cell neoplasms	Chronic lymphocytic leukaemia/small lymphocytic lymphoma
	B-cell prolymphocytic leukaemia
	Marginal zone lymphoma
	Hairy cell leukaemia
	Lymphoplasmacytic lymphoma (Waldenström macroglobulinaemia)
	Heavy chain diseases
	Plasma cell neoplasms
	Follicular lymphoma
	Mantle zone lymphoma
	Diffuse and other large B-cell lymphoma
	Primary effusion lymphoma
	B-cell lymphoma, unclassifiable
Mature T-cell and NK cell neoplasms	T-cell leukaemias
	Hepatosplenic T-cell lymphoma
	Mycosis fungoides/Sézary syndrome
	Primary cutaneous T-cell lymphomas
	Peripheral T-cell lymphoma, NOS
	Angioimmunoblastic T-cell lymphoma
	Anaplastic large cell lymphoma
Hodgkin lymphoma	Nodular lymphocyte predominant Hodgkin lymphoma (NLPHL)
	Classic Hodgkin lymphoma (CHL)
	Nodular sclerosis CHL
	Lymphocyte-rich CHL
	Mixed cellularity CHL
	Lymphocyte-depleted CHL
Histiocytic and dendritic cell neoplasms	Histiocytic sarcoma
	Langerhans cell sarcoma
	Interdigitating dendritic cell sarcoma
	Follicular dendritic cell sarcoma
	Fibroblastic reticular cell tumour
	Indeterminate dentritic cell tumour
	Disseminated juvenile xanthogranuloma
Post-transplant lymphoproliferative disorders (PTLD)	Early lesions
	Polymorphic PTLD
	Monomorphic PTLD
	Classic Hodgkin lymphoma-type PTLD

Lymphoblastic leukaemia/lymphoma

- B-lymphoblastic leukaemia/lymphoma, not other wise specified (B-ALL-NOS) is a disease of B-cell precursors. As leukaemia, it is most common in children (around 10% is lymphoblastic lymphoma). B-lymphoblastic leukaemia with t(9;22) is a neoplasm of precursors of B-cell lineage characterised by recurrent abnormalities, composed of lymphoblasts similar to other types of ALL
- T-lymphoblastic leukaemia (T-ALL) comprises around 15% of childhood and 25% of adult leukaemias. It presents with a high leukocyte count, large mediastinal mass or other tissue mass
- Lymphoblastic lymphomas are neoplasms of lymphoblasts committed to the B- or T-cell lineage with nodal or extranodal involvement. T-lymphoblastic lymphoma often shows mediastinal and thymic involvement, with no or minimal evidence of peripheral blood or bone marrow involvement

Cytological findings (Figs 7.15–7.19)

B-lymphoblastic leukaemia/lymphoma, not otherwise specified

- Small or medium-sized to larger blasts with round, irregular or convoluted nuclei; cytoplasm is scant or light blue with moderate amounts, occasionally vacuolated, some with presentation of coarse azurophilic granules or pseudopods (hand mirror cells); chromatin is homogenous with inconspicuous to prominent nucleoli
- Several lymphoblasts have high nuclear/cytoplasmic ratio

T-lymphoblastic leukaemia/lymphoma

- Medium-sized blasts with high nuclear/cytoplasmic ratio (some cases vary in size from large to small); nuclei are round, irregular or convoluted with inconspicuous nucleoli

Differential diagnosis

- Acute leukaemias of ambiguous lineage – undifferentiated leukaemias
- Acute undifferentiated leukaemias
- Acute myeloid leukaemia with minimal differentiation
- Embryonal rhabdomyosarcoma
- Neuroblastoma
- Ewing's sarcoma/PNET

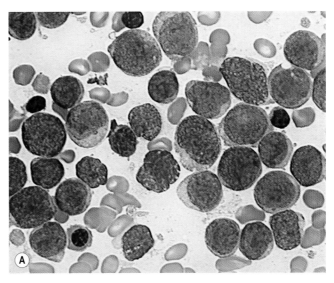

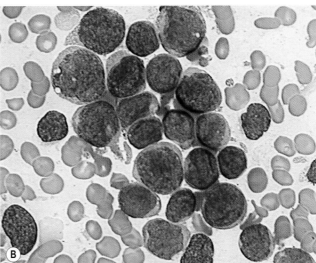

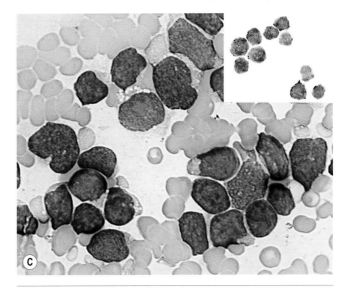

Fig. 7.15 B-lymphoblastic leukaemia. Bone marrow aspirate. (A,B,C) Lymphoblasts vary from small blasts with scant cytoplasm to larger cells with moderate amounts of basophilic cytoplasm (MGG). (Inset, C) Blasts immunostained for CD10 (LSAB).

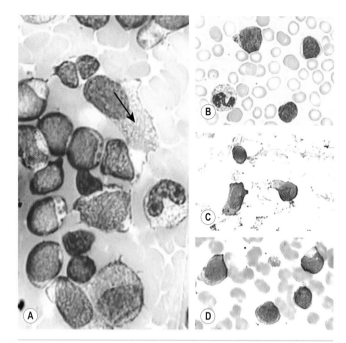

Fig. 7.16 B-lymphoblastic leukaemia. (A) Bone marrow aspirate shows lymphoblasts with coarse azurophilic granules (*arrow*). (B) Peripheral blood smear also presents granulated lymphoblast (MGG). (C) Blast immunostained for CD10 (LSAB). (D) Blasts are cytochemically negative for myeloperoxidase (cytochemistry).

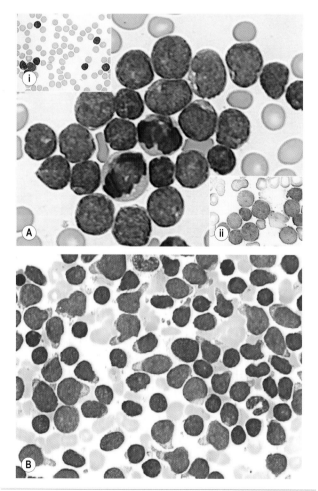

Fig. 7.17 T-lymphoblastic leukaemia. (A) Bone marrow aspirate with very high nuclear to cytoplasmic ratio, scant cytoplasm and nuclear convolution, mitotic figures are present (MGG). (Inset i) Peripheral blood smear with small lymphoblast (MGG). (Inset ii) CD3 positive blasts (LSAB). (B) 'Hand mirror-like' lymphoblasts in bone marrow aspirate (MGG).

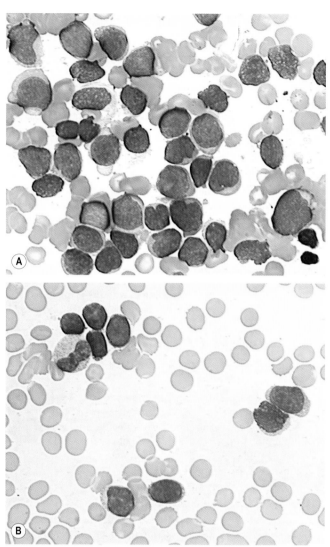

Fig. 7.18 B-lymphoblastic leukaemia with t(9;22). (A) Bone marrow smear presenting features of lymphoblasts which are similar to lymphoblasts of other acute lymphoblastic leukaemias. (B) Peripheral blood smear with small lymphoblasts (MGG).

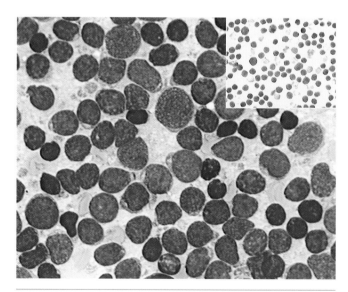

Fig. 7.19 T-lymphoblastic lymphoma. Small to medium-sized lymphoblasts (MGG). (Inset) CD3-positive lymphoblasts (LSAB).

Chronic lymphocytic leukaemia/small lymphocytic lymphoma (CLL/SLL)

- Chronic lymphocytic leukaemia is a lymphoid neoplasm with $\geq 5 \times 10^9$/L B lymphocytes in peripheral blood and more than 30% in bone marrow aspirate. A typical B-CLL shows the morphology of small mature lymphocytes in peripheral blood, bone marrow and lymph nodes, expression of CD19, CD5 and CD23 antigens, and low proliferative activity

- Atypical CLL (variants of CLL) represents around 15% of CLL cases and comprises two major subtypes: chronic lymphocytic leukaemia/prolymphocytic leukaemia (CLL/PLL) and CLL with lymphoplasmacytoid differentiation (CLL/LP). CLL/PLL is defined by more than 10% but less than 55% of prolymphocytes in peripheral blood. The cases that show lymphoplasmacytoid morphology are called atypical CLL with lymphoplasmacytoid differentiation

- The term small lymphocytic lymphoma (SLL) is used to indicate a non-leukaemic form with morphology and immunophenotype of CLL. This neoplasm presents with lymphadenopathy, without cytopenias and $<5 \times 10^9$/L B lymphocytes in peripheral blood

- Approximately 2–8% of CLL cases develop diffuse large B-cell lymphoma and less than 1% classic Hodgkin lymphoma

Cytological findings (Figs 7.20–7.24)

- CLL/SLL consists of monomorphic small lymphocytes admixed with prolymphocytes (small to medium-sized with clumped chromatin and small nuclei) and paraimmunoblasts (larger cells with round nuclei, central nucleoli and basophilic cytoplasm)

- Richter's syndrome has the same findings as DLBCL (large transformed lymphoid B cells) or Hodgkin lymphoma with typical Hodgkin and Reed–Sternberg cells. The presence of Reed–Sternberg cells in the background of CLL cannot be diagnosed as Hodgkin lymphoma

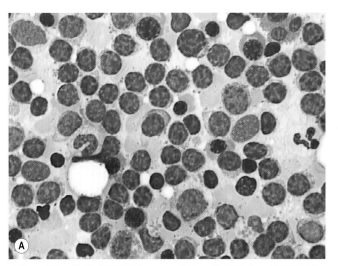

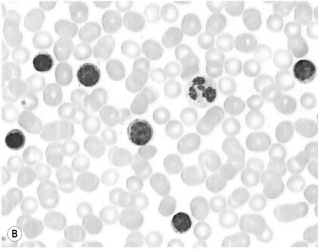

Fig. 7.20 Typical B-chronic lymphocytic leukaemia with small mature lymphocytes. (A) Bone marrow aspirate (MGG); (B) peripheral blood smear (MGG).

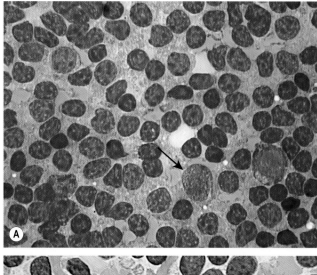

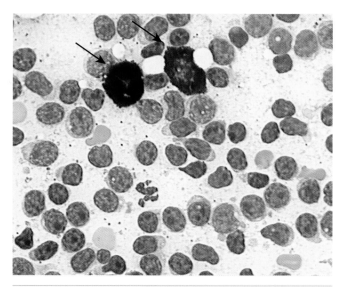

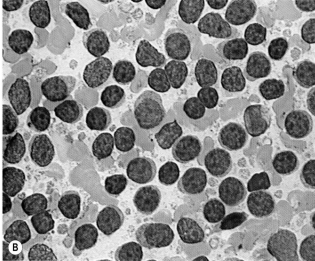

Fig. 7.23 Differential diagnosis includes lymphoplasmacytic NHL (Waldenström's macroglobulinaemia). There is monotonous proliferation of small lymphocytes, lymphoplasmacytoid cells and plasma cells with mast cells (*arrows*) (MGG).

Fig. 7.21 FNA of lymph node - SLL. (A) Small lymphocytes with some prolymphocytes and paraimmunoblasts (*arrow*). (B) SLL with lymphoplasmacytoid features (MGG).

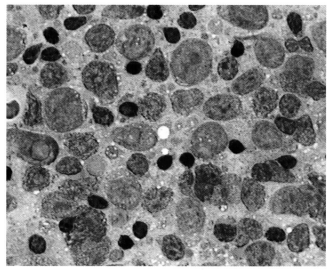

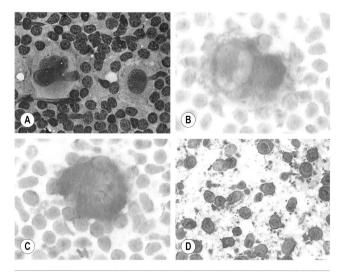

Fig. 7.24 FNA of lymph node. Richter syndrome (DLBCL) (MGG).

Fig. 7.22 (A) Reed–Sternberg-like cells in the background of small lymphocytic lymphoma (MGG). (B) CD30-positive Reed–Sternberg-like cell. (C) CD15-positive Reed–Sternberg-like cell. (D) CD20-positive small lymphocytes in background (LSAB).

Marginal zone lymphoma (MZL)

Marginal zone lymphoma includes three subtypes depending on the site of lymphoma involvement:

- Splenic MZL
- Extranodal marginal zone B-cell lymphoma of mucosa-associated lymphoid tissue (MALT-lymphoma)
- Nodal MZL

Cytological findings (Figs 7.25–7.28)

Splenic MZL

- Two cell types (small lymphocytes and marginal zone cells), epithelioid histiocytes may be present
- Peripheral blood tumours cells have polar villi

Extranodal marginal zone B-cell lymphoma of mucosa-associated lymphoid tissue (MALT-lymphoma)

- Lymphoma cells resembling centrocytes
- Plasmacytic differentiation is present as well as monocytoid appearance

Nodal MZL

- Variable number of centrocyte-like or monocytoid B-cells, plasma cells and transformed B-cells
- Immunophenotype:
  - The tumour cells express IgM, CD20, CD79a and are CD5, CD10, CD23, BCL-6 negative

Differential diagnosis

- Small lymphocytic lymphoma/chronic lymphocytic leukaemia
- Hairy cell leukaemia
- Follicular lymphoma
- Mantle cell lymphoma
- Lymphoplasmacytoid lymphoma

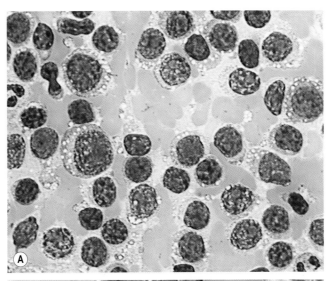

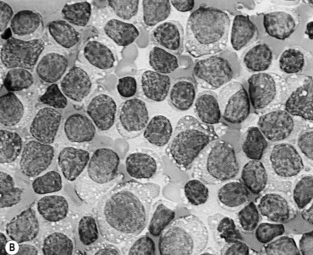

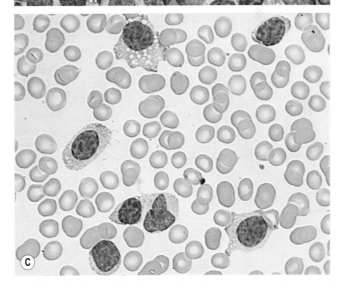

Fig. 7.25 Splenic marginal zone lymphoma. (A,B) FNA of spleen with large cells of marginal zone. (C) Peripheral blood smear also shows atypical large cells (MGG).

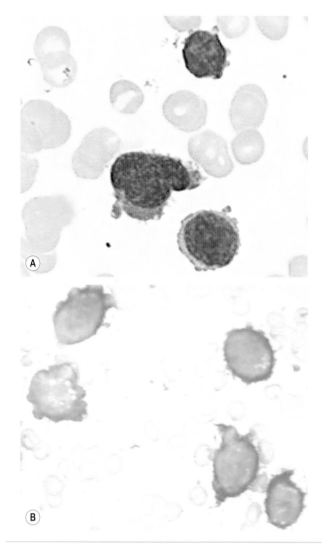

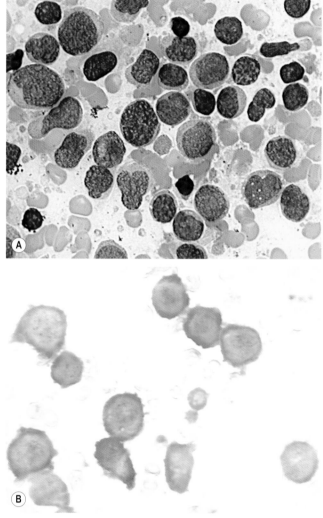

Fig. 7.26 Splenic marginal zone lymphoma with villous lymphocytes. (A) Peripheral blood smear and atypical large cells, lymphoma with villous lymphocytes (MGG). (B) Lymphoid cells immunostained for DBA 44 (LSAB).

Fig. 7.28 Nodal marginal cell lymphoma. (A) FNA of lymph node and medium-sized, partially monocytoid lymphoid cells (monocytoid B-cell lymphoma) (MGG). (B) CD20-positive lymphoid cells (LSAB).

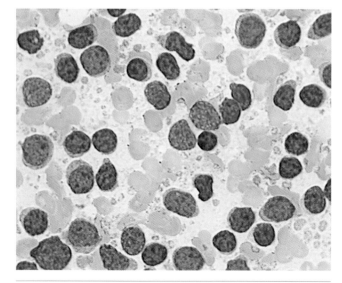

Fig. 7.27 Mucosa associated lymphoid tissue lymphoma, (MALT). FNA of intraparotid lymph node with small to medium-sized lymphoid and lymphoplasmacytoid cells (MGG).

Plasma cell myeloma and primary amyloidosis

The diagnosis of plasma cell myeloma is made by a combination of morphological (bone marrow clonal plasma cells), radiological (lytic bone lesions), laboratory (M-protein in serum and/or urine) and clinical (presence of end-organ damage – renal insufficiency, anaemia) features.

Primary amyloidosis is associated with abnormal immunoglobulin light or rarely heavy chain deposits in various tissues (bone marrow, kidney, ventricle, etc.).

Cytological findings (Figs 7.29–7.30)

Plasma cell myeloma

- Monoclonal plasma cells usually exceed 10%
- Mature and immature forms:
  - plasma cells of mature are oval with round eccentric nucleus and abundant basophilic cytoplasm
  - immature with plasmablastic or pleomorphic features, dispersed chromatin, prominent nucleoli and high nuclear to cytoplasmic ratio

Primary amyloidosis

- Amorphous waxy substance (amyloid deposition)
- Mild increase in plasma cells
- Macrophages and foreign-body giant cells found around deposits

Clinical variants of plasma cell myeloma

- Asymptomatic (smouldering) plasma cell myeloma
  - 10–20% plasma cells in bone marrow
  - medium level of serum M-protein
  - stable disease
- Non-secretory myeloma
  - absence of M-protein
- Plasma cell leukaemia
  - in peripheral blood $> 2 \times 10^9$/L or 20% clonal plasma cells

Further investigations

- Plasma cell myeloma
  - immunophenotype: CD79a+, CD138+, CD38+, CD56± (PCL CD56–)
  - genetics: immunoglobulin heavy and light chain genes are clonally rearranged, numerical and structural abnormalities, monosomy or partial deletion of chromosome 13 etc.
- Primary amyloidosis
  - positive Congo red
  - immunophenotype: monoclonal kappa or lambda, amyloid P component
  - genetics: similar to other plasma cell neoplasms

Differential diagnosis

- Polyclonal plasmacytosis
- Secondary amyloidosis

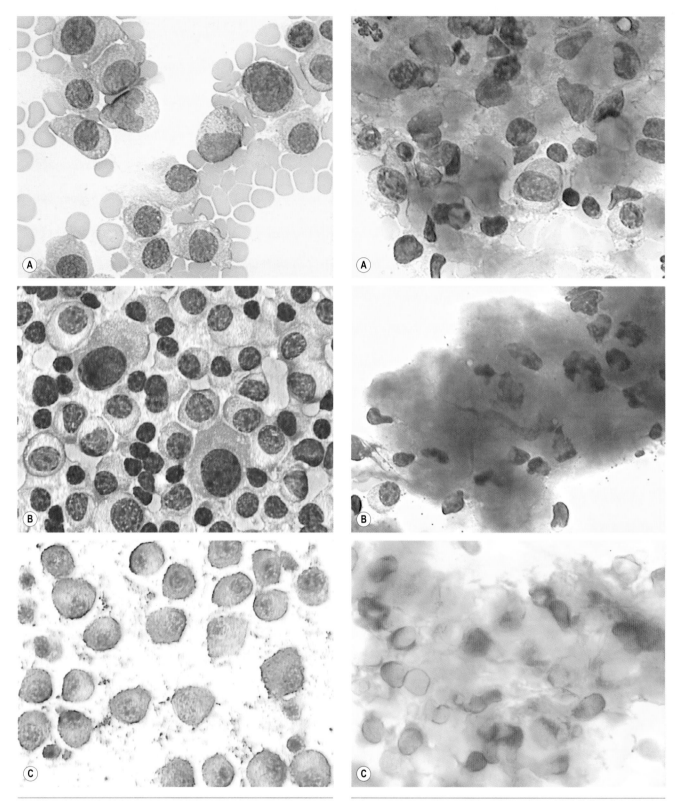

Fig. 7.29 Plasma cell neoplasms. (A) Bone marrow aspirate – plasma cell myeloma showing atypical plasma cells. (B) Solitary plasmacytoma of bone (MGG). (C) CD138-positive plasma cells (LSAB).

Fig. 7.30 Amyloidosis. (A,B) Plasma cells with amyloid deposits (MGG). (C) Congo red-positive amyloid, (cytochemistry).

Mantle cell lymphoma

Mantle cell lymphoma (MCL) comprises 3–10% of NHL, and includes several morphological variants (typical, blastoid, pleomorphic).

Cytological findings (Fig. 7.31)

- Typical (classic) variant
    - small to medium-sized cells
    - most cells with markedly irregular nuclear contours as centrocytes, dispersed chromatin and inconspicuous nucleoli
- Blastoid variant
    - cells resemble lymphoblasts
    - high mitotic rate
- Pleomorphic variant
    - large pleomorphic cells
    - irregular nuclear contours
    - prominent nucleoli
    - high proliferative index

Differential diagnosis

- Small lymphocytic lymphoma
- Follicular lymphoma
- Marginal zone lymphoma

Table 7.2 Immunocytochemistry markers in distinguishing lymphomas composed of small lymphocytes

	Mantle cell lymphoma	Follicle centre lymphoma	Small lymphocytic lymphoma
CD5	Positive	Negative	Positive
CD10	Negative	Positive	Negative
CD23	Negative	Negative	Positive
Light chain	$\lambda > \kappa$	$\kappa > \lambda$	$\kappa > \lambda$
Cyclin D1	Positive	Negative	Negative

From Mason, D, Gatter, K. Lymphoma Classification, DAKO Denmark, 1999.

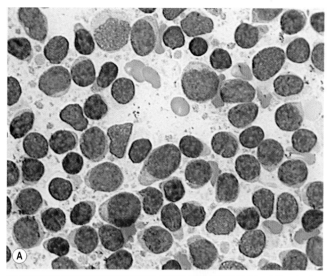

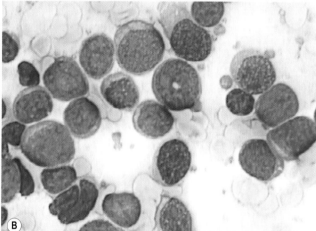

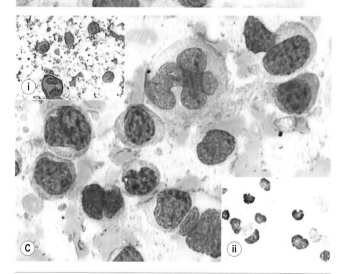

Fig. 7.31 Mantle cell lymphoma. (A) Typical variant (MGG). (B) Blastoid variant (MGG). (C) Pleomorphic variant (MGG). (Inset i) CD20-positive cell (LSAB). (Inset ii) Ki-67-positive cells (HRP).

Follicular lymphoma (FL)

Follicular lymphoma is one of the most common NHLs. It is composed of centrocytes and centroblasts, and usually has at least a partially follicular pattern. FL is graded histologically (I, II and III) by counting the absolute number of centroblasts in 10 neoplastic follicles, expressed per 40× high-power microscopic fields (hpf). This grading can be performed on cytological smears as well.

Cytological findings (Figs 7.32–7.33)

- Follicular lymphoma grade I
  - monotonous population of centrocytes – small cells with irregular nuclei, 1 or more basophilic nucleoli and moderate amount
  - rare centroblast (<5%) – large cell with usually round nuclei, occasionally indented or multilobated, vesicular chromatin, 1–3 peripheral nucleoli and narrow rim of basophilic cytoplasm
- Follicular lymphoma grade II
  - predominance of centrocytes and only few centroblasts (6–15/hpf)
- Follicular lymphoma grade III
  - have >15 centroblasts/hpf
  - grade IIIA – centrocytes are still present
  - grade IIIB – large cells are centroblasts and immunoblasts

Differential diagnosis

- Follicular lymph node hyperplasia
- Other low-grade non-Hodgkin lymphoma (see Table 7.2, p. 191)
  - mantle cell lymphoma
  - marginal zone lymphoma
  - atypical chronic lymphocytic leukaemia

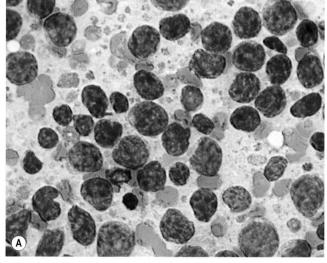

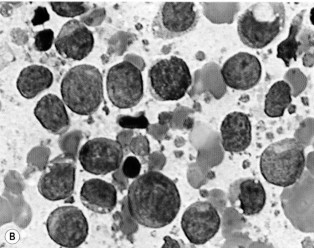

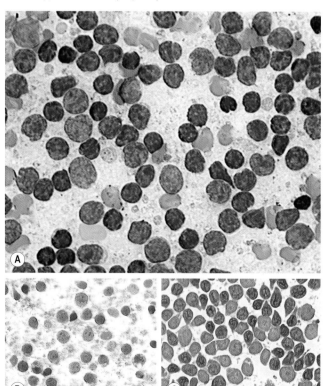

Fig. 7.32 Follicular lymphoma grade I – monotonous population of centrocytes. (A) MGG. (B) CD 20-positive cells. (C) BCL 2-positive cells (LSAB).

Fig. 7.33 Follicular lymphoma grade II – many centrocytes with some centroblasts (MGG). (B) Follicular lymphoma grade III – centroblasts without centrocytes.

Diffuse large B-cell lymphoma (DLBCL)

DLBCL is an NHL consisting of large B-lymphoid cells and diffuse growth pattern. It is one of the most common NHLs. It is a biologically heterogeneous group with morphologically, molecularly, immunophenotypically and clinically distinct entities.

Cytological findings (Fig 7.34–7.38)

- Morphological variants:
  - *centroblastic* – medium-sized to large transformed lymphoid cell with round or oval nuclei, basophilic cytoplasm and peripherally localised 1–3 nucleoli
  - *immunoblastic* – large deeply basophilic cells with centrally situated single nucleolus and sometimes plasmacytoid differentiation
  - *anaplastic* – very large lymphoid cells with anaplastic (some multinucleated – Hodgkin or Reed–Sternberg-like) nuclei and basophilic cytoplasm
- Rare morphological variant:
  - T-cell/histiocyte-rich B-cell lymphoma – single large B cells and a background of small T-cell lymphocytes
- Immunophenotype
  - The tumour cells express B-cell markers (e.g. CD19, CD20, CD22, CD79a), surface and/or cytoplasmic Ig and in a variable way BCL-6, CD10 and IRF4/MUM1

Differential diagnosis

- Seminoma
- Rhabdomyosarcoma
- Amelanotic melanoma
- Sarcoma
- Poorly differentiated carcinoma

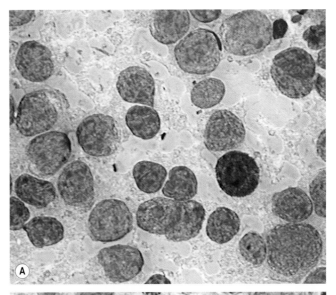
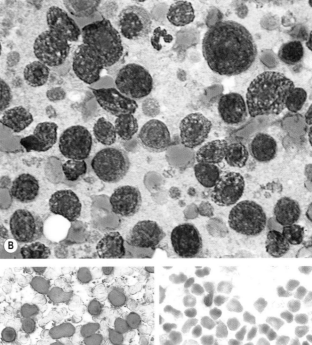
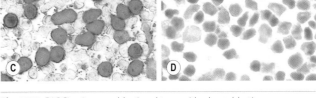

Fig. 7.34 DLBCL – immunoblastic subtype with plasmablastic differentiation. (A,B) Large immunoblasts with prominent single centrally placed nucleoli (MGG). (C) CD20-positive and (D) CD3-negative cells (LSAB).

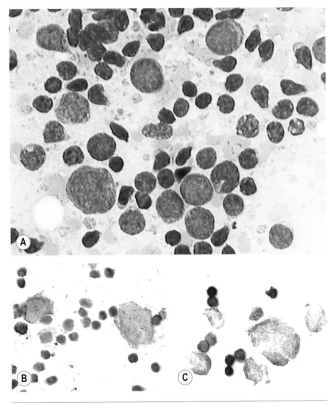

Fig. 7.35 DLBCL T-cell rich. (A) Large lymphoid cells admixed with small lymphocytes (MGG). (B) CD20-positive large lymphoid cells. (C) CD3-negative large cells and positive small reactive lymphocytes (LSAB).

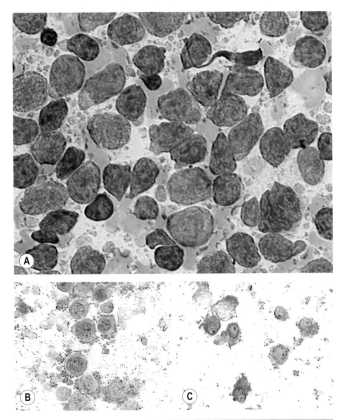

Fig. 7.37 DLBCL – CD30-positive. (A) Monomorphous population of large cells (MGG). (B) CD20- and (C) CD30-positive lymphoid cells (LSAB).

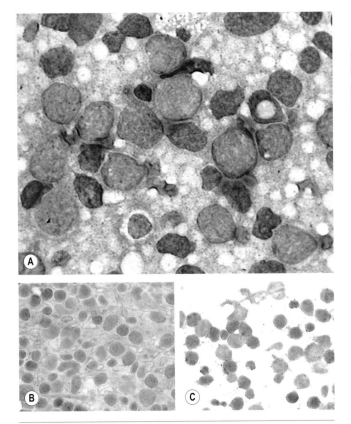

Fig. 7.36 DLBCL – centroblastic type. (A) Medium-sized to large cells with oval or less irregular nuclear contour (MGG). (B) CD20 and (C) BCL positive lymphoid cells (LSAB).

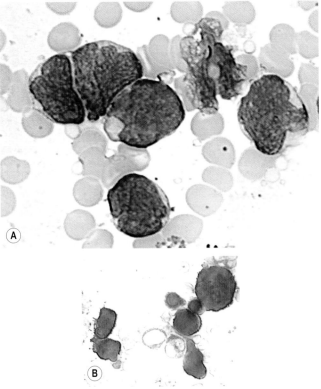

Fig. 7.38 DLBCL – pleomorphic type. (A) Large pleomorphic cells with irregular nuclei (MGG). (B) CD20-positive large lymphoid cells (LSAB).

Primary effusion lymphoma

Primary effusion lymphoma is a high-grade B-cell lymphoma presenting in pleural, pericardial or peritoneal serous effusions most commonly without any other organ involvement. It is associated with immunodeficiency (HIV) in co-infection with EBV virus as well as in the absence of immunodeficiency (HHV-8 virus infection).

Cytological findings (Figs 7.39–7.45)

- Large basophilic, immunoblastic, plasmablastic or anaplastic cells
- Some cases contain Reed–Sternberg-like cells
- Immunophenotype: the tumour cells often lack pan-B-cell markers and often express CD45, CD30, CD138 and EMA. They are EBER positive (as demonstrated by *in situ hybridisation*)

Differential diagnosis

- Anaplastic poorly differentiated carcinoma, melanoma or sarcoma
- Tumours of germ cell origin
- Hodgkin lymphoma

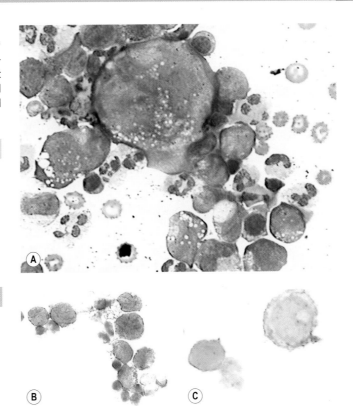

Fig. 7.40 Primary effusion lymphoma in pleural effusion. (A) Large basophilic lymphoid cells with anisocytosis (MGG). (B) CD20- and (C) CD30-positive cells (LSAB).

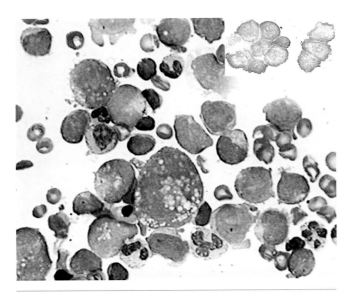

Fig. 7.39 Primary effusion lymphoma in a pleural effusion. Atypical lymphoid cells with prominent vacuolation (MGG). (Inset) CD20-positive cells (LSAB).

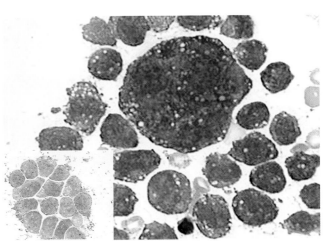

Fig. 7.41 Burkitt's lymphoma in ascitic effusion. Numerous medium-sized vacuolated blast cells with a single multinucleated cell (MGG). (Inset) Lymphoma cells positive for CD20 (LSAB).

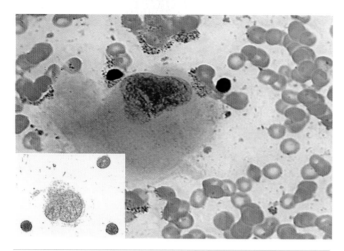

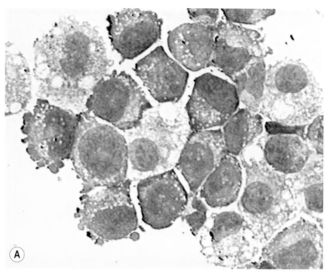

Fig. 7.42 Differential diagnosis of PEL with similar features in effusions. Reed–Sternberg cell of Hodgkin lymphoma in pleural effusion (MGG). (Inset) CD30-positive Reed–Sternberg cell (LSAB).

(A)

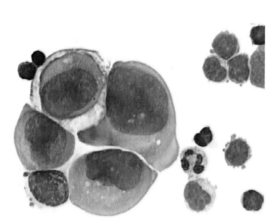

(B)

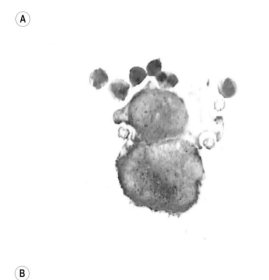

(A)

(B)

Fig. 7.43 Differential diagnosis of PEL with similar features in effusions. (A) Rhabdomyosarcoma in ascitic effusion (MGG). (B) Desmin-positive malignant cells (LSAB).

Fig. 7.44 Differential diagnosis of PEL with similar features in effusions. (A) Malignant epithelial cells in ascitic effusion (MGG). (B) BerEp4-positive malignant cells (LSAB).

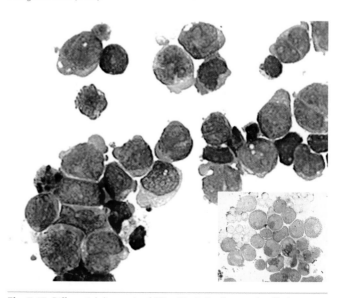

Fig. 7.45 Differential diagnosis of PEL with similar features in effusions. Blasts of acute myeloid leukaemia in ascitic effusion (MGG). (Inset) Myeloperoxidase-positive myeloblasts (cytochemistry).

Burkitt's lymphoma/leukaemia

Burkitt's lymphoma (BL) presents as three clinical variants: sporadic; endemic and immunodeficiency-associated, each with either the extranodal or acute leukaemia presentation.

Burkitt's leukaemia is a leukaemic phase of Burkitt's cell lymphoma, but rare cases present purely as acute leukaemia with bone marrow and peripheral blood involvement.

Cytological findings (Figs 7.46–7.47)

- Uniform medium-sized transformed cells
- The nuclei are round, except they are more irregular with multiple medium-sized nucleoli paracentrally situated
- Cytoplasm is deeply basophilic with abundant lipid vacuoles
- 'Starry sky' pattern with numerous benign macrophages
- Immunophenotype: The tumour cells express B-cell associated markers and are CD10, BCL-6, CD38 positive but usually lack BCL-2. A characteristic feature of BL is the presence of MYC translocation

Differential diagnosis

- Other large B-cell lymphomas
- B-cell lymphoma, unclassifiable (features between DLBCL and Burkitt's lymphoma)
- T-cell lymphoblastic lymphoma with extremely cytoplasmic vacuolation

Further investigations

See Chapter 13, p. 13-22, Figs 13.53–13.56.

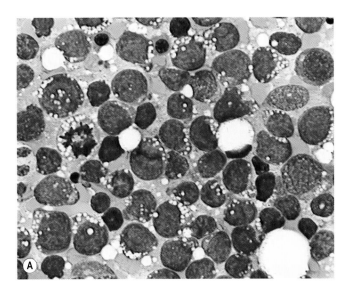

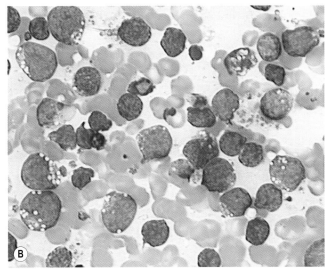

Fig. 7.46 Burkitt's lymphoma/leukaemia show vacuolated medium-sized cells. (A) Lymph node aspirate. (B) Bone marrow smear (MGG).

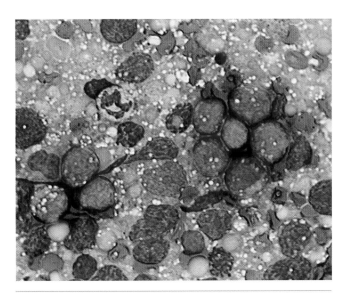

Fig. 7.47 Atypical features of lymphoma cells cytologically classified as Burkitt's lymphoma and histopathologically as follicular lymphoma. Cytogenetically present both t(8;14) and t(14;18) (MGG).

Hepatosplenic T-cell lymphoma

This is a rare extranodal and systemic lymphoma (<1% of all non-Hodgkin lymphoma) associated with chronic immune suppression and presentation with hepatosplenomegaly without lymphadenopathy.

Cytological findings (Fig. 7.48)

- Medium-sized lymphoid cells
- Monomorphic nuclei with small nucleoli
- Rim of pale basophilic cytoplasm
- Blastic variant may be seen in disease progression

Differential diagnosis

- Other indolent T-cell lymphoma (like peripheral T-cell lymphoma NOS)

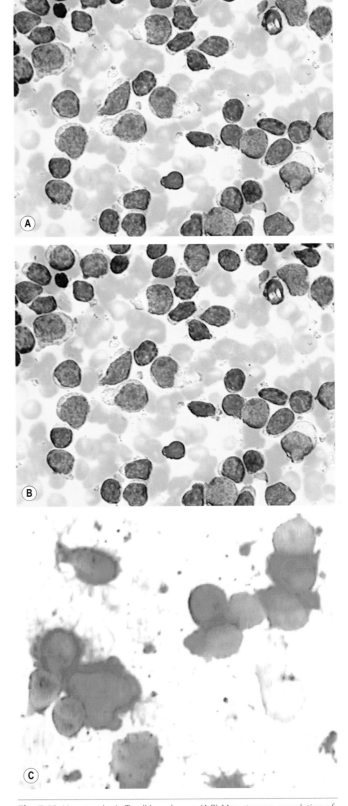

Fig. 7.48 Hepatosplenic T-cell lymphoma. (A,B) Monotonous population of medium-sized lymphoid cells with medium-sized nuclei (MGG). Strong positivity in neoplastic cells for CD3 (LSAB).

Peripheral T-cell lymphoma, not otherwise specified (NOS)

These lymphomas are a heterogeneous group of nodal and extra-nodal diseases (30% of all peripheral T-cell lymphomas). They present with lymphadenopathy, B symptoms and paraneoplastic features (eosinophilia, haemophagocytic syndrome or pruritus).

Cytological findings (Figs 7.49–7.50)

- Malignant cells are medium-sized to large with polymorphous nuclei, prominent nucleoli and basophilic cytoplasm, sometimes with Reed–Sternberg-like cells
- Small cell variant presents with atypical, irregular nuclei
- Background consists of eosinophils, plasma cells, epithelioid histiocytes and large B cells
- Lymphoepithelioid cell variant with numerous epithelioid histiocytes

Differential diagnosis

- Adult T-cell leukaemia/lymphoma
- Angioimmunoblastic lymphoma
- Anaplastic large cell lymphoma
- T-cell-rich large B-cell lymphoma
- T-zone hyperplasia

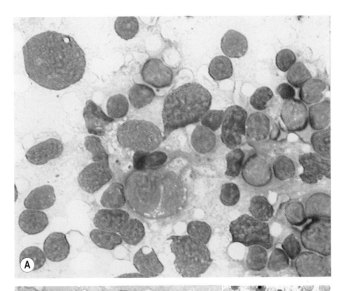

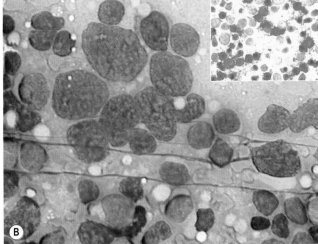

Fig. 7.49 Peripheral T-cell lymphoma, NOS. (A, B) Large lymphoid cells with large nuclei admixed with small to medium-sized cells (MGG). (Inset) CD3-positive lymphoma cells (LSAB).

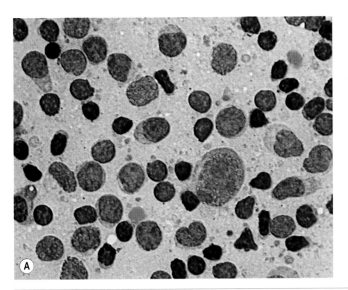

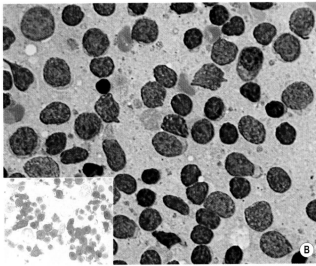

Fig. 7.50 Small cell variant of peripheral T-cell lymphoma, NOS. (A,B) MGG. (Inset) CD3-positive lymphoma cells (LSAB).

Mycosis fungoides/Sézary syndrome

Mycosis fungoides is a primary cutaneous T-cell lymphoma. Sézary syndrome is a generalised disease with lymphadenopathy and erythroderma. Both of these diseases contain clonal neoplastic Sézary cells (T cells).

Cytological findings (Figs 7.51–7.54)

- Sézary cells are small to medium-sized atypical cells with cerebriform nuclei and a narrow rim of cytoplasm

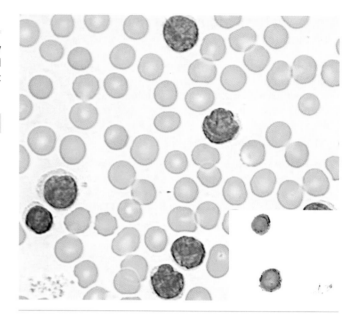

Fig. 7.52 Mycosis fungoides/Sézary syndrome. Peripheral blood smears. Sézary cells with cerebriform nuclei (MGG). (Inset) CD3-positive atypical lymphoid cells (LSAB).

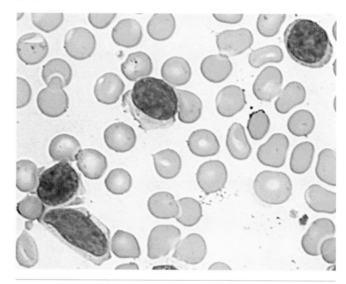

Fig. 7.53 Peripheral blood smear. Atypical large cells of T-cell prolymphocytic leukaemia (MGG).

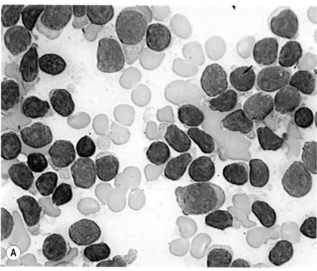

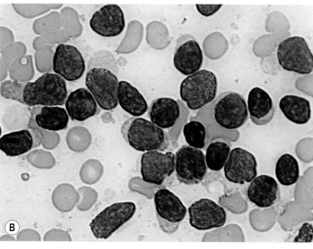

Fig. 7.51 Mycosis fungoides/Sézary syndrome. FNA of lymph node. (A, B) Proliferation of lymphocytes with some atypical irregular cerebriform forms (MGG).

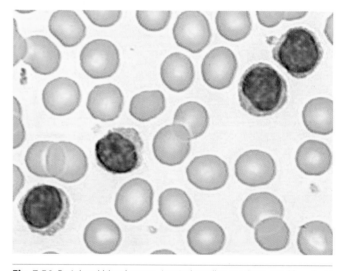

Fig. 7.54 Peripheral blood smear. Atypical small to medium-sized lymphoid cells of prolymphocytic T-cell leukaemia (MGG).

Angioimmunoblastic T-cell lymphoma (AITL)

AITL is a systemic peripheral T-cell lymphoma with generalised lymphadenopathy, hepatosplenomegaly, B symptoms and polyclonal hypergammaglobulinaemia, histologically characterised by the proliferation of endothelial venules and follicular dendritic cells.

Cytological findings (Figs 7.55–7.56)

- Polymorphic pattern consists of small and medium-sized cells with minimal atypia to large lymphoid cells (B-immunoblasts) admixed with eosinophils, plasma cells and histiocytes; in some cases Reed–Sternberg-like cells may be presents
- Proliferation of endothelial venules and dendritic cells
- At relapse, EBV-positive B-cell proliferations including diffuse large B-cell lymphoma, classic Hodgkin lymphoma or plasmacytoma

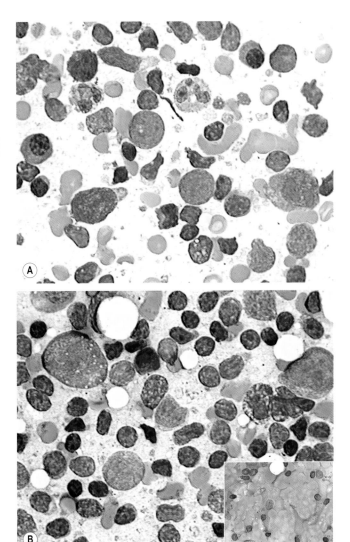

Fig. 7.55 Angioimmunoblastic T-cell lymphoma. (A,B) Small, medium-sized lymphoid cells, immunoblasts, eosinophils and plasma cells (MGG). (Inset) PAS-positive extracellular matrix.

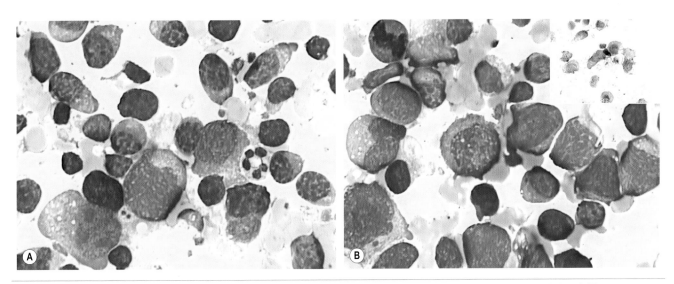

Fig. 7.56 AITL transformation into diffuse large B-cell lymphoma (DLBCL). (A,B) Proliferation of large clonal B-immunoblasts (MGG). (Inset) CD20-positive large lymphoid cells (LSAB).

Anaplastic large cell lymphoma (ALCL)

Systemic CD30-positive T cell lymphoma usually composed of cohesive large cells with abundant cytoplasm and pleomorphic nuclei; half or more express anaplastic lymphoma kinase (ALK1):

- ALK positive
- ALK negative ALCL
- Primary cutaneous (C-ALCL) anaplastic large cell lymphoma

Cytological findings and variants of ALK-positive ALCL (Figs 7.57–7.60)

- Depending on the variant:
  - large (hallmark 'horseshoe') cells with irregular, eccentric kidney-shaped, U-shaped or C-shaped, nuclei
  - pleomorphic giant cells
  - Reed–Sternberg like cells
  - signet ring cells
- Immunophenotype and genetics: CD30+, Ki-1+, ALK+, CD2−, CD4+/−CD5+/−, CD3−/+, t(2;5), EMA+, EBV−
- Variants:
  - common type
  - lymphohistiocytic pattern
  - small cell pattern
  - composite pattern
  - Hodgkin-like pattern
  - other morphological patterns: monomorphic large cell, pleomorphic large cell and rich in signet ring cells

Differential diagnosis

- DLBCL with immunoblastic/plasmablastic features
- Some non-haemopoietic neoplasms (rhabdomyosarcoma and inflammatory myofibroblastic tumours
- Peripheral T-cell lymphoma, NOS
- Classic Hodgkin lymphoma
- Anaplastic carcinoma

Cytological findings and variants of ALK-negative ALCL

- Similar morphological spectrum to ALK-positive ALCL (small cell variant is not recognised)
- The neoplastic cells in ALK-negative ALCL tend to be larger and more pleomorphic and have a higher nuclear/ cytoplasmic ratio than ALK-positive
- Immunophenotype: CD30+, CD5+, CD43+, CD2−, CD3−

Cytological findings of C-ALCL

- C-ALCL has large CD30-postive tumour cells with morphology of anaplastic cells or non-anaplastic (pleomorphic or immunoblastic) appearance
- Immunophenotype: CD30+, CD4+, CD2−, CD5−, CD3−, EMA−, ALK−, CD15−

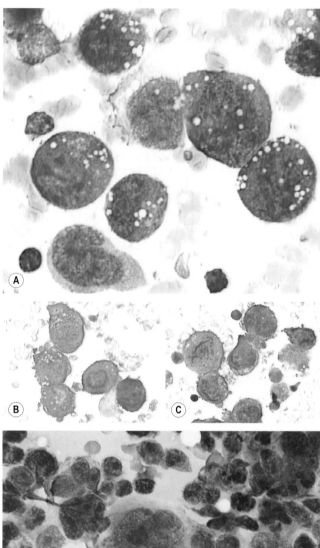

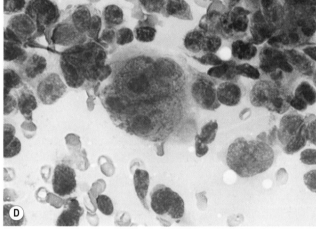

Fig. 7.57 FNA of axillary lymph node – anaplastic large cell lymphoma, ALK-positive. (A) Large anaplastic basophilic and vacuolated cells (MGG). (B) CD30-positive cells. (C) ALK-positive cells. (D) Cutaneous variant of ALCL has similar morphological features but a more indolent clinical course.

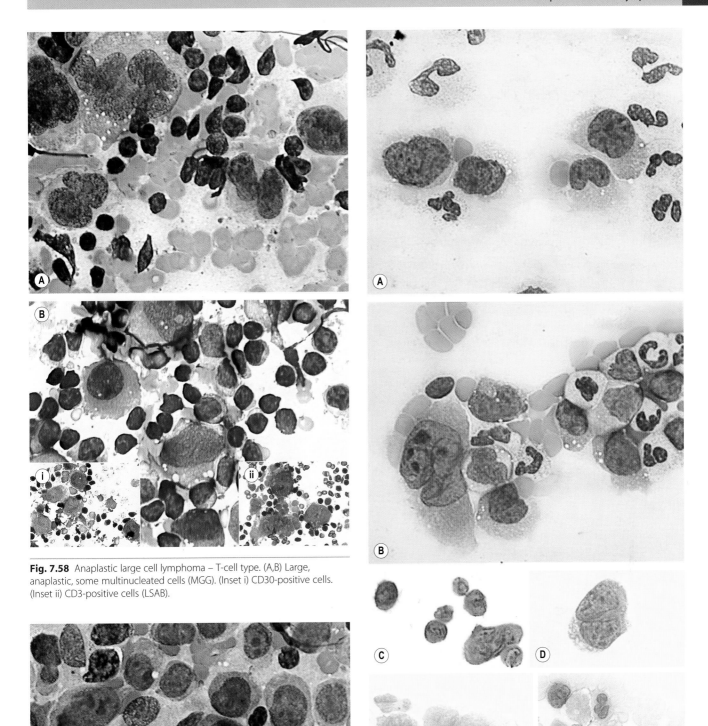

Fig. 7.58 Anaplastic large cell lymphoma – T-cell type. (A,B) Large, anaplastic, some multinucleated cells (MGG). (Inset i) CD30-positive cells. (Inset ii) CD3-positive cells (LSAB).

Fig. 7.59 Primary cutaneous anaplastic ALK-positive large cell lymphoma. Large anaplastic cells with anisocytosis and anisonucleosis (MGG). (Inset i) CD30-positive cells. (Inset ii) Strong positivity for CD4 (LSAB).

Fig. 7.60 Leukaemic phase of anaplastic large cell lymphoma. (A,B) Atypical large anaplastic lymphoid cells with lobulated nuclei and prominent nucleoli in peripheral blood smears (MGG). (C) CD30-positive cells. (D) Negative for CD3. (E) CD20 and (F) CD15 (polymorphs positive for CD15) (LSAB).

Hodgkin lymphoma

According to WHO classification, Hodgkin lymphoma comprises two disease entities (see Table 7.3):

- Nodular lymphocyte predominant Hodgkin lymphoma (NLPHL)
- Classic Hodgkin lymphoma (CHL) which includes four subtypes:
    - nodular sclerosis (CNS)
    - mixed cellularity (CMC)
    - lymphocyte-rich (CLR)
    - lymphocyte-depleted (CLD)

Cytological findings and immunophenotype of NLPHL

- Monoclonal B-cell neoplasm
- Infiltrate of small lymphocytes, histiocytes and epithelioid histiocytes
- LP cells – popcorn (large cell with large multilobated nucleus, multiple basophilic nucleoli and scant cytoplasm)
- Immunophenotype: CD20+, CD45+, PAX5+, BCL6+, OCT2+, CD79a+, CD15–, CD30–

Cytological findings and immunophenotype of CHL (Fig. 7.61)

- Rich inflammatory background (depends on histological subtype): lymphocytes, histiocytes, epithelioid histiocytes and eosinophils
- Classic diagnostic Reed–Sternberg cells: large bi- or multinucleated cells with large prominent basophilic nucleoli
- Mononuclear Hodgkin cells
- Immunophenotype: CD30+, CD15+/–, CD45–, CD20–/+, PAX5(+)/–, OCT2+/–, EBER+/–, CD3–

Differential diagnosis

- Diffuse large B-cell lymphoma
- T-cell rich diffuse large B-cell lymphoma
- Anaplastic large cell lymphoma

Table 7.3 Immunocytochemistry panel that helps distinguish between Classic and NLP Hodgkin lymphoma

Immunocytochemistry	Classic HL	NLPHL
CD30	Positive (nearly all cases)	Negative
CD15	Positive (75%)	Negative
CD45	Negative	Positive
CD20	Negative	
J chain CD75	Negative	Positive in nearly all cases
BCL 6	Negative	Positive
EMA	Negative	Positive in approx half

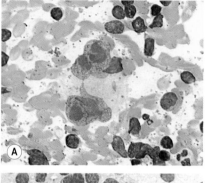
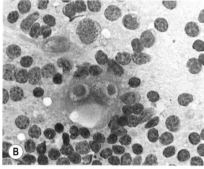
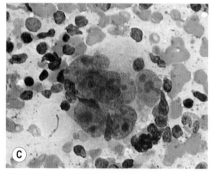
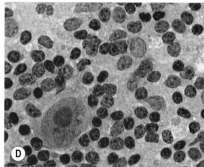
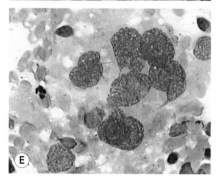

Fig. 7.61 Types of Reed–Sternberg cells. (A) Diagnostic multilobated classic. (B) Diagnostic bilobated. (C) Popcorn cell with folded and extreme multilobated. (D) Mononuclear Hodgkin cell. (E) Pleomorphic LD forms (MGG).

Immunodeficiency-associated lymphoproliferative disorders

Lymphoma associated with HIV infection

These lymphomas include Burkitt's lymphoma, diffuse large B-cell lymphoma (DLBCL), primary effusion lymphoma (PEL), plasmablastic lymphoma and Hodgkin lymphoma (HL).

Cytological findings (Figs 7.62–7.65)

- Depend of type of lymphoma:
  - Burkitt's lymphoma – 2/3 cases have plasmacytoid differentiation
  - DLBCL – 90% of cases are the immunoblastic variant
  - Hodgkin lymphoma – classic HL (mixed cellularity, lymphocytes depleted or nodular sclerosis)
  - PEL – plasmablastic variant

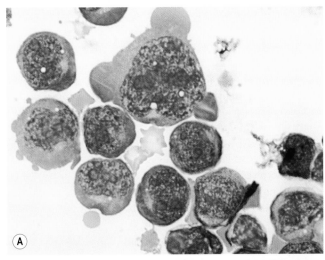
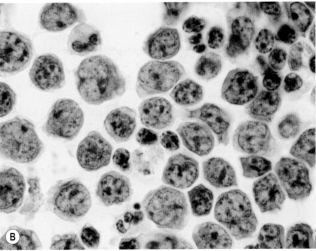

Fig. 7.64 Primary effusion lymphoma in HIV-positive patient. Large basophilic cells (MGG). (Inset) PAP staining shows irregular chromatin pattern and cell pleomorphism.

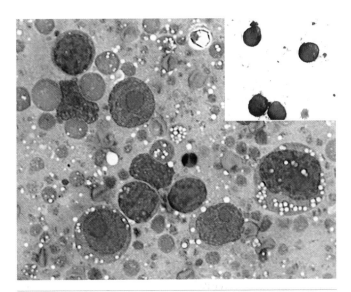

Fig. 7.62 FNA of diffuse large cell lymphoma in cervical lymph node in HIV-positive patient. Immunoblastic subtype with large cells with prominent nucleoli (MGG). (Inset) CD20-positive cells (LSAB).

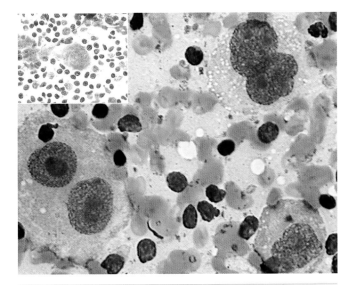

Fig. 7.63 Hodgkin lymphoma in HIV-positive patient (FNA of inguinal lymph node). Smear includes typical Reed–Sternberg cells (MGG). (Inset) CD30-positive Reed–Sternberg cell (LSAB).

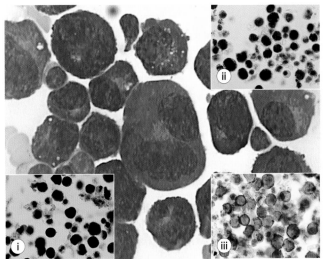

Fig. 7.65 Primary effusion lymphoma – plasmablastic variant – in HIV-positive patient. Strong basophilic atypical mono- and binucleated lymphoid cells. (Inset i) EBER-positive cells. (Inset ii) KSHV-positive cells. (Inset iii) CD 138- positive cells.

Post-transplant lymphoproliferative disorders (PTLD)

Post-transplant lymphoproliferative disorders may develop in post-transplant patients (due to transplantation of solid organs, bone marrow or stem cell allograft), after immunosuppression (HIV and non-HIV) and in the majority of patients with EBV infection. These disorders present either as:

- Early lesions (plasmacytic hyperplasia or infectious mononucleosis-like lesion)
- Polymorphic PTLD;
- Monomorphic PTLD (B- and T-cell lymphoma) or
- Classic Hodgkin lymphoma-type PTLD

Cytological findings (Figs 7.66–7.68)

Depend on the disease stage
- Early lesions – plasmacytic hyperplasia with plasma cells and small lymphocytes or infectious mononucleosis-like lesion with immunoblastic and plasma cell proliferation
- Polymorphic – with full range of B-cell maturation from immunoblasts to plasma cells admixed with small and medium-sized lymphocytes
- Monomorphic PTLD – B-cell (neoplasms with criteria for DLBCL, Burkitt's lymphoma, plasmacytoma or myeloma) or T-cell (peripheral T-cell lymphoma – NOS, hepatosplenic or other)
- Hodgkin lymphoma – classic HL (with CD30- and CD15-positive Reed–Sternberg cells)

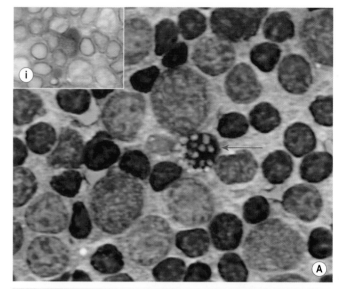

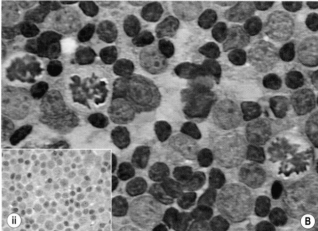

Fig. 7.67 Polymorphic PTLD – mixed proliferation of immunoblasts, plasma cells, small and medium-sized lymphocytes. (A) Mott cell (*arrow*) and (Inset i) numerous mitoses (MGG). (B) PAS-positive Mott cell (cytochemistry, ×1000). (Inset ii) CD20-positive cells (LSAB).

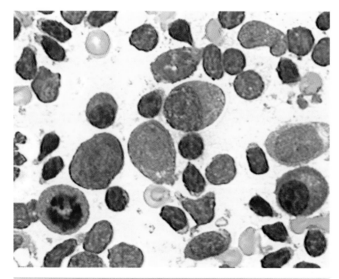

Fig. 7.66 Early lesion, infectious mononucleosis-like PTLD: mixed proliferation of immunoblasts, plasma cells, and small and medium-sized lymphocytes (MGG).

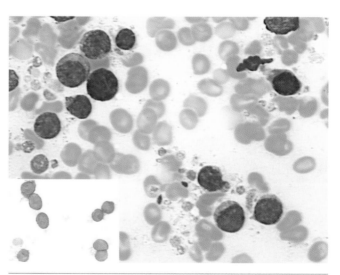

Fig. 7.68 Monomorphic PTLD. Diffuse large B-cell lymphoma (MGG). (Inset) CD20-positive large lymphoid cells (LSAB).

Lymph node metastases (Figs 7.69–7.77)

Fine needle aspiration (FNA) is a preferred method for evaluating a variety of pathologic processes in lymph node, including reactive changes, malignant or benign neoplasms and metastases. FNA has high sensitivity, specificity, and diagnostic accuracy in identification of the lymph node metastases as well as in determining a primary tumour site by immunocytochemistry.

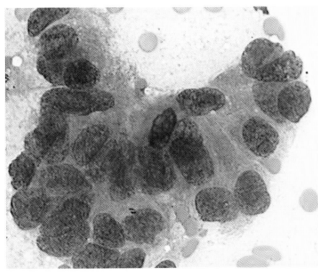

Fig. 7.71 Metastatic adenocarcinoma of colon shows palisading columnar cells (MGG).

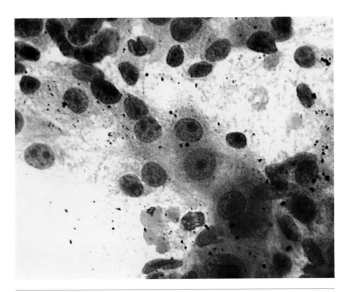

Fig. 7.69 Metastatic well-differentiated hepatocellular carcinoma in a cervical lymph node – cells similar to normal hepatocytes with slight atypia, visible nucleoli and biliary pigment in some cells (MGG). This is extremely rare.

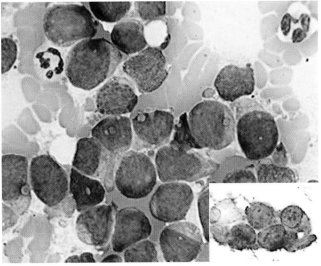

Fig. 7.72 Metastatic small cell carcinoma of the lung. The aspirate shows cohesive clusters of tumour cells with moulding effect (MGG). (Inset) BerEP4-positive malignant cells (LSAB).

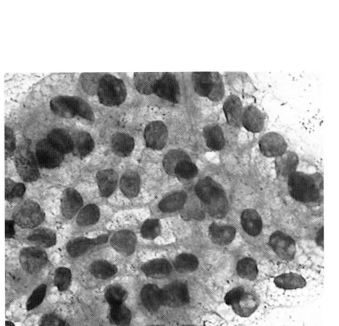

Fig. 7.70 FNA of cervical lymph node. Metastatic acinar cell carcinoma of the pancreas. Cohesive clusters of polygonal cells with round nuclei, similar to benign acinar cells (MGG). This is extremely rare.

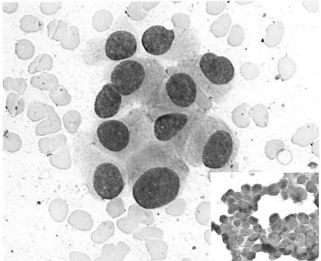

Fig. 7.73 FNA of intra-abdominal lymph node. Carcinoid tumour cells with round nuclei of variable size and polygonal, weakly granular cytoplasm (MGG) (Inset) Cells immunostained for chromogranin (LSAB).

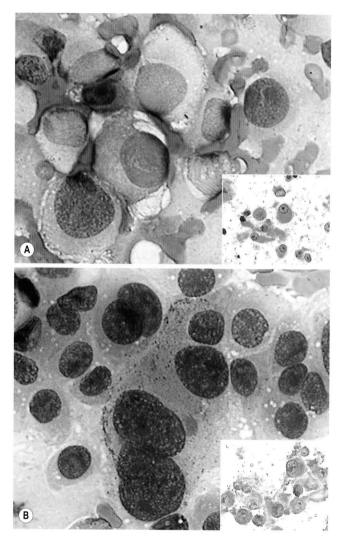

Fig. 7.74 FNA of cervical lymph nodes. (A) Metastatic amelanotic melanoma – large single cells with round eccentrically placed nuclei and abundant basophilic cytoplasm without visible pigment (MGG). (Inset) HMB45-positive large cells. (B) Melanotic melanoma – bi- and multinucleated cells with fine cytoplasmic vacuolation and cytoplasm pigment granules (MGG). (Inset) S100-positive malignant cells (LSAB).

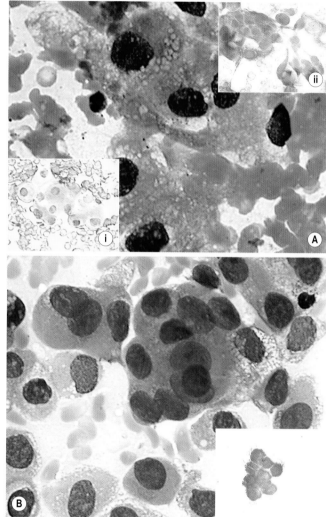

Fig. 7.76 Metastatic renal cell carcinoma (RCC). (A) FNA of cervical lymph node, clear cell RCC: cluster of uniform cells with small nuclei and abundant vacuolated cytoplasm (MGG). (Inset i) Oil red-positive cells (cytochemistry, ×400). (Inset ii) Vimentin-positive cells (LSAB). (B) FNA of intra-abdominal lymph node, chromophobe RCC: some clusters and isolated cells with well-defined borders (MGG). (Inset) Cells immunostained for pan-cytokeratin (LSAB).

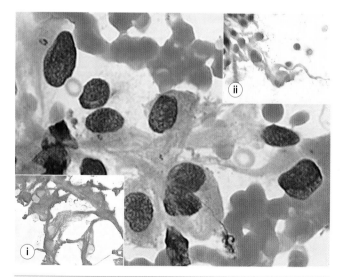

Fig. 7.75 Intra-abdominal lymph node. Leiomyosarcoma – cells with elongated abundant cytoplasm (MGG). (Inset i) Vimentin- and (Inset ii) SMA-positive malignant cells (LSAB).

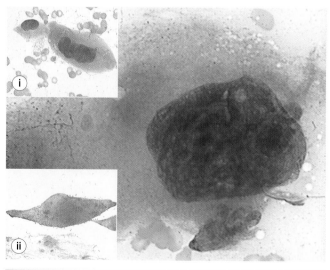

Fig. 7.77 Axillary lymph node. Metastatic malignant peripheral nerve sheath tumour (MPNS) – pleomorphic cells with large nuclei, prominent nucleoli (Inset i) and fibrillary, abundant cytoplasm (MGG). (Inset ii) Vimentin-positive cells (LSAB).

Myeloid neoplasms

The World Health Organization (WHO) classification of myeloid neoplasms (Table 7.4) is based on morphology, cytochemistry and immunophenotype to establish their lineage and degree of maturation, and to decide whether proliferation is cytologically normal or dysplastic, effective or ineffective. These findings are presented together with the genetic or molecular and clinical findings in an integrated report.

Table 7.4 WHO classification of myeloid neoplasms

Myeloproliferative neoplasms	Chronic myelogenous leukaemia, *BCR/ABL* 1 positive
	Chronic neutrophilic leukaemia
	Polycythaemia vera
	Primary myelofibrosis
	Essential thrombocythaemia
	Chronic eosinophilic leukaemia, NOS
	Mastocytosis
	Myeloproliferative neoplasm, unclassifiable
Myelodysplastic/myeloproliferative neoplasms	Chronic myelomonocytic leukaemia
	Atypical chronic myeloid leukaemia, *BCR/ABL* 1 negative
	Juvenile myelomonocytic leukaemia
	Myelodysplastic/myeloproliferative neoplasm, unclassifiable
Myelodysplastic syndromes	Refractory cytopenia with unilineage dysplasia
	Refractory anaemia with ring sideroblasts
	Refractory cytopenia with multilineage dysplasia
	Refractory anaemia with excess blasts
	Myelodysplastic syndrome associated with isolated del(5Q)
	Childhood Myelodysplastic syndrome
Acute myeloid leukaemia (AML)	AML with recurrent genetic abnormalities
	AML with t(8;21) – *RUNX1-RUNX1T1*
	AML with inv(16) or t(16;16) – *CBFB-MYH11*
	Acute promyelocytic leukaemia with t(15;17) – *PML-RARA*
	AML with t(9;11) – *MLLT3-MLL*
	AML with t(6;9) – *DEK-NUP214*
	AML with inv(3) or t(3;3) – *RPN1-EVI1*
	AML (megakaryoblastic) with t(1;22) – *RBM15-MKL1*
	Other
	AML with Myelodysplastic-related changes
	Therapy-related myeloid neoplasms
	Acute myeloid leukaemia, NOS
	AML with minimal differentiation
	AML without maturation
	AML with maturation
	Acute myelomonocytic leukaemia
	Acute monoblastic and monocytic leukaemia
	Acute erythroid leukaemia
	Acute megakaryoblastic leukaemia
	Acute basophilic leukaemia
	Acute panmyelosis with myelofibrosis
	Myeloid sarcoma
	Myeloid proliferation related to Down syndrome
	Blastic plasmacytoid dendritic neoplasm
Acute leukaemias of ambiguous lineage	

Chronic myeloid leukaemia, BCR-ABL 1 positive (CML)

Chronic myeloid leukaemia, BCR-ABL 1 positive, is a myeloproliferative neoplasm of abnormal pluripotent BM stems cell with abnormal BCR-ABL 1 fusion gene and consequently chromosomal abnormality – t(9;22) – Philadelphia chromosome (Ph). This disease includes the initial chronic phase, the accelerated and the blast phases.

Cytological findings (Figs 7.78–7.80)

- Chronic phase
  - hypercellular bone marrow aspirate due to neutrophilic proliferation with all stages of maturation, prominent eosinophils and smaller megakaryocytes (often mononuclear forms)
  - 'megakaryocyte rich' cases have numerous megakaryocytes in BM and greater platelet count in PB ($>1000\times10^9$/L)
  - leukocytosis due to neutrophils in all stages of maturation, without significant dysplasia, blasts <2%, prominent eosinophilia and basophilia, usually <3% monocytes
- Accelerated phase
  - 10–19% myeloblasts in BM or PB; $\geq$20% basophils in PB: additional chromosomal abnormalities; increasing splenomegaly; persistent or increasing platelets ($>1000\times10^9$/L) or WBC count during therapy
- Blast phase
  - $\geq$20% blasts (neutrophilic, basophilic, eosinophilic, megakaryocytic, monocytic, erythroid or lymphoblastic) in PB or of the nucleated cells of BM

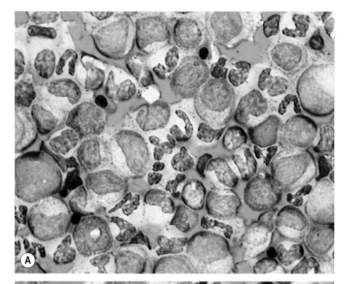

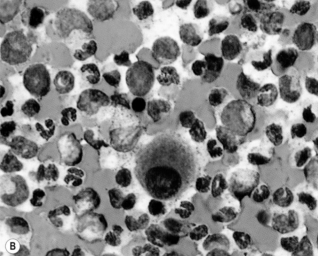

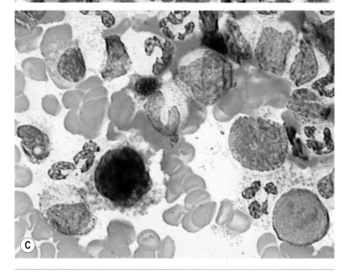

Fig. 7.78 Chronic myeloid leukaemia, *BCR-ABL 1* positive. (A) Hypercellular bone marrow smear with granulocytic proliferation in different stages. (B,C) Mononuclear form of megakaryocytes (MGG).

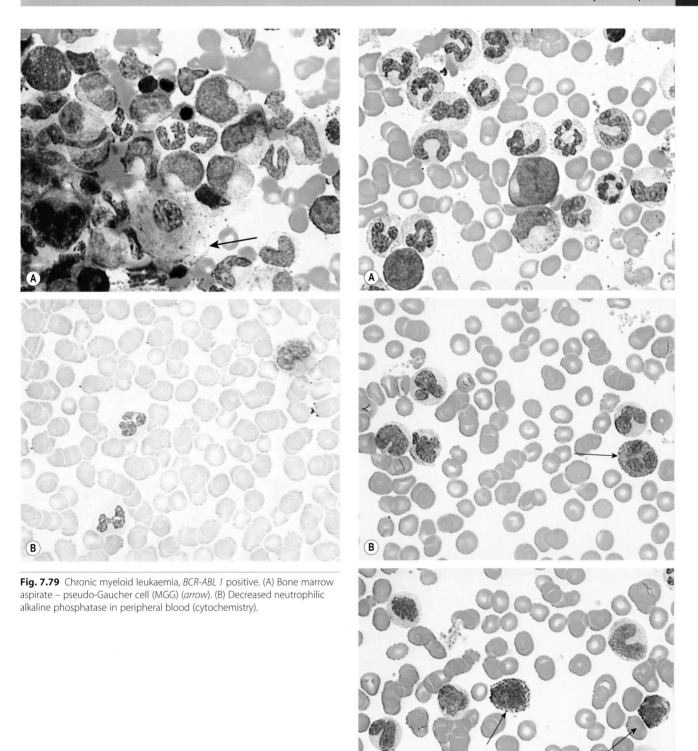

Fig. 7.79 Chronic myeloid leukaemia, *BCR-ABL 1* positive. (A) Bone marrow aspirate – pseudo-Gaucher cell (MGG) (*arrow*). (B) Decreased neutrophilic alkaline phosphatase in peripheral blood (cytochemistry).

Fig. 7.80 Chronic myeloid leukaemia, *BCR-ABL 1* positive. (A) Peripheral blood smears – leucocytosis due to neutrophils with all stages of maturation without significant dysplasia. (B) Increased number of eosinophils (*arrow*) and (C) basophils (*arrows*) (MGG).

Polycythaemia vera (PV)

Polycythaemia vera is a myeloproliferative neoplasm with primarily a proliferation of red blood cells, independent of the mechanisms that normally regulate erythropoiesis, which include the pre-polycythaemic, overt polycythaemic and post-polycythaemic myelofibrosis phases.

Cytological findings (Fig. 7.81)

- Morphological findings of BM and PB must be correlated with other clinical and laboratory findings (JAK2 mutation, serum erythropoietin level, bone marrow biopsy)
- Pre-polycythaemic and overt polycythaemic phase
  - effective proliferation of erythroid, granulocytic and megakaryocytic lineages – panmyelosis – in BM and PB
  - megakaryocytes show increased pleomorphism without maturation defects (nuclear/cytoplasmic ratio differentiation)
- 'Spent' or post-polycythaemic myelofibrosis phase
  - abnormal megakaryocytic proliferation and depletion of erythroid and granulocytic lineages
  - leukoerythroblastosis in peripheral blood smear with numerous teardrop-shaped red blood cells
  - elevated leukocytic alkaline phosphatase

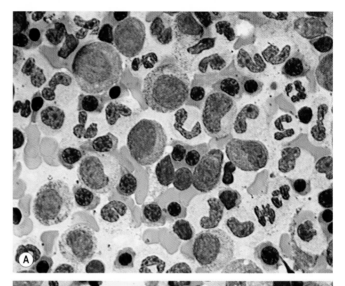

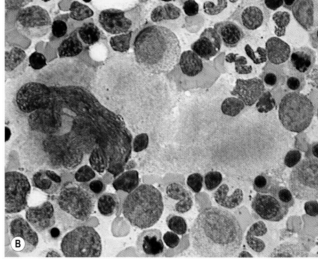

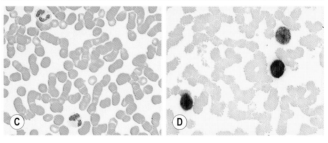

Fig. 7.81 Polycythaemia vera. (A) Bone marrow shows proliferation of erythroid and granulocytic cells. (B) Atypical, pleomorphic megakaryocyte. (C) Peripheral blood smear – normochromic and normocytic 'sticky' erythrocytes (MGG). (D) Increased expression of leukocytic alkaline phosphatase (cytochemistry).

Primary myelofibrosis (PM)

Primary myelofibrosis is a myeloproliferative neoplasm with proliferation of megakaryocytic and granulocytic lineage, reactive deposition of fibrous tissue in the bone marrow, and extramedullary haemopoiesis with consequent splenomegaly.

Cytological findings (Figs 7.82–7.83)

- Bone marrow
  - cellularity depends on stage of the disease (prefibrotic or fibrotic)
  - usually is hypocellular with abnormal megakaryocytes, clusters ('nests') of erythroid precursors and mild left shift in granulopoiesis (but metamyelocytes, bands and segmented forms predominate)
- Peripheral blood
  - leukoerythroblastocytosis and anisopoikilocytosis-dacryocytes: red blood cell with a single, tear-shaped spicule; observed in fragmentation anaemia and myelofibrosis
- Spleen
  - infiltration by erythroid, granulocytic and megakaryocytic precursors

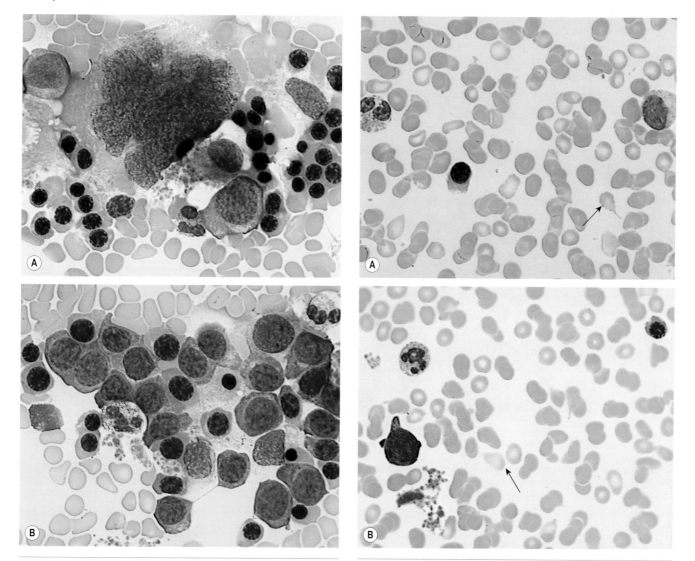

Fig. 7.82 Primary myelofibrosis. (A) Bone marrow aspirate with abnormal megakaryocyte and clusters of erythroid precursors. (B) Nests of erythroid precursors (MGG).

Fig. 7.83 Primary myelofibrosis. (A,B) Peripheral blood smears. Leukoerythroblastocytosis with anisopoikilocytosis and dacryocytes (*arrows*) (MGG).

Essential thrombocythaemia (ET)

Essential thrombocythaemia is a myeloproliferative neoplasm with primarily proliferation of megakaryocytic lineage and sustained thrombocytosis amounting to $\geq 450 \times 10^9$/L.

Cytological findings (Fig. 7.84)

- Bone marrow
  - proliferation of large to giant forms of megakaryocytes with lobulated and hyperlobulated nuclei
  - megakaryocytes show increased pleomorphism with maturation defects (nuclear/cytoplasmic ratio differentiation)
  - phenomenon of emperipolesis (active penetration by one cell into and through a larger cell: in ET, the incorporation of other marrow cells, mostly erythroblasts and granulocytes, into megakaryocytes)
  - no significant increase in erythropoiesis and granulopoiesis
- Peripheral blood
  - thrombocytosis with anisocytosis and atypical giant platelets
  - white blood cell count and leukocyte differential count are normal, or slightly elevated WBC
  - basophilia absent or minimal
  - leukocytic alkaline phosphatase is usually elevated
- Red blood cells are normal or microcytic

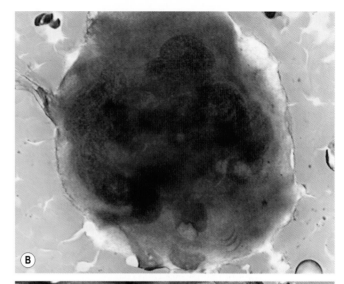

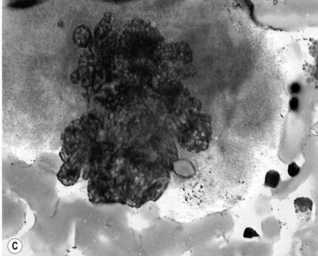

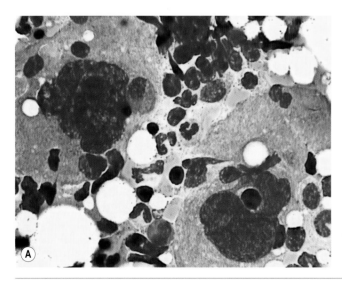

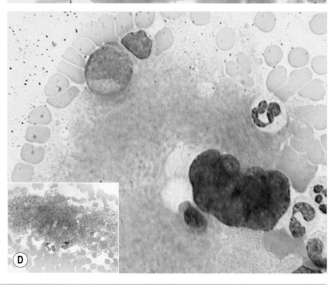

Fig. 7.84 Essential thrombocythaemia. (A) Bone marrow aspirate shows megakaryocytes increased in number and size. (B,C) Large, giant multinuclear form of megakaryocytes. (D) Phenomenon of emperipolesis: erythroblast and granulocytes in the cytoplasm of the megakaryocyte. (D, Inset) Aggregates of thrombocytes in peripheral blood smear (MGG).

Chronic eosinophilic leukaemia, not otherwise specified (CEL-NOS)

Chronic eosinophilic leukaemia is a myeloproliferative neoplasm with clonal, autonomous proliferation of eosinophils in BM, PB and peripheral tissues and <20% blasts in PB or BM.

Cytological findings (Figs 7.85–7.86)

- Bone marrow
  - hypercellular with eosinophilic proliferation
  - increased number of myeloblasts (5–19%) supports diagnosis of CEL
  - Charcot–Leyden crystals are often present
- Peripheral blood
  - mature and small number of immature eosinophils are present
  - eosinophil abnormalities including sparse granulation, cytoplasmic vacuolation, nuclear hyper- or hyposegmentation
  - neutrophilia, mild basophilia and monocytosis may be present
  - blasts may also be present, but less than 20%

Differential diagnosis

- Idiopathic hypereosinophilic syndrome
  - without an increase in blast cells
  - eosinophilia $\geq 1.5 \times 10^9$/L persisting for at least 6 months
  - involvement and dysfunction of organs
  - without evidence of clonality

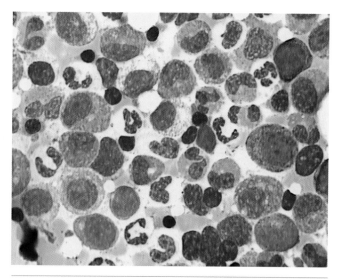

Fig. 7.85 Chronic eosinophilic leukaemia, not otherwise specified. Bone marrow aspirate consists of immature and mature eosinophils (MGG).

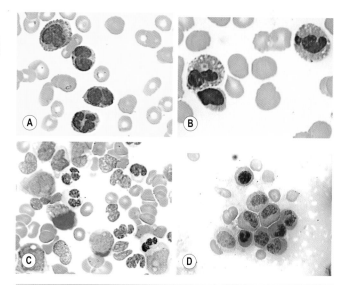

Fig. 7.86 Chronic eosinophilic leukaemia, not otherwise specified. Peripheral blood smears. (A,B) Abnormal mature and immature eosinophils (MGG). (C) ASD-chloroacetate-positive eosinophils in bone marrow. (D) peripheral blood smears (cytochemistry).

Mastocytosis

Mastocytosis is a heterogeneous group of disorders (cutaneous, indolent or aggressive systemic mastocytosis, mast cell leukaemia, mast cell sarcoma and extracutaneous mastocytoma), with clonal proliferation of mast cells.

Cytological findings (Fig. 7.87)

- Clustered or diffuse pattern of mast cells depend on type of mastocytosis
- Medium-sized or oval cells with round or oval nuclei, plentiful cytoplasm containing toluidine blue-positive metachromatic granules
- Atypical immature mast cells (metachromatic blast cells) are present in mast cell leukaemia
- Cytomorphological atypia, bi- or multinucleated nuclei, and mitotic figures all point to an aggressive mast cell proliferation

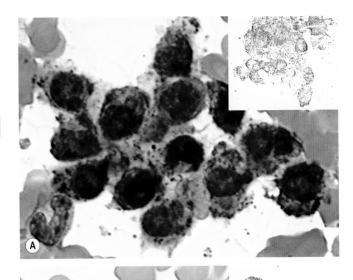

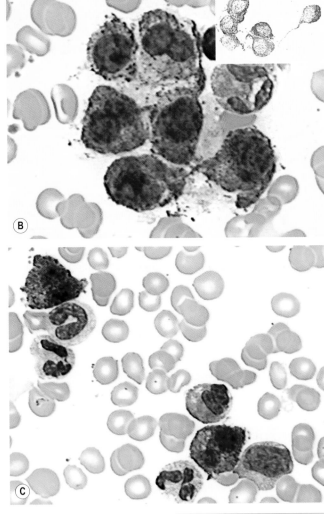

Fig. 7.87 Mastocytosis. (A) FNA of lymph node shows cluster of mast cells (MGG). (Inset) Toluidine blue-positive reaction of metachromatic granules in lymph node smear. (B) Bone marrow aspirate with metachromatic granules (MGG). (Inset) Cohesive infiltrates of mast cells positive for toluidine blue on bone marrow smear. (C) Atypical mast cells in peripheral blood smear (MGG).

Chronic myelomonocytic leukaemia (MDS/MPN-CMML)

Chronic myelomonocytic leukaemia comprises approximately 30% of all cases of MDS/MPN, and is characterised by features of both MDS and MPN.

Cytological findings (Fig. 7.88)

- Monocytosis in PB, $>1 \times 10^9$/L
- Monocytes are always >10% of WBC
- Lack of *BCR/ABL* gene or Ph chromosome
- Blasts (which include myeloblasts, monoblasts and promonocytes) are <20% of all nucleated cells in BM and PB
- Dysplasia in one or more myeloid lineages
- Lack of rearrangement of PDGFRA or PDGFRB

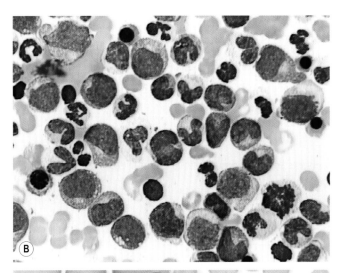

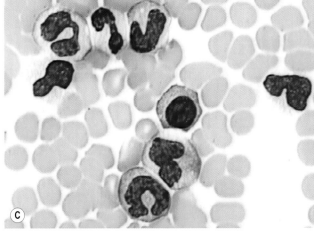

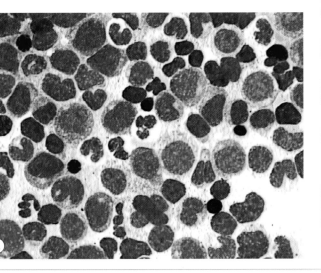

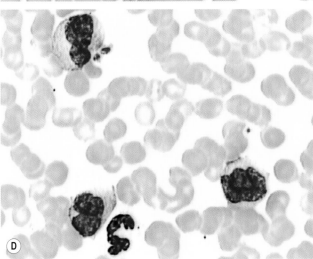

Fig. 7.88 Chronic myelomonocytic leukaemia. (A,B) Bone marrow aspirate with dysplastic granulocytic cells and increased monocytic component. (C,D) Peripheral blood smears show monocytosis (MGG).

Juvenile myelomonocytic leukaemia (MDS/MPN-JMML)

Juvenile myelomonocytic leukaemia comprises approximately 20–30% of all cases of MDS/MPN in children <14 years (75% of cases in patients <3 years of age) and 2–3% of all children's acute leukaemia in children.

Cytological findings (Figs 7.89–7.90)

- Blasts and promonocytes <20% of nucleated cells in BM and PB
- Monocytosis in PB, $>1 \times 10^9$/L
- Lack of *BCR/ABL* gene or Ph chromosome
- Two or more of the following criteria:
  - WBC count $>10 \times 10^9$/L
  - granulocytic precursors in PB
  - increased synthesis of haemoglobin F
  - chromosomal abnormalities
  - aberrant molecular mutation of the RAS/MAPK signalling pathway

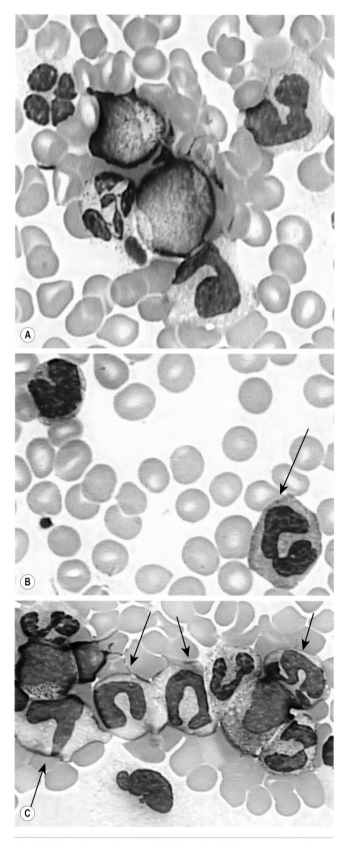

Fig. 7.90 Juvenile myelomonocytic leukaemia. (A,B) Bone marrow aspirate – monocytes are a prominent component (*arrow*). (C) Monocytosis in peripheral blood smear (*arrows*) (MGG).

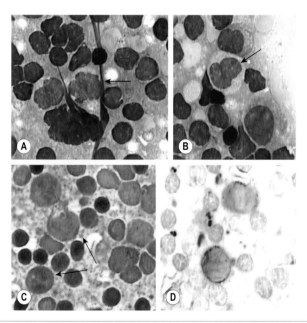

Fig. 7.89 Juvenile myelomonocytic leukaemia. (A,B) Lymph node aspirate with infiltration of monocytes (*arrow*) (MGG). (C) CD68-positive monocytes (*arrows*) (immunocytochemistry, LSAB). (D) Cells positive for non-specific esterase (cytochemistry).

Myelodysplatic/myeloproliferative neoplasms, unclassifiable (MDS/MPN-U)

Unclassifiable myelodysplastic/myeloproliferative neoplasms are characterised by dysplastic changes and effective proliferation, both in one or more myeloid lineages without criteria for other MDS/MPN categories.

Cytological findings (Fig. 7.91)

- Clinical, laboratory and morphological features with overlapping MDS and MPN criteria
- *De novo* disease, without history of underlying MPN or of MDS
- Thrombocytosis $\geq 450 \times 10^9$/L, or leukocytosis $\geq 13 \times 10^9$/L
- Blasts represent <20% in PB and BM
- Simultaneous presentation of proliferative and dysplastic features in at least one cell line
- Lack of cytogenetic or molecular abnormalities specific for this group
- Sometimes *JAK2 V617F* mutation may help for diagnosis of haematological neoplasm

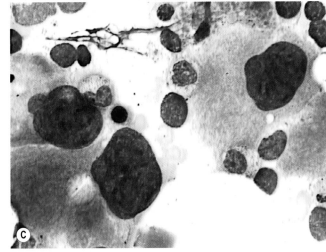

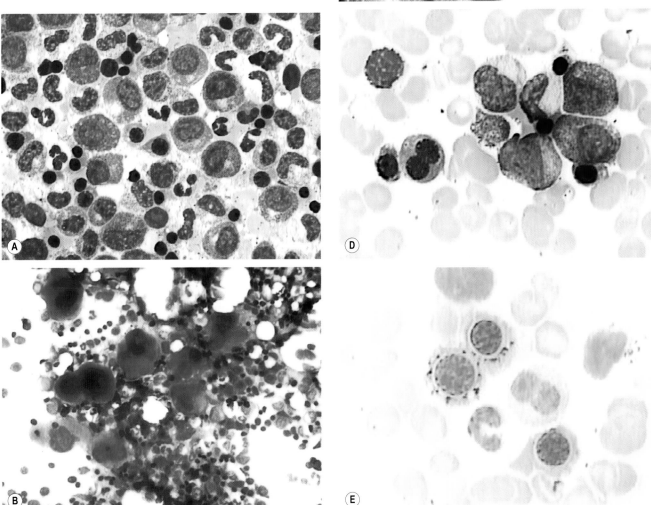

Fig. 7.91 Myelodysplastic/myeloproliferative neoplasms – unclassifiable. (A) Hypercellular bone marrow aspirate. (B,C) Increased number of abnormal megakaryocytes. (D) Presence of abnormal erythroid precursors (MGG) and (E) ring sideroblasts (cytochemistry).

Refractory cytopenia with unilineage dysplasia (RCUD)

Refractory cytopenia with unilineage dysplasia comprises approximately 10–20% of all cases of MDS, and includes refractory anaemia (RA), refractory neutropenia (RN) and refractory thrombocytopenia (RT).

Cytological findings (Fig. 7.92)

- Refractory anaemia (RA)
  - dyserythropoiesis of ≥10% erythroid precursors in BM including karyorrhexis, multinucleation, nuclear megaloblastoid changes, vacuolated cytoplasm
  - none or minimal dysplasia of neutrophils and megakaryocytes
- Refractory neutopenia (RN)
  - ≥10% dysplastic neutrophils in the BM or PB including cytoplasmic hypogranulation and nuclear hypolobulation
  - <10% dysplastic changes of erythroid and thrombocytic precursors
- Refractory thrombocytopenia (RT)
  - ≥dysplastic megakaryocytes showing hypolobulation, binucleation or multinucleation and presence of micromegakaryocytes
  - <10% dysplastic changes of other myeloid cell lines

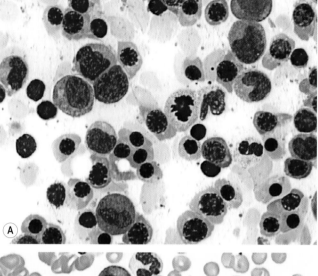
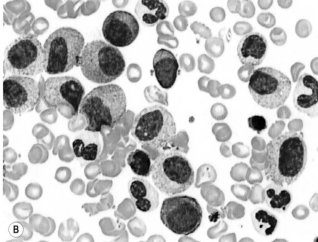
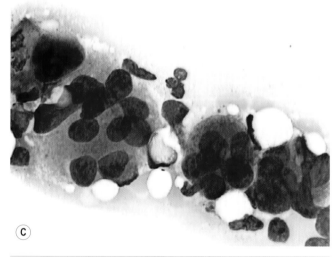

Fig. 7.92 Refractory cytopenia with unilineage dysplasia. (A) Bone marrow aspirate. Dysplastic features in erythroid precursors (RA). (B) Hypogranulation and hypolobulation of neutrophils known as pseudo-Pelger anomaly or 'pince-nez' bilobed appearance of neutrophils (RN). (C) Multinucleation of megakaryocytes (RT) (MGG).

Refractory anaemia with ring sideroblasts (RARS)

Refractory anaemia with ring sideroblasts comprises approximately 3–11% of all cases of MDS. It is characterised by abnormal iron deposits in erythroid precursors.

Cytological findings (Figs 7.93–7.94)

- Erythroid proliferation with dysplastic erythroblasts: macroblastosis, megaloblastosis, nuclear lobulation, multinucleation
- ≥15% of BM erythroid precursors are ring sideroblasts
- <10% dysplastic granulocytes and megakaryocytes
- <5% of all nucleated BM cells are myeloblasts
- Abundant haemosiderin-laden macrophages

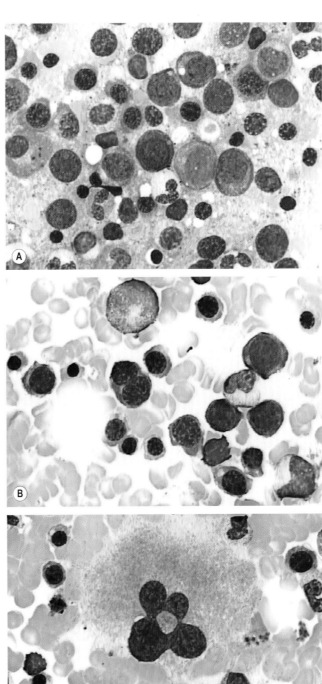

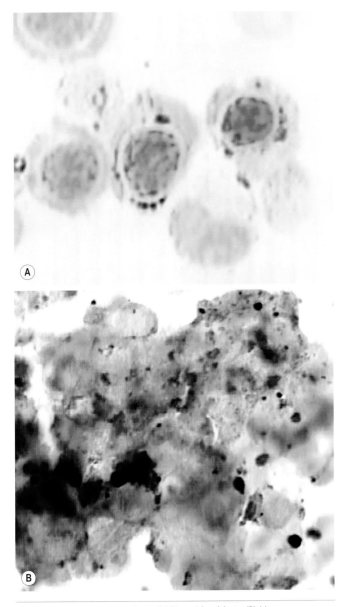

Fig. 7.93 Bone marrow aspirate. (A) Ring sideroblasts. (B) Many siderophages and extracellular iron, iron stain (cytochemistry).

Fig. 7.94 Bone marrow aspirate. (A) Erythroid proliferation. (B) Dysplastic features in erythroid precursors: macro- and megaloblastoid changes, binucleation. (C) Normal granulocytes and megakaryocytes (MGG).

Refractory cytopenia with multilineage dysplasia (RCMD)

Refractory cytopenia with multilineage dysplasia comprises approximately 30% of all cases of MDS and occurs in patients between 70 and 80 years of age.

Cytological findings (Fig. 7.95)

- BM is hypercellular
- <5% blasts in BM
- Dyserythro- dysgranulo- and dysthrombocytopoiesis
- Diffuse or granular cytoplasmic positivity of erythroid precursors
- Presentation of Pappenheimer bodies* in peripheral blood and ring sideroblasts in BM smears

*Pappenheimer bodies are abnormal granules of iron found inside red blood cells on routine blood stain. They are a type of inclusion body formed by phagosomes that have engulfed excessive amounts of iron. They appear as dense, blue-purple granules within the red blood cell and there are usually only one or two, located in the cell periphery. They are seen in diseases such as sideroblastic anaemia, haemolytic anaemia, and sickle cell disease as well as in the condition described here. They can interfere with platelet counts when the analysis is performed by electro-optical counters.

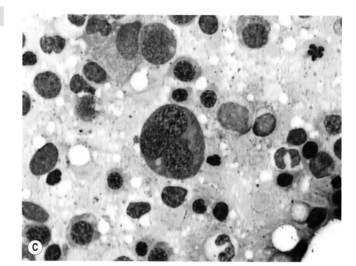

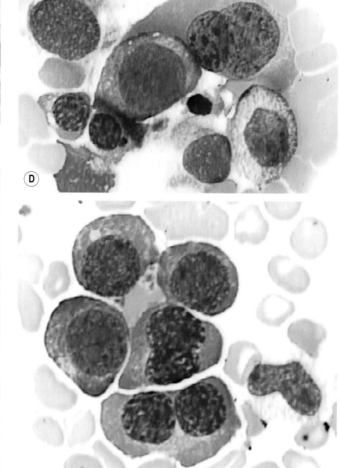

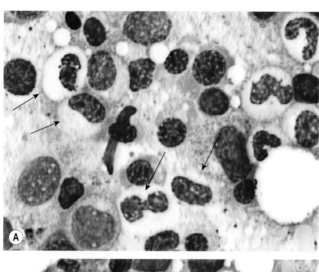

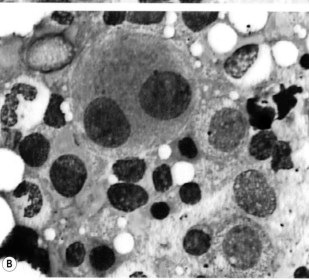

Fig. 7.95 Bone marrow aspirate. (A) Dysplastic features in granulocytic precursors: hypolobulation and hypogranulation (*arrows*). (B) Binucleation of megakaryocytes. (C,D,E) Multinucleation, macro- and megaloblastoid changes of erythroid precursors (MGG, × 1000).

Refractory anaemia with excess blasts (RAEB)

Refractory anaemia with excess blasts comprises approximately 40% of all cases of MDS, and is of unknown aetiology. Patients present with anaemia, thrombocytopenia and neutropenia.

Cytological findings (Figs 7.96–7.97)

- Usually hypercellular BM. In a minority of cases, normocellular or hypocellular BM
- Dyserythro- dysgranulo- and dysthrombocytopoiesis are present and show variable degrees of dysplasia
- The number of blasts is increased
  - 5–9% in the BM or 2–4% in PB of RAEB-1
  - 10–19% in the BM or PB of RAEB-2
- RAEB with fibrosis
  - significant degree of reticulin fibrosis
  - dysplasia in at least two cell lineages

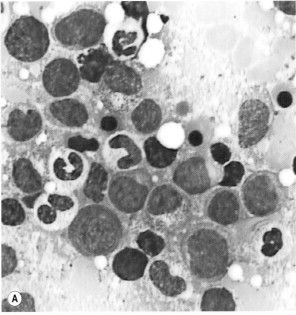

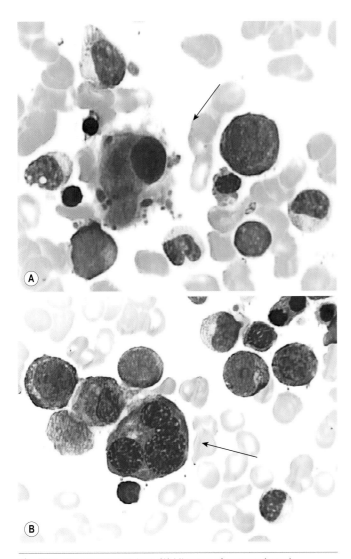

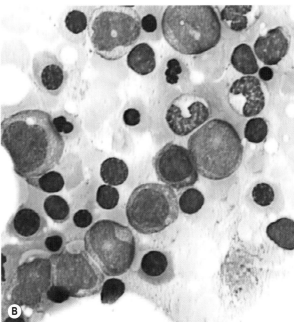

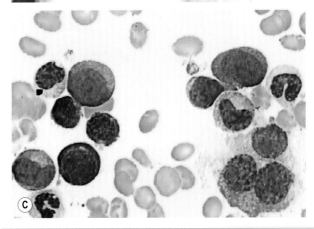

Fig. 7.96 Bone marrow aspirate. (A) Micromegakaryocyte (*arrow*). (B) Multinucleation of erythroblasts (*arrow*) (MGG).

Fig. 7.97 Bone marrow aspirate. (A,B,C) Increased number of blasts (MGG).

Myelodysplastic syndrome with isolated del(5q)

Myelodysplastic syndrome with isolated del(5q) is very rare. It includes anaemia with or without leukopenia and with or without thrombocytosis.

Cytological findings (Fig. 7.98)

- Normal or dysplastic megakaryocytes with hypolobated or non-lobated nuclei
- Erythroid and granulocytic dysplasia are uncommon
- <1% blasts in PB smears
- <5% blasts in BM smears
- Auer rods* are absent

*Auer rods are clumps of azurophilic granular material that form elongated needles seen in the cytoplasm of leukaemic blasts. They can be seen in the leukaemic blasts of M2 and M3 acute myeloid leukaemia and in high-grade myelodysplastic syndromes and myeloproliferative syndromes. They are composed of fused lysosomes/primary neutrophilic granules and contain peroxidase, lysosomal enzymes, and large crystalline inclusions. They are also used to distinguish the pre-leukaemia myelodysplastic syndromes: refractory anaemia with excess blasts 2 (which has Auer rods) from RAEB 1 (which does not) (see p. 225).

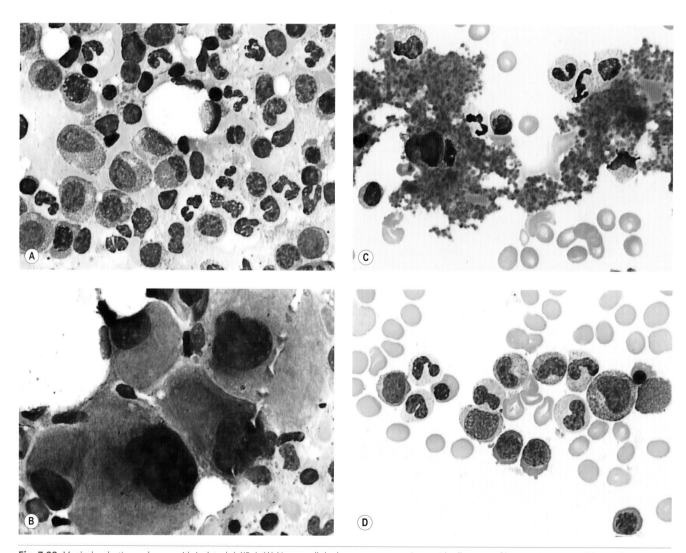

Fig. 7.98 Myelodysplastic syndrome with isolated del(5q). (A) Normocellular bone marrow aspirate with all stages of haemocytopoiesis. (B) Megakaryocytes with non-lobated and hypolobated nuclei. (C) Aggregates of platelet. (D) Erythroblasts and granulocytes without dysplasia (MGG).

Myelodysplastic syndrome, unclassifiable (MDS-U)

Myelodysplastic syndrome, unclassifiable is MDS with unknown incidence, which lacks findings for classification into a known MDS category.

Cytological findings (Fig. 7.99)

- Hyper- or normocellular BM
- No specific morphological findings
- Pancytopenia in cases of MDS with unilineage dysplasia
- RCUD with 1% blasts in PB
- Persistent cytopenia(s) without increased number of blasts, dysplasia in less than 10% of cells in one or more myeloid lineages and with cytogenetic abnormalities which are characteristic for MDS

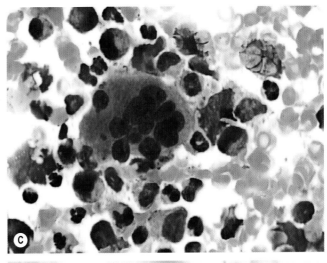

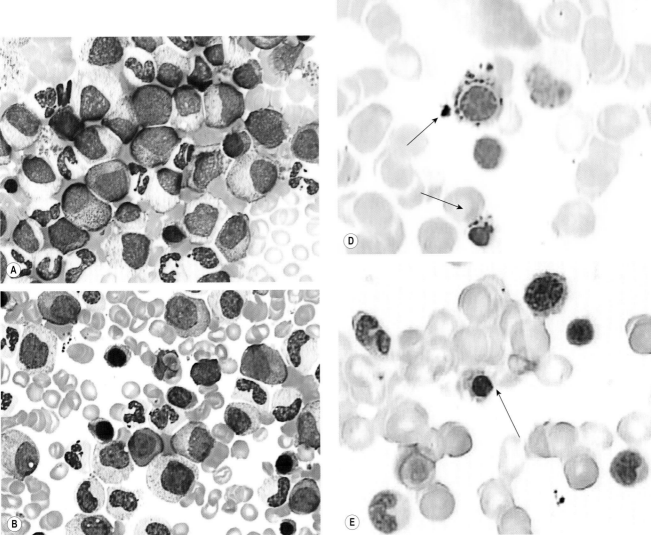

Fig. 7.99 Myelodysplastic syndrome, unclassifiable. (A) Normo/hypercellular smear of bone marrow aspirate shows: (B) hypogranulation and hypolobulation of neutrophils, (C) multinucleation of megakaryocytes (MGG), (D) ring sideroblasts (*arrows*) and (E) diffuse PAS-positive erythroblasts (*arrow*) (cytochemistry).

Refractory cytopenia of childhood (RCC)

Childhood myelodysplastic syndrome is very rare, representing <5% of all haematological neoplasms in children and includes many forms observed in adult patients with MDS.

Cytological findings (Fig. 7.100)

- Refractory cytopenia of childhood
  - cytopenia with <5% blasts in BM and <2% blasts in PB
  - dyserythrocytopoiesis (dysplastic and/or megaloblastoid changes in at least 10% of erythroid precursors; dysthrombocytopoiesis (micromegakaryocytes); dysgranulopoiesis (at least 10% dysplastic granulocytic precursor and <5% blasts in BM)
  - normo- or hypercellular BM aspirates, 5–10% hypocellular
  - differential diagnosis includes aplastic anaemia (in cases of hypocellular BM), paroxysmal nocturnal haemoglobinuria (PNH)

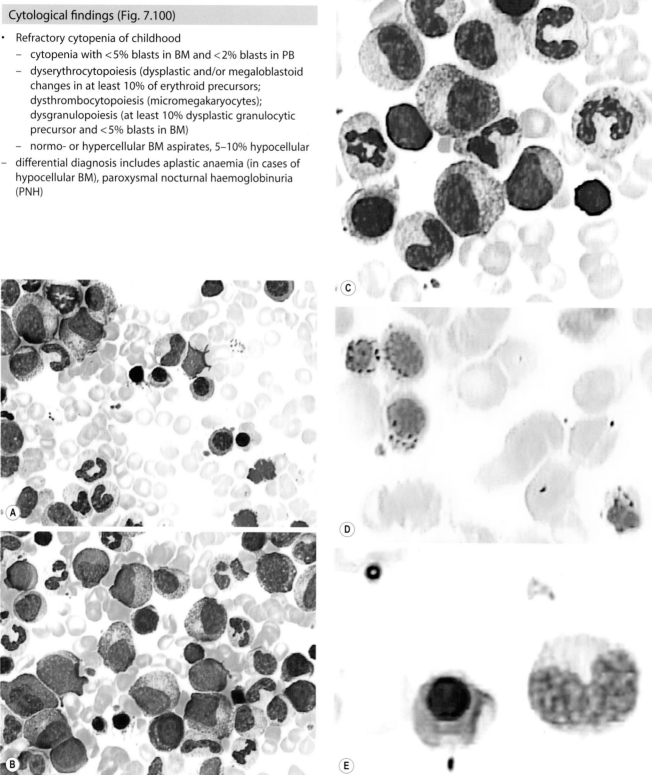

Fig. 7.100 Childhood myelodysplastic syndrome – refractory cytopenia of childhood. (A) Bone marrow aspirate with hypocellular smear with dysplastic granular and erythroid precursors. (B) Normocellular smear with slightly increased number of blasts, amounting to <5%. (C) Dysplastic features of neutrophils (MGG). (D) Abnormal sideroblasts and (E) PAS-positive erythroblast (cytochemistry).

Acute myeloid leukaemia

Acute myeloid leukaemia with recurrent genetic abnormalities – acute myeloid leukaemia with t(8;21)

Acute myeloid leukaemia with t(8;21) comprises approximately 5% of all cases of AML, and has maturation in the neutrophil lineage.

Cytological findings (Fig. 7.101)

- Abnormal blasts with myeloid differentiation
- Eosinophil precursors without cytological or cytochemical abnormalities
- Variable dysgranulopoiesis as hypogranulation and pseudo-Pelger–Hüet* anomalies
- Hypergranulation, presentation of pseudo-Chediak–Higashi granules** in large blasts with abundant basophilic cytoplasm and Auer rods*** in mature neutrophils
- With minimal or absent monocytic component
- Without dyserythropoiesis and dysthrombocytopoiesis

*Pelger–Hüet anomaly: Nucleus of a neutrophil is mature with 2 lobes connected by thin chromatin filament.
**Pseudo-Chediak–Higashi granules: Giant cytoplasmic inclusions in myeloblasts or myeloid precursors, resembling those seen in the Chediak–Higashi syndrome (CHS).
***Auer rods: See p. 224.

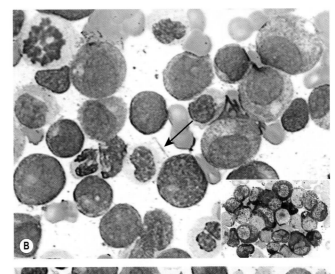

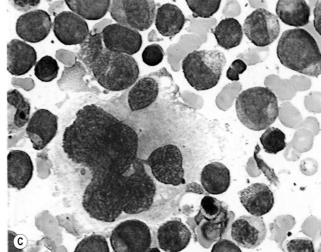

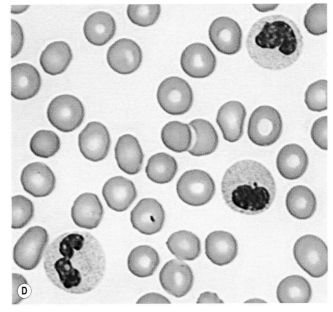

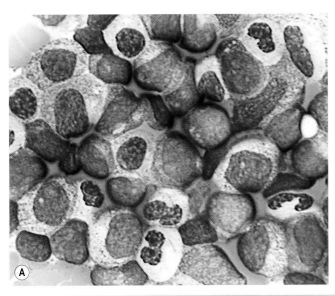

Fig. 7.101 Bone marrow aspirate. Acute myeloid leukaemia with t(8;21). (A,B) Myeloid blasts with maturation, hypogranulation of cytoplasm and Auer rods in mature neutrophils (*arrow*). (B, Inset) Myeloperoxidase cytochemically strong positive blasts. (C) Megakaryocytes are morphologically normal. (D) Peripheral blood smear with pseudo-Pelger–Hüet abnormalities*, namely bilobed neutrophils resembling spectacles, hence called 'pince-nez' cells, hypo- or hypergranulation of cytoplasm (MGG).

Acute myeloid leukaemia with recurrent genetic abnormalities – acute promyelocytic leukaemia (PML)

PML comprises 5–8% of AML; both hypergranular (typical) and microgranular (hypogranular) types are associated with disseminated intravascular coagulation. The leukocyte count is very high in microgranular APL, unlike typical APL with low leukocyte count.

Cytological findings (Fig. 7.102)

- Hypergranular (typical) type
    - irregular, kidney-shaped or bilobed nuclei
    - intense azurophilic granulation
    - Auer rods ('faggot cells') (see p. 224)
- Microgranular (hypogranular) type
    - bilobed, almost cerebriform nuclei
    - distinct small azurophilic granules (or submicroscopic size of the granules)
    - small number of typical abnormal promyelocytes with granules and/or Auer rods ('faggot cells')

Further investigations

- Strongly positive myeloperoxidase (MPO) – both types
- t(15;17)
- PML-RARA fusion gene
- Immunophenotype: HLA-DR–, CD34–/+, CD33+ (homogenous, bright), CD 13 (heterogeneous), CD117+/–, CD15–, CD56–

Differential diagnosis

- Acute basophilic leukaemia (hypergranular type of APL)
- Acute monocytic leukaemia (microgranular type of APL)

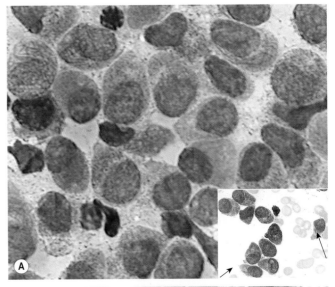

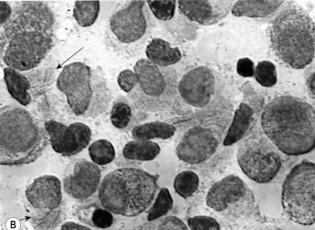

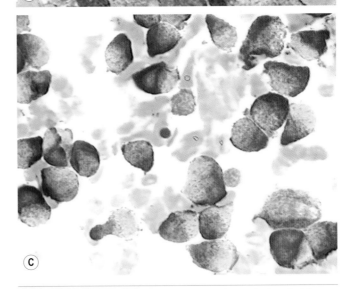

Fig. 7.102 Bone marrow aspirate. Acute promyelocytic leukaemia. (A) Hypergranular type with oval to round nuclei and numerous granules. (Inset) Hypergranular type with Auer rods (*arrows*) (MGG). (B) Hypergranular type with Auer rods (*arrows*) ('faggot cells'). (C) MPO-positive cells (cytochemistry).

Acute myeloid leukaemia with recurrent genetic abnormalities – acute myeloid leukaemia with inv(16) or t(16;16)

Acute myeloid leukaemia with inv(16) or t(16;16) comprises approximately 5–8% of all cases of AML, and consists of blasts with myelomonocytic differentiation and abnormal eosinophils.

Cytological findings (Figs 7.103–7.104)

- Morphological features like other cases of acute myelomonocytic leukaemia in bone marrow and peripheral blood
- Myeloid cells are positive for MPO (≥3%)
- Monoblasts and promonocytes show non-specific esterase (NSE) reactivity
- Variable number of eosinophils (usually increased, sometimes <5%) at all stages of maturation with immature eosinophilic granules
- In some eosinophils granules are basophilic coloured, positive for chloroacetate esterase (CAE)

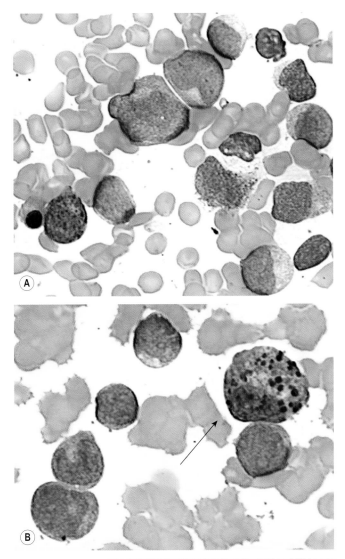

Fig. 7.103 Bone marrow aspirate. Acute myeloid leukaemia with inv(16) or t(16;16). (A,B) Myeloid blasts with monocytic component and abnormal eosinophils (*arrow*) (MGG).

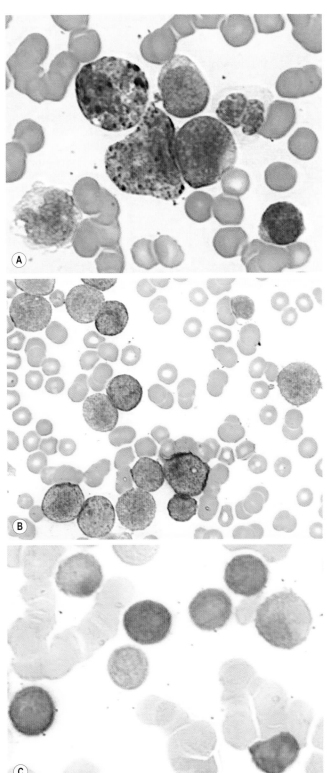

Fig. 7.104 Acute myeloid leukaemia with inv(16) or t(16;16). (A) Myeloid blasts and abnormal eosinophils with large coloured granules (MGG). (B) MPO-positive blasts. (C) NSE-positive blast cells (cytochemistry).

Acute myeloid leukaemia with myelodysplastic-related changes

Acute myeloid leukaemia with myelodysplastic-related changes comprises 24–35% of all cases of AML, and consists of ≥20% PB or BM blasts with myelodysplastic morphological features; prior history of MDS or MDS/MPN; MDS-related cytogenetic abnormalities without specific genetic abnormalities of AML with recurrent genetic abnormalities.

Cytological findings (Fig. 7.105)

- Cytological evidence of dysplasia in at least 50% of the cells in at least two BM cell lines
- Dyserythro-, dysgranulo- and dysthrombopoiesis are characterised by megaloblastosis, karyorrhexis, fragmentation or multinucleation of erythroblasts; hypogranulation, hyposegmentation (pseudo-Pelger–Hüet anomaly) of neutrophils*; micromegakaryocytosis or dysmegakaryocytosis with non-lobulated or multiple nuclei

*Pseudo-Pelger–Hüet anomaly: See p. 229.

Differential diagnosis

- Other types of AML such as acute megakaryoblastic leukaemia, acute erythroid leukaemia
- MDS-RAEB

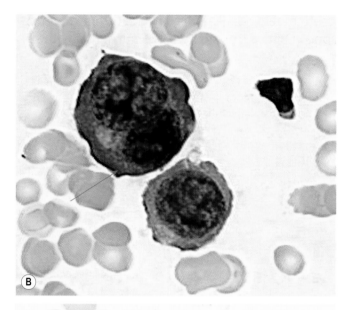
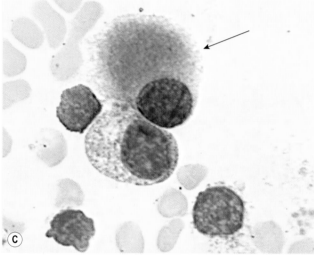
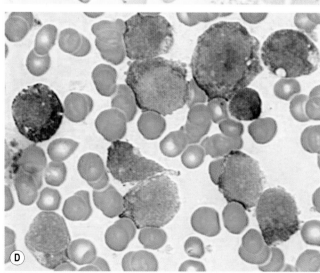
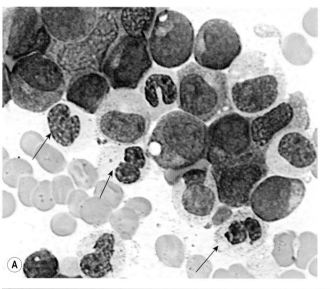

Fig. 7.105 Bone marrow aspirate. (A) Increased myeloblasts with features of dysgranulopoiesis – pseudo-Pelger–Hüet anomaly and hypogranulation (*arrows*). (B) Dyserythropoiesis – binuclear megaloblastoid erythroblast (*arrow*). (C) Dysthrombocytopoiesis – micromegakaryocyte (*arrow*) (MGG, ×1000). (D) MPO-positive cells (cytochemistry).

Acute myeloid leukaemia, not otherwise specified – acute myeloid leukaemia with minimal differentiation

Acute myeloid leukaemia (AML) with minimal differentiation comprises <5% of all cases of AML, and consists of poorly differentiated blasts, without morphological or cytochemical features of myeloid differentiation. Blasts express early myeloid-associated antigens, without expression for B and T lymphoid markers.

Cytological findings (Figs 7.106–7.107)

- Blasts vary in size without differentiating features
- Round or slightly indented nuclei with inconspicuous nucleoli
- Agranular cytoplasm resembling lymphoblasts
- Negative cytochemical reaction for myeloperoxidase (MPO), alpha-naphthyl acetate esterase (ANAE), Sudan Black B (SBB) and chloracetate esterase (CAE)

Differential diagnosis

- Other types of AML such as megakaryoblastic leukaemia
- Mixed phenotype acute leukaemia
- Acute lymphoid leukaemia
- Leukaemic phase of large cell lymphoma

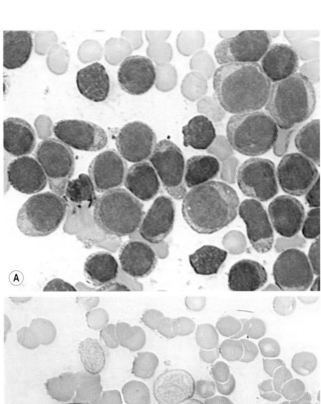

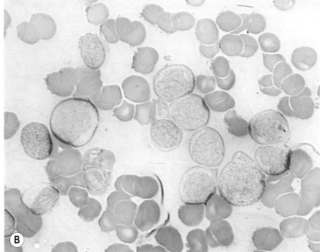

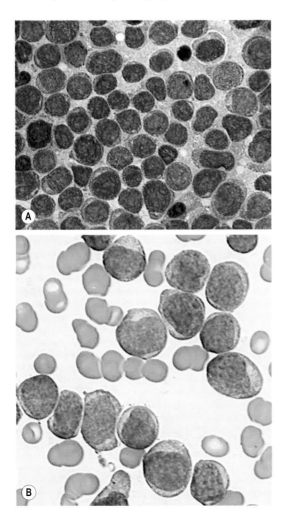

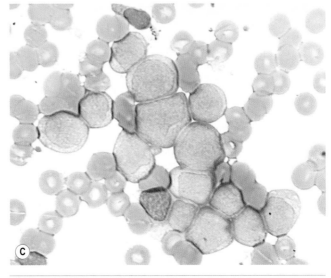

Fig. 7.106 Acute myeloid leukaemia with minimal differentiation. (A,B) Hypercellular smears with blasts without morphological myeloid differentiation (MGG).

Fig. 7.107 Acute myeloid leukaemia with minimal differentiation. Cytochemical features. (A) MPO-negative blasts. (B) NSE-negative blasts. (C) PAS-negative blasts (cytochemistry).

Acute myeloid leukaemia, not otherwise specified – acute myeloid leukaemia without maturation

Acute myeloid leukaemia without maturation comprises 5–10% of all cases of AML, and consists of ≥90% blasts of the non-erythroid cells.

Cytological findings (Fig 7.108–7.109)

- The cells are predominantly myeloblasts, some contain azurophilic granules or Auer rods (see p. 224)
- No evidence of maturation beyond the myeloblast stage (<10%)
- Variable number of myeloperoxidase (MPO) and Sudan black B (SBB) positive blasts

Differential diagnosis

- Other acute myeloid leukaemias such as AML with minimal differentiation and AML with maturation
- Acute lymphoid leukaemia

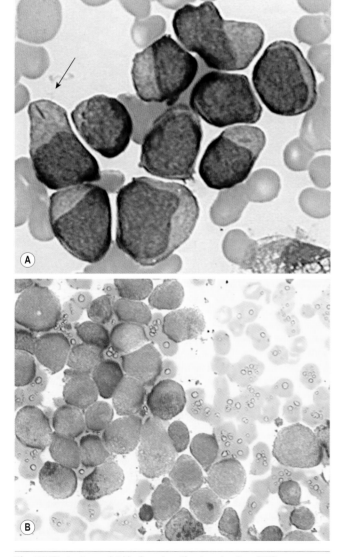

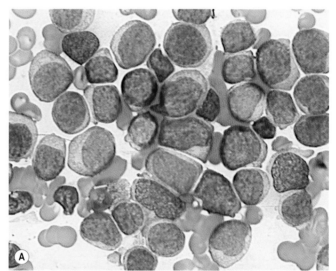

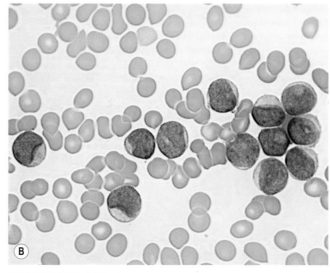

Fig. 7.108 Acute myeloid leukaemia without maturation. (A) Bone marrow smear. Uniform blasts with Auer rods (*arrow*) (MGG). (B) Blasts are both negative and positive for myeloperoxidase reaction (cytochemistry).

Fig. 7.109 Acute myeloid leukaemia without maturation. (A) Bone marrow smear. Predominant population are myeloblasts. (B) Peripheral blood smear also shows uniform population of myeloblasts.

Acute myeloid leukaemia, not otherwise specified – acute myeloid leukaemia with maturation

Acute myeloid leukaemia (AML) with maturation comprises approximately 10% of all cases of AML, and features ≥20% blasts in the bone marrow or peripheral blood, and ≥10% maturing cells of myeloid lineage.

Cytological findings (Figs 7.110–7.111)

- Blasts with or without azurophilic granulation and Auer rods
- Promyelocytes, myelocytes and mature neutrophils represent ≥10% of the bone marrow cells
- Variable degree of dyserythro-, dysgranulo- or dysthrombopoiesis
- Eosinophils and basophils without abnormalities (cytological or cytochemical) are frequently increased

Differential diagnosis

- Myelodysplastic syndrome with excess blasts (RAEB)
- Acute myeloid leukaemia without maturation
- Acute myelomonocytic leukaemia

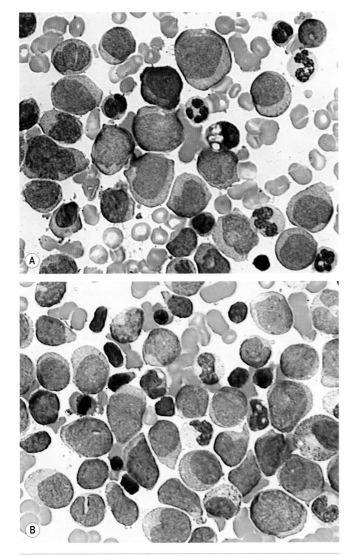

Fig. 7.110 Acute myeloid leukaemia with maturation. (A,B) Bone marrow smears. Myeloid blasts with some more mature neutrophils and very rare monocytic form (MGG).

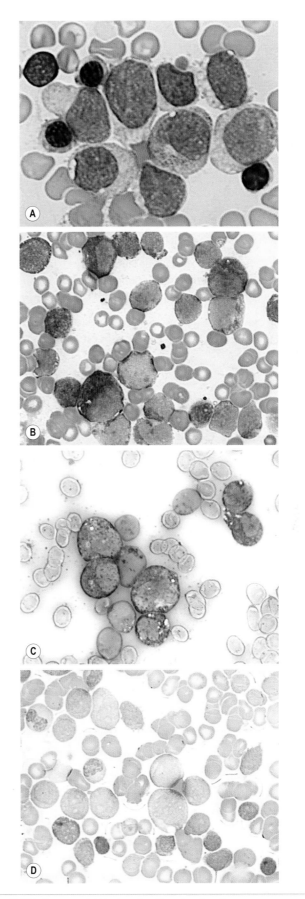

Fig. 7.111 Acute myeloid leukaemia with maturation. Bone marrow smears. (A) Blasts with and without granules are present (MGG). (B) Myeloperoxidase positive. (C) Sudan black reaction positive in many blasts. (D) Blasts are negative for non-specific esterase (NSE) (cytochemistry).

Acute myeloid leukaemia, not otherwise specified – acute myelomonocytic leukaemia

Acute myelomonocytic leukaemia is characterised by the proliferation of both granulocyte and monocyte precursors.

Cytological findings (Figs 7.112–7.113)

- ≥20% blasts (including promonocytes) in BM or PB
- Monocytes and their precursors (promonocytes and monoblasts) and granulocytes and their precursors each comprise ≥20% in BM
- Positivity for MPO (>3%) and NSE (>20%) or double staining for NSE/CAE or NSE/MPO

Differential diagnosis

- Other acute myeloid leukaemias such as AML with maturation or acute monocytic leukaemia
- Myelodysplastic syndrome/myeloproliferative neoplasm as chronic myelomonocytic leukaemia

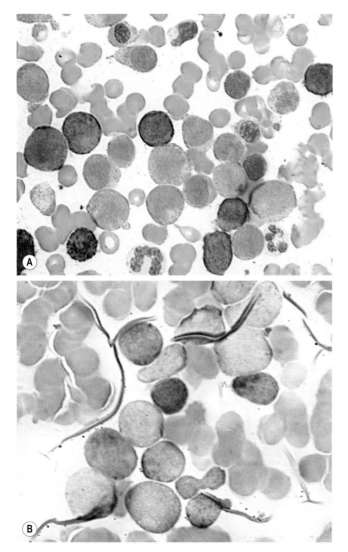

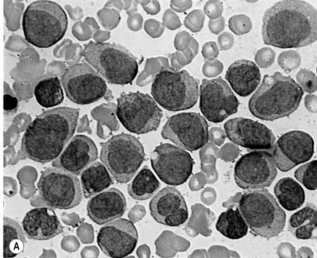

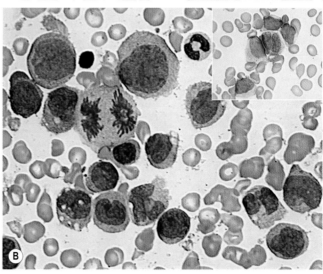

Fig. 7.112 Acute myelomonocytic leukaemia. Bone marrow smears. (A) Cells are positive as well as negative for MPO. (B) NSE-positive and -negative cells (cytochemistry).

Fig. 7.113 Acute myelomonocytic leukaemia. (A,B) Bone marrow smears show myelo- and monocytic blasts and promonocytes (MGG). (Inset) Monoblasts and myeloblasts in peripheral blood.

Acute myeloid leukaemia, not otherwise specified – acute monoblastic and monocytic leukaemia

Acute myeloid leukaemia without maturation comprises <5% of all cases of AML, and consists of ≥80% blasts of monocytic lineage.

Cytological findings (Figs 7.114–7.115)

- ≥80% of blasts are of monocytic lineage (monocyte, promonocytes and monoblasts), in some cells erythrophagocytes
- <20% are neutrophils and their precursors, Auer rods are rare (usually in cells identifiable as myeloblasts)
- Monoblastic leukaemia – ≥80% monoblasts
- Monocytic leukaemia – <80% are monoblasts; the majority of the cells are promomocytes
- Myeloperoxidase (MPO) negative, non-specific esterase (NSE), a spectrum ranging from intense to weakly or negative activity

Differential diagnosis

- Other acute myeloid leukaemias such as AML with minimal differentiation, AML without maturation, megakaryocytic leukaemia, microgranular APL or prolymphocytic leukaemia

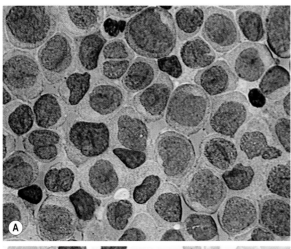
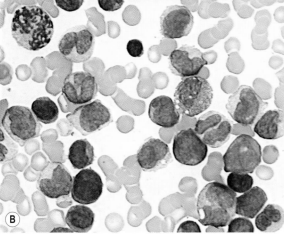

Fig. 7.114 Acute monocytic leukaemia. (A) Bone marrow aspirate where the majority of the cells are promonocytes. (B) Peripheral blood smears with numerous promonocytes (MGG).

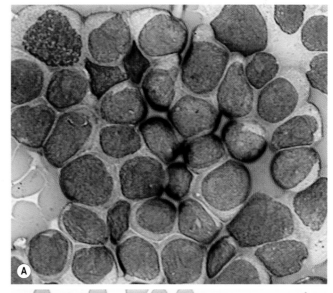
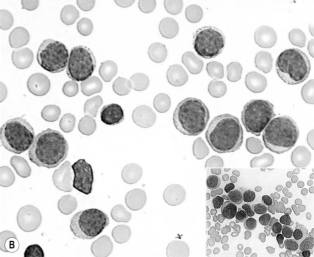

Fig. 7.115 Acute monoblastic leukaemia. (A) Bone marrow smear shows monomorphous blast population without differentiation to promonocytes. (B, Inset) Peripheral blood smears with numerous monoblasts (MGG).

Acute myeloid leukaemia, not otherwise specified – acute erythroid leukaemia

Acute erythroid leukaemia comprises 5–10% of all cases of AML, and consists of the predominant erythroid population, positive for PAS, NSE and AF, and negative for MPO and SBB. There are two types: erythroleukaemia (erythroid/myeloid) and pure erythroid leukaemia.

Cytological findings (Figs 7.116–7.117)

- Erythroleukaemia (erythroid/myeloid)
  - ≥50% erythroid precursors, which are of all maturation stages and dysplastic with megaloblastoid nuclei (bi- or multinucleated)
  - ≥20% myeloblasts of non-erythroid cells
- Pure erythroid leukaemia
  - ≥80% immature (undifferentiated or proerythroblastic) erythroid population without significant myeloblastic component. Erythroblasts are medium to large sized, occasionally are smaller like lymphoblasts

Differential diagnosis

- Other acute myeloid leukaemias as with maturation, megakaryoblastic leukaemia and AML myelodysplasia-related, MDS (RAEB), ALL/lymphoma
- Megaloblastic anaemia or reactive erythroid hyperplasia following therapy of erythropoietin

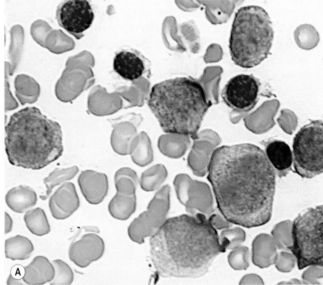

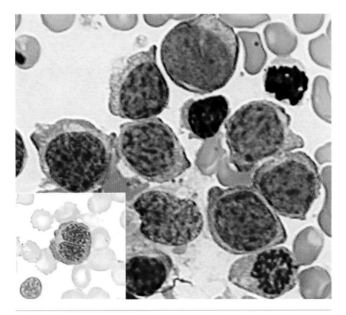

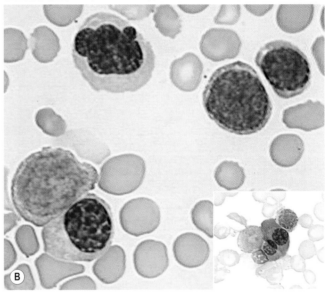

Fig. 7.116 Pure erythroid leukaemia. Bone marrow smear shows immature erythroid population without significant myeloblastic component. Some mitotic figures are present. (Inset) PAS-positive atypical erythroblasts (cytochemistry).

Fig. 7.117 Erythroleukaemia (erythroid/myeloid). (A,B) Bone marrow aspirate shows myeloblasts and erythroid precursor with dyserythropoiesis. (B, Inset) PAS-positive atypical erythroblast (cytochemistry).

Acute myeloid leukaemia, not otherwise specified – acute megakaryoblastic leukaemia

Acute myeloid leukaemia without maturation comprises 5–10% of all cases of AML, and consists of ≥20% blasts of which at least 50% blasts are of megakaryoblastic lineage. At the genetic level, there seem to be 3 types of acute megakaryocytic leukaemia: Down syndrome-associated, t(1;22)(p13;q13)-associated, and those with other abnormalities.

Cytological findings (Figs 7.118–7.119)

- Varying degree of reticulin fibrosis results in hypocelullarity of bone marrow aspirates
- Megakaryoblasts are medium- to large-sized blasts with round, irregular or indented nuclei
- Cytoplasm is basophilic, agranular with distinct blebs or pseudopod formations
- Occasionally blasts occur in small clusters, negative for SSB, MPO and CAE, but may show PAS, AF and focal NSE reactivity
- Immunophenotyping using MoAb to megakaryocyte-restricted antigen (CD41 and CD61) may be diagnostic

Differential diagnosis

- Other acute myeloid leukaemias such as AML with minimal differentiation, AML with myelodysplasia-related changes, acute panmyelosis with myelofibrosis, pure erythroblastic leukaemia, blastic transformation of CML or megakaryoblastic acceleration of MPN or ALL

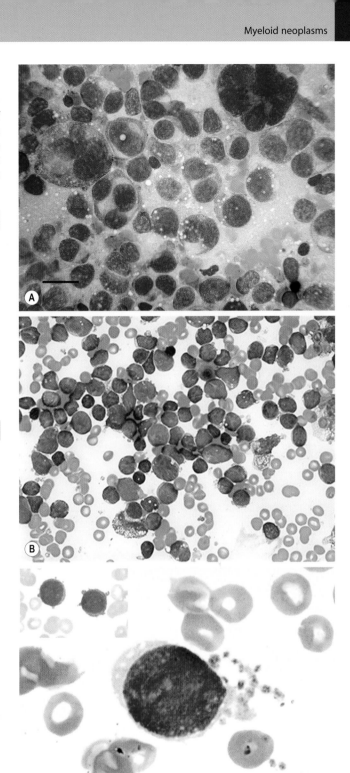

Fig. 7.118 Acute megakaryoblastic leukaemia. (Inset) CD61 immunostained megakaryoblasts (LSAB).

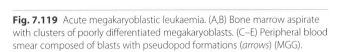

Fig. 7.119 Acute megakaryoblastic leukaemia. (A,B) Bone marrow aspirate with clusters of poorly differentiated megakaryoblasts. (C–E) Peripheral blood smear composed of blasts with pseudopod formations (*arrows*) (MGG).

Acute leukaemia, not otherwise specified – acute basophilic leukaemia

Acute basophilic leukaemia is a very rare neoplasm (<1% of all cases of AML) with primary differentiation into basophils.

Cytological findings (Figs 7.120–7.121)

- Medium-sized blasts with high nuclear/cytoplasmic ratio
- Oval, round or bilobed nucleus
- Basophilic cytoplasms with coarse basophilic metachromatic granules
- Blasts positive for toluidine blue and negative for SBB, MPO, CAE and non-specific esterase
- Dyserythopoiesis may be present

Differential diagnosis

- Other types of AML with basophilia
- Blast phase of MPN-CML
- Mast cell leukaemia
- ALL with prominent granules

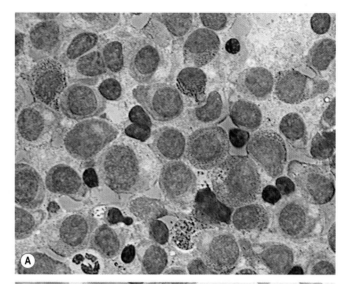

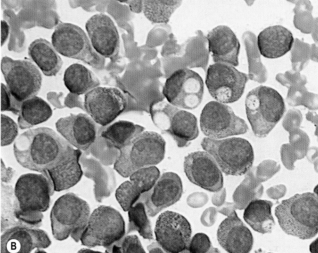

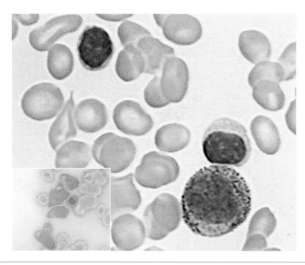

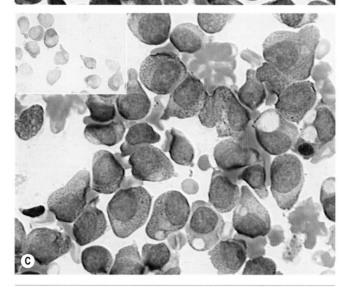

Fig. 7.120 Acute basophilic leukaemia. Peripheral blood smears. Leukopenia with basophils (MGG). (Inset) Myeloperoxidase-negative cells (cytochemistry).

Fig. 7.121 Acute basophilic leukaemia. Bone marrow aspirate. (A,B,C) Hypercellular smears with atypical blasts and immature basophils (MGG). (C, Inset) Toluidine blue-positive cells (cytochemistry).

Acute myeloid leukaemia, not otherwise specified – acute panmyelosis with myelofibrosis

Acute panmyelosis with myelofibrosis is an acute leukaemia with bone marrow fibrosis and increased proliferation of erythroid, myeloid and megakaryocytic precursors in the foci within a diffusely fibrotic stroma.

Cytological findings (Figs 7.122–7.123)

- Hypocellular (unsuccessful) bone marrow aspiration
- Dysplastic changes in myeloid cells
- Dysplastic megakaryocytes (micromegakaryocytes with hypolobulated or non-lobulated nuclei)
- Pancytopenia in peripheral blood

Differential diagnosis

- Other types of AML with fibrosis (acute megakaryoblastic leukaemia)
- Primary myelofibrosis
- Secondary myelofibrosis (myelofibrotic phase of myeloproliferative neoplasms such as polycythaemia vera, and essential thrombocythaemia)
- Metastatic malignancies with a desmoplastic stromal reaction

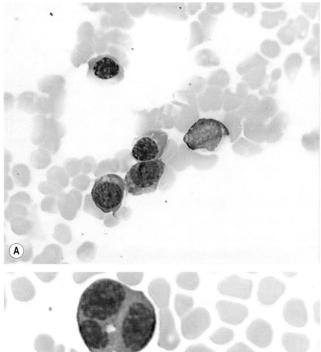

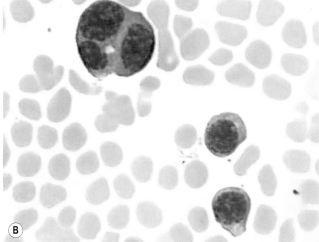

Fig. 7.122 Acute panmyelosis with myelofibrosis. (A) Bone marrow aspirate. Hypocellular smears with several erythroid and myeloid precursors. (B) Atypical megaloblastoid and multinucleated erythroblasts (MGG).

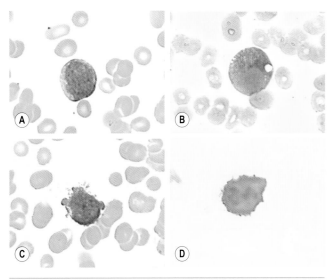

Fig. 7.123 Acute panmyelosis with myelofibrosis. Peripheral blood smears. (A) Myeloblast (MGG). (B) MPO-positive blast (cytochemistry). (C) Megakaryoblast (MGG). (D) CD61-positive megakaryoblast (LSAB).

Acute leukaemias of ambiguous lineage

Acute leukaemias of ambiguous lineage constitute less than 4% of all cases of acute leukaemias. They include undifferentiated leukaemias (unusual lineages) and mixed phenotype acute leukaemias (separate blast population of more than one lineage or single blast population with coexpressing antigen of more than one lineage). Diagnosis is based on immunophenotyping by flow cytometry or immunohistochemistry/immunocytochemistry and cytochemical stains for myeloperoxidase (MPO), non-specific esterase (NSE), PAS, etc. on smears to detect myeloid, B or T lymphoid or other components.

Cytological findings (Fig. 7.124)

- Depend on type of acute leukaemia of ambiguous lineage
- Some cases have a dysmorphic blast population (myeloblasts and lymphoblasts or other), blasts without distinguishing features, or have morphology resembling ALL

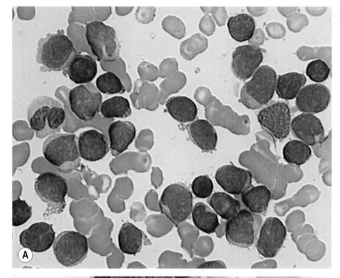

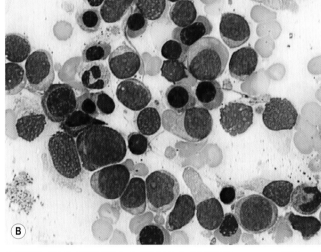

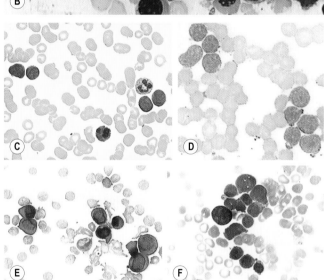

Fig. 7.124 Acute leukaemias of ambiguous lineage. (A,B) Bone marrow aspirate shows dismorphic blast populations, one resembling lymphoblasts and the other myeloblasts (MGG). (C) Peripheral blood smear with small blasts resembling lymphoblasts (MGG). (D) Granular positivity for PAS. (E) Blasts strongly positive for CD10. (F) Majority of blasts are cytochemically negative for myeloperoxidase (only one positive).

Myeloid sarcoma

Myeloid sarcoma is an extramedullary tumour consisting of blasts of myeloid differentiation.

Cytological findings (Figs 7.125–7.126)

- Myeloid blasts with or without maturation
- Myelomonocytic or pure monoblastic morphology
- Very rare with trilineage haemopoiesis

Differential diagnosis

- Malignant lymphoma
  - lymphoblastic lymphoma
  - Burkitt's lymphoma
  - diffuse large B-cell lymphoma
  - small round cell lymphoma
  - blastic plasmacytoid dendritic cell neoplasm

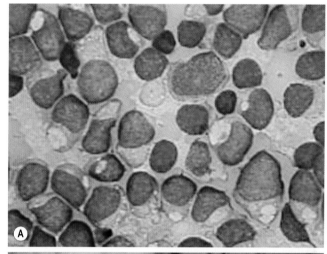

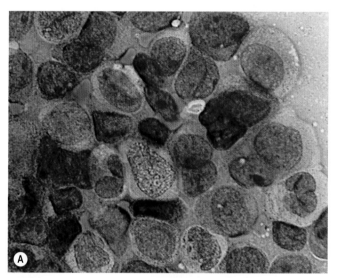

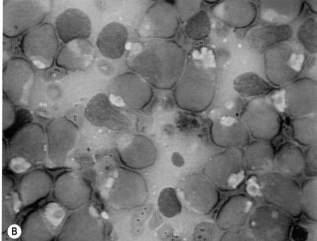

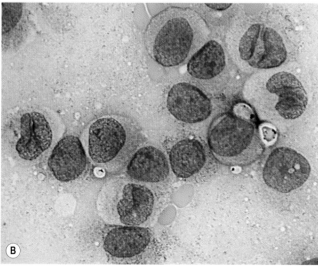

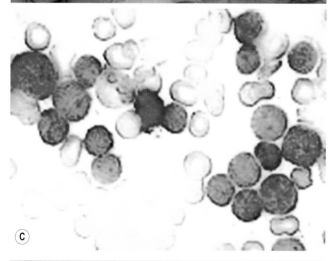

Fig. 7.125 Myeloid sarcoma. FNA of lymph node. Myeloid sarcoma with monoblastic and promonocytic morphology of blasts (MGG).

Fig. 7.126 Myeloid sarcoma. FNA of breast. (A) Myeloid sarcoma with undifferentiated blasts (MGG). (B) Myeloperoxidase-negative blast cells (cytochemistry). (C) Blast cells positive for myeloperoxidase (LSAB).

Histiocytic and dendritic cell neoplasms

This group of neoplasms consists of tumours of histiocytes or mononuclear phagocytes (myeloid-derived macrophages and myeloid-derived dendritic cells) and stromal-derived dendritic cells.

Histiocytic sarcoma (HS)

Histiocytic sarcoma is a malignant proliferation of mature tissue histiocytes (morphological and immunophenotypic).

Cytological findings (Figs 7.127–7.128)

- Large monomorphic or pleomorphic cells with abundant slightly basophilic and vacuolated cytoplasm
- Nuclei are round, oval or irregular
- Background consists of small lymphocytes, plasma cells, eosinophils and benign histiocytes

Differential diagnosis

- Anaplastic large cell lymphoma (especially ALK negative)
- Other T, B or NK cell neoplasms
- Poorly differentiated epithelial, stromal or melanocytic tumours

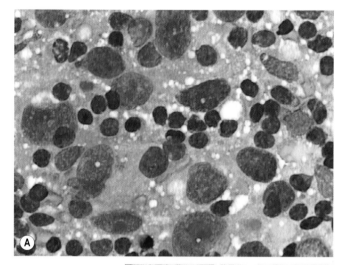

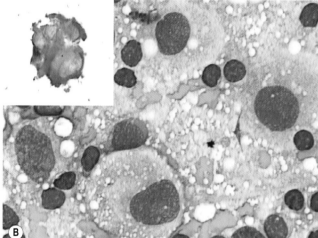

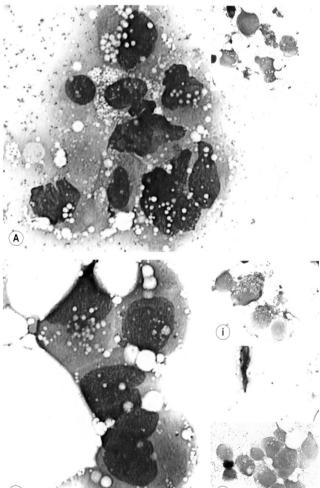

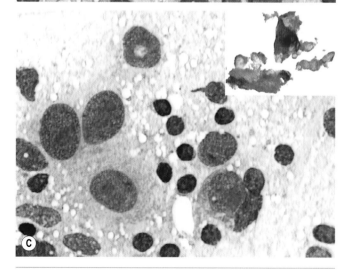

Fig. 7.127 Differential diagnosis of HS. (A,B) Anaplastic large cell lymphoma shows pleomorphic, anaplastic large cells (MGG). (A, Inset) CD30-positive malignant cells. (B, Inset i) CD68-positive cells. (B, Inset ii) Negative reaction for ALK (LSAB).

Fig. 7.128 Histiocytic sarcoma. (A,B,C) There are large atypical reticular cells (MGG). (B, Inset) Malignant cells positive for CD68. (C, Inset) Lysozyme-positive histiocytic cells (LSAB).

Langerhans cell histiocytosis

Langerhans cell histiocytosis (LCH) is a clonal proliferation of Langerhans cells that can present as a solitary lesion (eosinophilic granuloma), multiple lesions (Hand–Schüller–Christian disease) or disseminated or visceral lesions (Letterer–Siwe disease).

Cytological findings (Fig. 7.129)

- LCH cells are oval with folded or lobulated nuclei, inconspicuous nucleoli, minimal atypia and variable mitotic figures
- Multinucleated LCH and osteoclast-like giant cells
- Background consists of small lymphocytes, neutrophils and eosinophils
- Cells immunostain for CD1a

Differential diagnosis

- Lymphomas
- Sarcomas

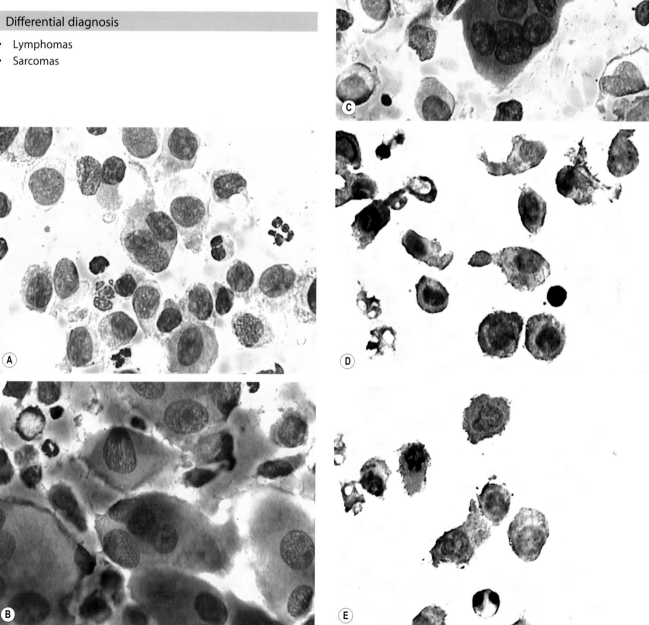

Fig. 7.129 FNA tumour mass of the gluteal region. (A) LCH mono- and multinucleated cells. (B) Large multinucleated LCH cells. (C) Osteoclast-like multinucleated cells (MGG). (D) Vimentin-positive and (E) CD1a-positive LCH cells (LSAB).

Other rare dendritic cell tumours

Fibroblastic reticular cell tumour

This is a rare type described as cytokeratin-positive interstitial reticulum cell tumour, which can occur in lymph node, spleen or soft tissues with variable clinical outcome.

Cytological findings (Fig. 7.130)

- Spindle cells with delicate cytoplasmic extensions and features reminiscent of myofibroblasts
- Tumour cells are variably positive for smooth muscle actin (SMA), desmin, cytokeratin and CD68

Differential diagnosis

- Follicular dendritic cell sarcoma
- Interdigitating dendritic cell sarcoma

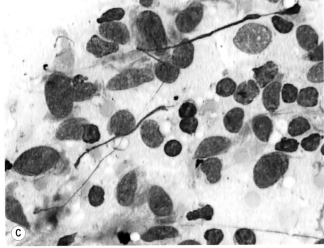

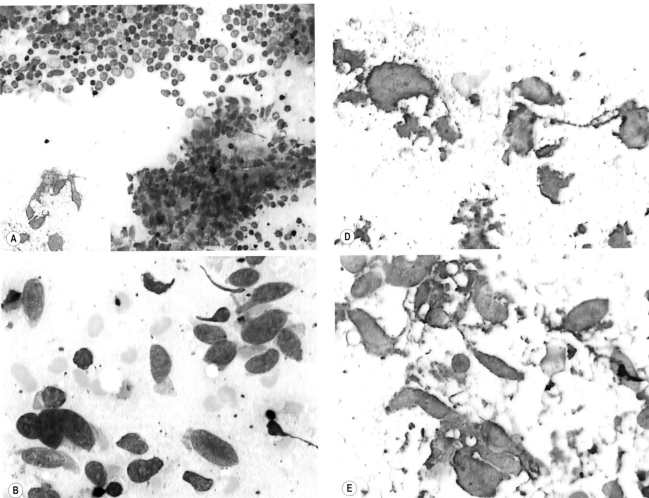

Fig. 7.130 Fibroblastic reticular cell tumour. (A) Small and transformed lymphoid cells and clusters of spindle cells (MGG). (A, Inset) CD68-positive spindle cells (LSAB). (B,C) Spindle cells with some lymphoid cells (MGG). (D) Cells immunostained for SMA. (E) Malignant cells show positivity for pan-cytokeratin (LSAB).

CHAPTER 8

Breast

Contents

The normal breast   245

Inflammatory conditions   249

Benign breast changes   253

Benign tumours and tumour-like lesions   255

Epithelial hyperplasia and tumour-like lesions   261

Complex sclerosing and fibrocystic lesions   262

Borderline epithelial lesions   263

Common malignant breast epithelial tumours   265

Uncommon malignant breast epithelial tumours   270

Primary sarcomas, lymphomas and metastatic tumours   275

Reporting breast FNAs: the role of FNA in management   277

The normal breast

The normal mature breast is histologically composed of regularly arranged, radially disposed, independent glandular units with duct and lobules surrounded by connective and adipose tissue (Fig. 8.1).

FNA from normal, adult breast tissue will contain variable amounts of ductal epithelial cell groups, small stromal fragments and fatty tissue. The epithelial cell yield is usually higher in younger age groups.

Cytological findings: normal breast (Figs 8.2–8.5)

- Normal epithelial cells
- Small cohesive groups
- Monolayer sheets
- Occasional complete terminal duct lobular unit (TDLU)
- Oval nuclei with regular outlines, 8–10 µm in diameter
- Inconspicuous nucleolus
- Evenly distributed chromatin
- Scanty cytoplasm
- Myoepithelial cells appear as ovoid, dense nuclei at the periphery and above (on a different focus plane) of ductal sheets and groups
- Naked, bipolar (myoepithelial cell) nuclei in the background

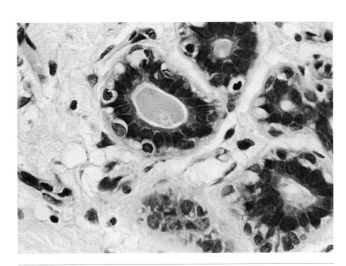

Fig. 8.1[†] The histology of normal breast lobules (H&E). Normal mature breast and changes during lactation.

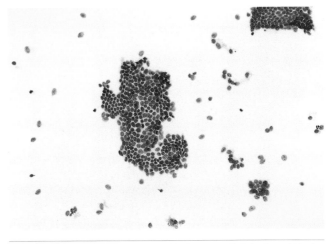

Fig. 8.2[†] Normal pattern with sheets of cohesive epithelial cells and bipolar nuclei in the background (H&E).

Differential diagnosis

- Missed target (Fig. 8.3)
- Pregnancy-related changes (see Figs 8.7, 8.8)
  - the aspirate may be moderately or markedly cellular
  - the cells are single and well dispersed in a lipid-rich foamy or granular background
  - the cells and their nuclei are large
  - there is abundant vacuolated or wispy cytoplasm
  - bare nuclei are common
  - the nuclei are round and uniform with active granular or vesicular, but evenly distributed chromatin
  - single prominent nucleoli

Further investigations

- Triple assessment (clinical, radiological and cytological) is mandatory.
- Any discordance between cytopathological results and clinical and/or radiological findings needs to be investigated further, usually by histopathological study of a core needle biopsy.
- It is important for the cytopathologist to be informed about pregnancy or lactation when the aspirate is performed by others, to lessen the likelihood of interpretive errors; one must also remember that foci of lactational change can occur unassociated with pregnancy and generalised lactation.

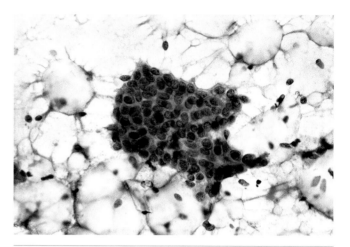

Fig. 8.3[†] Normal breast: a group of benign ductal cells surrounded by bipolar nuclei in the background (PAP).

FNA of palpable lesions: capillary technique (Fig. 8.6)

- Fix the lump between the second and the third fingers of the non-dominant hand
- Insert the needle without the syringe (unless aspirating a cyst), ideally at a 90° angle (Fig. 8.6), adapting this to take account of structures that are normally avoided, such as pleura and areola
- Move the needle to and fro in a fan-shaped manner to sample as many parts of the lump as feasible
- Unless a cyst is being drained, stop when material or blood appears in the needle hub
- If using syringe, release the negative pressure before the needle is withdrawn from the breast
- Express the solid material from the needle on the glass slide, or fluid into a container
- Make direct spreads on the glass slides and either fix them in 90% alcohol or air dry them, depending on the laboratory's preference for PAP or MGG stains (for further details see Ch 13)

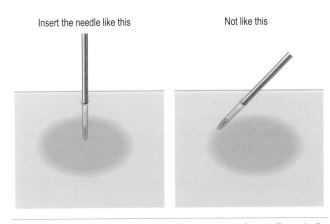

Fig. 8.6† Aspiration technique: it is important to insert the needle vertically. Small lesions may be missed if the needle is inserted obliquely.

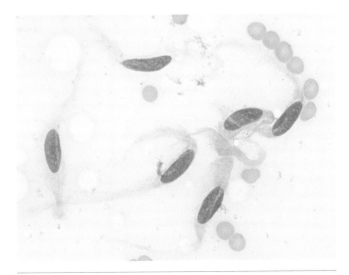

Fig. 8.4 Myoepithelial cells seen at the periphery and above ductal sheet (MGG).

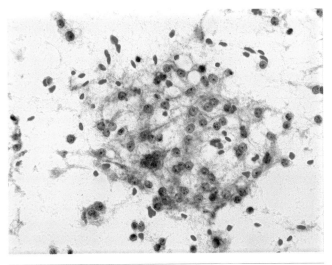

Fig. 8.7† Typical lactation pattern with a granular-vacuolated background due to cytoplasmic rupture of the fragile epithelial cells. Nucleoli are large, larger than in most breast carcinomas.

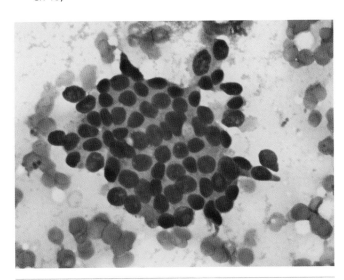

Fig. 8.5 Rare fibroblasts may be seen in the background (MGG).

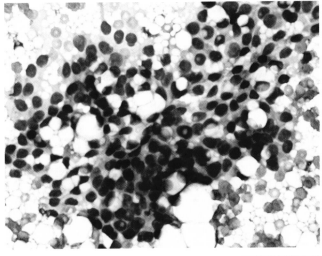

Fig. 8.8 Lactation pattern with loose cellular sheets and widespread vacuolation.

Galactocele

- Galactoceles are often easily diagnosed clinically without need for further investigation
- Occasionally, a galactocele can accumulate abundant inspissated milk to form a large mass, even up to 80 mm in diameter, which can be clinically worrying

Cytological findings: galactocele

- The aspirated material is composed of milk
- Abundant granular, secretory material
- Foamy macrophages
- Calcified debris in 'old', long-standing lesions

Gynaecomastia (Figs 8.9–8.11)

Gynaecomastia is the enlargement of the male breast due to hypertrophy and hyperplasia of both the glandular and stromal components.

Cytological findings: gynaecomastia

- Scanty or moderately cellular smears
- Small to medium-sized epithelial fragments that may be hyperplastic and three-dimensional
- Small to moderate numbers of bipolar cells

Differential diagnosis: gynaecomastia

- In florid hyperplasia, there may be marked anisokaryosis that can be misinterpreted as atypia
- Fibrocystic change may rarely occur in the male breast as can most benign/reactive and malignant lesions that occur in the female breast

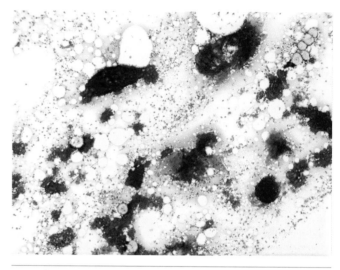

Fig. 8.9[†] Gynaecomastia. A typical pattern of benign ductal sheets and aggregates and stroma fragments.

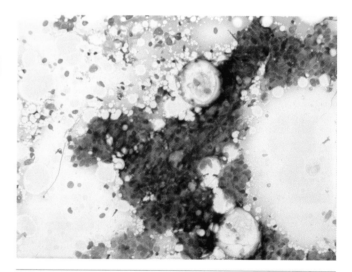

Fig. 8.10[†] Gynaecomastia. Cohesive and complex aggregate of ductal epithelial cells and a moderate number of naked nuclei.

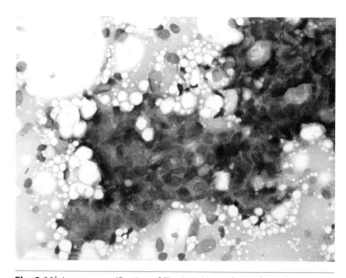

Fig. 8.11[†] Larger magnification of Fig. 8.10. Hyperplastic, three-dimensional aggregate with benign ductal nuclei and scattered myoepithelial cell nuclei.

Inflammatory conditions

Fat necrosis

Fat necrosis: Trauma and extravasation of duct contents can give rise to fat necrosis and various types of mastitis.

Cytological findings (Figs 8.12–8.14)

- Foamy macrophages and multinucleate giant cells with foamy cytoplasm
- Small irregular groups of (reactive) histiocytic cells
- Fragments of normal as well as degenerate fatty tissue
- Variable numbers of other inflammatory cells but usually sparse
- Few if any epithelial cells
- Free lipid droplets, seen as empty spaces that may be surrounded by blood or as empty spaces in a granular background
- Granular background debris

Differential diagnosis

- Aspirates from tuberculosis or other causes of panniculitis may be mistaken for fat necrosis
- Epithelioid cells in fat necrosis and granulation tissue can closely imitate carcinoma
- Vacuolated histiocytic cells may be mistaken for lobular carcinoma cells

Fat necrosis is often found in the periphery of a tumour in areas where the carcinoma cells infiltrate fatty tissue. If the aspirated cells are from the periphery only, cells from the underlying tumour may not be seen.

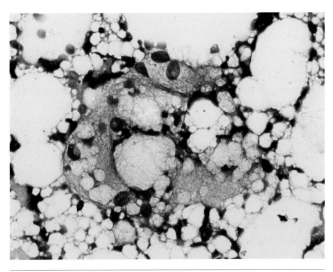

Fig. 8.12 Fat necrosis: typical aspect consisting of macrophages with foamy cytoplasm, lipid droplets and granular debris.

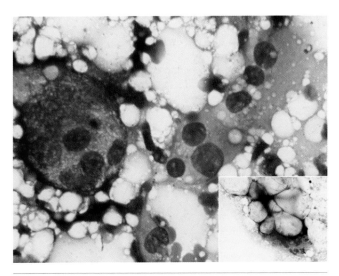

Fig. 8.13 Fat necrosis: multinucleated cells, histiocytes and degenerate fatty tissue. (Inset) PAP stain shows multinucleate giant cells.

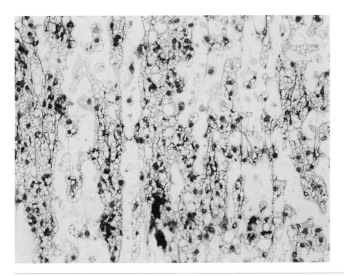

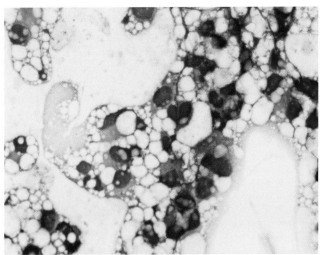

Fig. 8.14 Diagnostic pitfall. Invasive carcinoma may sometimes present with a pattern of single cell infiltration of the fat so that epithelial cells appear as histiocytes. In these cases, it is necessary to use epithelial markers.

Periductal mastitis (Fig. 8.15)

Clinically, this lesion may mimic carcinoma, as there can be retraction of the nipple associated with a well-defined lesion:

- Usually centrally located; in one-fifth of cases there is nipple discharge
- Mammography may show calcifications

Cytological findings

- Abundant, thick-spreading pasty aspirate
- Loss of much of the material on smears because of dissolution in the methanol fixative
- Abundant amorphous debris in smears
- Foamy macrophages, occasional giant cells and plasma cells
- Scant epithelium which may show reactive atypia

Differential diagnosis

- As with fat necrosis, the clinical features can falsely raise the index of suspicion
- If epithelium is included, it can appear atypical because of the inflammation
- Necrotic carcinomas, including comedo ductal carcinoma in situ, can be mistaken for duct ectasia

Subareolar abscess (Figs 8.16, 8.17)

There is often a history of the recurrent formation of a tender mass in the subareolar region, sinus tract formation and discharge with partial healing.

Cytological findings

- Numerous polymorphs
- Anucleate squames
- Multinucleate giant cells
- Macrophages
- Epithelium showing reactive atypia

Diagnostic pitfalls

- Other inflammatory conditions including tuberculosis
- Sometimes the reactive atypia in the epithelial component of the aspirate is such that it may be confused with a more significant lesion

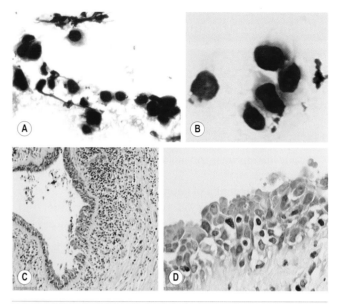

Fig. 8.15 Periductal mastitis. (A,B) Epithelium showing reactive atypia. (C,D) Histology of periductal mastitis/duct ectasia showing inflammatory exudate including lymphocytes and plasma cells and reactive epithelial atypia.

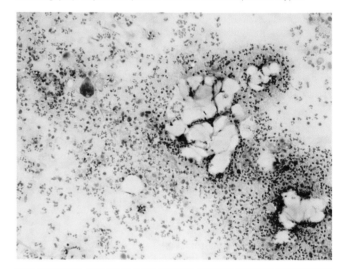

Fig. 8.16 Subareolar abscess with a mixed inflammatory infiltrate with many neutrophilic granulocytes, anuclear squames, macrophages and multinucleated histiocytic giant cells.

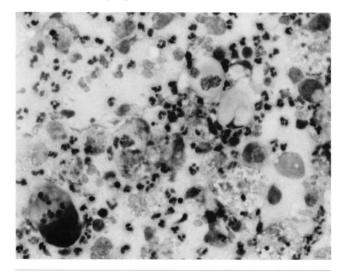

Fig. 8.17 Higher-power view of subareolar abscess shows squamous cells surrounded by many neutrophilic granulocytes, anuclear squames, macrophages and multinucleated histiocytic giant cells.

Granulomatous mastitis (Figs 8.18–8.21)

Cytological findings

- Sheets or clusters of epithelioid cells with abundant cytoplasm and elongated nuclei
- Multinucleate giant cells associated with epithelioid cells
- The giant cells often have epithelioid cell characteristics
- Langhans-type giant cells may be identified
- A variable number of inflammatory cells: lymphocytes, plasma cells, neutrophilic granulocytes
- In tuberculosis and fungal infections, a mixture of necrotic debris and inflammatory cells is often the dominant finding

Differential diagnosis

- Nuclear features in histiocytic/epithelioid cells may give the impression of pleomorphism and these cells may be mistaken for carcinoma cells
- Necrosis, as in tuberculosis, may add to this suspicion
- Carcinomas or lymphomas may rarely elicit a granulomatous response
- Carcinoma with osteoclast-type giant cells must be considered
- A largely necrotic carcinoma can occasionally give the misleading appearance of a granulomatous condition
- Reactive/reparative epithelial cells with additional degenerative nuclear changes may be interpreted as atypical and reported as suspicious. Cells with degenerative nuclear changes should never be the basis of an unequivocal malignant diagnosis

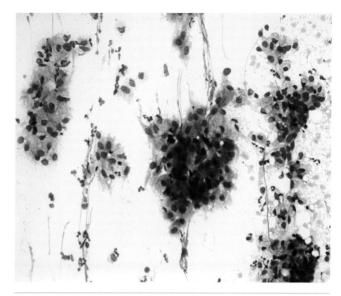

Fig. 8.19[†] Irregular histiocytic aggregates in a case of granulomatous mastitis in a woman with SLE.

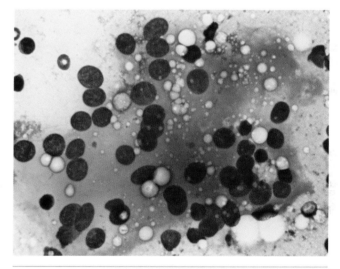

Fig. 8.20 Typical silicone granuloma showing multinucleated cells and silicone droplets.

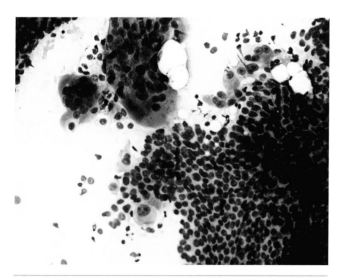

Fig. 8.18 A rare case of mammary carcinoma with multinucleated osteoclast-like giant cells.

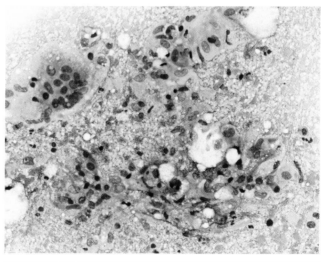

Fig. 8.21 Tuberculous mastitis. This aspirate contained numerous groups of epithelioid histiocytes and occasional giant cells. Cultures and histology confirmed a diagnosis of tuberculous mastitis.

Abscess and acute mastitis (Fig. 8.22)

- Breast abscesses and acute mastitis occur most commonly, but not invariably, in the puerperium
- The diagnosis is usually made clinically
- The possibility of an inflammatory carcinoma has to be considered

Sclerosing lymphocytic lobulitis (Fig. 8.23)

- Also known as lymphocytic or diabetic mastopathy
- Histologically, dense lobulocentric lymphoid infiltration associated with marked stromal fibrosis
- It can present as a lump
- The cytological features are not specific: a paucicellular benign pattern with lymphocytes
- These lesions can be clinically suspicious

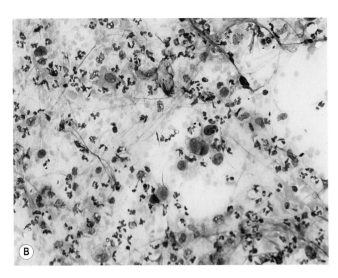

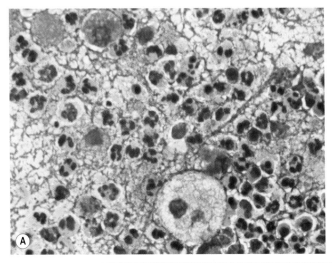

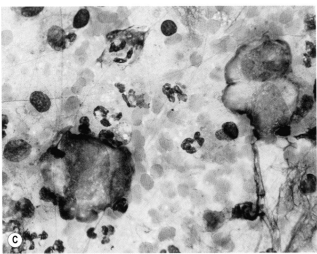

Fig. 8.22 PV image. Acute mastitis with numerous leucocytes and few macrophages. (B) Carcinomas may sometimes have an acute inflammatory background. The epithelial detail has to be examined carefully (C).

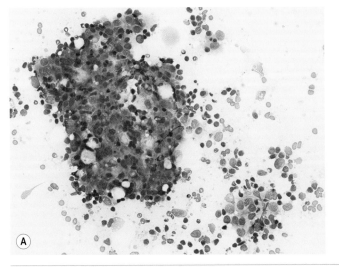

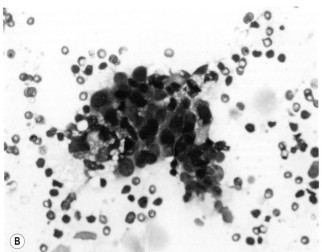

Fig. 8.23 Sclerosing lymphocytic lobulitis. The cytological features are not specific, a paucicellular benign pattern with lymphocytes including lymphoid follicle centre cells. (A) Lymphoid infiltrate. (B) Benign breast epithelium surrounded by lymphocytes.

Benign breast changes (Figs 8.24–8.32)

The spectrum of histological appearances generally included under the heading of 'benign breast changes' is very wide. The basic histological elements are:

- The formation of cysts
- Apocrine metaplasia of cyst lining cells and of duct and lobular epithelium
- Rupture of the cyst lining with extravasation of contents and associated inflammation
- Fibrosis of the stroma
- Chronic inflammation of non-specific type
- Epithelial hyperplasia of various types
- Fibroadenomatoid change

Cytological findings: breast cysts

- Cysts usually show foamy macrophages, proteinaceous granular debris and apocrine cells
- The spectrum of fibrocystic changes includes: formation and/or rupture of cysts, apocrine metaplasia, fibrosis, inflammation and epithelial hyperplasia of various types

Differential diagnosis

- Apocrine cells may present various aspects and degenerative changes mimicking high-grade carcinoma
- The epithelial hyperplasia should be differentiated from a low-grade in situ or infiltrative carcinoma

Further investigations

- Close cooperation between the clinician, the radiologist and the cytopathologist (triple test) is highly recommended
- In case of any discordance, core-needle biopsy or surgical excision is mandatory

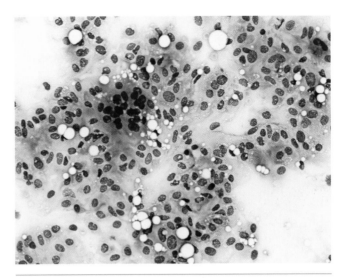

Fig. 8.24 Foamy macrophages in benign fibrocystic change.

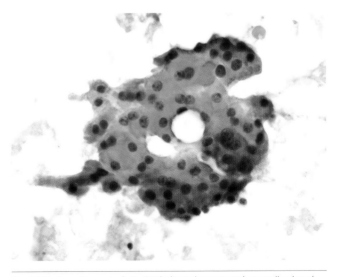

Fig. 8.25[†] Foamy macrophages in benign fibrocystic change.

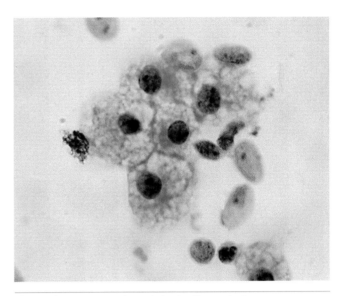

Fig. 8.26 Apocrine metaplasia. Epithelium shows round, centrally placed nuclei and a dense, well-defined cytoplasm.

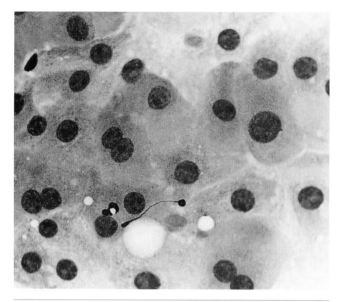

Fig. 8.27† Benign apocrine cells from fibrocystic change.

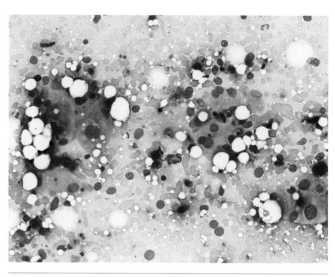

Fig. 8.30 Apocrine carcinoma. Apocrine cells are scattered singly and in sheets, showing anisonucleosis and prominent nucleoli.

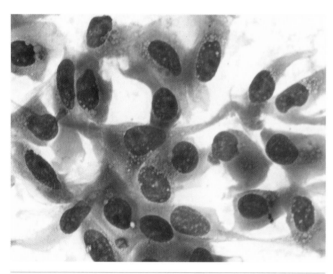

Fig. 8.28 Apocrine cells in benign fibrocystic change can assume spindle shapes and cause concern about their nature.

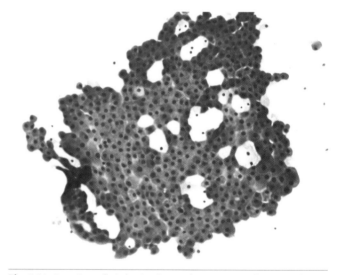

Fig. 8.31 Apocrine cells in benign breast change are usually arranged in cohesive flat sheets.

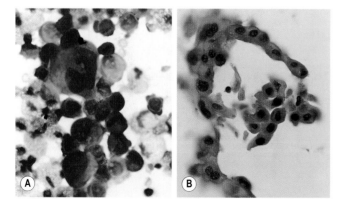

Fig. 8.29† Apocrine cells. (A) Cyst fluid containing atypical apocrine cells which were deemed suspicious. (B) Apocrine cyst lining from the same case as in (A). This histological section shows that the atypical apocrine epithelium showed only degenerate change with no evidence of premalignancy.

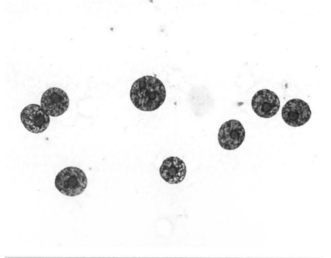

Fig. 8.32 Apocrine cells in benign breast change may present as bare nuclei with very prominent nucleoli. Care should be taken not to confuse these with apocrine carcinoma.

Benign tumours and tumour-like lesions

Fibroadenoma (Figs 8.33–8.41)

Fibroadenoma is by far the commonest benign lesion. It usually presents in women between the age of 20 and 35 years.

Cytological findings

- Moderate or high cellularity, but may be scanty in older or fibrotic lesions
- Cohesive sheets with an antler-like appearance containing recognisable myoepithelial cell nuclei
- Many naked bipolar cell nuclei in the background
- If apocrine or foamy cells are present, they are few

Differential diagnosis

Misdiagnosis of fibroadenoma is the commonest cause of false-positive diagnoses, although these are rare.

- High cellularity should not be interpreted as suspicious
- Reduced cellular cohesion and significant nuclear enlargement with anisonucleosis and prominent nucleoli may risk a false-positive diagnosis of carcinoma
- A very myxoid stroma, particularly when associated with over-spread dissociate epithelium, may mimic mucinous carcinoma
- Phyllodes tumour shares some cytological features with fibroadenoma

Further investigations

- Cytological diagnosis of fibroadenoma is usually straightforward.
- However, unusual clinical or radiological presentations, as well as atypical cytological features, may require a core needle biopsy or a surgical excision of the lesion.

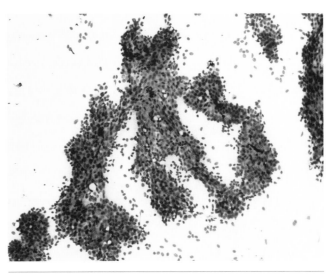

Fig. 8.33 Fibroadenoma: monolayer sheet of epithelial cells showing antler horn branching, associated with myoepithelial cells.

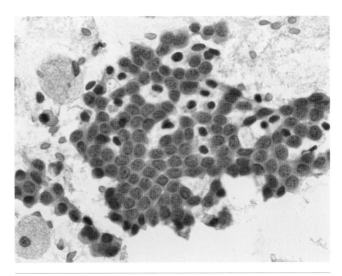

Fig. 8.34 Fibroadenoma: monolayer sheet of epithelial cells with some smaller and darker myoepithelial nuclei (PAP).

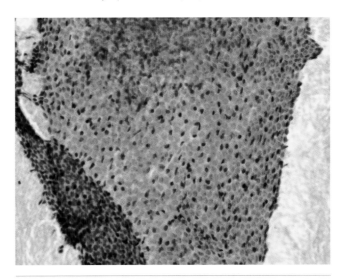

Fig. 8.35 Fibroadenoma: sheet of regular epithelial cells associated with myoepithelial cells, which appear as 'sesame seeds', smaller, darker and on a different plane of focus.

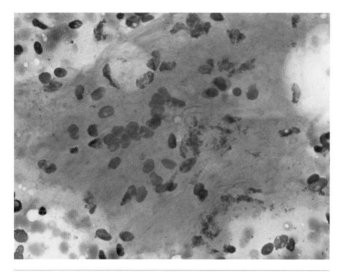

Fig. 8.36 Fibroadenoma: stromal fragment (MGG).

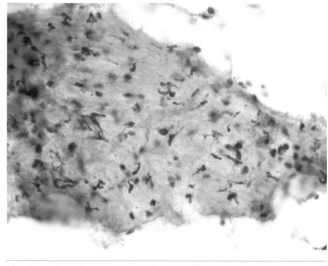

Fig. 8.39 Fibroadenoma: stromal fragment (PAP).

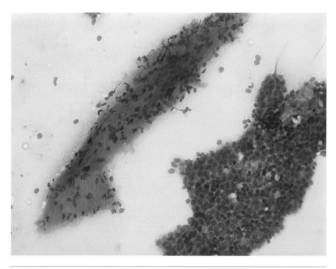

Fig. 8.37† Fibroadenoma. Stromal fragment and cohesive sheet of epithelial cells and a few naked nuclei in the background.

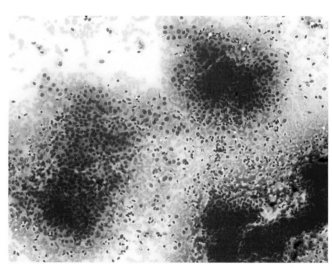

Fig. 8.40 Fibroadenoma: apocrine change in the epithelium with single epithelial cells in the background may appear worrying.

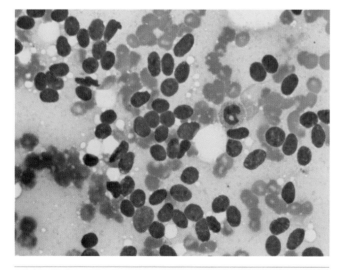

Fig. 8.38 Fibroadenoma: bipolar naked nuclei in the background.

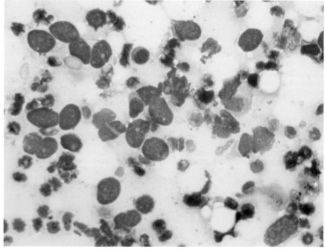

Fig. 8.41 Fibroadenoma: focal area of atypia in a benign lesion, probably caused by the smearing artefact.

Benign phyllodes tumour (Figs 8.42–8.46)

Phyllodes tumours form a spectrum of fibroepithelial tumours from benign with a strong resemblance to fibroadenomas, through borderline with notable stromal overgrowth and proliferation, to malignant, in which the stroma is frankly sarcomatous.

Cytological findings

- Cellular smears with occasional large sheets of benign epithelium
- Numerous plump, single stromal cells with little cellular pleomorphism
- The prominence and number of bipolar cells are usually greater than in fibroadenomas
- Obvious stromal fragments, some large and with high cellularity
- Fragments composed entirely of bipolar cells containing pink or purple ground substance in MGG preparations

Differential diagnosis

- Frequently impossible to distinguish from a fibroadenoma, particularly juvenile fibroadenoma which has a pronounced stromal component
- Cytologically, borderline lesions are difficult to differentiate from benign

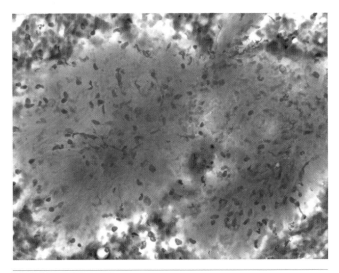

Fig. 8.44 Benign phyllodes tumour: stromal component (MGG).

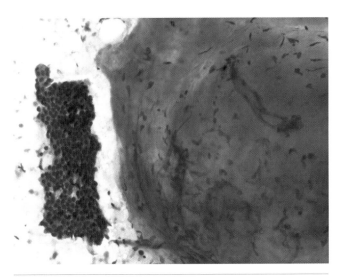

Fig. 8.45 Benign phyllodes tumour: stromal and epithelial components (MGG).

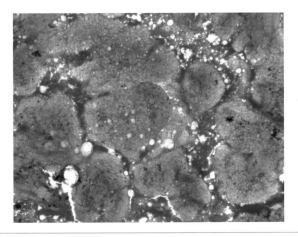

Fig. 8.42 Benign phyllodes tumour: stromal component in large, leaf-like fragments (MGG).

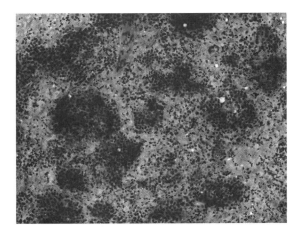

Fig. 8.43 Juvenile fibroadenoma has numerous naked nuclei in the background and is cytologically indistinguishable from phyllodes tumour.

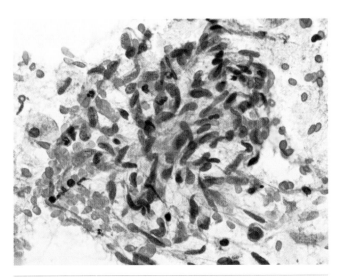

Fig. 8.46 Low-grade phyllodes tumour with spindle cells in groups (PAP). The final diagnosis was made histologically.

Tubular adenoma (Fig. 8.47)

- Histologically, consist of a mass of densely packed benign tubular structures with a double layer of epithelial and myoepithelial cells
- Very little stroma between the tubules part of the spectrum of fibroepithelial neoplasms where the stromal component is minimal

Cytological findings

- Moderate to highly cellular aspirate with a basic benign pattern
- No large antler-like groups are seen
- The epithelial cells are cytologically benign and in small groups, some displaying a microacinar arrangement
- Bipolar cells are fewer than seen in fibroadenomas

Differential diagnosis

- Tubular carcinoma

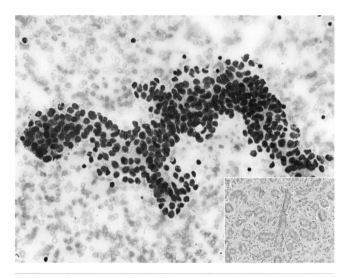

Fig. 8.47 Tubular adenoma. The epithelial cells are cytologically benign and in small groups, some displaying a microacinar arrangement. (Inset) Histology: densely packed tubular structures with epithelial and myoepithelial cells.

Lactating adenoma and lactational changes in benign lesions (Figs 8.48, 8.49)

- Moderately cellular aspirates composed of dispersed cells singly or in small groups in a foamy background containing cell fragments and lipid droplets
- The cytoplasm is vacuolated or wispy and stripped epithelial nuclei may be present
- The nuclei are uniform and show fine, stippled chromatin and a prominent nucleolus

Differential diagnosis

- As for pregnancy-related changes
- Benign breast lumps in lactation and pregnancy can feel suspicious clinically
- If the secretory background and cytological features are not appreciated, there is a significant risk of false-positive diagnosis of malignancy or unwarranted suspicious diagnosis
- When a non-pathologist is taking the aspirate, failure to supply the essential clinical information of pregnancy makes this more likely

Mammary hamartoma

- Consists of varying amounts of breast parenchyma and adipose tissue
- Cytologically, cannot be reliably distinguished from normal breast tissue, fibroadenoma or other cellular benign lesions

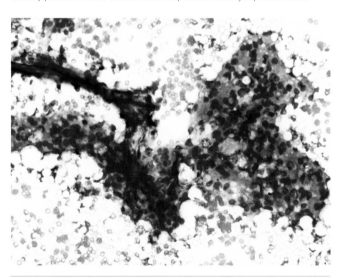

Fig. 8.48 Fibroadenoma with lactation change. Note vacuolated cytoplasm.

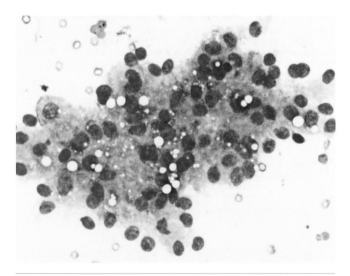

Fig. 8.49 Fibroadenoma in lactatation. Cells are larger, have prominent nucleoli, more dispersed. The association with myoepithelium is not always immediately apparent.

Other benign lesions (Figs 8.50–8.55)

Cytological findings and differential diagnosis of epidermoid cyst

This is an inclusion cyst derived from the skin overlying the mammary gland rather than a true mammary cyst. Anucleate squames (Fig. 8.51), sometimes associated with acute or subacute inflammation or even with multinucleated giant cells, may be seen.

Metaplastic apocrine cells in a true cyst of the breast may be reminiscent of keratinising cells but they usually contain a clearly defined nucleus.

Other benign lesions include:

- Duct ectasia (see also periductal mastitis) (Fig. 8.50)
- Intramammary lymph node (Fig. 8.52)
- Granular cell (Abrikossov) tumour
- Epidermoid cyst
- Adenomyoepithelioma

Cytological findings and differential diagnosis of duct ectasia

- Duct ectasia usually consists of proteinaceous substance in the background with crystals and metaplastic cells
- The proteinaceous substance may mimic extensive necrosis seen in a high-grade intraductal carcinoma and may be associated with a papillary lesion

Cytological findings and differential diagnosis of intramammary lymph node

- Intramammary lymph node is usually composed of normal mature lymphoid cells. Under certain circumstances reactive lymphoid cells may also be seen (see lymphocytic lobulitis, page 252)
- Differential diagnosis includes primary and secondary non-Hodgkin lymphoma

Cytological findings and differential diagnosis of granular cell tumour

- Derived from nerve sheath cells, granular cell tumour usually presents as a firm, painless mass composed of cells with a large granular cytoplasm. These granules are also seen in the background
- Granular cells should not be interpreted as histiocytes or malignant ductal cells

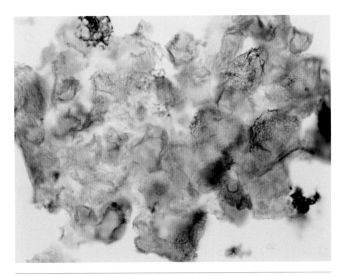

Fig. 8.50 Epidermoid cyst: anucleate squames without associated inflammatory component (PAP).

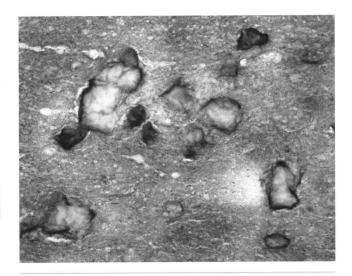

Fig. 8.51 Epidermoid cyst stained with MGG and containing anucleate squames.

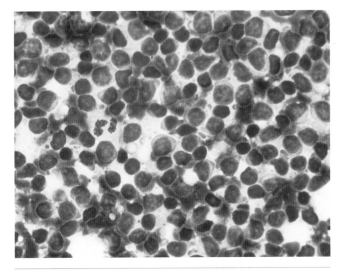

Fig. 8.52 Reactive intramammary lymph node.

Cytological findings: adenomyoepithelioma

- Bundles of spindle cells with an admixture of epithelial cells
- Spherical structures can also be found
- They are translucent or slightly light-green with Papanicolaou staining and metachromatic with Giemsa staining (collagenous spherulosis)
- Differential diagnosis is adenoid cystic carcinoma of the breast

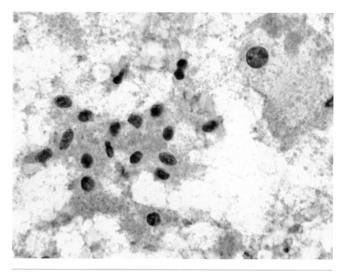

Fig. 8.53 Duct ectasia: proteinaceous substance with crystals (MGG).

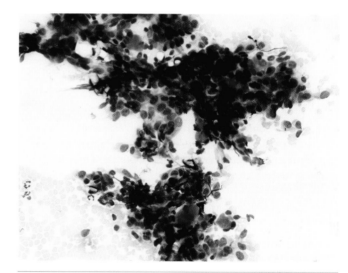

Fig. 8.54 Adenomyoepithelioma: spindle cells, epithelial cells and round globules. The appearance is known as 'collagenous spherulosis'.

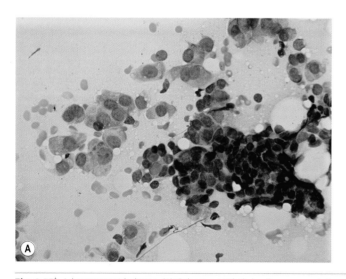

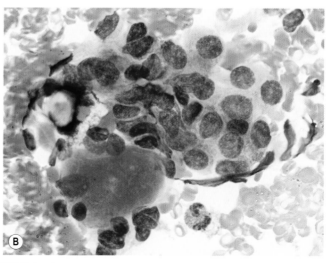

Fig. 8.55† Adenomyoepithelioma. (A) Cohesive epithelial cell groups and dissociated (myoepithelial) cells. (B) Higher-power view of the image in Fig. 8.54 shows collagenous globules.

Epithelial hyperplasia and tumour-like lesions

Epithelial hyperplasia without atypia (Figs 8.56–8.58)

Cytological findings: epithelial hyperplasia

- Low or moderate cellularity with small epithelial groups or high cellularity with large flat or folded sheets and three-dimensional aggregates of cohesive regular cells
- Adenosis lesions may show a microacinar appearance in smears as well as true tubular structures
- Nuclei may be enlarged, but the chromatin pattern is fine and nucleoli inconspicuous
- The epithelial groups contain the smaller, darker ovoid nuclei of myoepithelial cells
- Variable numbers of bipolar nuclei between the groups
- Any separate epithelial cells present also have a fine chromatin pattern and small nucleoli
- The nuclear membrane, often difficult to see in compact groups, has a smooth profile
- Macrophages and apocrine cells may be present
- An absence of nuclear atypia, widespread loss of cell cohesion or necrotic debris

Differential diagnosis: epithelial hyperplasia

- Epithelial hyperplasia may be difficult to distinguish from low-grade intraductal carcinoma or low-grade ductal carcinomas, especially tubular carcinoma
- Apocrine cells may be worrisome

Cytological findings: microglandular adenosis

- Abundant cellularity
- Epithelial cells in small groups and cohesive three-dimensional elongated tubular arrays
- The cells have scant cytoplasm, but round uniform nuclei with fine evenly dispersed chromatin and single nucleoli
- No bipolar cells

Differential diagnosis: microglandular adenosis

- Possible confusion with tubular carcinoma

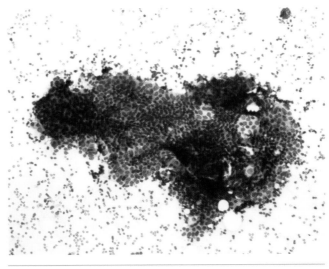

Fig. 8.56 Large sheet of mainly monolayered epithelial cells (MGG).

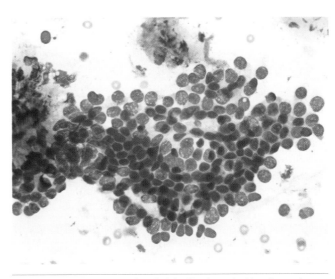

Fig. 8.57 Cohesive groups of epithelial cells admixed with collagen tissue (MGG).

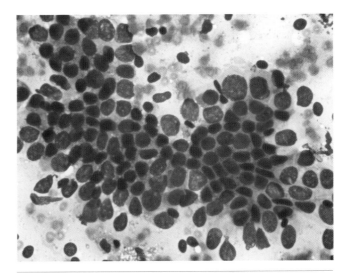

Fig. 8.58 Naked nuclei are seen in the background of this benign hyperplasia (MGG).

Complex sclerosing and fibrocystic lesions (Figs 8.59–8.61)

Cytological findings: radial sclerosing lesions

- Variable cellularity from scanty to abundant
- Cohesive three-dimensional epithelial aggregates without recognisable myoepithelial nuclei
- Small groups of uniform or slightly pleomorphic epithelial cells and dispersed bipolar cells
- Apocrine and/or columnar cells may be present, usually in small numbers
- Stromal fragments, partly as cell-poor elastoid fragments
- Single fibroblasts, histiocytic cells, macrophages and mucoid material

Differential diagnosis: radial sclerosing lesions

- Mild cell pleomorphism, single cells and absence of myoepithelial nuclei on the groups and aggregates may lead to a false-positive or false-suspicious cytological diagnosis

Benign papillary lesions

- Nipple adenoma
- Papilloma of the nipple ducts
- Erosive adenosis of the nipple
- Subareolar papillomatosis

Cytological findings: nipple adenoma, papilloma of the nipple ducts, erosive adenosis of the nipple, subareolar papillomatosis

- Moderate or high cellularity with a basic benign pattern
- Dispersed epithelial cells and small groups
- Little anisonucleosis, the uniform nuclei showing finely distributed chromatin and small nucleoli
- Occasional hyperchromatic nuclei possible
- Adenosquamous nests may be apparent
- Small amount of debris, inflammatory cells and siderophages may be a feature
- Apocrine cells may be present

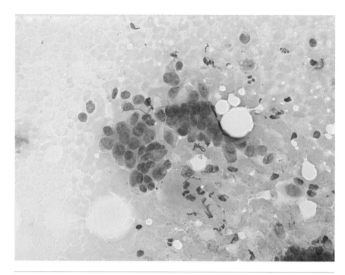

Fig. 8.59[†] Complex sclerosing lesion: smaller, cohesive epithelial groups, a few single cells and a stromal fragment.

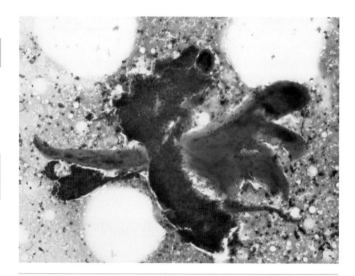

Fig. 8.60 The presence of large sheets of epithelial cells intimately mixed with dense connective tissue against a background of macrophages may raise the possibility of a papilloma.

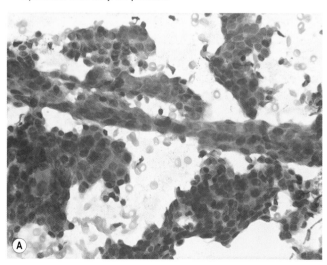

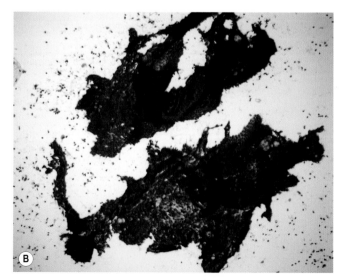

Fig. 8.61[†] Benign papilloma. (A) Cohesive papillary clusters with epithelial and myoepithelial cells clearly visible. (B) Overview showing complex folded sheets.

Differential diagnosis: nipple adenoma, papilloma of the nipple ducts, erosive adenosis of the nipple, subareolar papillomatosis

- Clinically, may be mistaken for Paget's disease of the nipple
- Low-grade papillary carcinoma may be difficult to exclude except by local excision, which is in any case appropriate

Borderline epithelial lesions (Figs 8.62–8.67)

Columnar cell lesions (CCL)

Hyperplasia with atypia

- A group of conditions characterised by dilatation of terminal duct lobular units (TDLU) lined by columnar epithelial cells
- CCL can be subdivided according to the extent of cellular proliferation and atypia
- CCL with hyperplasia: the acini are lined by more than two layers of columnar-type epithelial cells
- CCLs with cytological atypia encompass lesions also described as low-grade clinging carcinoma or flat epithelial atypia

Cytological findings: columnar cell lesions

- Columnar cell changes, hyperplasia with atypia and cellular papillary lesions show overlapping features
- A spectrum ranging from benign, monolayer sheets and crowded strips to three-dimensional aggregates resembling low-grade ductal carcinoma in situ (DCIS)

Differential diagnosis: columnar cell lesions

- Columnar cell changes, hyperplasia with atypia and cellular papillary lesions may mimic low-grade carcinoma

Cytological findings: hyperplasia with atypia

- Increased crowding and overlapping of cells within the groups
- Three-dimensional epithelial aggregates
- Obvious papillary groups
- Decreased cohesion of epithelial cells
- More variation in nuclear size
- More prominence of nucleoli
- Less evidence of cells of apocrine type

Differential diagnosis: hyperplasia with atypia

- ALH and LCIS cannot be differentiated cytologically or chromosomally, and can have the same FNA appearances as invasive lobular carcinoma
- CCL, ADH and low-grade DCIS cannot be differentiated cytologically or chromosomally
- Fibroepithelial neoplasms may appear atypical when the clinical and mammographic features are not available and the cytology is viewed under a high-power lens
- Low-grade and lobular carcinomas may be mistaken for a hyperplastic process
- Inflammatory lesions may cause quite marked reactive atypia
- Previous radiotherapy may cause atypia

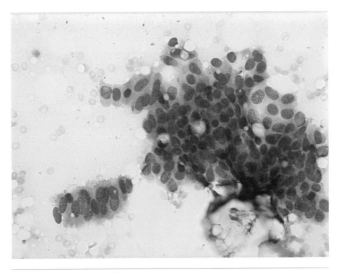

Fig. 8.62† Columnar cell lesion: palisading strip and monolayer sheet. Cohesive, micropapillary epithelial groups, a few single cells and minimal pleomorphism in a cellular papillary lesion.

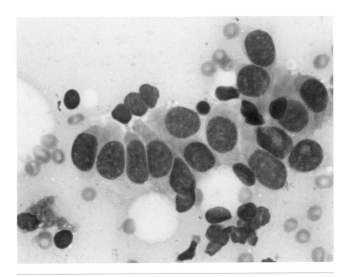

Fig. 8.63 Apocrine cells may give an impression of anisonucleosis and be rather worrisome (MGG).

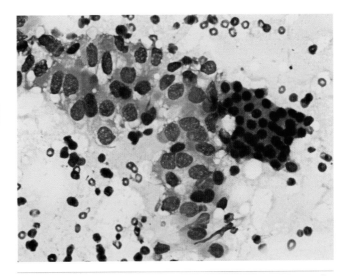

Fig. 8.64 Anisocytosis and anisonucleosis may be due to the presence of apocrine epithelial cells. Note cytoplasmic vacuolation. A sheet of benign ductal epithelium on the right is reassuring.

Cellular (florid) papillary lesions

- Intracystic/intraductal papillary tumours may have growth patterns that range from a 'simple' benign papilloma to very cellular lesions with a marked epithelial proliferation and hyperplasia, that resemble epithelial hyperplasia with and without atypia as well as fully diagnostic papillary intracystic carcinoma

Cytological features: cellular papillary lesions

- Cellular lesions
- Moderate to distinct cellular/nuclear pleomorphism
- Papillary fragments and fibrovascular stalks
- Usually, the epithelial fragments are rather cohesive
- Population of single cells is almost always present as well
- Apocrine cells, macrophages and intracystic debris is common

Differential diagnosis: cellular papillary lesions

- On cytology, it may be impossible to give a confident diagnosis of benign versus malignant lesion of a papillary lesion since most papillary, intracystic carcinomas are low-grade and show a discrete atypia
- Papillary lesions should all be excised.

Cytological findings: mucocele-like lesions

- Abundant mucin
- Scant to moderate cellularity with cohesive, monolayer clusters and sheets of epithelial cells
- Variable nuclear atypia
- No or only few single cells

Differential diagnosis

- Overdiagnosis of mucinous carcinoma

Lobular intraepithelial neoplasia

- Characterised by a proliferation of small and often loosely cohesive cells originating in the TDLU
- May or may not show pagetoid involvement of the terminal ducts
- Lesions are usually not palpable and have no radiologic appearance
- Sampled on FNA, they are an incidental finding to a radiological and/or clinical abnormality

Cytological findings: lobular neoplasia

- Loosely cohesive groups
- Uniform cells with occasional intracytoplasmic lumina
- Slightly irregular and eccentric nuclei

Diagnostic pitfalls: lobular neoplasia

- May be mistaken for benign cells
- More pleomorphic tumour cells may be diagnosed as carcinoma

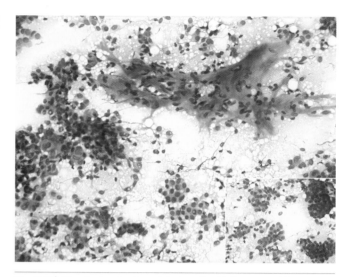

Fig. 8.65[†] Discohesive sheets and single cells with few atypical features and stromal capillary fragment. (Inset) Cohesive and micropapillary epithelial groups with a few single cells showing minimal pleomorphism and fine chromatin (MGG).

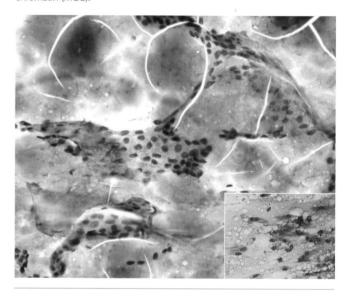

Fig. 8.66[†] Mucocele-like lesion consisting of abundant mucin and monolayer sheets of apocrine cells.

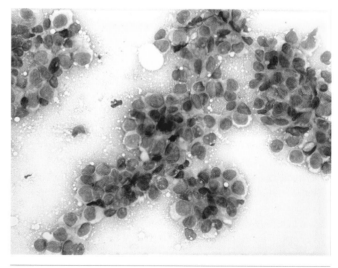

Fig. 8.67[†] Lobular neoplasia. Loosely lobuloid arrangement of monomorphic epithelial cells with a discrete atypia.

Common malignant breast epithelial tumours (Table 8.1, Box 8.1)

- The vast majority of malignant breast lesions are of epithelial origin
- Ductal carcinomas are more frequent than lobular carcinomas
- Differentiating invasive from in situ lesions by cytology is unreliable

Table 8.1 General diagnostic criteria for the recognition of benign and malignant conditions in FNA cytology of the breast

Morphological criteria	Benign	Malignant
Cellularity	Poor or moderate	Usually high
Cell-to-cell cohesion	Good, with large defined clusters of cells	Dissociated cells
Cell arrangement	Even, usually in flat sheets	Irregular, overlapping, often three-dimensional
Cell types	Mixture of epithelial, myoepithelial and other cells, e.g. stromal	Usually uniform cell population
Bipolar (elliptical) bare nuclei	Present	Not conspicuous
Background	Generally clean	Occasionally with necrosis and macrophages
NUCLEAR CHARACTERISTICS		
Size (in relation to RBCs)	Small	Variable, often large, depending on tumour type and grade
Pleomorphism	Rare	Common
Nuclear membranes (PAP)	Smooth	Irregular with indentations
Nucleoli (PAP)	Indistinct or small and single	Variable, may be prominent
Chromatin	Smooth or fine	Clumped, may be irregular
Additional features	Apocrine metaplasia, foamy macrophages	Mucin, intracytoplasmic lumina

Modified from Guidelines for non-operative diagnostic procedures and reporting in breast cancer screening. Non-operative Diagnosis Subgroup of the National Coordinating Group for Breast Screening Pathology. NHSBSP Publication 2001; 50:15.

Box 8.1   The 2003 World Health Organization (WHO) classification of tumours of the breast which includes benign (harmless) tumours and malignant (cancerous) tumours, recommends the following pathological types*

Invasive breast carcinomas
- Invasive ductal carcinoma
  - Most are 'not otherwise specified'
  - The remainder are given subtypes:
    - Mixed-type carcinoma
    - Pleomorphic carcinoma
    - Carcinoma with osteoclast giant cells
    - Carcinoma with choriocarcinoma features
    - Carcinoma with melanotic features
- Invasive lobular carcinoma
- Tubular carcinoma
- Invasive cribriform carcinoma
- Medullary carcinoma
- Mucinous carcinoma and other tumours with abundant mucin
  - Mucinous carcinoma
  - Cystadenocarcinoma and columnar cell mucinous carcinoma
  - Signet ring cell carcinoma
- Neuroendocrine tumours
  - Solid neuroendocrine carcinoma (carcinoid of the breast)
  - Atypical carcinoid tumour
  - Small cell/oat cell carcinoma
  - Large cell neuroendocrine carcinoma
- Invasive papillary carcinoma
- Invasive micropapillary carcinoma
- Apocrine carcinoma
- Metaplastic carcinomas
  - Pure epithelial metaplastic carcinomas
    - Squamous cell carcinoma
    - Adenocarcinoma with spindle cell metaplasia
    - Adenosquamous carcinoma
    - Mucoepidermoid carcinoma
  - Mixed epithelial/mesenchymal metaplastic carcinomas
- Lipid-rich carcinoma
- Secretory carcinoma
- Oncocytic carcinoma
- Adenoid cystic carcinoma
- Acinic cell carcinoma
- Glycogen-rich clear cell carcinoma
- Sebaceous carcinoma
- Inflammatory carcinoma
- Bilateral breast carcinoma

Mesenchymal tumours (including sarcoma)
- Hemangioma
- Angiomatosis
- Hemangiopericytoma
- Pseudoangiomatous stromal hyperplasia
- Myofibroblastoma
- Fibromatosis (aggressive)
- Inflammatory myofibroblastic tumour
- Lipoma
  - Angiolipoma
- Granular cell tumour
- Neurofibroma
- Schwannoma
- Angiosarcoma
- Liposarcoma
- Rhabdomyosarcoma
- Osteosarcoma
- Leiomyoma
- Leiomyosarcoma

Tumors of the male breast
- Gynaecomastia (benign)
- Carcinoma
  - In situ
  - Invasive

Malignant lymphoma
- Non-Hodgkin lymphoma

Metastatic tumours to the breast from other places in the body

Precursor lesions
- Lobular neoplasia
  - Lobular carcinoma in situ
- Intraductal proliferative lesions
  - Usual ductal hyperplasia
  - Flat epithelial hyperplasia
  - Atypical ductal hyperplasia
  - Ductal carcinoma in situ
- Microinvasive carcinoma
- Intraductal papillary neoplasms
  - Central papilloma
  - Peripheral papilloma
  - Atypical papilloma
  - Intraductal papillary carcinoma
  - Intracystic papillary carcinoma

Benign epithelial lesions
- Adenosis, including variants
  - Sclerosing adenosis
  - Apocrine adenosis
  - Blunt duct adenosis
  - Microglandular adenosis
  - Adenomyoepithelial adenosis
- Radial scar/complex sclerosing lesion
- Adenomas
  - Tubular adenoma
  - Lactating adenoma
  - Apocrine adenoma
  - Pleomorphic adenoma
  - Ductal adenoma

Myoepithelial lesions
- Myoepitheliosis
- Adenomyoepithelial adenosis
- Adenomyoepithelioma
- Malignant myoepithelioma

Fibroepithelial tumours
- Fibroadenoma
- Phyllodes tumour
  - Benign
  - Borderline
  - Malignant
- Periductal stromal sarcoma, low grade
- Mammary hamartoma

Benign tumors of the nipple
- Nipple adenoma
- Syringomatous adenoma
- Paget's disease of the nipple

Malignant tumors of the nipple
- Paget's disease of the nipple

*Peter Devilee; Fattaneh A. Tavassoli (2003). World Health Organization: Tumours of the Breast and Female Genital Organs. Oxford University Press. ISBN 92-832-2412-4.

Ductal carcinoma (Figs 8.68–8.78)

Cytological findings: invasive ductal carcinoma

- Varying cellularity from abundant to scanty
- The epithelial cells present as single cells, loose aggregates and cohesive groups often three-dimensional in appearance
- Varying cellular and nuclear atypia according to histological grade
- Cells may be vacuolated and occasional signet ring cells are seen
- Microcalcification is quite common
- Mitoses are uncommon, but may be seen in high-grade lesions
- Necrosis is not common

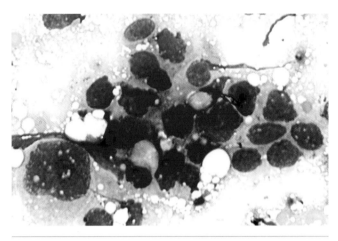

Fig. 8.70 High-grade ductal carcinoma with marked cytological atypia.

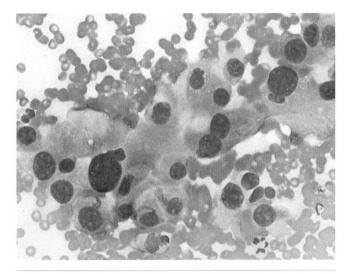

Fig. 8.68 High-grade ductal carcinoma. Tumour cells show large variations in size and shape (MGG).

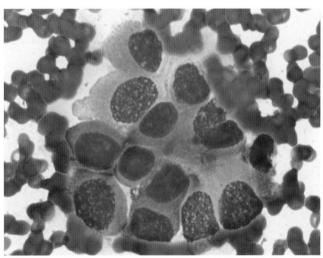

Fig. 8.71 High-grade ductal carcinoma with large tumour cells.

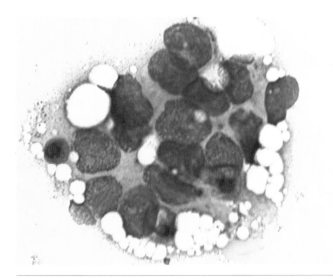

Fig. 8.69 High-grade ductal carcinoma with an attempt at glandular formation.

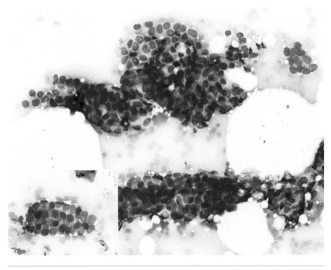

Fig. 8.72 Low-grade ductal carcinoma mimicking fibroadenoma, with tightly cohesive cell clusters. (Inset) Higher-power view of the same tumour.

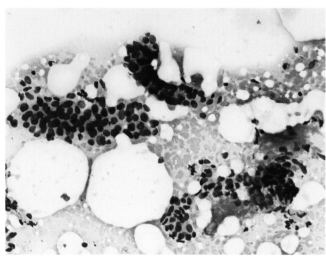

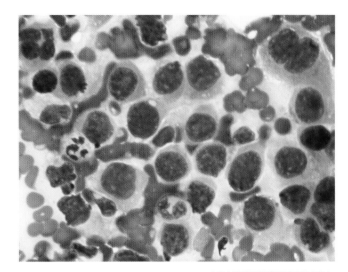

Fig. 8.73 High-grade ductal carcinoma with dissociated malignant cells (MGG).

Fig. 8.76 Low-grade ductal carcinoma mimicking fibroadenoma. No myoepithelial cells. Bare nuclei in the background may be mistaken for stromal cells.

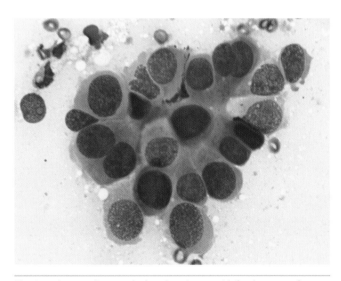

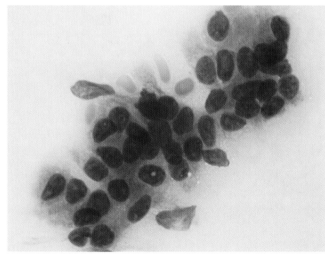

Fig. 8.74 Intermediate-grade ductal carcinoma with focal aspects of glandular differentiation (MGG).

Fig. 8.77 Low-grade ductal carcinoma with the presence of a gland (MGG).

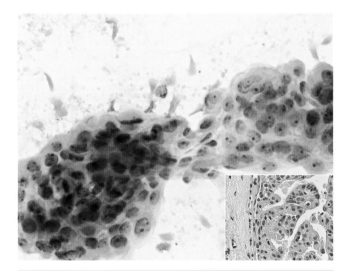

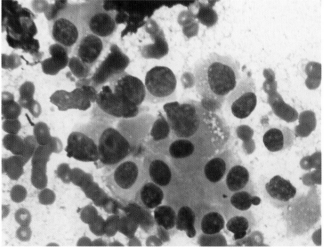

Fig. 8.75 Ductal carcinoma in situ. Cytologically, cannot be diagnosed. May have a bland cell appearance with necrotic background. (Inset) Histology of DCIS from the same patient.

Fig. 8.78 Low-grade ductal carcinoma. Note the small size of tumour cells (MGG).

Invasive lobular carcinoma (Figs 8.79–8.83)

Cytological findings

- Scanty aspirates are common
- Tumour cells are usually dispersed and mainly single or in small groups of two to five cells
- Cells are small, nuclei have an abnormal appearance with irregular outline
- Occasional single-file 'chains', usually containing only three or four cells, may be seen
- Cytoplasm is scanty, with the nucleus eccentrically placed and some cells may contain an intracytoplasmic lumen with a signet ring appearance
- Nuclei show slight but definite variation in size but tend to be round in shape
- The chromatin is stippled but not coarse
- The nucleolus is inconspicuous in the classic type

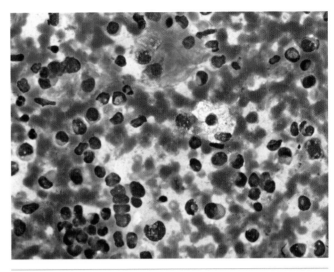

Fig. 8.81 Classic lobular carcinoma. Note that tumour cells are small and dissociated (MGG).

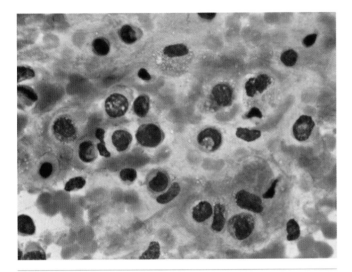

Fig. 8.79 Classic lobular carcinoma. Note that tumour cells are embedded in dense collagen (MGG).

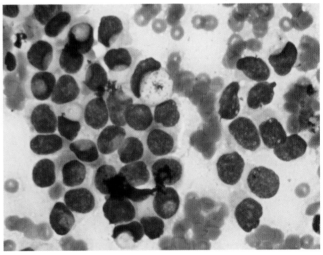

Fig. 8.82 Intracytoplasmic vacuoles in a lobular carcinoma (MGG).

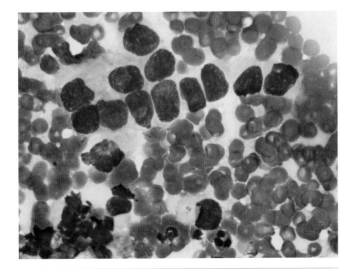

Fig. 8.80 'Indian files' may be seen but are not diagnostic of the lobular type of adenocarcinoma. Note nuclear molding (MGG).

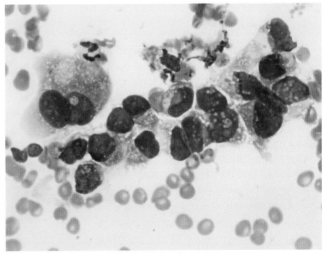

Fig. 8.83 Pleomorphic type of lobular carcinoma with intracytoplasmic microvacuoles (MGG).

Differential diagnosis

- Lobular carcinomas account for many of the false-negative cases in most series
- It is not always possible to distinguish lobular carcinomas from ductal carcinomas
- Cases with prominent intracytoplasmic lumina may be mistaken for signet ring carcinoma
- High-grade or 'pleomorphic' lobular carcinoma resembles high-grade ductal carcinoma
- Because of the diffusely infiltrative nature of these tumours, it is common for lobular carcinoma cells to be seen together with a variety of benign epithelial changes

Uncommon malignant breast epithelial tumours

Tubular carcinoma (Figs 8.84, 8.85)

Cytological findings

- Aspirates may be poorly cellular, but with an optimal technique, they may yield a more cellular and diagnostic material
- Epithelial cells in cohesive clusters and sheets that have a recognisable acinar structure, but abnormal rigid finger-like groups and cell balls also may be seen
- Monolayer sheets, often folded and with part of an intact tubular structure in one end
- True tubular structures, often broken with sharp angles
- There is slight anisonucleosis and mild hyperchromasia
- The chromatin is finely granular and evenly distributed
- Nucleoli are indistinct or small

Differential diagnosis

- Bland appearances may be mistaken for epithelial hyperplasia or fibroadenoma, giving a false-negative diagnosis

Medullary carcinoma with lymphoid stroma (Fig. 8.86)

Cytological findings

- Very cellular smears are easily obtained
- Poorly cohesive large malignant cells with abundant pale-staining cytoplasm, some forming syncytial aggregates
- Large angular nuclei with coarse chromatin and prominent nucleoli
- Mitotic figures are not unusual
- The background of small lymphocytes and plasma cells is a vital feature but their number is very variable and they can be so few that they are overlooked
- These cells may be entirely separate from the epithelial cells or intimately mixed with the syncytial groups
- Tumour giant cells are sometimes a feature

Differential diagnosis

- Although the diagnosis of carcinoma is not usually difficult, the presence of lymphoid cells and the clinical features of a circumscribed round nodule can cause difficulty in distinguishing a primary carcinoma high in the axillary tail from a lymph node metastasis

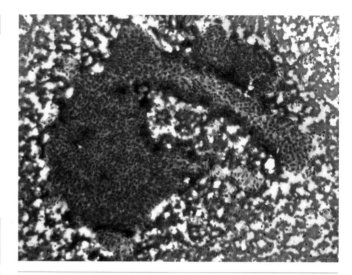

Fig. 8.84 Tubular carcinoma. Large sheet of cells with tubular architecture (MGG).

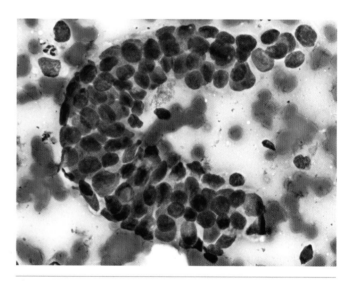

Fig. 8.85 Tubular carcinoma showing an intact tubule (MGG).

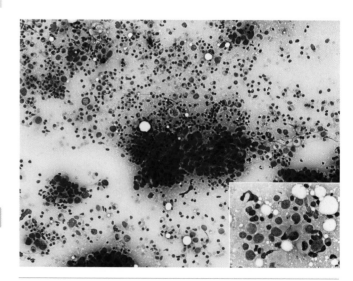

Fig. 8.86 Medullary carcinoma: high-grade tumour epithelial cells are intermixed with lymphocytes and plasma cells.

Mucinous (colloid) carcinoma (Fig. 8.87)

- Relatively rare
- Typically occurs at an age of 60 years or more
- Most mucinous carcinomas are low grade, slow growing and have a favourable prognosis with a 5-year survival of up to 86%
- High-grade mucinous carcinomas do occur

Cytological findings

- On spreading, the aspirate is quite glairy, hinting at a high mucin content
- The smear is usually cellular
- The epithelial cells present as single cells, loose aggregates and cohesive groups often three-dimensional in appearance
- The cells are small, with small, uniform, round nuclei, smooth nuclear outlines, bland, possibly granular, chromatin and inconspicuous nucleoli
- The cells are bathed in mucin of variable density. This is more obvious in MGG preparations, where they stain violet
- Cells may be vacuolated and occasional signet ring cells are seen
- Some cases contain microcalcifications

Differential diagnosis

- As cytologically bland, they may be misdiagnosed as benign, particularly when they occur in younger women
- Some ductal carcinomas of no special type can contain large foci of mucinous carcinoma
- Cell-poor samples with ample mucin and scanty tumour cells may mimic mucocele/mucocele-like lesions (see Fig. 8.66, p. 264)

Neuroendocrine carcinoma (Figs 8.88, 8.89)

- Clinically, these tumours present like a ductal carcinoma
- They are often well circumscribed, both clinically and radiologically
- They express neuroendocrine markers in over 50% of the tumour cell population

Cytological findings

- Cellular aspirates contain dispersed single cells and cells in small groups
- The cells are remarkably uniform with an eccentrically placed nucleus resembling plasma cells
- The chromatin is stippled and thickening of the nuclear border may be noted
- Cytoplasmic (endocrine) granules may be seen in a few tumour cells

Diagnostic pitfalls

- Lymphoplasmacytoid lymphoma or plasmacytoma can form deposits in soft tissue and breast
- Lymphoma usually displays complete absence of cell cohesion

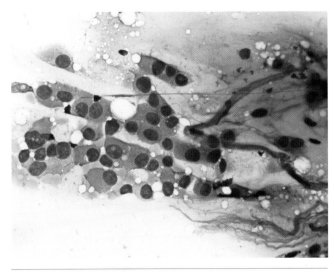

Fig. 8.87 Mucin producing (colloid) carcinoma: malignant glandular cells are intermixed with mucinous substance.

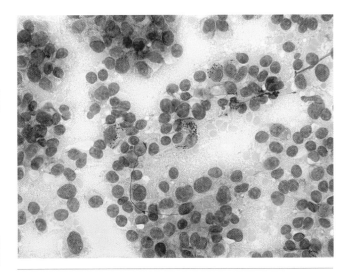

Fig. 8.88† Neuroendocrine carcinoma cells with some of the cells showing pink endocrine cytoplasmic granules.

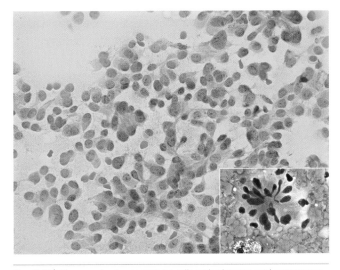

Fig. 8.89† Neuroendocrine carcinoma cells with plasmacytoid appearance. (Inset) Neuroendocrine carcinoma with a rosette.

Papillary carcinoma (Figs 8.90, 8.91)

- Pure papillary carcinoma has a better prognosis than invasive ductal carcinoma (80% 5-year survival rate)
- FNA diagnosis of the subtype can be of benefit in deciding the extent of surgery

Cytological findings

- May be cystic on aspiration
- The cell material is usually abundant
- Epithelial cells are monotonous and appear 'clonal'
- Anisonucleosis, hyperchromasia, coarse chromatin and prominent nucleoli are uncommon
- Benign bipolar cells are absent from the background and myoepithelial cells are not seen within the groups
- Large papillary cell clusters forming arborising arrays bearing overlapping, palisaded cells on a fibrovascular core may be present as with papillomas
- Cells may be dispersed and the fibrovascular cores denuded
- The cells are often distinctly columnar in appearance, although this feature is shared with papillomas

Differential diagnosis

- Intraductal papilloma may have greater anisonucleosis but usually cells in papilloma are in cohesive sheets and in papillary carcinoma dispersed
- Background in papilloma is cystic but 'clean' whilst papillary carcinoma has necrotic background with apoptotic debris

Apocrine carcinoma (Fig. 8.92)

Cytological findings

- Aspirates tend to be cellular and the cells dispersed
- The cells are large with abundant acidophilic cytoplasm that may be granular but this is less marked than in benign apocrine epithelium
- The cell borders tend to be indistinct or ragged in contrast to the well-defined borders of benign apocrine cells
- This is an important feature if low-grade apocrine carcinoma is suspected
- The nucleus is also large and the chromatin coarse and unevenly distributed
- The single nucleolus is very large, sometimes spectacularly so
- Multiple nucleoli are also seen in the higher-grade tumours

Differential diagnosis:

- Apocrine carcinoma may be mistaken, with apocrine metaplasia or atypical apocrine cells sometimes observed in a benign cyst

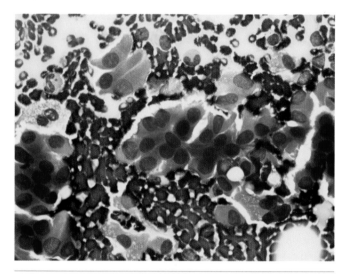

Fig. 8.90 Papillary adenocarcinoma: relatively large cells with eccentric nuclei (MGG).

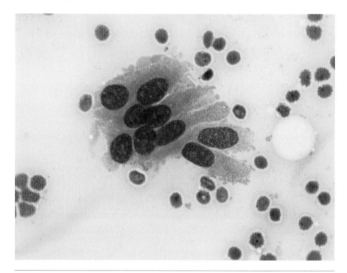

Fig. 8.91 Papillary adenocarcinoma: note the cylindrical appereance of adenocarcinoma cells (MGG).

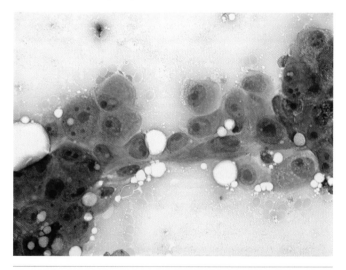

Fig. 8.92[†] Cells from a high-grade carcinoma with apocrine differentiation with abundant dense cytoplasm and prominent nucleoli. Cytoplasmic borders are indistinct or ragged compared to normal apocrine cells (see Figs 8.26–8.32, pp. 253–254).

Glycogen-rich (clear cell) carcinoma (Fig. 8.93)

Cytological findings

- Abundantly cellular aspirate
- Tumour cells in groups, clusters and as single cells
- Large dispersed cells with plentiful clear or eosinophilic, finely granular to vacuolated cytoplasm and centrally placed nuclei
- Fragile cytoplasm that may smear out and appear as a granular background material
- Moderate to marked nuclear pleomorphism

Diagnostic pitfalls

- May resemble signet ring carcinoma but the prognosis is, in any case, similar
- Metastatic renal cell carcinoma

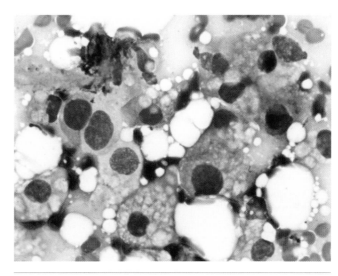

Fig. 8.93 Glycogen-rich carcinoma (MGG).

Carcinoma with osteoclast-like stromal giant cells (Fig. 8.94)

- Some otherwise unremarkable ductal carcinomas are associated with osteoclast-like stromal giant cells. The stromal cells are not malignant and are thought to be a reaction to the tumour

Cytological findings

- Aspirates are cellular, containing malignant ductal epithelial cells of any grade
- Can look very bland and be mistaken for fibroadenoma with giant cells
- The giant cells have abundant basophilic cytoplasm and variable numbers of nuclei but are not cytologically malignant

Diagnostic pitfalls

- Occasional cases may be dominated by the giant cells and there is a risk that they may be diagnosed as granulomatous inflammation, fat necrosis or foreign body reaction (see Figs 8.18–8.21, p. 251)

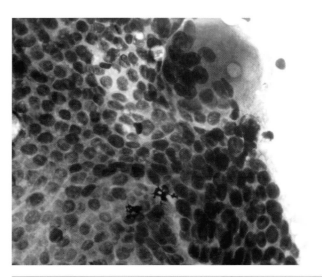

Fig. 8.94 Carcinoma with osteoclast-like giant cells. Note bland epithelium which was misdiagnosed as benign.

Paget's disease of the nipple (Fig. 8.95)

- Malignant cells from an intraductal or invasive ductal carcinoma can spread to the nipple
- Irritation of the nipple may be a first sign of disease
- Nipple scraping or nipple discharge should be examined carefully for presence of classic malignant cells

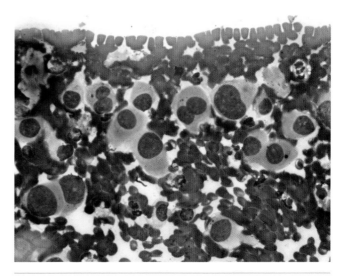

Fig. 8.95 Paget's disease of the nipple: adenocarcinoma cells were obtained by scraping (MGG).

Metaplastic carcinoma/carcinosarcoma (Figs 8.96–8.98)

- High-grade carcinoma
- Tumour undergoes metaplastic change, producing a sarcomatous pattern

Cytological findings

- The aspirates are usually cellular
- The cells may be indistinguishable from those of a high-grade ductal carcinoma of breast depending on the area aspirated
- Additional features depending on the extent and type of the metaplastic malignancy may include:
  - Large, malignant multinucleated giant cells
  - Malignant cells associated with fragments of amorphous metachromatic material
  - Large malignant spindle cells singly or in syncytial clusters
  - Squamous cell differentiation

Differential diagnosis

- The extent and degree of metaplasia are variable and so some cases may be diagnosed as ductal carcinoma without special features on cytological assessment
- The aspirate may contain only spindle cells and may be diagnosed as a sarcoma
- High-grade malignant phyllodes tumour has similar sarcomatous elements

Malignant myoepithelioma

- An infiltrating tumour composed purely of myoepithelial, predominantly spindle cells

Cytological findings

- Single and small groups of spindle cells which may reveal a distinct pleomorphism
- Metachromatic ground substance as well as metachromatic stromal fragments
- Admixed benign ductal epithelial cells and lymphocytes

Differential diagnosis

- May resemble metaplastic carcinoma where only the non-epithelial component has been aspirated or another non-epithelial lesion

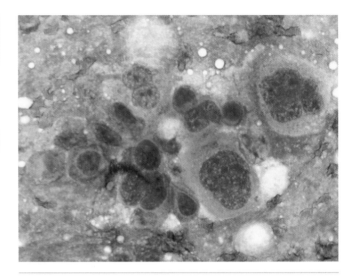

Fig. 8.96 Metaplastic carcinoma (MGG).

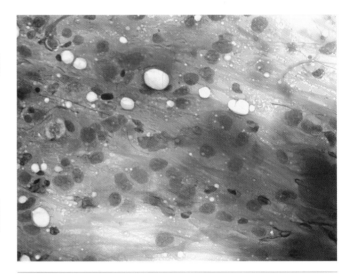

Fig. 8.97† Metaplastic carcinoma. Chondro-myxoid material and high-grade malignant cells from a metaplastic carcinoma.

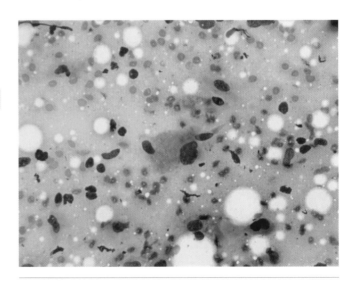

Fig. 8.98† Pleomorphic spindle and polygonal cells from a malignant myoepithelioma.

Primary sarcomas, lymphomas and metastatic tumours (Figs 8.99–8.107)

Cytological findings

- Primary sarcomas mainly correspond to malignant phyllodes tumour or to angiosarcoma following irradiation of the breast
- Primary lymphomas are rare and more often secondary sites of involvement (see Chapter 7)
- Other metastatic lesions to the breast may originate from the contralateral breast or from tumours such as small cell lung cancer, melanoma, renal carcinoma

Differential diagnosis

- Primary breast sarcomas should be differentiated from radiation-induced changes in the breast
- Primary breast low-grade lymphomas from normal intra-mammary lymph node
- Metastatic small cell carcinoma and lymphoma to the breast can imitate ductal and lobular carcinoma, and amelanotic melanoma may mimic high-grade ductal carcinoma

Further investigations

- Considering the rarity of these tumours, the use of ancillary techniques such as immunocytochemical methods on cell blocks and/or immunohistochemical analysis on a biopsy are usually required

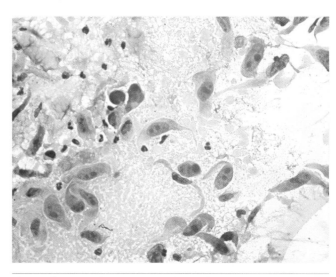

Fig. 8.99[†] High-grade malignant spindle cells from a malignant phyllodes tumour (MGG).

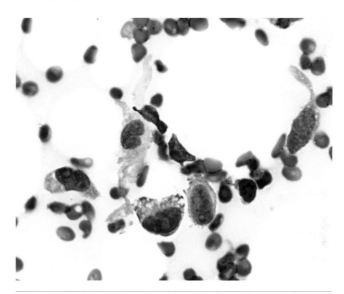

Fig. 8.100[†] Spindle and polygonal cells with high-grade atypia and large abnormal nucleoli from a post-irradiation angiosarcoma (MGG).

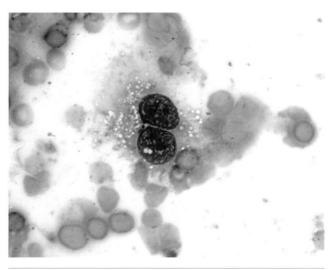

Fig. 8.101[†] Irradiation atypia with enlarged (benign) nuclei with degenerative chromatin pattern and vacuolated, fuzzy cytoplasm.

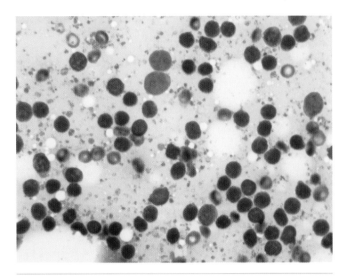

Fig. 8.102 Primary breast mantle cell lymphoma: note the presence of lymphoglandular bodies in the background (MGG).

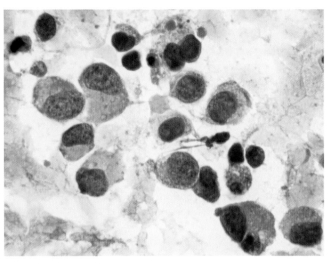

Fig. 8.105 Metastatic melanoma to the breast (PAP).

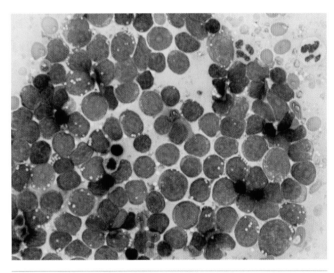

Fig. 8.103 Metastasis to the breast of a Diffuse large B-cell lymphoma (MGG).

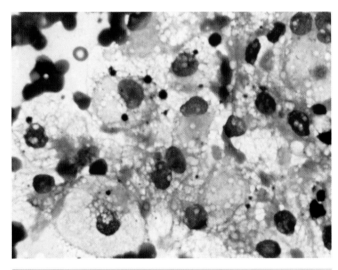

Fig. 8.106 Metastasis to the breast of a renal clear cell carcinoma (MGG).

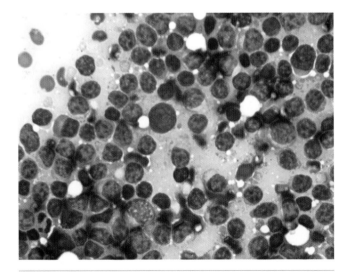

Fig. 8.104 Metastasis to the breast of a lymphoplasmacytic lymphoma (MGG).

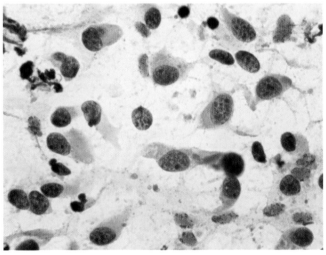

Fig. 8.107 Metastasis to the breast of a stromal endometrial sarcoma (PAP).

Reporting breast FNAs: the role of FNA in management

The use of breast FNA cytology differs. When used, cytology forms part of the triple assessment approach (clinical, imaging and pathology) to breast diagnosis.

The role of the multidisciplinary team

- Management of patients with cancer or suspected cancer is coordinated through a multidisciplinary team (MDT) of surgeons, oncologists, radiologists, pathologists, specialist nurses and other support services
- MDT provides a forum for discussing individual patients and deciding which options of treatment should be recommended
- MDT agrees protocols for initial surgical treatment following FNA and radiological diagnosis
- Good communication between the cytologist and the clinical and imaging teams is crucial
- Written communication can be helped by the use of standardised reporting systems such as C1–C5, used in Europe (Table 8.2)
- The report should be provided in writing even in the one-stop clinic
- Unusual, complicated and malignant cases should be discussed by the MDT prior to surgery
- Local (cytopathological and radiological) expertise is one of the major factors influencing the extent of FNA use. In well-trained hands, FNA is cheap, reliable and the least invasive method for obtaining a preoperative diagnosis
- Whenever possible, the cytopathologists should be active participants wherever samples are taken, both in the aspiration process and in the preparation of the aspirated material

The role of FNA in management of breast lesions (Fig. 8.108)

- Cytology forms part of the triple assessment approach (clinical, imaging and pathology) to breast diagnosis
- It is the first-line pathological investigation in symptomatic and some screening populations (with the exception of cases with microcalcifications)
- The majority of centres practice a degree of one-stop diagnosis with a cytopathologist present in the out-patient clinic
- Image guidance (ultrasonography and stereotactic device) is used in most centres and is an important part of the modern approach to FNA in non-palpable lesions
- Stereotactic core biopsy is usually performed in cases of microcalcifications
- **When triple assessment is concordant, final treatment may proceed on the basis of FNA, without a tissue biopsy**
- ER and PR assessment can be done safely on FNA material, provided there is local expertise, as can investigation of HER-2 status by in situ hybridisation
- The absence of cytology expertise is the most common cause for using the core biopsy as the first line investigation and should be discouraged since most palpable lesions are benign

Table 8.2 Modified reporting categories in breast FNA according to NHSBSP guidelines

Reporting category	Description
C1	**Inadequate.** Assessment is subjective and based on the presence of a sufficient number of epithelial cells to provide sample adequate for confident assessment. Aspirates from cysts, abscesses, fat necrosis and nipple discharge should not be classified as inadequate. Apart from hypocellularity, crush, air-drying, blood and thickness of smear could cause inadequate sample. It is helpful to comment on the cause of inadequate specimens.
C2	**Benign.** Adequate sample without evidence of atypia, composed of regular epithelial cells, usually in monolayers; background composed of dispersed individual or paired nuclei. A specific diagnosis, such as fibroadenoma, fat necrosis, granulomatous mastitis, breast abscess or lymph node, can be given if sufficient features are present.
C3	**Atypia, probably benign.** In addition to benign features, certain features not commonly seen in benign aspirates may be present: nuclear pleomorphism, loss of cell cohesion, nuclear or cytoplasmic changes (pregnancy, contraceptive pill, hormone replacement therapy) and increased cellularity.
C4	**Suspicious of malignancy.** This category should be used for aspirates with highly atypical features, such that the pathologist is almost certain that they come from a malignant lesion, although a confident diagnosis cannot be made due to the following: (a) specimen is scanty, (b) the sample shows some malignant features in the absence of overt malignant features, (c) the sample has an overall benign pattern with large numbers of naked nuclei and/or cohesive sheets of cells but with occasional cells showing distinct malignant features. Definitive therapeutic surgery SHOULD NOT be undertaken on the basis of C3 or C4 report.
C5	**Malignant.** Adequate sample containing cells characteristic of carcinoma. Malignancy should not be diagnosed on the basis of a single criterion.

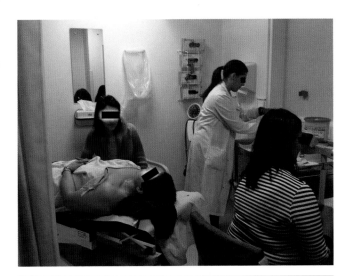

Fig. 8.108 The 'one-stop' breast clinic gives an opportunity to examine the patient, take and prepare samples, and check material adequacy under the microscope. In many cases, the final report can be given straight away and the patient discharged from the hospital care.

CHAPTER 9

Salivary gland

Contents

Introduction   279

Normal salivary gland   280

Tumours of the salivary gland   281

Non-neoplastic conditions   300

Salivary gland cysts   302

Diagnostic approach to salivary gland FNA   308

Introduction (Figs 9.1–9.3)

Clinical management of salivary gland masses increasingly relies on pre-treatment diagnosis based on microscopic FNA findings. FNA can reduce the rate of salivary gland surgery in one-third to one-half of cases.

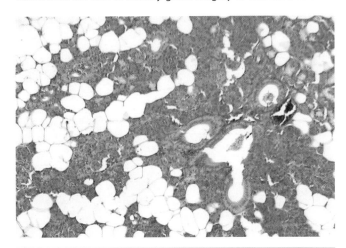

Fig. 9.1 Salivary gland histology. Normal salivary gland acini and ducts separated by adipose tissue.

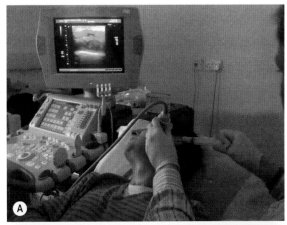

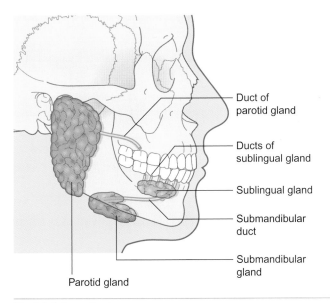

Fig. 9.2 Salivary glands.

Duct of parotid gland

Ducts of sublingual gland

Sublingual gland

Submandibular duct

Submandibular gland

Parotid gland

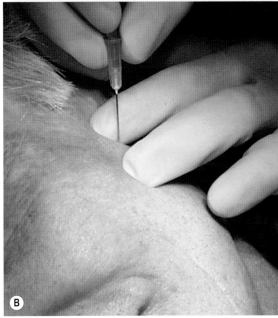

Fig. 9.3 FNA of salivary gland. (A) Image-guided FNA. Deep lesions that are less than 1 cm in diameter are best aspirated under ultrasonographic or CT scanning guidance. Ultrasound cannot reliably distinguish benign from malignant lesions. (B) Capillary FNA technique. The nodule is immobilised and the needle tip is rapidly directed through the skin. Once the needle enters the mass, it is continuously moved in and out for a few seconds.

Normal salivary gland (Figs 9.4–9.6)

Cytological findings

- Acinar cells:
  - large cells, often in lobulated groups
  - abundant cytoplasm
  - small round uniform nuclei
  - cytoplasm finely granular in serous glands
  - clear or lightly vacuolated in mucous glands
  - fragile and easily disrupted by smearing
  - bare dispersed nuclei in the background
- Ductal cells:
  - arranged in flat sheets
  - displaying good cohesion
  - uniform morphology
  - myoepithelial cell nuclei are small and pointed

Differential diagnosis

- Acinic cell carcinoma: cellular, lacking ductal cells
- Myoepithelial sialadenitis or MALT (if lymphoid cells from intraparotid lymph node are present)

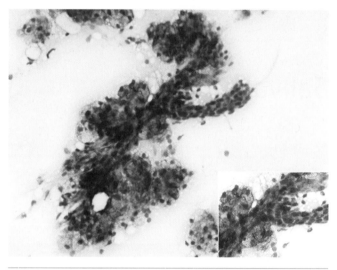

Fig. 9.4 Low-power view of the normal salivary gland FNA. (Inset) Ductal and acinar epithelium join imperceptibly together.

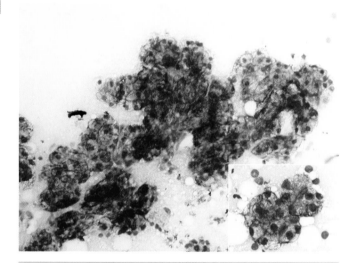

Fig. 9.5 Normal salivary gland FNA at medium power showing acinar epithelium. (Inset) Acinal cells have small, round, eccentrically placed nuclei and vacuolated, granular cytoplasm which is very fragile so that the cells often show only as bare nuclei in the background.

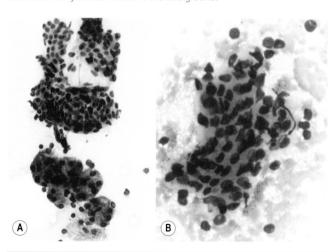

Fig. 9.6 Normal salivary gland epithelium. (A) Acinar epithelium below, ductal epithelium above. (B) Ductal epithelium in tightly cohesive flat sheets of cuboidal cells.

Tumours of the salivary gland

The majority of primary epithelial tumours occur in the parotid gland.

The smaller the involved salivary gland, the higher is the possibility of the tumour being malignant.

Most common tumour types (WHO classification 2005*)

Benign tumours

- Pleomorphic adenoma (Figs 9.7, 9.10–9.17)
- Warthin's tumour (adenolymphoma) (Figs 9.8, 9.18–9.26)
- Basal cell adenoma (Fig. 9.27)
- Myoepithelioma (myoepithelial adenoma) (Fig. 9.28)
- Other benign tumours (Figs 9.29–9.31)

Malignant tumours

- Adenoid cystic carcinoma (Figs 9.9, 9.48–9.53)
- Acinic cell carcinoma (Figs 9.32–9.38)
- Mucoepidermoid carcinoma (Figs 9.39–9.47)
- Polymorphous low-grade adenocarcinoma (terminal duct adenocarcinoma) (Figs 9.61–9.63)
- Salivary duct carcinoma (Figs 9.64–9.66)
- Adenocarcinoma (not otherwise specified)
- Rare types of salivary gland malignant tumours (Figs. 9.67–9.69)
- Other carcinomas (Figs 9.70–9.75)

*Barnes L, Eveson JW, Reichart P, et al. Pathology and genetics of head and neck tumors. World Health Organization Classification of Tumours. Lyon: IARC Press; 2005:209–281.

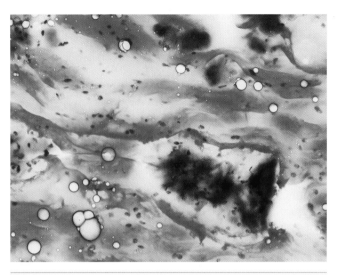

Fig. 9.7† Pleomorphic adenoma is the most common benign salivary gland tumour. It shows a characteristic fibrillary myxoid background in which cells are immersed.

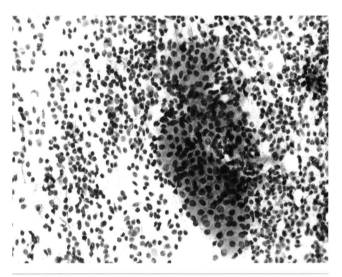

Fig. 9.8† Adenolymphoma (Warthin's tumour) is the second most common benign salivary gland tumour. Typically, it contains oncocytic epithelium surrounded by lymphoid cells.

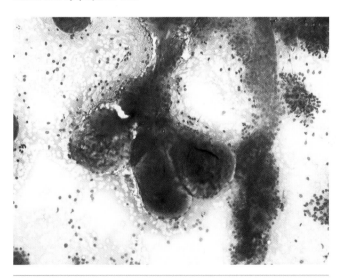

Fig. 9.9 Adenoid cystic carcinoma is the most common malignant salivary gland tumour in adults. Globules of myxoid matrix are a helpful pointer towards the diagnosis.

Pleomorphic adenoma

Normal salivary gland is usually sampled by fine needle aspiration (FNA) unintentionally, when trying to establish the origin and nature of a lump in the neck. The FNA of normal gland can be painful unless local anaesthetic is applied.

- Pleomorphic adenoma (mixed tumour) is the commonest salivary gland neoplasm, accounting for 60% of all tumours
- Most (80%) occur in the parotid gland but it is occasionally encountered in the nasal cavity, paranasal sinuses, upper respiratory tract and gastrointestinal tract
- Histologically, the typical tumour consists of glandular structures composed of a double layer of epithelial and myoepithelial cells embedded in myxoid stroma

Cytological findings (Figs 9.7, 9.10–9.17)

- Cellular aspirates with large amount of myxoid background matrix
- Myoepithelial cells singly or in sheets
- Epithelial cells in form of tubules or as squamous or oncocytic cells
- Cell nuclei vary in size but have uniform chromatin
- Spindle-shaped mesenchymal cells
- Chondroid or other metaplastic changes sometimes seen

Differential diagnosis

- Dominance of one cell type: myoepithelioma (Fig. 9.28)
- Cytological atypia: carcinoma ex pleomorphic adenoma (Figs 9.67, 9.68)
- Globules of basement membrane material: adenoid cystic carcinoma (see Figs 9.102–9.106)
- Cystic change: retention cyst, Warthin's tumour
- Mucin production: mucoepidermoid carcinoma
- Squamous, mucinous, sebaceous metaplasia, squamous cell carcinoma or mucoepidermoid carcinoma

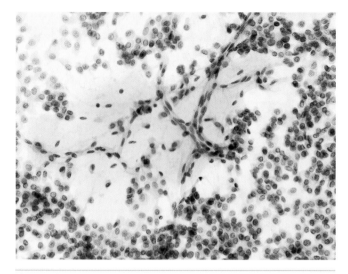

Fig. 9.11[†] Pleomorphic adenoma. Appearances in PAP-stained samples show better nuclear detail.

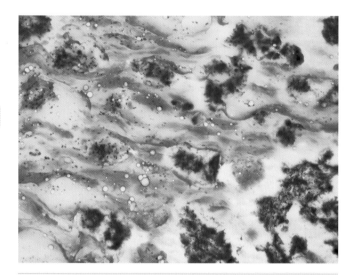

Fig. 9.12 Pleomorphic adenoma. Myxoid matrix often dominates the picture, most of the cells being immersed in it.

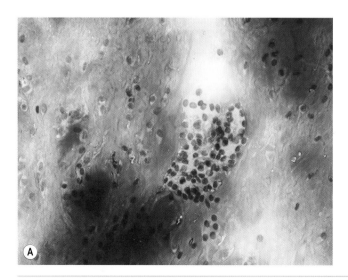

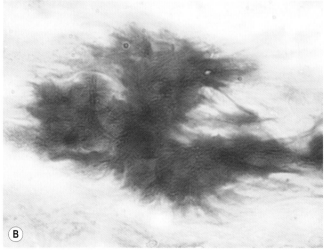

Fig. 9.10 Pleomorphic adenoma. (A) Low-power view shows fibrillary myxoid background material, epithelial and myoepithelial cells. [†] (B) High-power view shows the fibrillary quality of the stroma, sometimes describes as sun rays.

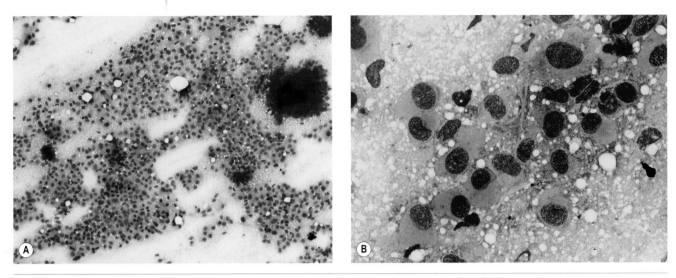

Fig. 9.13 Pleomorphic adenoma. Sometimes, a sample can be very cellular (A) and myxoid stroma present only focally. Myoepithelial cells (B, high-power view) show plasmacytoid features, are arranged singly and have bland oval nuclei.

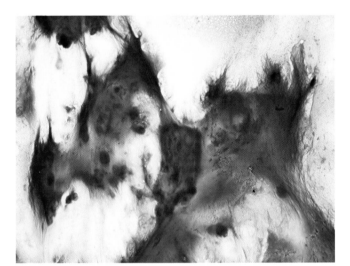

Fig. 9.14 Pleomorphic adenoma. Chondroid stroma sometimes dominates the findings.

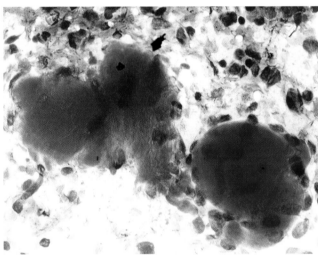

Fig. 9.16 Pleomorphic adenoma. Myxoid stroma may sometimes appear as cylindromatous hyaline globules such as seen in adenoid cystic carcinoma.

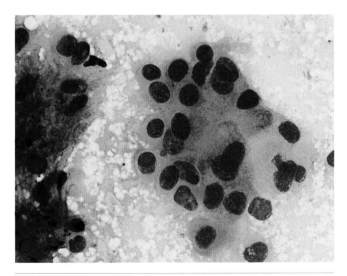

Fig. 9.15 Pleomorphic adenoma. Epithelial cells may show squamous metaplasia.

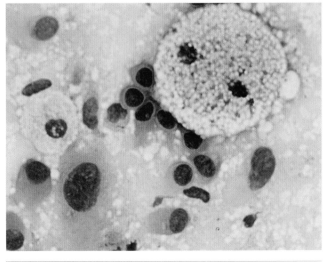

Fig. 9.17 Pleomorphic adenoma. Cystic change, as shown here by a macrophage, is not an uncommon feature of PA.

Warthin's tumour (adenolymphoma)

- The second most common salivary gland tumour
- More common in males than in females
- Most occur in the middle-aged or elderly
- Associated with smoking
- Slow growing, often fluctuant
- Can be bilateral or unilaterally multicentric
- Composed of glandular, often cystic, papillary structures with a lymphoid stroma
- The epithelium is double-layered and predominantly oncocytic but mucus or goblet cells and areas of squamous metaplasia may be present

Cytological findings (Figs 9.18–9.26)

- Watery or mucoid aspirate
- Sheets of oncocytic epithelial cells
- Admixture of lymphocytes
- Background debris

Differential diagnosis

- **Cystic change:** benign lymphoepithelial lesions, mucus retention cyst, branchial cleft cyst, chronic sialadenitis, cystadenoma, cystic low-grade mucoepidermoid carcinoma, cystic metastasis of a squamous cell carcinoma, cystic pleomorphic adenoma, lymphangioma, cystadenocarcinoma, cystic acinic cell carcinoma, polycystic disease of the parotid gland and lymphoma
- **Oncocytic cells:** oncocytoma, degenerate oncocytes (pyknocytes), possess pseudokeratinised, orangeophilic cytoplasm masquerading as squamous cells
- **Squamous metaplasia** and cystic degeneration: metastatic squamous carcinoma with cystic change
- **Extracellular or intracellular mucin:** mucoepidermoid carcinoma (see Mucoepidermoid carcinoma, p. 290)
- **Other factors:** may show I-131 increased uptake, despite a negative Tc-99m pertechnetate salivary gland scintigraphy, which may be misleading in patients investigated for thyroid carcinoma

For diagnostic approach and differential diagnosis of salivary gland FNA please see Fig. 9.112 and Table 9.1.

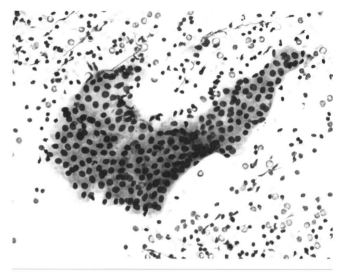

Fig. 9.18 Warthin's tumour. Aspirates are composed of flat sheets of oncocytic epithelium with variable number of lymphoid cells.

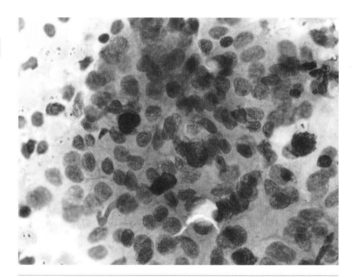

Fig. 9.19 Warthin's tumour. The epithelium is double-layered and predominantly oncocytic. Mast cells can be seen associated with epithelium.

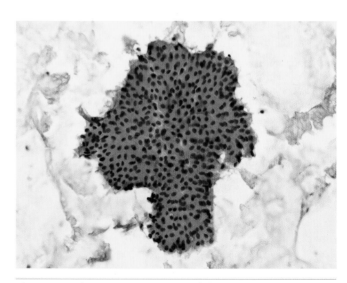

Fig. 9.20 Warthin's tumour. Oncocytic epithelium shows a bright orange or pink colour on PAP stain. Note the uniformity of cell architecture.

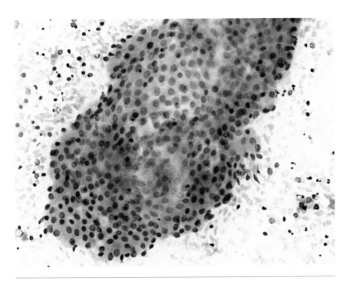

Fig. 9.21 Warthin's tumour. Regularly spaced oval nuclei and dense well-outlined cytoplasm are characteristic.

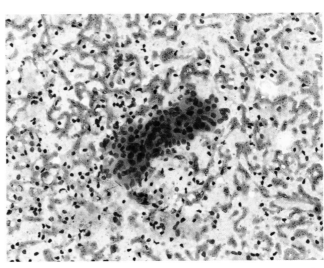

Fig. 9.24 Salivary duct epithelium showing squamous metaplasia in chronic sialadenitis may resemble Warthin's tumour.

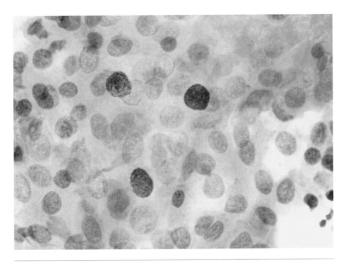

Fig. 9.22 Warthin's tumour. Mast cells may be appreciated in some of the poorly stained parts of the sample.

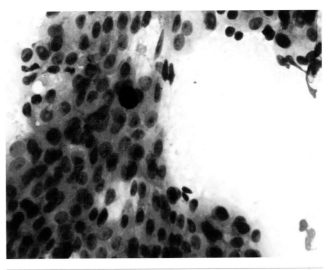

Fig. 9.25 Oncocytic epithelium has to be differentiated from oncocytoma.

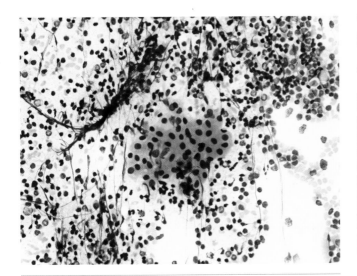

Fig. 9.23 Warthin's tumour. Oncocytic cells surrounded by numerous lymphoid cells may be mistaken for a metastatic carcinoma.

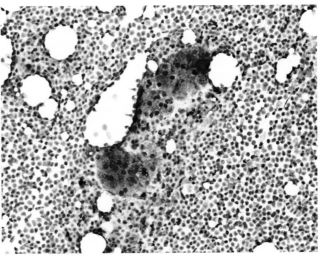

Fig. 9.26 FNA parotid gland. Intraparotid lymph node containing lymphoid cells and contaminant salivary gland acinar and ductal epithelium may be a pitfall in the diagnosis of Warthin's tumour.

Benign salivary gland tumours: basal cell adenoma and myoepithelioma

Basal cell adenoma (BCA) and myoepithelioma are both rare benign epithelial tumours of the salivary gland.

Both tumours are seen most frequently in the parotid gland and less commonly in the submandibular gland and minor glands of the upper lips, oral cavity and hard palate.

Cytological findings: basal cell adenoma (Fig. 9.27)

- Well-polarised basaloid cells, often with peripheral palisading
- Accompanying hyaline stroma, may have cylindromatous globules

Differential diagnosis: basal cell adenoma

- Adenoid cystic carcinoma (ACC): hyaline globules in BCA are smaller and fewer than those seen in ACC; in BCA, the collagenous stroma interdigitates with adjacent cells, whereas in ACC, the two are separated by a sharp, smooth border. The stroma of BCA can contain rare spindle cells or capillaries, but the cylinders of ACC are acellular (see Figs 9.102–9.105)
- Basal cell adenocarcinoma

Cytological findings: myoepithelioma (Fig. 9.28)

- Loosely cohesive fusiform or spindle cells
- Epithelioid, clear cell or hyaline (plasmacytoid) cells may be a component or predominate
- Ovoid nuclei with finely dispersed chromatin
- Little or no epithelial cell population
- Absent or scant stromal component

Differential diagnosis: myoepithelioma

- Cellular pleomorphic adenoma
- Benign spindle cell tumour

For diagnostic approach and differential diagnosis of salivary gland FNA please see Fig. 9.112 and Table 9.1.

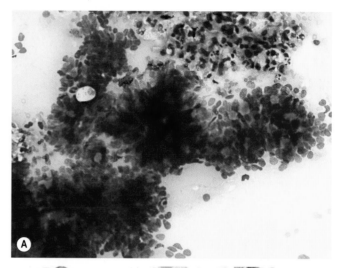

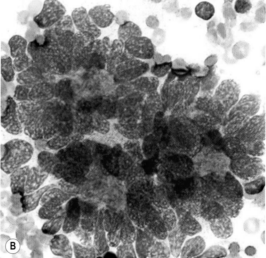

Fig. 9.27 Basal cell adenoma. (A) Hyaline globules surrounded by basal cells. (B) High-power view of basal cells.

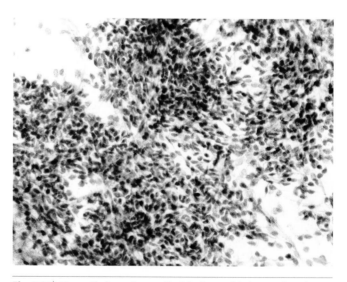

Fig. 9.28[†] Myoepithelioma (myoepithelial adenoma) in its pure form is a rare, benign tumour composed exclusively of myoepithelial cells, devoid of any stromal component.

Other benign salivary gland tumours

Oncocytic adenoma, sebaceous adenoma and intraductal papilloma are rare salivary gland tumours.

It is important to be aware of their existence since they may pose difficulties in differential diagnosis with other benign tumours or their own malignant counterparts.

Differential diagnosis: oncocytic adenoma (Fig. 9.29)

- Squamous metaplasia, especially if accompanied by atypia and necrosis
- Benign oncocytic cells may exhibit a worrisome degree of nuclear atypia
- Malignant oncocytes may appear deceptively monomorphic
- Degenerate oncocytes (pyknocytes) with pseudokeratinised, orangeophilic cytoplasm masquerading as squamous cells
- Clear cell change: metastatic renal, thyroid and apocrine mammary carcinoma
- Besides Warthin's tumour, oncocytic cells occur in other conditions (see Figs 9.107–9.111)

Differential diagnosis: sebaceous adenoma (Fig. 9.30)

- Sebaceous differentiation may infrequently be seen in normal salivary parenchyma, pleomorphic adenoma, Warthin's tumour, myoepithelioma and mucoepidermoid carcinoma

Differential diagnosis: intraductal papilloma (Fig. 9.31)

- Three-dimensional epithelial clusters, some with a papillary configuration, may mimic other papillary tumours including papillary adenocarinoma (see Fig. 9.31)
- Histiocytes and cystic change can be seen in other tumours
- May have mucoid globules surrounded by single cells mimicking adenoid cystic carcinoma
- Oncocytic differentiation and benign-appearing ductal cells in honeycomb sheets can mimic other oncocyte-containing tumours (see p. 307)

For diagnostic approach and differential diagnosis of salivary gland FNA please see Fig. 9.112 and Table 9.1.

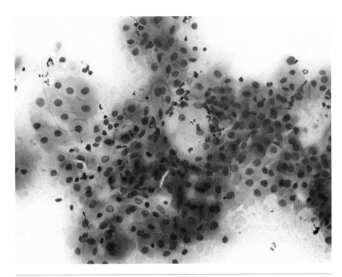

Fig. 9.29 Oncocytic adenoma. Oncocytic epithelium has abundant dense cytoplasm and centrally placed, round nuclei.

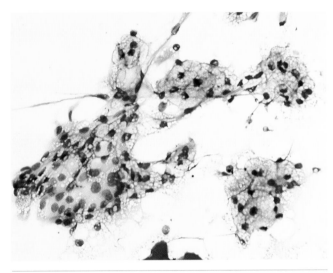

Fig. 9.30 Differential diagnosis of sebaceous adenoma. Cells filled with lipid globules are indistinguishable from a case of sialosis shown here.

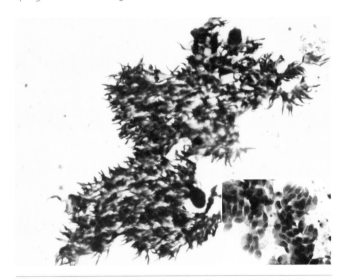

Fig. 9.31 Papillary clusters of intraductal papilloma is indistinguishable from intracystic papillary adenocarcinoma, as shown here. (Inset) High-power view shows columnar epithelium.

Malignant salivary gland neoplasms: acinic cell carcinoma (Figs 9.32–9.38)

- Malignant tumours are more common in submandibular and minor salivary glands than parotid glands
- Most are slow growing
- Present as a lump with no distinctive features
- Pain, facial nerve involvement, rapid growth or associated lymphadenopathy, suggestive of malignancy

Cytological findings

- Cellular smears
- Background containing bluish cytoplasmic granules and many bare nuclei
- Loose, linear oracinar aggregates of uniform epithelial cells
- Bland, eccentric nuclei with small nucleoli
- Granular or clear cytoplasm

Histological variation:

- Architectural
  - solid/lobular, microcystic, papillary-cystic, follicular type
- Cellular
  - acinar, intercalated ductal, vacuolated, clear, non-specific glandular cell patterns
  - Diagnostic feature: (at least focal) acinar cell differentiation

Differential diagnosis

- Normal salivary gland tissue: normal acinar cell groups are smaller, tightly cohesive with well-defined, rounded outlines. They do not display variation in size and shape
- Tumours containing ductal epithelium are difficult to classify as acinic cell but are recognisable as neoplastic
- Poorly differentiated or dedifferentiated variant shows pleomorphism and can be diagnosed as carcinoma
- Papillary-cystic variant of acinic cell carcinoma:
  - Cystic background with monolayered sheets or branching papillary clusters of uniform epithelial cells; differential diagnosis includes:
    - retention cyst
    - Warthin's tumour
    - mucoepidermoid carcinoma
    - cystadenocarcinoma
  - Clear cell tumours:
    - clear cell oncocytoma, mucoepidermoid carcinoma
    - primary clear cell carcinoma
    - epithelial-myoepithelial carcinoma
    - metastatic renal cell carcinoma

For diagnostic approach and differential diagnosis of salivary gland FNA please see Fig. 9.112 and Table 9.1.

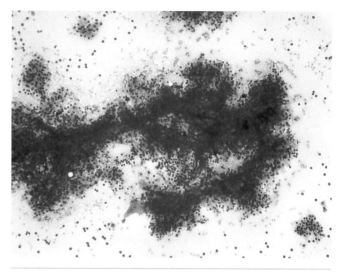

Fig. 9.32[†] Acinic cell carcinoma. Loosely cohesive clusters of cells with vascular stroma in a clean background.

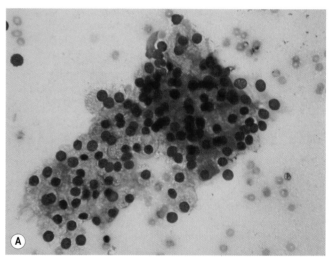

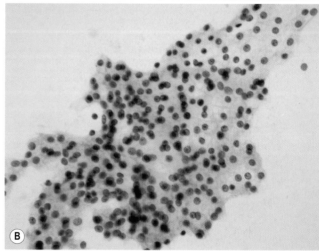

Fig. 9.33[†] Acinic cell carcinoma. (A,B) Cells with acinar differentiation showing finely vacuolated cytoplasm and uniform nuclei. Note the finely granular background ((A) MGG, (B) PAP).

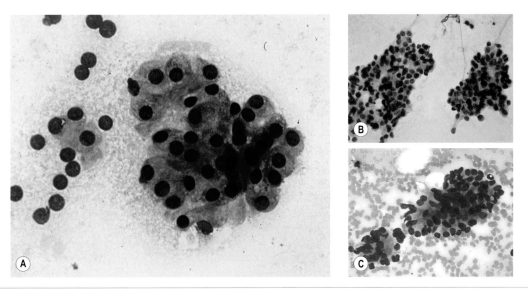

Fig. 9.34† Acinic cell carcinoma. (A) Non-specific acinar cells (MGG). (B) PAP stain of acinic cell carcinoma, where recognition as a carcinoma is easy but classification as acinic cell carcinoma difficult. (C) Acinar differentiation may be better appreciated at low-power view.

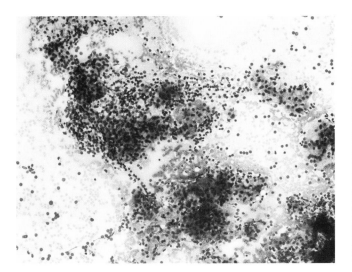

Fig. 9.35 Acinic cell carcinoma resembles normal salivary gland aspirate but is usually very cellular with numerous bare nuclei in the background and no ductal epithelium.

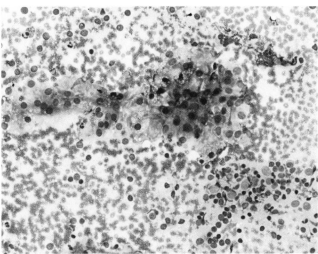

Fig. 9.37 Acinic cell carcinoma may contain a prominent lymphoid cell component. Clear cells may mimic other tumours (see p. 288).

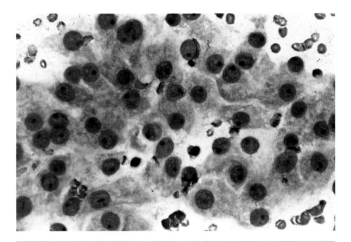

Fig. 9.36 Acinic cell carcinoma. Epithelial cells may show prominent nucleoli.

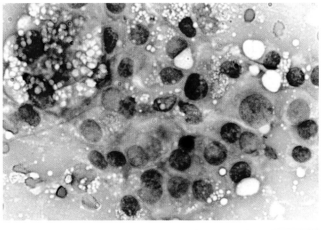

Fig. 9.38 Cystic variant of acinic cell carcinoma may be particularly difficult to recognise due to degenerative changes in acinar cells and a dirty background.

Mucoepidermoid carcinoma (Figs 9.39–9.47)

- Mucoepidermoid carcinoma is the most common salivary gland tumour
- Architectural and cellular heterogeneity
  - Cystic and solid areas
  - Mucous, intermediate and squamous cells
  - Clear and oncocytic cells may occur
- Histologically:
  - A three-tier grading system (low, intermediate or high grade) according to cystic change, pleomorphism, mitoses, neural invasion and necrosis, but not the proportions of different cell types

Cytological findings

- Variably cellular smears
  - depends on proportion of solid or cystic areas aspirated
- 'Dirty background'
  - Variably contains mucin, evidence of cystic change (inflammatory cells, macrophages and cell debris) or necrosis
- Mixture of epithelial cells: mucous, squamous and intermediate
  - Mucous cells in cohesive honeycombed sheets, often with finely vacuolated cytoplasm and basally situated nuclei
  - Squamous cells have abundant, 'plate-like' cytoplasm, almost never keratinised
  - Intermediate cells occur in cohesive sheets and have features in between mucous and squamous cells

Differential diagnosis

- **Sialadenitis:** Low-grade mucoepidermoid carcinoma may mimic inflammatory lesions: inflammatory cells and macrophages may predominate, epithelial cells may be in the minority and mimic macrophages
- **Salivary duct carcinoma and adenocarcinoma** can be indistinguishable from high-grade mucoepidermoid carcinoma; if keratinised cells present, a metastatic squamous cell carcinoma should be considered
- **Warthin's tumour:** The background of mucin and cell debris along with groups of intermediate and squamous cells may mimic Warthin's, which usually has granular cytoplasm and generally shows nuclear uniformity
- **Mucinous cyst.** In tumours with sparse epithelium, the content may be mistaken for a mucinous cyst

For diagnostic approach and differential diagnosis of salivary gland FNA please see Fig. 9.112 and Table 9.1.

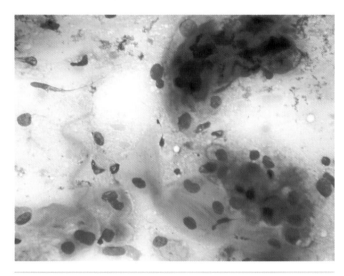

Fig. 9.39[†] Mucoepidermoid carcinoma. The squamous cells have plate-like, turquoise-blue cytoplasm. The mucous cells contain faintly eosinophilic mucin vacuoles.

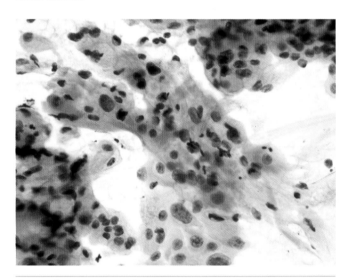

Fig. 9.40[†] Mucoepidermoid carcinoma. A mixture of squamous, mucous and intermediate cells.

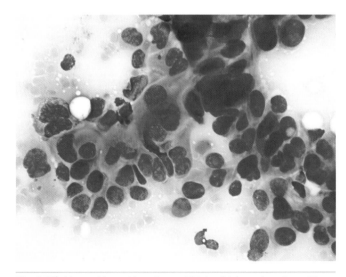

Fig. 9.41[†] Mucoepidermoid carcinoma. This is a high-grade variant with nuclear atypia and a suggestion of squamous differentiation.

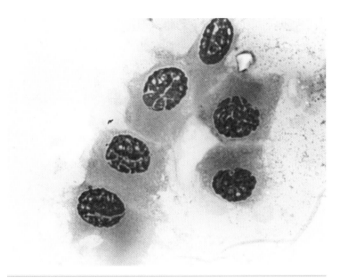

Fig. 9.42 Mucoepidermoid carcinoma. Some of the cells have polygonal, relatively well-defined cytoplasm, giving them a 'squamoid' appearance though they are not keratinised (see pp. 294, 295).

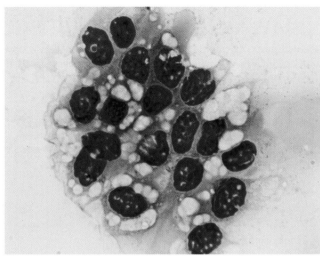

Fig. 9.45 Mucoepidermoid carcinoma. Vacuolated cytoplasm in which mucin can be demonstrated is often diagnostic.

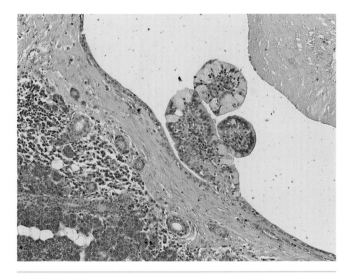

Fig. 9.43 Mucoepidermoid carcinoma. Histology shows bland mucin-secreting epithelium in the wall of a cystic lesion.

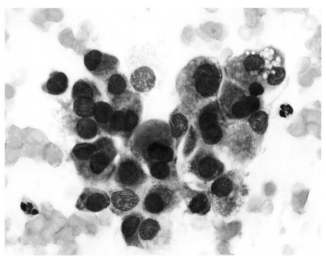

Fig. 9.46 Mucoepidermoid carcinoma. Cells are often poorly preserved and autolysed.

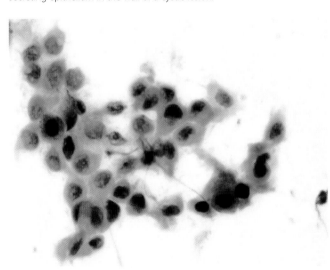

Fig. 9.44 Mucoepidermoid carcinoma. PAP staining of cuboidal epithelium shows dense cytoplasm without keratinisation (see pp. 294, 295).

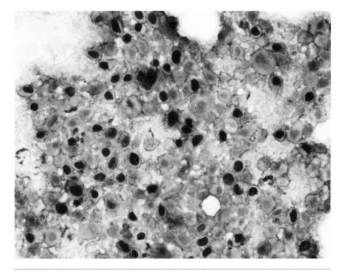

Fig. 9.47 Mucoepidermoid carcinoma. Tumour cells in a partly necrotic background can be difficult to recognise. They can be also mistaken for a mucocele (see Figs 9.86, 9.87).

Adenoid cystic carcinoma (Figs 9.48–9.53)

Adenoid cystic carcinoma represents 10% of all salivary gland tumours but 30% of epithelial tumours in *minor* salivary glands. It is malignant but usually slow growing.

Histologically:

- Three architectural patterns: cribriform, tubular and solid (often coexisting)
- Two cell types: basal cells (modified myoepithelial cells) and epithelial cells
- Characteristic myxoid stroma

Cytological findings

- Cellular smears
- Uniform basaloid cells
- Characteristic stroma made up of sharply demarcated globules and cylinders of basement membrane material

Differential diagnosis

- Salivary tumours containing hyaline globules:
  - pleomorphic adenoma: hyaline globules in PA are smaller and with less well-defined outlines
  - basal cell neoplasms
  - epithelial-myoepithelial carcinoma
  - polymorphous low-grade adenocarcinoma (see Figs 9.102–9.106)
- Salivary gland tumours containing basaloid cells:
  - cellular pleomorphic adenoma: contains myoepithelial cells with intact cytoplasm in the background (Fig. 9.13)
  - basal cell neoplasms (Fig. 9.27)
  - polymorphous low-grade adenocarcinoma (Figs 9.61–9.63)
  - epithelial-myoepithelial carcinoma (Fig. 9.69)
  - differentiation from pleomorphic adenoma may be possible (fibrillary stroma and single myoepithelial cells)
  - differentiation from other basal cell containing tumours may not be possible, particularly in poorly differentiated tumours which are composed of solid sheets of cells and may lack hyaline material

For diagnostic approach and differential diagnosis of salivary gland FNA please see Fig. 9.112 and Table 9.1.

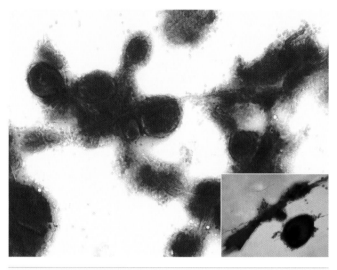

Fig. 9.48[†] Adenoid cystic carcinoma. Hyaline globules and finger/plate-like stromal material (MGG).

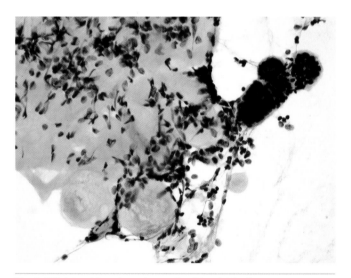

Fig. 9.49[†] Adenoid cytsic carcinoma. Small basaloid cells are present adherent to the stroma.

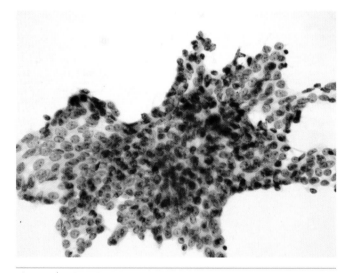

Fig. 9.50[†] Adenoid cystic carcinoma. The aspirates contain predominantly basaloid (myoepithelial) cells, which are present in tight clusters, rosette-like formations or adhering to globules.

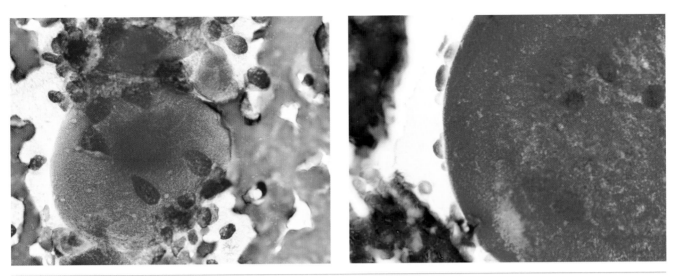

Fig. 9.51 Adenoid cystic carcinoma. Globules of basement membrane material are well defined and may be associated with epithelial cells.

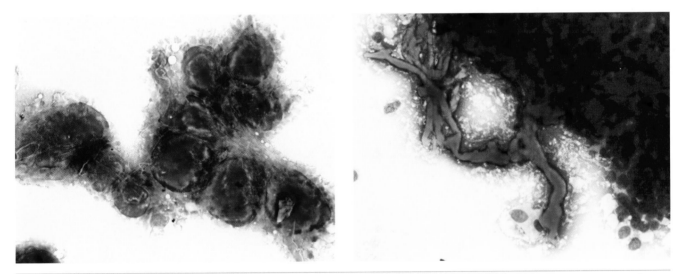

Fig. 9.52 Adenoid cystic carcinoma. This demonstrates the hyaline globules and finger/plate-like stromal material. Small basaloid cells are present, adherent to the stroma.

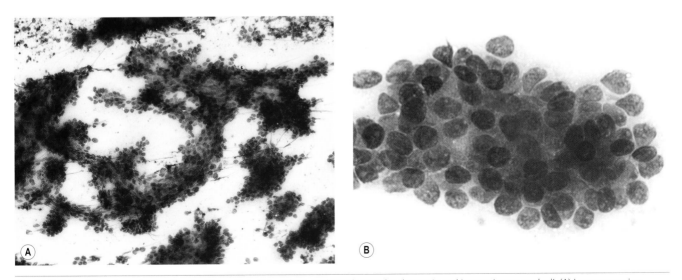

Fig. 9.53 Adenoid cystic carcinoma, basal cell type. Note the uniform nuclei with granular chromatin and inconspicuous nucleoli. (A) Low-power view, (B) high-power view. Note no hyaline globules are seen. A coarse chromatin pattern may be helpful.

Squamous cells in salivary gland aspirates

Squamous cells, although not a constituent of a normal salivary gland or its tumours – except in a rare instances of primary or metastatic sqaumous cell carcinoma – can nevertheless be found in several salivary gland lesions, both benign and malignant, as a result of squamous metaplasia.

Cytological findings (Figs 9.54–9.59)

- Warthin's tumour
- Lymphoepithelial cyst
- Chronic sialadenitis
- Pleomorphic adenoma
- Mucoepidermoid carcinoma
- Squamous cell carcinoma

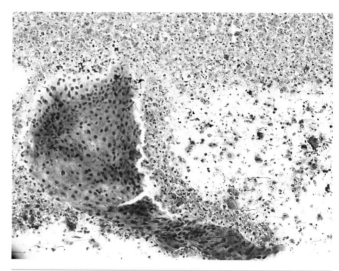

Fig. 9.56[†] Chronic sialadenitis. Ductal cells may show squamous metaplasia with possible atypia (MGG).

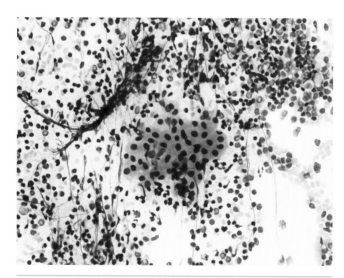

Fig. 9.54 Squamous metaplasia in Warthin's tumour may mimic metastatic squamous cell carcinoma.

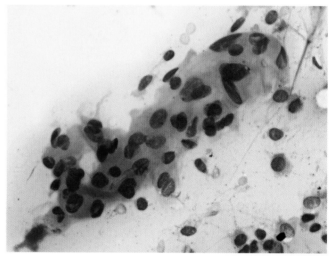

Fig. 9.57 Squamous metaplasia may be seen in pleomorphic adenoma.

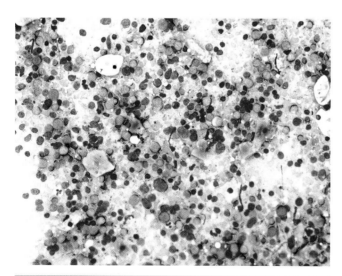

Fig. 9.55[†] Lymphoepithelial cyst. The aspirates contain foamy macrophages, lymphoid cells, epithelial (squamous) cells and, occasionally, multinucleated giant cells.

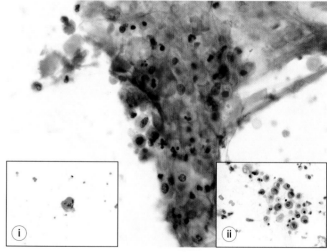

Fig. 9.58 Mucoepidermoid carcinoma. (Inset i) Occasional atypical keratinised cells are identified. (Inset ii) Numerous dyscohesive mucous cells.

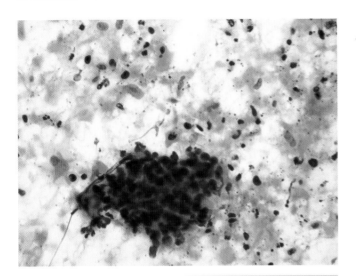

For diagnostic approach and differential diagnosis of salivary gland FNA please see Fig. 9.112 and Table 9.1.

Fig. 9.59[†] Metastatic squamous cell carcinoma. This degree of keratinisation is a feature of squamous cell carcinoma.

Case study

A 63-year-old male smoker with a long-standing history of neck swelling which yielded keratinous debris and inflammatory cells on repeated FNAs. Initially interpreted as an inflamed epidermoid cyst, the lesion was neglected for two years after which a repeat FNA revealed a metastatic squamous cell carcinoma. The delay in diagnosis was thought to have contributed to the poor clinical outcome.

Metastasis of a well-differentiated squamous cell carcinoma may clinically appear as a cystic lesion in the neck and microscopically contain mature squamous cells and keratin only. Any dyskaryotic nuclei may be pyknotic and discrete and therefore need to be searched for. In the absence of definite evidence of malignancy, a guarded report can be issued, suggesting repeat sampling of the wall of the lesion. Differentiation from a branchial cleft cyst is sometimes not possible.

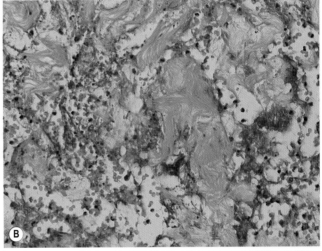

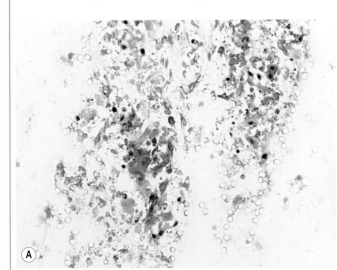

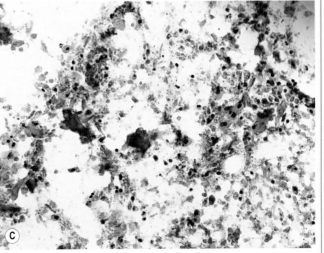

Fig. 9.60 (A,B) Keratinous debris and inflammatory cells which were initially misinterpreted as a ruptured epidermoid cyst. (C) Subsequent sample showed numerous dyskaryotic squamous cells which were diagnosed as metastatic squamous cell carcinoma.

Polymorphous low-grade adenocarcinoma (Figs 9.61–9.63)

Polymorphous low-grade adenocarcinoma (PLGA) is the second most common intraoral malignant salivary gland tumour, accounting for 26% of all carcinomas.

Histologically, tumours show a range of architectural patterns comprising sheets, cords, tubules, cribriform and papillary areas, composed of uniform, small to medium-sized cells with bland appearing nuclei. Variable amounts of myxoid, hyaline or myxo-hyaline stroma are present.

Cytological findings

- Cellular aspirates with branching papillary clusters and sheets of uniform cells
- Cells are basaloid with a small or moderate amount of cytoplasm
- The nuclei are regular, round to oval and with finely stippled chromatin
- Bare nuclei may be present
- Hyaline globules are often seen and fibrillary myxoid stromal material may be present in the background (see Figs 9.102–9.106, p. 306)

Differential diagnosis

- Cellular pleomorphic adenoma
- Basal cell neoplasms
- Adenoid cystic carcinoma
- Epithelial-myoepithelial carcinoma
- Papillary cystadenocarcinoma

For diagnostic approach and differential diagnosis of salivary gland FNA please see Fig. 9.112 and Table 9.1.

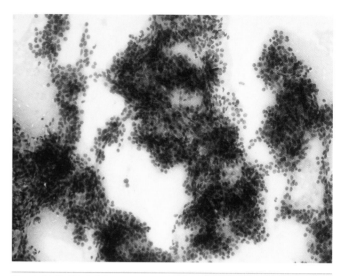

Fig. 9.61 PLGA. Cellular aspirates with branching papillary clusters and sheets of uniform cells.

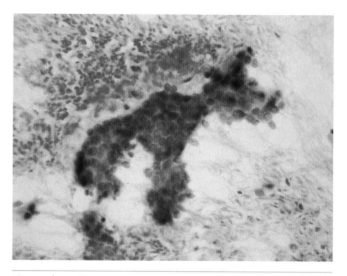

Fig. 9.62[†] Small hyaline globules are surrounded by uniform cells with delicate cytoplasm. Bland nuclear features are seen on Papanicolaou stain. (This case was kindly provided by Dr Ivan Robinson.)

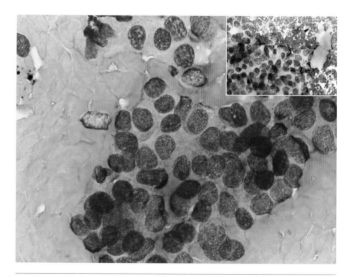

Fig. 9.63 PLGA. The nuclei are regular, round to oval with finely stippled chromatin. (Inset) A small amount of metachromatic stroma may be seen.

Salivary duct carcinoma (Figs 9.64–9.66)

Salivary duct carcinoma is a highly aggressive adenocarcinoma, histologically resembling high-grade intraductal and invasive breast carcinoma.

Cytological findings

- Cellular aspirates with loosely cohesive sheets of cytologically malignant epithelial cells
- Sieve-like pattern may be seen in cell sheets
- Necrosis often present in the background
- Most cells have uniform cytological features, though variation in nuclear size, coarse granular chromatin, giant nuclei and prominent nucleoli found
- Occasionally, squamous differentiation is seen

Differential diagnosis

- Differentiation from other high-grade carcinomas may not be possible
  - Mucoepidermoid carcinoma
  - Adenocarcinoma not otherwise specified
  - Metastatic carcinoma (breast)
  - Oncocytic carcinoma

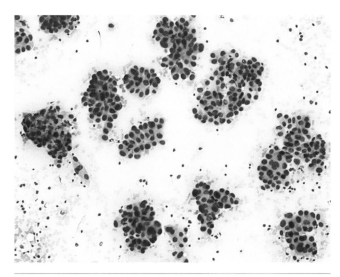

Fig. 9.64 Salivary duct carcinoma shows clusters of malignant epithelial cells in cribriform or pseudopapillary arrangement, often with necrotic background.

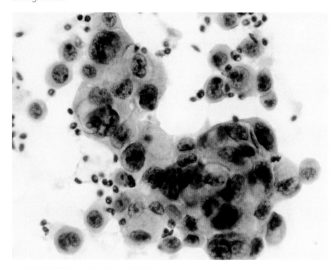

Fig. 9.65 Salivary duct carcinoma shows pleomorphism and may show signs of glandular and squamous differentiation.

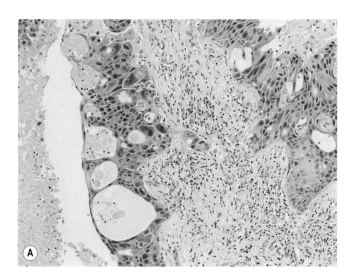

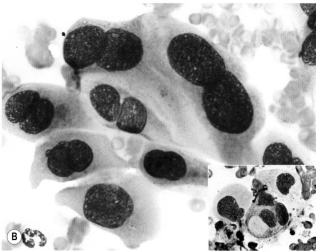

Fig. 9.66 Salivary duct carcinoma. (A) Expanded duct-like structures with a cribriform proliferation of cells and central necrosis are present along with an infiltrative (tubular, papillary, solid or cribriform) component. (B) Cells show high nuclear to cytoplasmic ratio, binucleation and prominent nucleoli reminiscent of breast or prostate carcinoma. (Inset) Cytoplasmic vacuoles may be present.

Carcinoma ex-pleomorphic adenoma (Fig. 9.67)

- Residual, benign pleomorphic adenoma must be identified in order to make this diagnosis
- Both benign (pleomorphic adenoma) and malignant (carcinomatous) elements are present, the former usually identified by its fibrillary, metachromatic stroma

Differential diagnosis

- Benign pleomorphic adenoma with atypia of myoepithelial cells (Fig. 9.68)

Epimyoepithelial carcinoma (Fig. 9.69)

- Cellular aspirates with cells arranged singly and in multilayered clusters, cohesive sheets or tubular structures
- Round, bland nuclei with scanty, ill-defined cytoplasm
- Myoepithelial cells may appear as small, bland basaloid cells or as larger cells with pale, fragile cytoplasm and show variable nuclear atypia
- A biphasic population may not always be present and myoepithelial cells may predominate
- Variable amounts of stroma, in the form of hyaline globules or chondromyxoid stroma

Differential diagnosis

- Similar chondromyxoid material can be seen
  - Pleomorphic adenoma (see pp. 282, 283)
  - Adenoid cystic carcinoma (see pp. 292, 293)
  - Polymorphous low-grade carcinoma (see p. 296)

Primary squamous cell carcinoma, basal cell carcinoma and myoepithelial carcinoma are some of the rare primary salivary gland carcinomas. Most common metastatic tumours are melanoma and squamous cell carcinoma. Spindle cell tumours, both benign and malignant, are rare. Salivary gland lymphomas are mainly low-grade MALT lymphoma associated with pre-existing MESA (see pp. 304–305); however, other primary lymphomas may occur (see Fig. 9.74).

For diagnostic approach and differential diagnosis of salivary gland FNA please see Fig. 9.112 and Table 9.1.

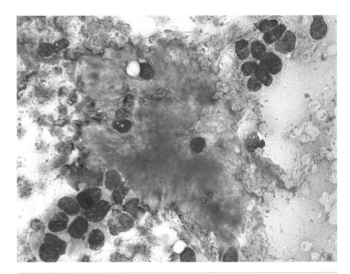

Fig. 9.67[†] Carcinoma ex pleomorphic adenoma. Malignant epithelial cells and fibrillary stroma.

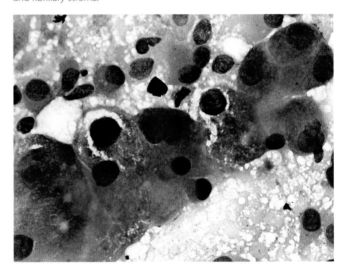

Fig. 9.68 Oncocytic metaplasia with atypia in pleomorphic adenoma should not be confused as carcinoma ex pleomorphic adenoma (see also Figs 9.10–9.17, pleomorphic adenoma).

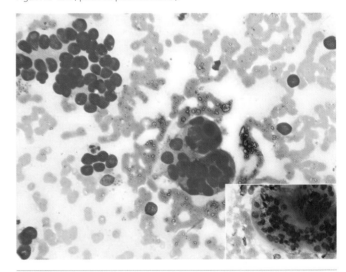

Fig. 9.69[†] Epimyoepithelial carcinoma shows myoepithelial cells with large pale cytoplasm surrounding an epithelial tubular structure with chondromyxoid stroma. Inset: A biphasic cell layer with pale, clear myoepithelial cells may be a helpful feature.

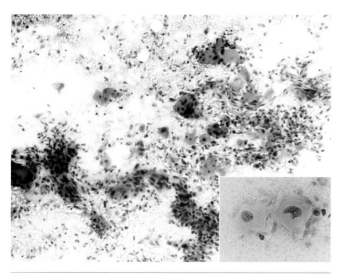

Fig. 9.70 Sqamous cell carcinoma is more frequently metastatic but can be a primary tumour of the salivary gland (PAP). (Inset) Keratinised cells stain orange in PAP and typical dense turquoise blue cytoplasm in MGG.

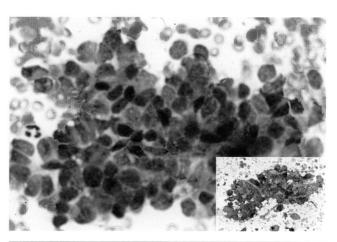

Fig. 9.73 Basal cell adenocarcinoma. (Inset) Laminin positive. Differential diagnosis includes adenoid cystic carcinoma (see Figs 9.9, 9.48–9.53) and basal cell adenoma (see Figs 9.27, 9.28, 9.48–9.53 and 9.102–9.106).

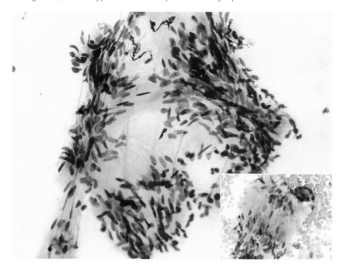

Fig. 9.71 Nerve sheath tumour composed of pallisading spindle cells and pale-staining background material (Antoni A and B areas). (Inset) High-power view, salivary gland acinus next to tumour cells.

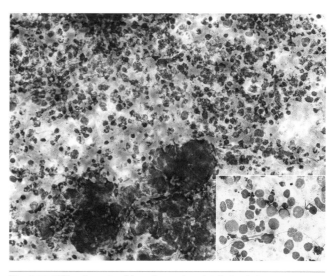

Fig. 9.74 Diffuse large B-cell lymphoma. (Inset) Cell detail shows a monotonous population of lymphoblasts.

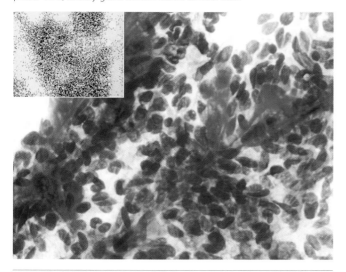

Fig. 9.72 Myoepithelial carcinoma. Spindle cells and metachromatic stroma. A definitive distinction from myoepithelioma (see Fig. 9.28) may not be possible on FNA. (Inset: PAP stain.)

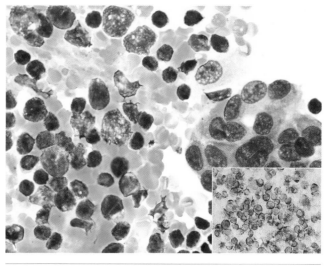

Fig. 9.75 Primary T-cell lymphoma. (Inset) CD3-positive cells. Diagnosis was made with the aid of PCR T-cell gene rearrangement.

Non-neoplastic conditions

- Acute sialadenitis (Figs 9.76, 9.77)
- Chronic sialadenitis/retention cyst (Figs 9.78–9.83)
- Granulomatous sialadenitis (Figs 9.82–9.85)

Pathogenesis and clinical findings

- *Acute sialadenitis* is due to a specific bacterial or viral infection such as mumps parotitis. It is usually clinically obvious and FNA is not indicated
- *Chronic sialadenitis* is most commonly caused by calculi (sialoliths) within the salivary ducts
- Clinically, calculi are associated with pain and swelling, and retrograde infection results in acute or chronic sialadenitis. Long-standing sialadenitis results in atrophy and fibrosis of acinar tissue (Kuttner tumour) and cystic change with a variety of crystalloids. However, chronic sialadenitis may be a primary disease as part of the anti-IgG4 spectrum of fibroses

Cytological findings: chronic sialadenitis

- Scanty aspirate
- Ductal cells with squamous metaplasia or atypia (see Fig. 9.56)
- Paucity of acinar cells
- Inflammatory cells and background debris
- Possible cystic change and crystalloids

For diagnostic approach and differential diagnosis of salivary gland FNA please see Fig. 9.112 and Table 9.1.

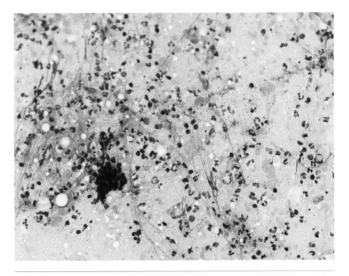

Fig. 9.77 Non-specific acute sialadenitis. Numerous polymorphs surround a cluster of ductal epithelium.

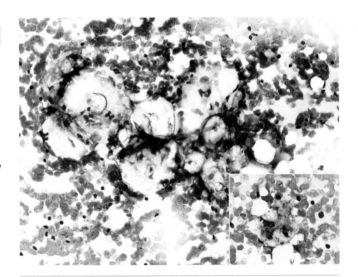

Fig. 9.78 Sialadenitis. Salivary gland acini show degenerative changes and may be replaced by globules of fat. (Inset) Acinar cell.

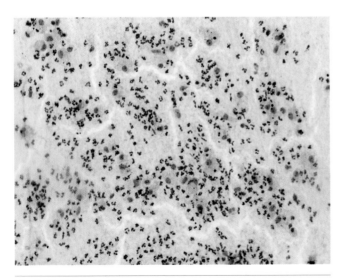

Fig. 9.76 Sialadenitis. Numerous inflammatory cells and macrophages.

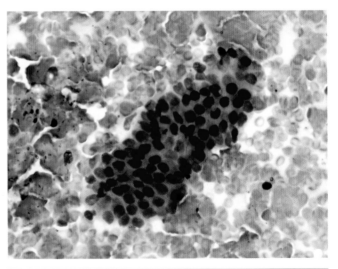

Fig. 9.79 Ductal epithelium in tightly cohesive clusters is often the only finding in chronic sialadenitis with acinar atrophy.

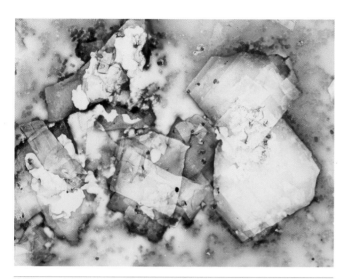

Fig. 9.80 Sialadenitis may contain large cholesterol crystals.

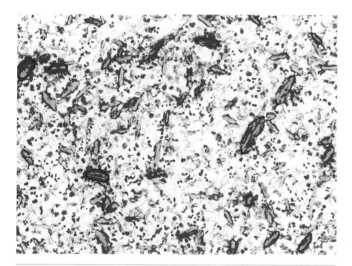

Fig. 9.81 Numerous amylase crystals are not commonly seen in chronic sialadenitis.

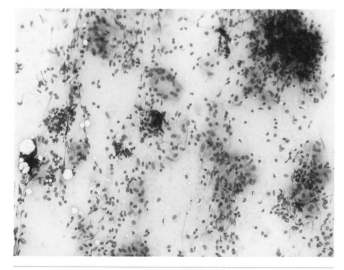

Fig. 9.82 Granulomatous sialadenitis. Salivary gland may be the first site of presentation of sarcoidosis. Note numerous epithelioid and giant cells.

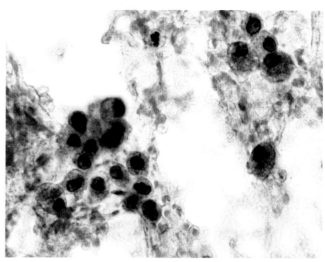

Fig. 9.83 Sialadenitis may resolve and result in a retention cyst containing numerous macrophages and debris, sometimes with variable number of inflammatory cells.

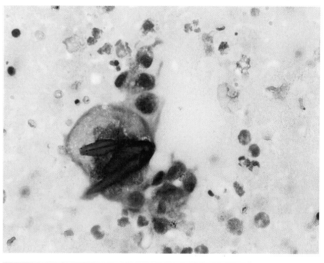

Fig. 9.84 Foreign body giant cell reaction to crystals may be seen in non-specific chronic sialadenitis.

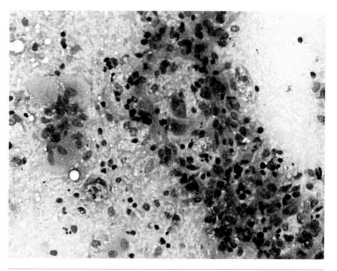

Fig. 9.85 Tuberculous sialadenitis contains giant cells of Langhans type, epithelioid cells and necrotic background.

Salivary gland cysts

Salivary cysts may originate from degenerative, inflammatory or neoplastic processes.

Mucus cyst (mucocele)

Mucocele (Figs 9.86–9.88)

- Caused by:
  - disruption of salivary ducts, often due to trauma, with salivary extravasation and reactive inflammation
  - ductal obstruction and accumulation of saliva in dilated ducts
- Mainly in minor salivary glands of the lip and oral cavity, sublingual
- Often target for FNA

Cytological findings

- Watery or viscous fluid
- Scanty cellularity
- Leucocytes and macrophages in variable numbers
- Few epithelial cells

Differential diagnosis

- Warthin's tumour
- Pleomorphic adenoma
- Acinic cell carcinoma
- High-grade carcinoma
- Low-grade mucoepidermoid carcinoma

For diagnostic approach and differential diagnosis of salivary gland FNA please see Fig. 9.112 and Table 9.1.

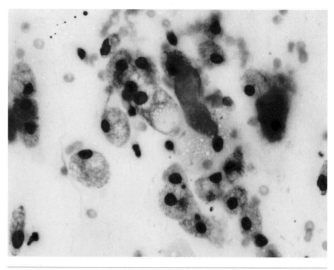

Fig. 9.86 Mucocele. Thick, viscous fluid contains macrophages and a few leucocytes against a mucinous background (MGG stain).

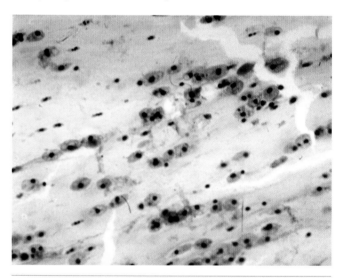

Fig. 9.87 Mucocele. Thick, viscous fluid contains macrophages and a few leucocytes against a mucinous background (Low-power view, PAP stain).

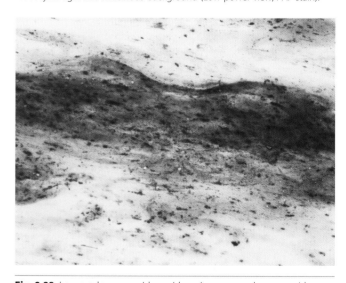

Fig. 9.88 Low-grade mucoepidermoid carcinoma may show mucoid background and absence of cells. It can be mistaken for a mucocele or a retention cyst (see Figs 9.39–9.47).

Lymphoepithelial and branchial cleft cyst

Bilateral and multiple lymphoepithelial cysts (LECs) of major salivary glands, in particular of parotid glands, are uncommon but are reported in human immunodeficiency virus (HIV)-infected patients with an incidence of about 3–6%.

Branchial cyst is a congenital squamous epithelium-lined cyst which becomes symptomatic in adulthood, usually as a result of acute inflammation. It can mimic squamous cell carcinoma.

Cytological findings: lymphoepithelial cyst (Figs 9.89–9.91)

- Cystic aspirates
- Foamy macrophages
- Lymphocytes including follicle centre cells
- A few squamous epithelial cells
- Occasionally multinucleated giant cells and crystalloids

Differential diagnosis

- Non-Hodgkin lymphoma
- Intraparotid lymph node
- Chronic sialadenitis
- Warthin's tumour
- Branchial cleft cyst (Fig. 9.92)

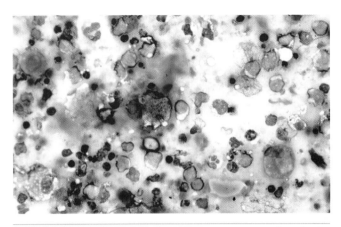

Fig. 9.90 Lymphoepithelial cyst is composed predominantly of lymphoid cells with occasional macrophages and anucleate squamous cells.

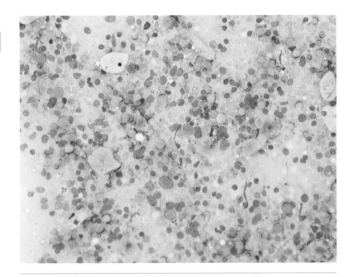

Fig. 9.91 Lymphoepithelial cyst. Low-power view of lymphoid cells may mimic non-Hodgkin lymphoma.

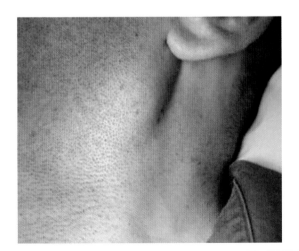

Fig. 9.89[†] Lymphoepithelial cyst. Patients usually present with unilateral or bilateral swellings at the angle of mandible.

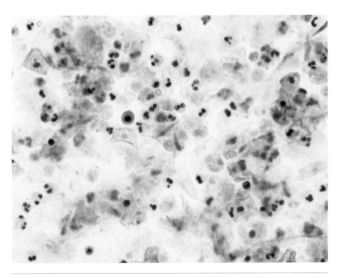

Fig. 9.92[†] Branchial cleft cyst contains mature squamous epithelium and usually acute inflammatory exudate but no lymphoid infiltrate.

Lymphoid lesions are uncommon and thus cytological experience on FNA is limited. A spectrum of diseases, ranging from benign lymphoepithelial lesions (localised myoepithelial sialadenitis or MESA) to systemic Sjögren's syndrome, are included in this benign sialadenopathy, believed to be of autoimmune origin.

Myoepithelial sialadenitis (MESA) is commonest in middle aged or elderly women and is usually bilateral and symmetrical. In cases of Sjögren's syndrome, other manifestations such as dryness of eyes and mouth, rheumatoid arthritis and hypergammaglobulinaemia are present.

Cytological findings: MESA

- Reactive lymphoid cells, plasma cells and histiocytes
- Clusters of myoepithelial cells are sometimes present

Mucosa associated lymphoid tissue (MALT) lymphoma (Figs 9.96–9.101)

Extranodal marginal zone B-cell lymphoma of MALT type is the most common type of primary salivary gland lymphoma. It is a low-grade lymphoma and therefore difficult to distinguish on morphology alone from MESA. Ancillary studies, in particular PCR, are recommended.

Cytological features: MALT lymphoma

- High cellularity
- Predominanace of medium-sized/centrocyte-like lymphoid cells
- Epithelial elements usually very sparse and usually ductal
- Presence of follicular dendritic cells and plasma cells is not a contraindication for diagnosis
- PCR or flow cytometry confirmation of clonality usually necessary for diagnosis

Differential diagnosis

- Chronic sialadenitis
- Warthin's tumour
- Lymphoepithelial cyst
- Mucoepidermoid carcinoma
- Acinic cell carcinoma
- Non-Hodgkin lymphoma
- Perisalivary lymph nodes

For diagnostic approach and differential diagnosis of salivary gland FNA please see Fig. 9.112 and Table 9.1.

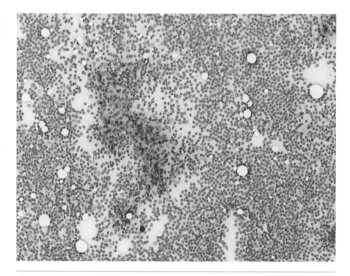

Fig. 9.93 Myoepithelial sialadenitis (MESA). Lymphoid cells are replacing normal salivary gland structures which are obscured.

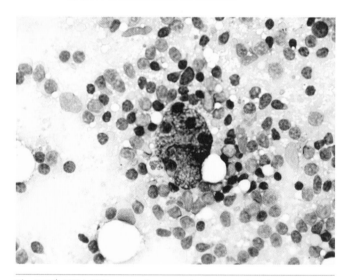

Fig. 9.94[T] MESA. FNA preparations contain numerous lymphocytes admixed with follicle centre cells, plasma cells and histiocytes. Acinar cells are seen trapped in the infiltrate.

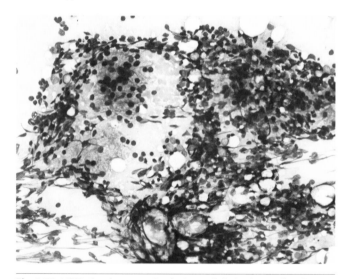

Fig. 9.95 MESA. Another example of acinar cells being 'trapped' in the lymphoid infiltrate.

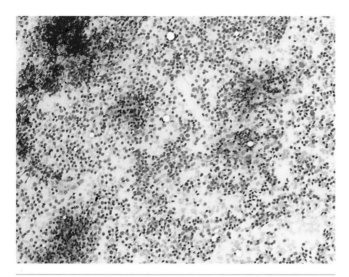

Fig. 9.96 Lymphoid infiltrate of the salivary gland is difficult to diagnose as MESA or MALT in some instances.

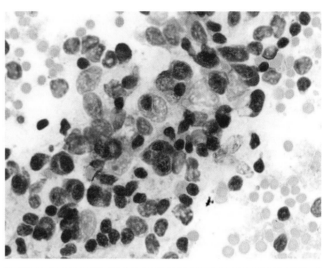

Fig. 9.99 MALT lymphoma may contain follicular dendritic cells and many plasma cells.

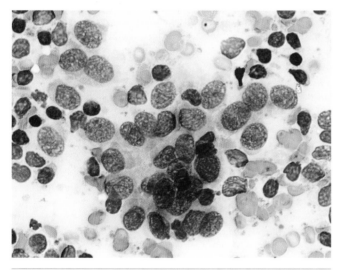

Fig. 9.97 A so-called 'lymphoepithelial lesion' where lymphoid cells infiltrate ductal salivary epithelium can be seen in both MALT and MESA.

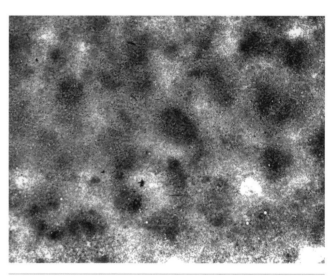

Fig. 9.100 MALT lymphoma shows a dense lymphoid population, which may contain residual follicle centre fragments.

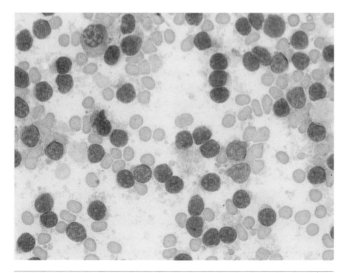

Fig. 9.98 Centrocyte-like cells in MALT lymphoma. Plasma cells are also present, sometimes in large numbers.

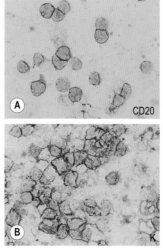

Fig. 9.101 MALT lymphoma immunocytochemistry. CD20-positive cells which are also lambda restricted support the diagnosis of lymphoma ((A) CD20, (B) kappa positive).

Hyaline globules and basaloid cells in salivary gland FNA

- Adenoid cystic carcinoma (Figs 9.102–9.104)
- Polymorphous low-grade carcinoma (Fig. 9.103)
- Pleomorphic adenoma (Fig. 9.105)
- Basal cell tumours (Fig. 9.106)
- Epimyoepithelial carcinoma

For diagnostic approach and differential diagnosis of salivary gland FNA please see Fig. 9.112 and Table 9.1.

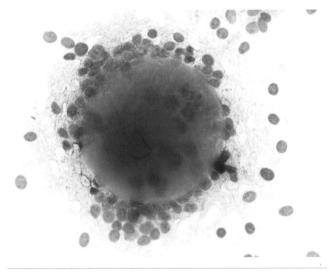

Fig. 9.104 Adenoid cystic carcinoma. Hyaline globules surrounded by epithelial cells.

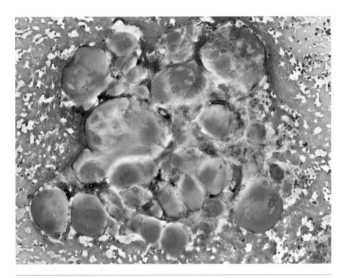

Fig. 9.102 Adenoid cystic carcinoma often, but not always, contains multiple, well-defined, dense hyaline globules.

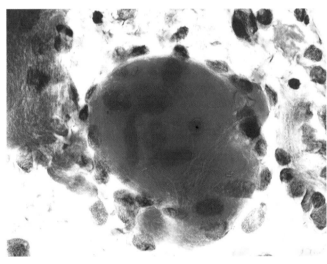

Fig. 9.105 Pleomorphic adenoma may contain hyaline globules similar to adenoid cystic carcinoma. They are usually fewer in number.

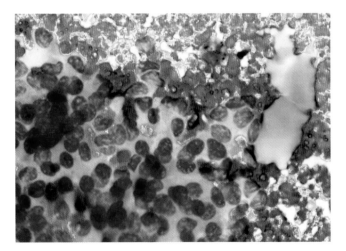

Fig. 9.103 Polymorphous low-grade carcinoma may show hyaline globules associated with epithelium. These are usually small and have well-defined edges.

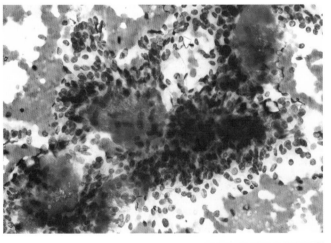

Fig. 9.106 Basal cell adenoma may contain cylindromatous hyaline globules. They are usually small and surrounded by basal cells.

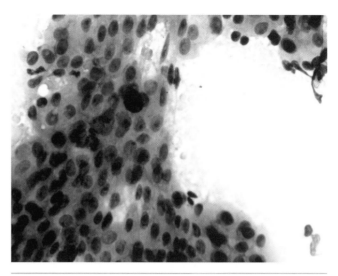

Oncocytic cells in salivary gland

- Oncocytic adenoma (Fig. 9.107)
- Oncocytic carcinoma (Fig. 9.108)
- Warthin's tumour (Fig. 9.109)
- Mucoepidermoid carcinoma (Fig. 9.110)
- Acinic cell carcinoma (Fig. 9.111)

For diagnostic approach and differential diagnosis of salivary gland FNA please see Fig. 9.112 and Table 9.1.

Fig. 9.109 Warthin's tumour has oncocytic epithelium associated with lymphoid cells in the background.

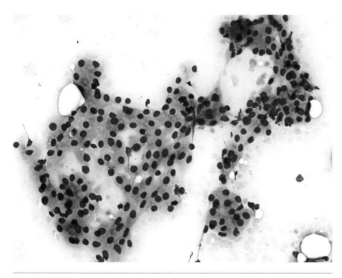

Fig. 9.107 Oncocytic adenoma. Oncocytic adenoma and oncocytic carcinoma may show similar features. Cells in the carcinoma are usually more dispersed.

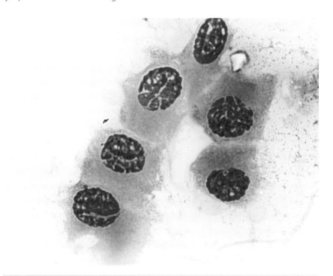

Fig. 9.110 Mucoepidermoid carcinoma may show oncocytic differentiation following the previous FNA.

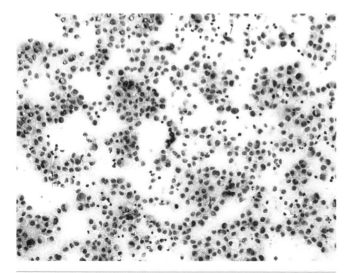

Fig. 9.108 Oncocytic carcinoma. Cells show relatively little pleomorphism or anisonucleosis. Distinction from adenoma on FNA is not usually possible.

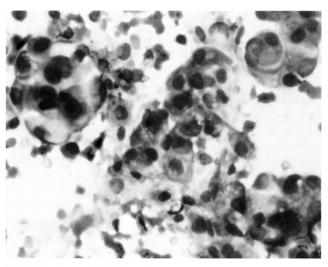

Fig. 9.111 Acinic cell carcinoma can show oncocytic change following previous FNA.

Diagnostic approach to salivary gland FNA

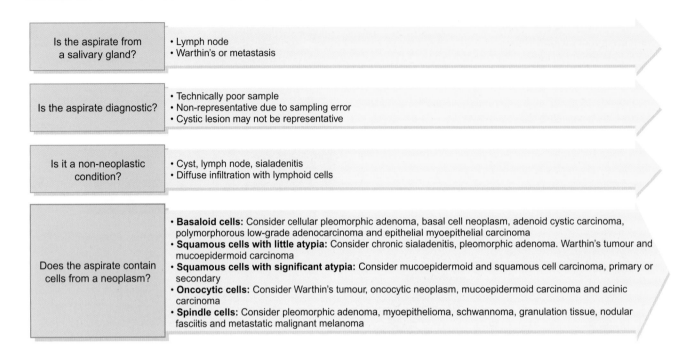

| Is the aspirate from a salivary gland? | • Lymph node
• Warthin's or metastasis |

| Is the aspirate diagnostic? | • Technically poor sample
• Non-representative due to sampling error
• Cystic lesion may not be representative |

| Is it a non-neoplastic condition? | • Cyst, lymph node, sialadenitis
• Diffuse infiltration with lymphoid cells |

| Does the aspirate contain cells from a neoplasm? | • **Basaloid cells:** Consider cellular pleomorphic adenoma, basal cell neoplasm, adenoid cystic carcinoma, polymorphorous low-grade adenocarcinoma and epithelial myoepithelial carcinoma
• **Squamous cells with little atypia:** Consider chronic sialadenitis, pleomorphic adenoma. Warthin's tumour and mucoepidermoid carcinoma
• **Squamous cells with significant atypia:** Consider mucoepidermoid and squamous cell carcinoma, primary or secondary
• **Oncocytic cells:** Consider Warthin's tumour, oncocytic neoplasm, mucoepidermoid carcinoma and acinic carcinoma
• **Spindle cells:** Consider pleomorphic adenoma, myoepithelioma, schwannoma, granulation tissue, nodular fasciitis and metastatic malignant melanoma |

Fig. 9.112 Algorithm showing a step-wise diagnostic approach to salivary gland FNA for ultimately deciding if the lesion is suitable for surgery or not.

Table 9.1 Common diagnoses based on type of salivary gland aspirate

Type of aspirate	Non-neoplastic			Neoplastic	
	Normal	**Pathological**	**Benign**	**Malignant**	
Solid	Intraparotid lymph node	Sialadenosis	See Benign neoplasms	See Malignant neoplasms	
Cystic		Sialadenitis			
Lymphoid	Intraparotid lymph node	Sialadenitis	Warthin's tumour	Reactive lymphoid infiltrate in primary salivary gland carcinoma	
Clean background	Normal gland	Sialadenosis	Basal cell neoplasms	Acinic cell carcinoma Adenoid cystic carcinoma	
Dirty background		Sialadenitis	Warthin's tumour	Mucoepidermoid carcinoma	

CHAPTER 10

Liver, biliary tree and pancreas

Chapter contents

Introduction   309

Liver   309

Gall bladder and extrahepatic bile ducts   326

Pancreas   332

The role of FNA in management of pancreatic lesions   350

Introduction

Cytology of the hepatobiliary tract (Fig. 10.1) has gained prominence with the development of new endoscopic imaging techniques making it possible to obtain samples from a wide variety of sites within the hepatobiliary tract. Since biopsies of the pancreas and biliary tract are often difficult and may be hazardous, cytology often provides the only pathology sample on which patient management is based. Since the prognosis of malignant disease in this area is still relatively poor, the importance of the cytopathologist being able to deliver an accurate diagnosis cannot be overstated.

Liver

Cytological analysis of the liver aims to establish the presence or absence of malignancy:

- Fine needle aspiration (FNA) of cells from focal mass lesions performed percutaneously or with endoscopic ultrasound guidance
- Brushing the lining of strictured intrahepatic ducts via endoscopic retrograde cholangiography (Fig. 10.2)

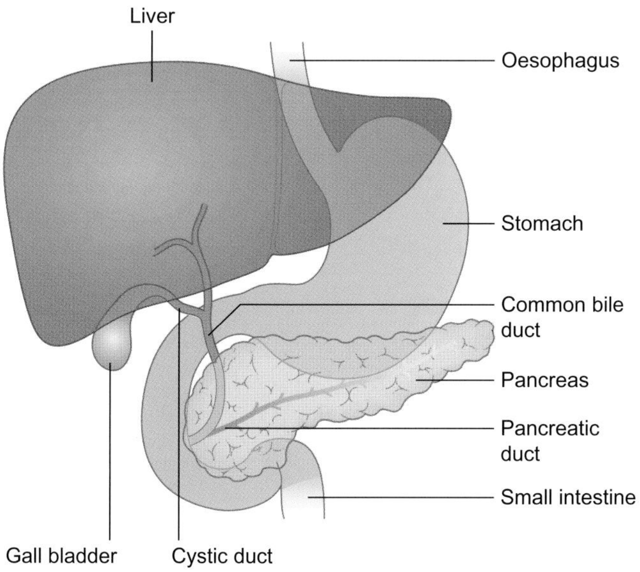

Routine use of FNA with a cell block of tissue fragments or core biopsy is better than either method alone, especially for benign neoplasms and poorly differentiated neoplasms that require ancillary studies.

In experienced hands, FNA of the liver is safe, minimally invasive, accurate, and cost effective. The specificity of FNA cytology of the liver approaches 100% and the sensitivity ranges from 67% to 100%, averaging about 85%.

Liver

Oesophagus

Stomach

Common bile duct

Pancreas

Pancreatic duct

Small intestine

Gall bladder   Cystic duct

Fig. 10.1 Normal anatomical relationships of liver, pancreas and bile ducts with the surrounding structures.

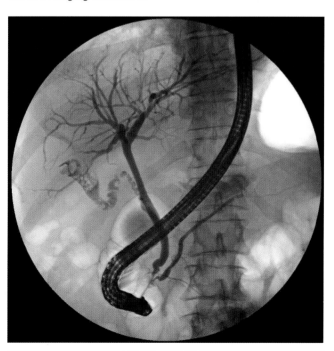

Fig. 10.2 Imaging, and in particular endoscopic retrograde pancreatography (ERCP) and endoscopic ultrasound (EUS) are complementary to pathology in diagnosis of hepatobiliary disease. This is ERCP image of the biliary tree including the main pancreatic duct.

Normal cytology of the liver

Cytological findings (Figs 10.3, 10.4)

- Hepatocytes: a large polygonal cell with:
  - abundant granular cytoplasm
  - one or two round to oval, centrally placed nuclei
  - even chromatin pattern
  - occasionally prominent nucleoli
  - generally appear as small clusters (Fig. 10.3) *or*
  - larger flat sheets with irregular jagged edges without endothelial cell wrapping (Fig. 10.4) *or*
  - single cells
- Biliary duct epithelium (see Figs 10.54–10.56)
  - picket fences with nuclear palisading
  - monolayered honeycomb sheets
  - cuboidal to columnar
  - scant pale cytoplasm

Complications of liver FNA

The occurrence of complications after hepatic FNA is rare:

- 0.5% minor complications
- 0.05% major complications requiring surgery
- Less than 0.01% mortality

Contraindications of liver FNA

Absolute contraindications include:

- Uncorrectable bleeding diathesis
- Lack of a safe access route, e.g. vascular structure in the biopsy path
- Uncooperative patients

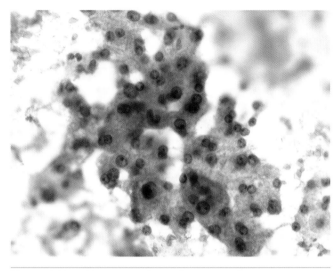

Fig. 10.3[†] Normal hepatocytes. Benign hepatocytes demonstrate a polygonal shape, abundant granular cytoplasm, focal steatosis and 1–2 round to oval centrally placed nuclei, with an even chromatin pattern and small nucleoli.

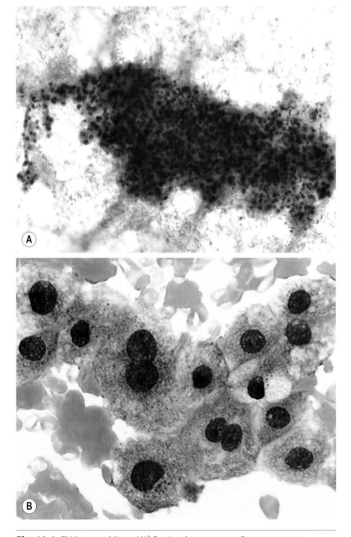

Fig. 10.4 FNA normal liver. (A)[†] Benign hepatocytes. Smear pattern includes jagged, irregularly shaped clusters of hepatocytes without peripherally wrapping endothelium. (B) High-power view shows large cells with round central nuclei and abundant granular cytoplasm.

Liver pigments and fatty change

- **Lipofuscin**: fine golden, granular, relatively non-refractile pigment in alcohol-fixed, Papanicolaou- (PAP) stained smears and is typically concentrated around the nucleus
- **Bile pigment** is produced by hepatocytes and is virtually pathognomonic of hepatocellular carcinoma when recognised within malignant cells. Bile appears as coarse, irregular, rather amorphous, non-refractile green to golden-brown globular intracytoplasmic and extracytoplasmic deposits on PAP stain (Figs 10.5, 10.6). With Giemsa–Romanowsky stain, bile has a dark green to black hue
- **Haemosiderin** is a coarse, brown-black refractile pigment with PAP stain and blue green on MGG stain. Malignant hepatocytes lose their ability to retain iron. It is helpful to use a special stain for iron like Prussian blue to highlight cells or clusters of cells without staining (Fig. 10.7)

Fatty change in hepatocytes is recognised as either one or two large vacuoles (macrovesicular) or multiple small vacuoles (microvesicular) (Fig. 10.8).

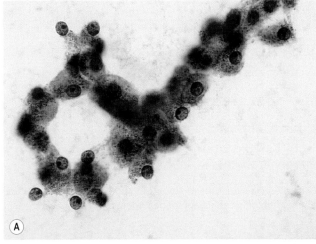

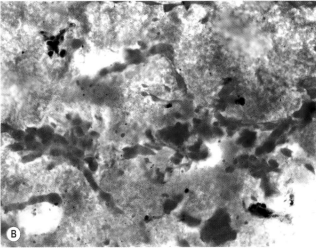

Fig. 10.7[†] Haemosiderin pigment. (A) This pigment appears as coarse, brown-black refractile pigment on the standard Papanicolaou stain (smear, PAP). (B) Iron stain distinguishes the benign cells that stain blue and the malignant cells that do not (smear, Prussian blue).

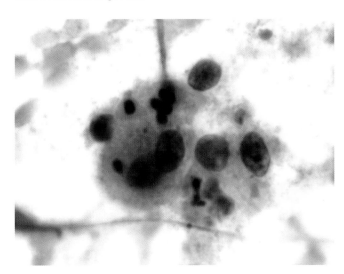

Fig. 10.5[†] Bile pigment. Although variable in colour, texture, size and density, bile is recognised by its globular, green-tinged non-refractile appearance.

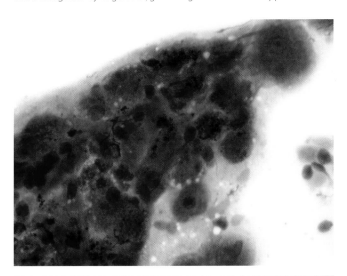

Fig. 10.6[†] Bile pigment. Canalicular bile plugs can be appreciated in cases of extrahepatic obstruction.

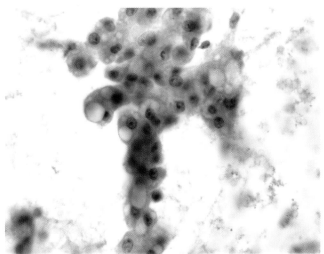

Fig. 10.8[†] Steatosis. Fatty change in hepatocytes is recognised as either one or two large vacuoles (macrovesicular) or multiple small vacuoles (microvesicular).

Liver infections

Organised abscesses can mimic hepatic tumours leading to FNA.

For therapeutic drainage, FNA is recommended only for small abscesses <50 mm; larger abscesses require percutaneous catheter drainage for complete management.

Pyogenic abscess

Non-specific acute inflammatory cells and cellular debris. Cultures are helpful for identification of bacterial organisms.

Amoebic abscess

Solitary liver mass in young patients, rarely requires drainage and responds to metronidazole therapy. The single-cell trophozoites of *E. histolytica* with round nucleus, condensed peripheral chromatin and central small nucleolus with foamy cytoplasm resemble histiocytes and can be easily overlooked.

Actinomyces spp. abscess

Contains characteristic 'sulphur granules'.

Echinococcus spp. (Figs 10.9–10.11)

Shows laminated cyst wall or necrotic background and may contain hooklets.

Granulomatous inflammation

Fungal or acid-fast organisms may be detected.

Granulomata (non-infectious)

Primary hepatobiliary disorders, sarcoidosis, tumours such as lymphoma and metastatic carcinoma (Fig. 10.12).

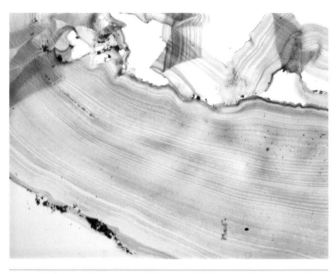

Fig. 10.10[†] Echinococcal cyst. The laminated cyst wall may be appreciated on both smears and cell block .

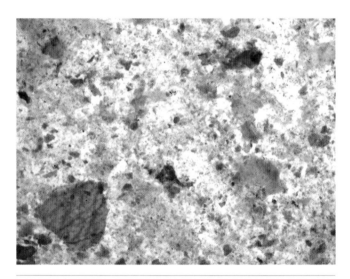

Fig. 10. 11[†] Echinococcal cyst. Aspirate smears of cyst contents can produce a thick and amorphous necrotic pattern often referred to as 'anchovy paste'.

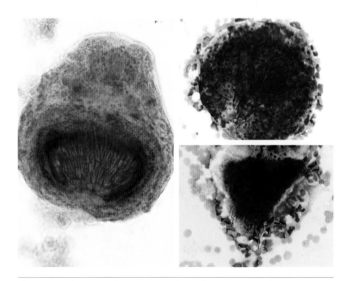

Fig. 10.9 Echinococcal cyst. Protoscolices of the organism demonstrate a crown of characteristic 'shark tooth-shaped ' hooklets (insets).

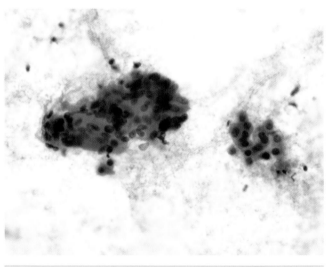

Fig. 10.12[†] Granulomatous hepatitis. Granulomas are composed of cohesive clusters of epithelioid histiocytes with oval to elongated, often twisted nuclei and indistinct but visible cytoplasm.

Lesions mimicking neoplasms

Bile duct hamartoma

Bile duct hamartoma may present as a mass lesion mimicking a neoplasm, and as a result, may be encountered on FNA.

Mesenchymal hamartoma

Hepatic mesenchymal hamartoma is a benign mass-forming lesion of malformed bile ducts and myxoid mesenchyme diagnosed in mostly male (70%) infants and children less than 5 years of age.

Inflammatory pseudotumour

Inflammatory pseudotumour (IPT) of the liver is an uncommon, benign, mass-forming proliferation of mixed inflammatory cells and histiocytes dominated by polyclonal plasma cells infiltrating a stroma of fibroblasts, myofibroblasts and collagen.

Cytological findings: bile duct hamartoma (adenoma) (Fig. 10.13)

* Benign-appearing glandular epithelium, often in flat monolayered sheets
* Round, uniform, evenly spaced nuclei
* Scant but visible, non-mucinous cytoplasm
* Uncharacteristically few to no hepatocytes in the background

Cytological findings: mesenchymal hamartoma (Fig. 10.14)

* Benign-appearing glandular epithelium, often in flat monolayered sheets
* Myxoid stroma
* Benign-appearing spindle cells
* Variable number of benign hepatocytes

Cytological findings: inflammatory myofibroblastic tumour (inflammatory pseudotumour) (Fig. 10.15)

* Mixed inflammatory proliferation
* Numerous plasma cells and foamy histiocytes
* Benign-appearing spindle cells in cohesive groups and singly

Diagnostic pitfall

Atypia, although usually focal and low grade, may suggest a spindle-cell neoplasm.

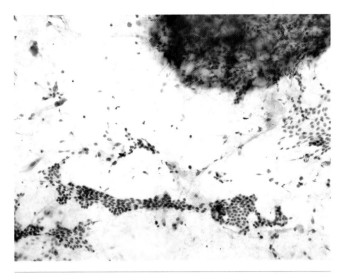

Fig. 10.13† Bile duct hamartoma. Aspirate smears are dominated by benign-appearing bile duct epithelial cells with uncharacteristically scant numbers of associated hepatocytes.

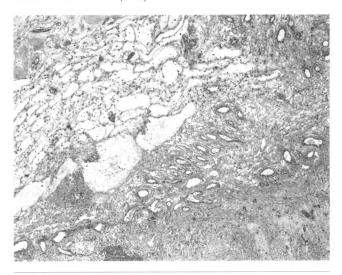

Fig. 10.14† Mesenchymal hamartoma. Disorganised loose, focally cystic myxoid mesenchymal tissue surrounds variably sized benign bile ducts and occasionally hepatocytes.

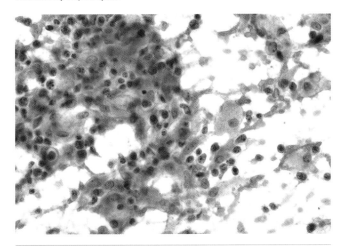

Fig. 10.15† Inflammatory myofibroblastic tumour (inflammatory pseudotumour). Xanthogranulomatous reaction composed of foamy histiocytes enmeshed with mixed inflammatory cells dominated by plasma cells and spindle mesenchymal cells is characteristic of this benign proliferation.

Miscellaneous benign lesions

- **Extramedullary haemopoiesis**
- **Hepatic splenosis**
- **Amyloidosis**

Cytological findings: extramedullary haemopoiesis (EMH) (Fig. 10.16)

- EMH is normal only within the first few weeks of life
- Commonly associated with hepatoblastomas and hepatic angiosarcomas
- Megakaryocytes, large cells with abundant granular cytoplasm and lobulated nuclei
- Normoblasts, and myelocytes

Cytological findings: hepatic splenosis (Fig. 10.17)

- Benign appearing haemopoietic cells: lymphocytes and neutrophils
- Lymphoid follicle
- Reticular network holding aggregates of cells together
- Bloody background

Cytological findings: amyloidosis (Fig. 10.18)

- Amorphous glassy or waxy extracellular material
- Rounded dense droplets on LBC
- Pink to green staining on Papanicolaou; magenta on Romanowsky
- Congo red stain is positive
- Apple-green birefringence with polarisation

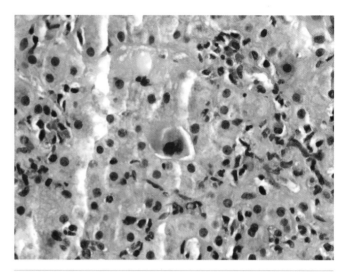

Fig. 10.16† Extramedullary haemopoiesis. This cell block preparation demonstrates a megakaryocyte in the centre surrounded by mixed haemopoietic cells infiltrating benign hepatic parenchyma.

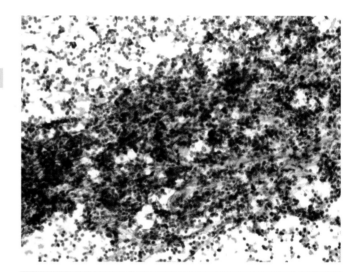

Fig. 10.17† Splenosis. Smears are cellular and composed of well-preserved mixed haemopoietic elements held together by a reticular network.

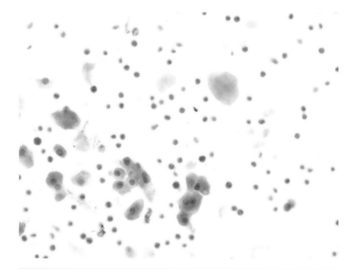

Fig. 10.18† Amyloid. In liquid-based processing, amyloid may form hard rounded droplets that are easy to overlook (ThinPrep®).

Benign neoplasms

- **Angiomyolipoma**
- **Haemangioma**
- **Hepatobiliary cystadenoma**

Cytological findings: angiomyolipoma (Fig. 10.19)

- Interlacing complex of smooth muscle, fat and blood vessels
- Immunocytochemical stain for confirmation: HMB-45

Diagnostic pitfalls: angiomyolipoma

- Smooth muscle may dominate smears and can demonstrate atypia
- Solid epithelioid areas may be dominant, can produce significant atypia and can lead to false-positive interpretations

Cytological findings: haemangioma (Fig. 10.20)

- Bloody, scantily cellular smears
- Coils of loose connective tissue and smooth muscle
- Generally few to no hepatocytes
- Smears commonly non-diagnostic; specific diagnosis dependent on cell block

Cytological findings: hepatobiliary cystadenoma (Fig. 10.21)

- Thin to mucoid cyst fluid
- Foamy histiocytes
- Benign-appearing mucinous glandular cells
- Subepithelial ovarian-type stroma is not aspirated
- Generally few to no hepatocytes

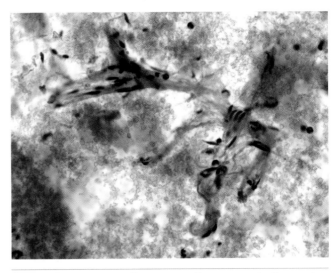

Fig. 10.20[†] Haemangioma. The presence of loose connective tissue and smooth muscle fragments associated with blood and few to no background hepatocytes, although considered non-diagnostic and often unsatisfactory for diagnosis, are typical findings in the aspiration of hepatic haemangioma.

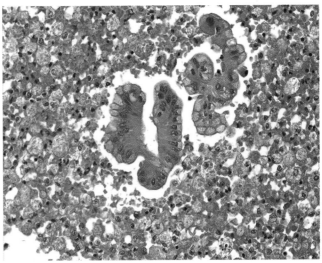

Fig. 10.21[†] Hepatobiliary cystadenoma. Mucinous glandular epithelium and foamy histiocytes characterise the contents of this benign hepatic cyst (cell block, H & E). (From Sidawy MK, Syed ZA. Liver. In: Goldblum JR (ed.) Fine Needle Aspiration Cytology. Foundations in Diagnostic Pathology series. London: Elsevier; 2007)

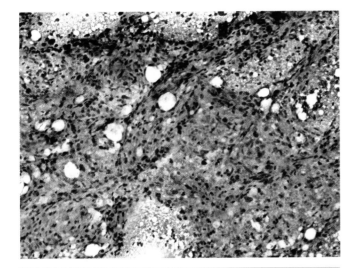

Fig. 10.19[†] Angiomyolipoma. A combination of vessels, smooth muscle and adipocytes allows for a specific diagnosis on FNA. (From Odze RD, Goldblum JR. Surgical Pathology of the GI tract, Liver, Biliary Tract and Pancreas, 1st edn. London: Elsevier; 2004)

- **Dysplastic nodule (DN)**
- **Focal nodular hyperplasia (FNH)**
- **Hepatocellular adenoma (HCA)**
  - all share many common cytological features
  - distinction between them on smear cytology alone is difficult if not impossible
  - all share the same differential diagnosis, namely well-differentiated hepatocellular carcinoma
  - cell blocks as well as radiological and clinical correlation are crucial in making a specific diagnosis

Dysplastic nodule

- In the clinical setting of a mass in a cirrhotic liver, clinically suspicious for hepatocellular carcinoma
- Subclassified as:
  - low-grade dysplasia (macroregenerative nodule)
  - high-grade dysplasia (small cell dysplasia)

Focal nodular hyperplasia

- Most commonly found in adult women in a non-cirrhotic liver
- Circumscribed, non-encapsulated mass

Hepatocellular adenoma

- Benign neoplasm of monoclonal hepatocytes arising in a non-cirrhotic liver
- Typically occurs in women between 15–45 years old with a history of oral contraceptive use

Cytological features: DN, FNH and HCA (Table 10.1)

- All three lesions share cellular features of 'reactivity ' which include an apparent hepatocytic pleomorphism rather than monomorphism (Figs 10.22–10.26)
- Increased number of binucleated cells which tend to be decreased in hepatocellular carcinoma
- Relatively low nuclear to cytoplasmic ratio
- Smooth nuclear membranes
- Prominent but not large nucleoli

Further investigations

- Cell block preparations of small tissue fragments or CNBs currently offer the best method of distinguishing between benign and malignant hepatocytic proliferations (See Table 10.1)
- Reticulin stain
- α-fetoprotein (AFP)
- Glypican-3, (GPC3)
- CD34

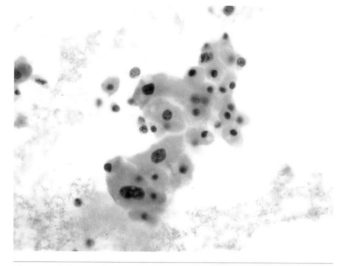

Fig. 10.22[†] Reactive hepatocytes. Cellular and nuclear pleomorphism or anisonucleosis of benign, reactive hepatocytes in contrast to the monomorphism demonstrated by hepatocellular carcinoma.

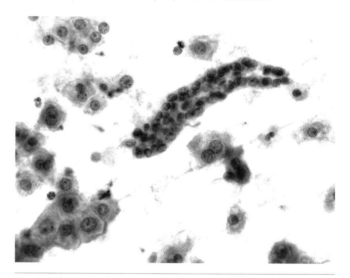

Fig. 10.23[†] Focal nodular hyperplasia. Smears are composed of benign hepatocytes and bile duct epithelial cells.

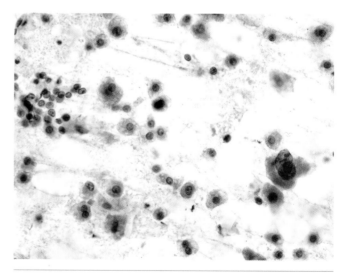

Fig. 10.24[†] Dysplastic nodule, low grade. Macroregenerative nodules contain hepatocytes that demonstrate significant atypia or large cell change (low-grade dysplasia), cells that are recognised as benign by their sporadic placement among otherwise benign and reactive-appearing hepatocytes. Note the bile duct cells in the upper left.

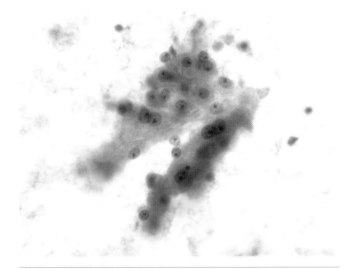

Fig. 10.25† Reactive hepatocytes. Reactive hepatocytes demonstrate a low nuclear to cytoplasmic ratio and nuclei with smooth nuclear membranes and prominent but not macro nucleoli.

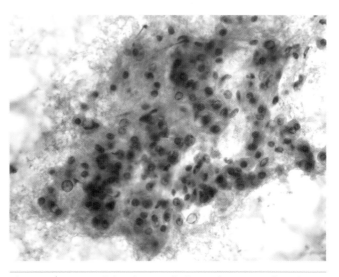

Fig. 10.26† Hepatocellular adenoma. The benign hepatocytes form clusters with irregular contours without associated peripherally wrapping endothelial cells.

Table 10.1 Features typical of benign hepatic nodules versus well-differentiated hepatocellular carcinoma

| | Benign hepatic nodules | | | |
	DN, low grade	HCA	FNH	WDHCC
Clinical				
Gender	Males and females	Females >>> males	Females >> males	Males > females
Age	Adults	15–45 years	All ages, mostly adult women	Adults
Cirrhosis	Yes	No	No	Yes
Other		Oral contraceptive use; glycogen storage diseases	Hepatic haemangiomas	Alcohol abuse, viral hepatitis
Radiology				
Nodule size	0.8–3 cm nodules	5–15 cm, solitary mass	5 cm mass; stellate scar	0.1 cm nodule
Serology				
AFP	Not elevated	Not elevated	Not elevated	Elevated
Cytology				
Hepatocytes	Irregular shaped clusters without peripheral or transgressing endothelial cells; single cells; bland appearing large hepatocytes ± cytoplasmic glycogen and/or fat; round regular nuclei without prominent nucleoli; scattered large dysplastic cells			Peripherally wrapping and transgressing vessels; monomorphic small hepatocytes; nucleoli, often macro; hyaline globules
Bile ducts	Yes	No	Yes	No
Ancillary tests				
Reticulin	Present, highlights normal 1 to 2-cell thick hepatic plates			Decreased to absent; highlights 0 to 3-cell thick plates when present
AFP	Negative	Negative	Negative	Present (30–40%)
Glypican-3	Negative	Negative (focal weak positive)	Negative	Positive
CD34	Negative	Positive, periportal/septal	Negative	Positive, diffuse

WDHCC, well-differentiated hepatocellular carcinoma; DN, dysplastic nodule; HCA, hepatocellular adenoma; FNH, focal nodular hyperplasia; AFP, alpha-fetoprotein.

Primary liver malignant neoplasms

Hepatocellular carcinoma

- **Low-grade** (well-differentiated)
- **High-grade** (moderately poorly differentiated) tumours

Cytological findings: well-differentiated hepatocellular carcinoma (Figs 10.27–10.30)

- Low-power smear pattern with smooth-edged clusters and thickened trabeculae with peripherally wrapping endothelial cells (pathognomonic)
- Low-power smear pattern with more than focal loosely cohesive sheets of hepatocytes with transgressing vessels (highly suspicious finding)
- Monotonous, uniform hepatocytic cell population with subtle malignant features
- Acinar formation in cell clusters
- Increased nuclear to cytoplasmic ratio compared to normal hepatocytes
- Macroeosinophilic nucleoli
- Reduced number of binucleated cells
- Background free of bile duct epithelial cells
- Reticulin stain demonstrates a loss of the normal 1–2-cell thick hepatic plate architecture
- Iron stain fails to stain tumour in cases of haemachromatosis
- Positive glypican-3 immunostaining; AFP

Cytological findings: moderately to poorly differentiated hepatocellular carcinoma (Figs 10.31–10.34)

- Peripherally wrapping endothelial smear pattern is virtually pathognomonic
- Transgressing vessels are suggestive but cannot distinguish hepatocellular from renal cell carcinoma
- Presence of intracytoplasmic bile is pathognomonic
- Polygonal cells with central nuclei and prominent nucleoli with visible, granular to clear cytoplasm in moderately differentiated tumours; scant to no cytoplasm in poorly differentiated tumours
- Immunophenotype:
  - low MW CK (Cam 5.2)
  - polyclonal CEA and CD10 (canalicular)
  - HepPar-1 positive
  - AFP variable
  - high MW CK (AE1) negative

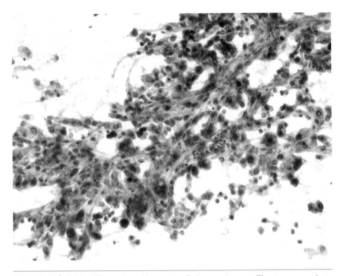

Fig. 10.27[†] Well-differentiated hepatocellular carcinoma. The transgressing endothelial pattern demonstrates an arborising, proliferating or transgressing meshwork of capillaries in a loosely cohesive sheet of neoplastic hepatocytes.

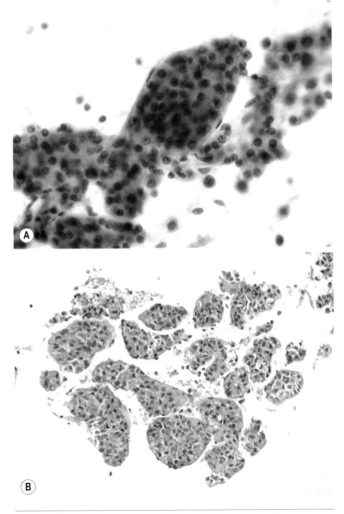

Fig. 10.28[†] Well-differentiated hepatocellular carcinoma. (A) The peripherally wrapping endothelial cell pattern demonstrates the capillarised endothelial cells of sinusoids wrapping around smooth-edged, rounded nests and thickened hepatic trabeculae of hepatocytes (smear, PAP). (B) This pathognomonic feature is also demonstrated in cell block preparations.

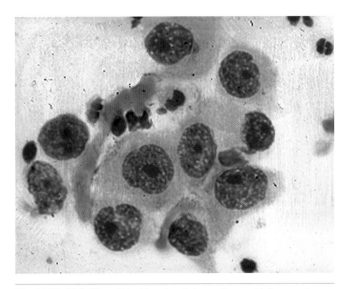

Fig. 10.29 Well-differentiated hepatocellular carcinoma. Malignancy is supported by the presence of macronucleoli.

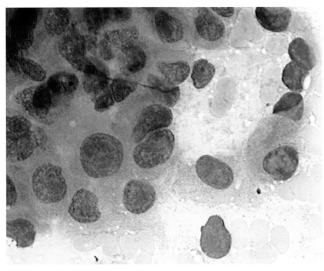

Fig. 10.32 Moderately differentiated hepatocellular carcinoma. This high-grade hepatocellular carcinoma maintains some hepatic preservation while displaying obvious malignant features.

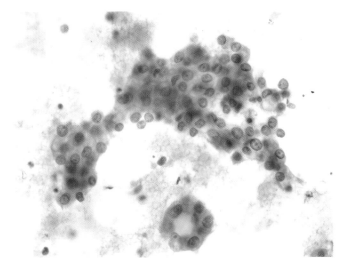

Fig. 10.30[†] Well-differentiated hepatocellular carcinoma. Malignancy is supported by the presence of cellular monotony resulting from a relatively uniform population of cells with an elevated nuclear to cytoplasmic ratio. Note the acinar architecture in the bottom centre of the image.

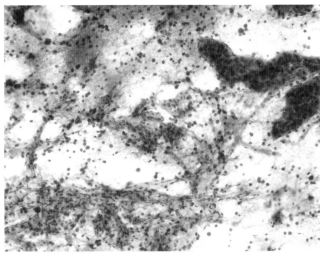

Fig. 10.33[†] Poorly differentiated hepatocellular carcinoma. Smear pattern is important in the recognition of high-grade hepatocellular carcinomas and its recognition can preclude the need for ancillary studies. Note here the peripherally wrapping endothelium, the transgressing endothelium and the numerous naked nuclei in the background.

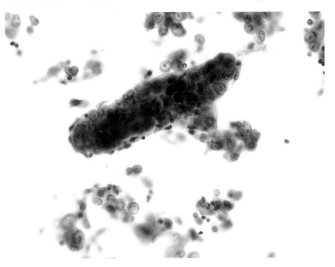

Fig. 10.31[†] Poorly differentiated hepatocellular carcinoma. This high-grade hepatocellular carcinoma appears as an obviously malignant high-grade carcinoma, and there is little to no hepatic preservation. Note the peripherally wrapping endothelium, a feature that supports hepatic origin.

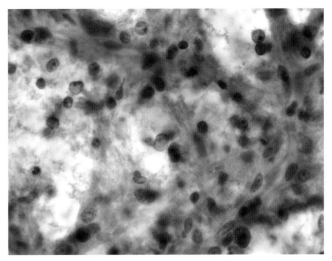

Fig. 10.34[†] Poorly differentiated hepatocellular carcinoma. The recognition of malignant epithelial cells producing bile is essentially diagnostic of hepatocellular carcinoma.

Hepatocellular carcinoma (cont'd)

Immunocytochemistry: Hepatocellular carcinoma and metastatic carcinoma (Fig. 10.35)

- Anti-hepatocyte antibody Hep-Par-1 (strong diffuse chunky staining pattern) (Fig. 10.35B)
- MOC-31
- GPC3 (Fig. 10.35C)
- AFP
- Low (CAM 5.2)and high (AE1) MWCK
- Polyclonal CEA
- Neprilysin (CD10) (Fig. 10.35D)

The hepatocytes markers Hep-Par-1 and GPC3 do not have 100% sensitivity or specificity for the diagnosis of malignancy of hepatic origin, so these markers should be used in a panel of markers to support the diagnosis of HCC.

The endothelial cell marker CD34 stains the sinusoids diffusely, indicating capillarisation of the sinusoids and supporting the diagnosis of hepatocellular carcinoma (see Fig. 10.35E). AFP staining is helpful if positive, but a negative stain does not rule out HCC as only about 40% of HCC are associated with a positive stain. AFP may occasionally be positive in reactive processes, so a positive stain does not in itself diagnose malignancy. Serum levels of AFP 400 ng/mL are strongly associated with the presence of hepatocellular carcinoma, but not all tumours are associated with elevated levels, particularly the fibrolamellar variant.

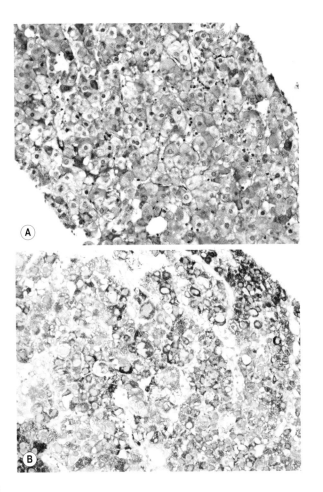

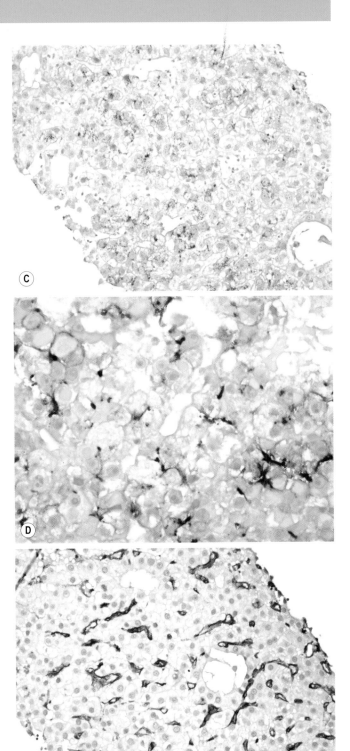

Fig. 10.35[†] Hepatocellular carcinoma. (A) A reticulin stain demonstrates the loss of reticulin staining typical of hepatocellular carcinoma. (B) Immunoperoxidase staining shows coarse, granular diffuse staining with anti-hepatocyte antibody (Hep-Par-1). (C) Malignant hepatocytes also stain with antibodies to glypican-3. (D) Polyclonal CEA antibodies demonstrate a linear canalicular staining pattern as does CD10. (E) CD34 highlights the capillarisation of the sinusoids diffusely in hepatocellular carcinoma.

Variants of hepatocellular carcinoma

Fibrolamellar variant

- Generally occurs in young patients as a solitary mass in a non-cirrhotic liver

Acinar cell variant

- Presents a diagnostic challenge on cell block preparations
- Frequently 'back-to-back' acini give the appearance of an adenocarcinoma

Clear cell variant

- Abundance of intracytoplasmic fat and/or glycogen
- Clear cell tumours metastatic from other sites

Cytological findings (Figs 10.36–10.39)

Fibrolamellar hepatocellular carcinoma

- Population of large hepatocytes singly and in loose clusters
- Smears may be paucicellular due to fibrosis
- Transgressing vessels may be seen, but no peripherally wrapping endothelial cells
- Deceptively low nuclear to cytoplasmic ratio
- Large, variably atypical nuclei with prominent nucleoli and frequent intranuclear inclusions
- Cytoplasm is characteristically abundant and oncocytic appearing

Acinar variant

- Back-to-back acini/rosettes of hepatocytes
- No mucin production

Clear cell variant

- Cells with abundant vacuolated, clear cytoplasm filled with glycogen and/or fat

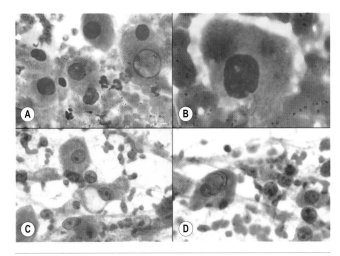

Fig. 10.37† Fibrolamellar variant of hepatocellular carcinoma. (A and B) Large discohesive tumour cells with abundant granular cytoplasm and low nuclear to cytoplasmic ratios. A well-defined cytoplasmic pale body is seen in (A). Papanicolaou-stained smears (C and D) demonstrate prominent nucleoli and naked nuclei. An intranuclear pseudoinclusion is also seen in (D). (From Crowe A et al. Diagnosis of metastatic fibrolamellar hepatocellular carcinoma by endoscopic ultrasound-guided fine needle aspiration. CytoJournal 2011, 8:2)

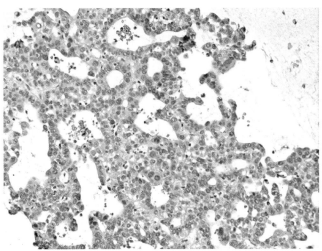

Fig. 10.38† Acinar variant of hepatocellular carcinoma. This variant becomes apparent on cell block preparations with the demonstration of numerous variably sized back-to-back glandular spaces.

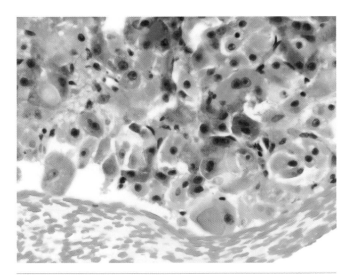

Fig. 10.36† Fibrolamellar hepatocellular carcinoma. This variant is characterised by large polygonal hepatocytes with dense oxyphilic cytoplasm often containing intracytoplasmic pale bodies and a deceptively low nuclear to cytoplasmic ratio (cell block, H & E. Courtesy of Dr Edmond Cibas, Brigham & Women's Hospital).

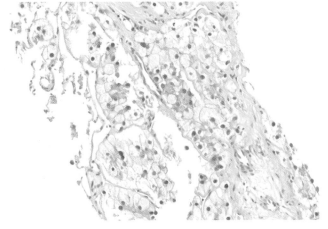

Fig. 10.39† Clear cell hepatocellular carcinoma. This variant demonstrates polygonal cells with abundant vacuolated cytoplasm, mimicking other clear cell tumours, especially renal cell carcinoma.

Hepatoblastoma

Hepatoblastoma is the most common tumour of children with 75% occurring in males and 90% occurring before the age of 5 years

- Strong association with familial adenomatous polyposis
- Serum AFP levels are almost always elevated
    - histologically, tumour recapitulates the developing liver and may contain heterologous mesenchymal or epithelial elements
- Hepatoblastomas are classified as either epithelial or mixed epithelial–mesenchymal

Cytological findings (Figs 10.40–10.43)

- Epithelial dominant smears
- Mesenchymal (spindle cell) component and/or heterologous elements, especially extramedullary haemopoiesis and osteoid, relatively scant
- Epithelial cells are either small hepatocytic (fetal type), smaller immature, pleomorphic cells (embryonal type) or smaller still undifferentiated blue cells (anaplastic type)
- Epithelial cells show acinar pattern, papillary pattern, or are arranged in sheets
- Immunophenotype: positive for low and high MW CK (CAM 5.2 and AE1), pCEA with variable canalicular/cytoplasmic staining, Hep-Par-1

Differential diagnosis

- Fetal-type hepatoblastoma and hepatocellular carcinoma
- Embryonal or anaplastic hepatoblastoma and other paediatric small round blue cell tumours

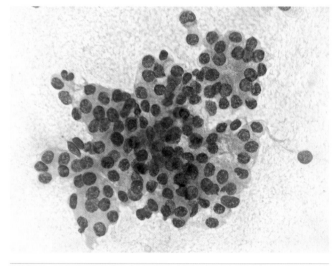

Fig. 10.41[†] Foetal hepatoblastoma. Sheets of uniform tumour cells with pseudo-acinar formations. Note the round central placed nuclei and the moderate amount of cytoplasm (MGG).

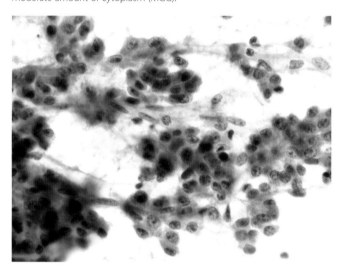

Fig. 10.42[†] The embryonal type is composed of more primitive cells with hyperchromatic nucleoli and scant cytoplasm.

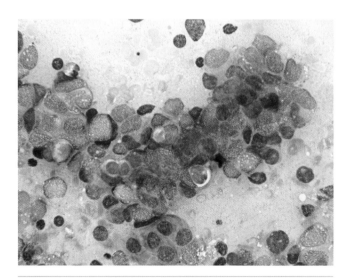

Fig. 10.40 Embryonal hepatoblastoma. Cluster of embryonal cells showing a scant cytoplasm and a high nuclear: cytoplasmic ratio. The nuclei are irregularly shaped (MGG). (From Edward G. Weir, Syed Z. Ali. Hepatoblastoma: cytomorphologic characteristics in serous cavity fluids. Cancer Cytopathol 2002, 96:267–74.)

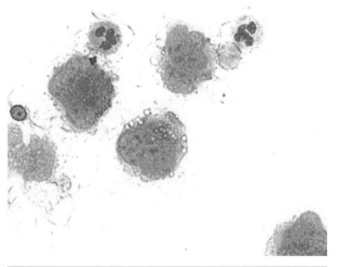

Fig. 10.43 Hepatoblastoma. Serous fluid specimen showing single, discohesive neoplastic cells with pleomorphic nuclei depicting cleft or lobulated nuclei. Note the small intracytoplasmic vacuoles. (From Edward G. Weir, Syed Z. Ali. Hepatoblastoma: cytomorphologic characteristics in serous cavity fluids. Cancer Cytopathol 2002, 96:267–74.)

Cholangiocarcinoma

- Adenocarcinoma of the bile ducts
- Occurs predominantly in the non-cirrhotic liver
- Elderly population most commonly affected
- South-east Asia due to the liver fluke
- Risk factors: primary sclerosing cholangitis (PSC) and cirrhosis due to hepatitis C

Cytological findings (Figs 10.44–10.47)

- Glandular cells in flat, angulated sheets
- Low-grade malignant nuclei with:
  - nuclear crowding
  - overlapping
  - slightly irregular nuclear membrane
  - parachromatin clearing
- A range of atypia may be seen from borderline malignant-appearing to obviously malignant-looking (see pp. 328, 329)
- Exaggerated honeycombed pattern from uneven nuclear distribution in the sheet
- Cell blocks can help by demonstrating sclerotic stroma and cribriform architecture
- Mucin stains positive at least focally in many cases
- Immunophenotype: keratin 7 and 19 positive; 20 negative; cytoplasmic pCEA, LeuM1, B72.3

Differential diagnosis: bile duct brushings

- Require more stringent set of criteria and a higher threshold for the interpretation of malignancy (see pp. 327–330)
- Difficulty in obtaining a specimen of quality and quantity sufficient for a confident diagnosis of malignancy
- Sclerosis and inflammation inherent to the tumour or secondary to an underlying condition (PSC, stent placement)
- Paucicellular sample, often preparation artefact from obscuring blood, crush and air drying artefact limit optimal interpretation

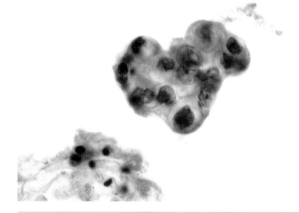

Fig. 10.45† Cholangiocarcinoma. Intraductal and periductal tumours sampled by bile duct brushing often have better preservation with liquid-based processing.

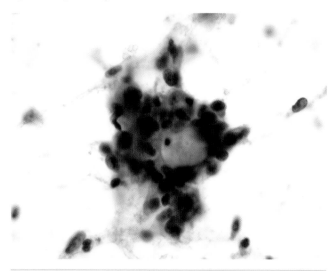

Fig. 10.46† Cholangiocarcinoma. The recognition of three-dimensional cell clusters with mucin vacuoles confirms the diagnosis of adenocarcinoma and excludes hepatocellular carcinoma.

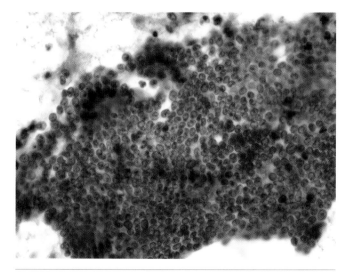

Fig. 10.44† Cholangiocarcinoma. This adenocarcinoma demonstrates irregular, variably sized sheets of atypical to malignant-appearing glandular cells that resemble bile duct epithelium.

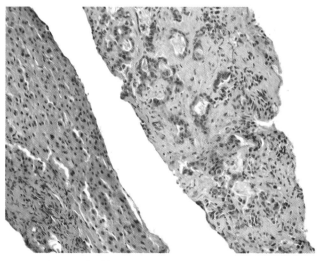

Fig. 10.47† Cholangiocarcinoma. Cell block preparations of tissue fragments often demonstrate the characteristic angulated glands invading dense sclerosis.

Angiosarcoma

- Most common primary sarcoma of the liver
- Occurs in the elderly
- Associated with exposure to vinyl chloride, Thorotrast, arsenic and anabolic steroids
- Single or multiple nodules of vascular channels lined by malignant endothelial cells

Cytological findings (Figs 10.48, 10.49)

- FNA smears are bloody and may be paucicellular
- Malignant endothelial cells can be seen interdigitating among reactive hepatocytes
- Elongated, spindled-shaped hyperchromatic nuclei easier to appreciate in small clusters than in large clusters where they tend to blend in with the hepatocytes
- Spindle cell malignancy possibly with blood lakes
- Immunocytochemistry stains: factor 8, CD31, CD34, Ulex Europeus lectin

Differential diagnosis

- Usually spindle cells but epithelioid appearance to the endothelial cells may also occur, creating a pitfall and misdiagnosis of a carcinoma (Fig. 10.49)

Embryonal sarcoma

- Embryonal sarcoma is a rare malignancy of children (6 to 10 years of age)
- Patients present with abdominal pain or with an abdominal mass
- Histologically, myxoid stroma embedded with spindle to stellate cells

Cytological findings (Fig. 10.50)

- Hypercellular smears
- Large, pleomorphic anaplastic cells with multinucleated giant cells and atypical spindle cells
- Intracytoplasmic globules that are PAS positive, diastase resistant
- Immunophenotype: vimentin, alpha-1-anti-trypsin and alpha-1-antichymotrypsin positive

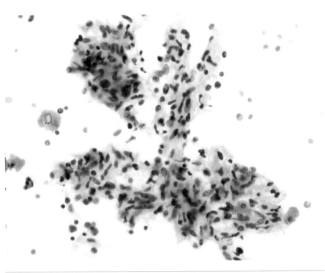

Fig. 10.48[†] Angiosarcoma. The malignant endothelial cells with elongated spindle-shaped hyperchromatic nuclei are enmeshed with benign hepatocytes.

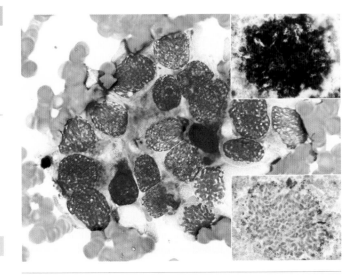

Fig. 10.49 Epithelioid angiosarcoma may mimic carcinoma. (Insets) CD31 positive (*above*), MNF 116 epithelial marker negative (*below*).

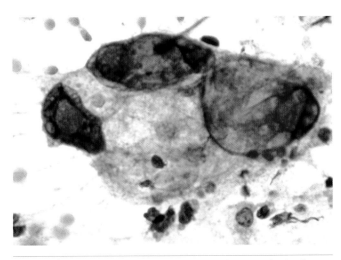

Fig. 10.50[†] Embryonal sarcoma. Tumour cells are large, anaplastic, often multinucleated tumour giant cells.

Metastatic liver tumours

- The majority of malignancies in the liver are metastases
- Adenocarcinoma from the colon is the most common metastasis to the liver
- Past medical history is of vital importance
- Adenocarcinoma presents the most difficulty in making a specific diagnosis as to site of origin
- Other metastatic malignancies commonly encountered in the liver are: pancreas (adenocarcinoma and neuroendocrine tumours), stomach (adenocarcinoma and gastrointestinal stromal tumours), breast, lung (adenocarcinoma, small cell carcinoma and much less commonly squamous cell carcinoma), skin (melanoma) and bladder

Cytological findings: colonic adenocarcinoma (Fig. 10.51)

- Cigar-shaped, often palisaded nuclei
- Variably prominent nucleoli but not macroeosinophilic nucleoli
- 'Dirty' necrotic background (KEY)
- Immunocytochemistry: CK20, CEA and CDX2 positive; CK7 negative

Cytological findings: well-differentiated neuroendocrine carcinoma (e.g. metastatic pancreatic endocrine neoplasm (PEN) and carcinoid tumour) (Fig. 10.52)

- Small uniform blue cells with visible cytoplasm that tends to be scant and more evenly perinuclear in carcinoid tumours and more abundant and eccentric in PEN
- Nuclei with coarse stippled chromatin, more obvious in carcinoids than PEN
- Nucleoli generally not present in carcinoid tumours but visible in PEN
- No nuclear moulding, much less crush artefact, and no significant necrosis/apoptosis compared with small cell undifferentiated carcinoma
- Immunocytochemistry: keratin, synaptophysin and chromogranin positive

Role of liver FNA in patient management

- FNA is the diagnostic procedure of choice for focal liver lesions
- When performed by experienced interventional radiologists and interpreted by experienced pathologists, the sensitivity of liver FNA is as high as 90% with specificity approaching 100%
- Sampling error is the reason for most false-negative results that are most often due to inexact needle localisation
- Concomitant core biopsy improves accuracy, specificity and sensitivity, and both are better than either alone
- The distinction between a primary and metastatic malignancy is important for proper patient care
- Access to the patient's past medical history is of vital importance
- Metastatic colon cancer is the most common malignancy in the liver (Fig. 10.53)

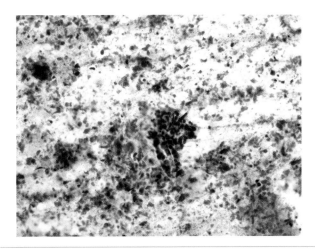

Fig. 10.51† Metastatic colonic carcinoma. This adenocarcinoma is recognised on smears by the background of dirty necrosis, a non-specific but characteristic feature. Viable aggregates of carcinoma may be few.

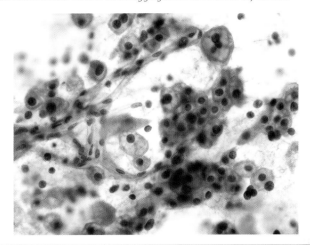

Fig. 10.52† Metastatic renal cell carcinoma. The classic appearance of renal cell carcinoma demonstrates large polygonal cells with clear to granular cytoplasm, central nuclei and large nucleoli. Note the transgressing endothelial pattern.

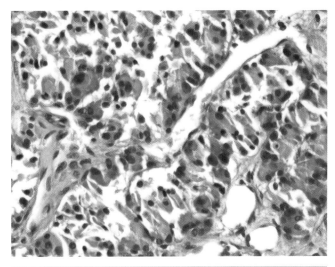

Fig. 10.53† Metastatic well-differentiated neuroendocrine carcinoma. Neuroendocrine tumours can mimic hepatocellular carcinoma architecturally on cell block with 'endothelial wrapping' as well as cytologically with polygonal cell shape and relatively low-grade malignant nuclear features (cell block).

Gall bladder and extrahepatic bile ducts

More than 80% of all cancers of the gallbladder and bile ducts are carcinomas. The list of all primary tumours in this area is shown in Box 10.1.

- Premalignant or non-invasive neoplastic lesions of bile ducts (biliary dysplasia or atypical biliary epithelium) have been replaced by the following nomenclature:
  - three-grade classification system (BilIN-1, BilIN-2 and BilIN-3) based on the degree of atypia
- Cholangiocarcinoma is a highly lethal disease with an overall 5-year survival of less than 5%
- Carcinoma of the hepatobiliary ducts is associated with the following:
  - cholelithiasis and chronic cholecystitis
  - hepatitis B and C
  - cirrhosis and alcohol abuse
  - primary sclerosing cholangitis (PSC)
  - biliary papillomatosis
  - biliary parasites such as liver flukes
  - ulcerative colitis
  - choledochal cysts

Procedures for collecting cytological material from the biliary tree

Bile sampling

- Three bile samples should be obtained on successive days from any patient undergoing percutaneous drainage
- Bile obtained from drainage bags shows bacterial overgrowth and loss of cell detail and is usually not suitable for cytological assessment
- In patients with external biliary drains, bile for cytology should be aspirated directly from the drainage catheter, or collected over a short period

Brush or catheter samples

- Obtained during ERCP
- A brush passed over the guide wire and drawn back and forth along the stricture
- Multiple samples improve sensitivity
- Washing the brushes in saline and cytocentrifuging the elutant may increase the yield

Liquid based cytology (LBC)

- Either alone or in combination with direct smears
- Reduces technical artefact
- Increases accuracy of biliary brushings cytology

FNA samples

- Obtained by EUS-FNA
- Multiple samplings may be necessary
- Multiple imaging procedures are of value
- The presence of the pathologist at the procedure for rapid on site evaluation (ROSE) can reduce the number of needle passes
- The practice of on-site cytology interpretation varies across endoscopic ultrasound (EUS) programmes in the USA and Europe but is generally considered beneficial to the level of diagnostic accuracy
- See Box 10.1 for tumour types in gall bladder and bile ducts

---

Box 10.1 Primary tumours of the gall bladder and extrahepatic bile ducts*

Epithelial neoplasms

Benign

- Adenoma
- Papillomatosis
- Cystadenoma
- Epithelial dysplasia and carcinoma in situ

Malignant

- Adenocarcinoma
- Papillary, intestinal, gastric foveolar
- Clear cell, mucinous, signet ring
- Cystadenocarcinoma
- Adenosquamous carcinoma
- Squamous cell carcinoma
- Small cell carcinoma (neuroendocrine, undifferentiated)
- Large cell neuroendocrine carcinoma
- Large cell undifferentiated carcinoma
- Spindle and giant cell/sarcomatoid
- With osteoclast-like giant cells
- Neuroendocrine neoplasms
- Carcinoid

- Adenocarcinoid (goblet-cell carcinoid)
- Carcinoid-adenocarcinoma (mixed)
- Paraganglioma, gangliocytic paraganglioma

Non-epithelial neoplasms

Benign

- Leiomyoma
- Lipoma
- Haemangioma
- Lymphangioma
- Osteoma
- Granular cell tumour
- Neurofibroma
- Ganglioneuroma

Malignant

- Rhabdomyosarcoma
- Malignant fibrous histiocytoma
- Angiosarcoma
- Leiomyosarcoma
- Kaposi's sarcoma
- Miscellaneous
- Carcinosarcoma

- Malignant melanoma
- Malignant lymphoma
- Germ cell tumours
- Tumour-like lesions
- Regenerative epithelial atypia
- Papillary hyperplasia
- Squamous metaplasia
- Adenomyomatous hyperplasia
- Mucocele
- Heterotopias
- Cholesterol polyp
- Inflammatory polyp
- Fibrous polyp
- Myofibroblastic proliferations
- Xanthogranulomatous cholecystitis
- Cholecystitis with lymphoid hyperplasia
- Malakoplakia
- Congenital cyst
- Amputation neuroma
- Primary sclerosing cholangitis
- Aspiration of gastric/duodenal contents

*Albores-Saveedra J, Henson DE, Klimstra DS. Armed Forces Institute of Pathology, 2000. ISBN 1 881041 58 1.Tumors of the Gallbladder, Extrahepatic Bile Ducts and Ampulla of Vater. Atlas of Tumor Pathology..

Normal cytology of bile ducts

Duodenal aspirates
- Biliary epithelium in monolayered sheets
- Duodenal cells with brush borders or goblet cell forms
- 'Matchstick' cells of gall bladder origin
- Cuboidal pancreatic acinar cells
- Degenerate cells of indeterminate origin

Bile
- Scanty cellular material
- Background of bile pigment and crystals
- Cholesterol crystals in some conditions
- Sheets of gall bladder epithelium, especially after saline irrigation

Bile duct brushings (Figs 10.54–10.56)
- Regular arrangement in flat sheets
- Sheets architecturally complex
- Cells tall, columnar
- Nuclei oval, round, basal
- Fine chromatin pattern
- Nucleoli inconspicuous

FNA samples
Epithelium of multiple types may be encountered as the needle traverses tissues such as:
- bowel mucosa
- liver
- pancreatic acinar and ductal tissue

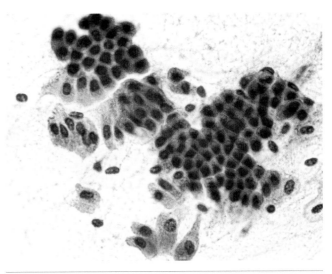

Fig. 10.54 Normal bile duct epithelium shows regular arrangement in flat sheets, cells are tall columnar, nuclei oval, round, basal with fine chromatin pattern and inconspicuous nucleoli.

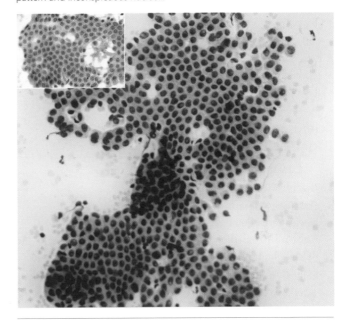

Fig. 10.55 Bile duct brushings. Monolayered sheet with enlarged nuclei and prominent nucleoli, but retained honeycomb structure and low nuclear to cytoplasmic ratio. Sheets may be architecturally complex and show 'holes'.

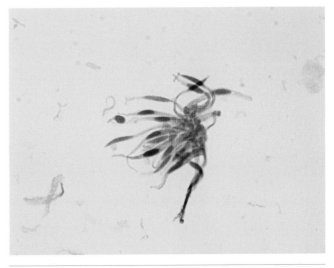

Fig. 10.56 Biliary epithelium. Slender columnar cells (matchstick cells) are often seen singly and in small clusters.

Inflammatory and reactive processes of the biliary ducts

Changes due to acute and chronic inflammation, primary sclerosing cholangitis (PSC), stent placement and postoperative effect are similar in all types of cytological samples and include a range of regenerative and degenerative alterations in bile duct epithelium which may mimic dysplasia and malignancy.

Cytological findings (Figs 10.57, 10.58)

- Slight overlapping of epithelial cells in sheets
- Small nucleoli
- Low nuclear to cytoplasmic ratio
- Variable inflammatory cell component
- Degenerative and regenerative changes in epithelial cells
- Extreme reactive changes may simulate malignancy

Parasitic infestation

- Parasitic ova
- Inflammatory and necrotic debris
- Worms, fragmented or entire
- Epithelial hyperplasia, metaplasia
- Late risk of cholangiocarcinoma

Sclerosing cholangitis and stent placement (Fig. 10.57B)

A range of regenerative and degenerative alterations in bile duct epithelium include:

- Squamous metaplasia
- Nuclear enlargement
- Nuclear size variation
- Prominent nucleoli
- Cellular disorganisation

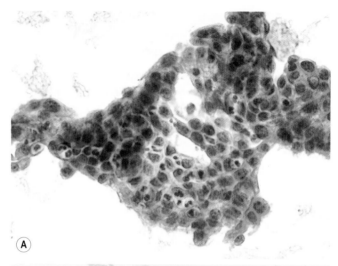

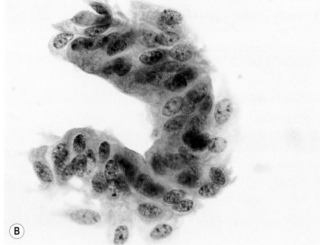

Fig. 10.57 (A) Biliary brushings. Inflammatory exudate and biliary epithelium showing mild cytological and architectural atypia. (B) Primary sclerosing cholangitis, nuclear enlargement, nuclear size variation, prominent nucleoli and cellular disorganisation.

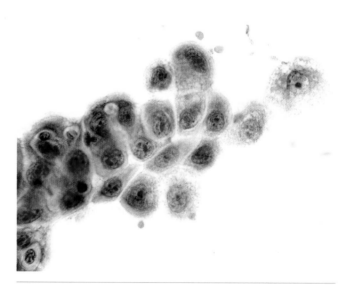

Fig. 10.58 Biliary duct epithelium showing reactive changes. Note polymorphs within the epithelium. Prominent nucleoli but regularly spaced cells and normal nuclear to cytoplasmic ratio.

Biliary Intraepithelial Neoplasia (BilIN) (previously dysplasia)

Premalignant changes are now recognised in the gall bladder and extrahepatic bile ducts (see p. 326, Box 10.1).

- Biliary dysplasia or atypical biliary epithelium) have been replaced by the following nomenclature:
  - three-grade classification system (BilIN-1, BilIN-2 and BilIN-3) based on the degree of atypia

Since biopsy of small mucosal lesions may be technically difficult, brushings are often the only way to diagnose premalignant lesions.

The main cytological criteria for detection of premalignant and malignant conditions of bile ducts are the following:

- Nuclear overlapping and crowding
- Small but distinct nucleoli
- Moderate nuclear to cytoplasmic ratio

Cytological findings: low-grade BilIN (Fig. 10.59)

- Sheets and clusters with nuclear crowding and overlapping
- Smooth nuclear outline, moderate nuclear to cytoplasmic ratio
- Granular chromatin with mild clumping
- 1–2 small distinct nucleoli

Cytological findings: high-grade BilIN (Figs 10.60, 10.61)

- Clusters and groups with prominent nuclear crowding and overlapping
- Irregular nuclear membranes, high nuclear to cytoplasmic ratio
- Coarse chromatin
- Distinct prominent nucleoli

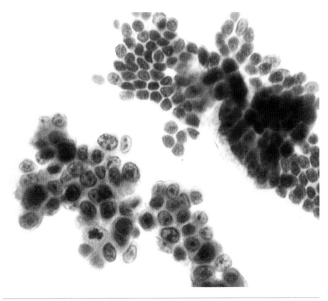

Fig. 10.59 Low-grade BilIN. The lower sheet of epithelium shows features of low-grade dysplasia. Differential diagnosis includes reactive conditions.

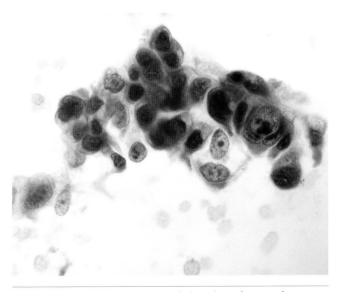

Fig. 10.60 Bile duct brushings. The epithelium shows features of high-grade BilIN. Features are suspicious for malignancy.

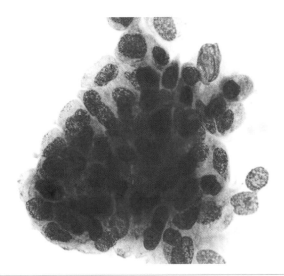

Fig. 10.61 High-grade BilIN. Epithelium shows crowding and overlapping.

Biliary papillomatosis/intraductal papillary tumour

Cytological findings: intraductal papillary tumour (Fig. 10.62)

- Hypercellular smear
- Very broad and often double-cell layered sheets of ductal epithelium
- Papillary configuration
- Preserved honeycomb pattern with even nuclear spacing
- Some nuclear overlapping but no frankly malignant nuclear features

Cholangiocarcinoma

Cytological findings: cholangiocarcinoma in biliary brush samples (Figs 10.63, 10.64 and Figs 10.44–10.47, p 323)

- Clusters of cells, disorganised sheets, loose aggregates, small acinar groups and single pleomorphic cells
- Marked overlapping and crowding
- Nuclear enlargement, moulding and irregular nuclear outlines
- Prominent nucleoli
- High nuclear to cytoplasmic ratio
- Coarse chromatin
- Background of necrotic debris

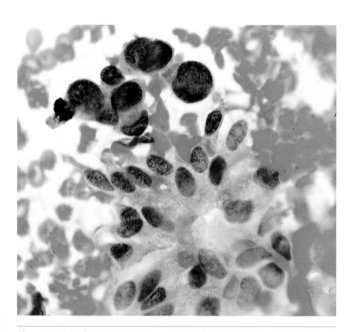

Fig. 10.63 Cholangiocarcinoma. A contrast between the benign (*bottom layer*) and malignant (*top layer*) bile duct epithelium. Malignant cells are arranged in clusters, and have coarse chromatin, and high nuclear to cytoplasmic ratio.

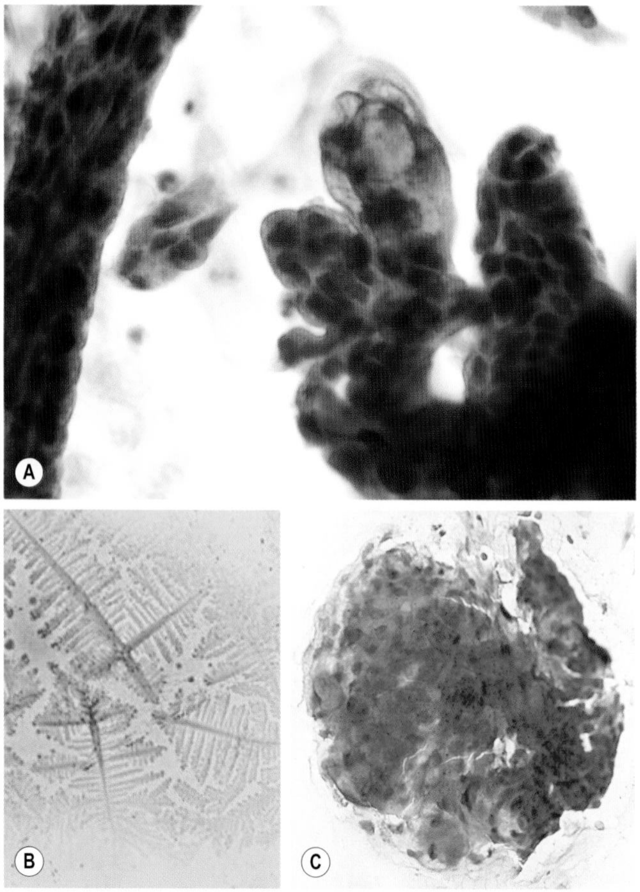

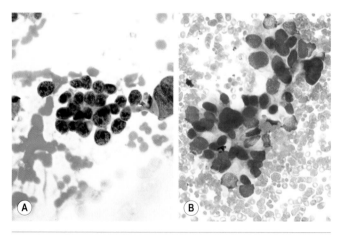

Fig. 10.62 (A) Intraductal papillary mucinous tumour showing dysplastic but not frankly malignant nuclear features. (B, C) Ferning effect of mucus, PASd positivity in the cytoplasm.

Fig. 10.64 Cholangiocarcinoma. Malignant epithelial cells showing marked nuclear pleomorphism, irregularity of nuclear outlines and prominent nucleoli.

Special tumour types

Adenosquamous and squamous cell carcinoma (Fig. 10.65)

Villous adenoma and well-differentiated papillary carcinoma

Cytological findings: villous adenoma

- Numerous clusters of hypercrowded columnar cells
- Irregular feathered edges
- Coarser chromatin than the surrounding normal bile duct epithelium

Sensitivity of biliary brushings for diagnosis of malignancy ranges from 35–47%. This area of diagnosis, perhaps more than any other, requires concentration of experience for optimal results.

Cystadenoma and cystadenocarcinoma

Cystic mucinous neoplasms of extrahepatic bile duct origin are morphologically identical to those described in the pancreas and intrahepatic ducts. (see Figs 10.113–10.116, p 349)

Cytological and clinical findings: cystadenoma and cystadenocarcinoma

- Biliary cystadenoma
  - Tends to occur in women
  - Has a well-known tendency for malignant transformation
  - Columnar or cuboidal mucin-secreting epithelium
  - Mostly uniform
- Mucinous cystadenocarcinoma (Fig. 10.66)
  - Cells differ in size
  - Nuclei show a coarse chromatin pattern
  - Haphazard arrangement

Differential diagnosis: biliary brushings

- Benign versus well-differentiated carcinoma
- Sclerosing cholangitis
- Dysplasia
- Carcinoma in situ
- Special tumour types, e.g. mucinous cystadenocarcinoma
- Papillary adenocarcinoma versus adenoma of the ampulla

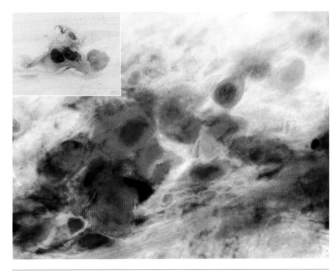

Fig. 10.65 Keratinous debris and malignant cells from an adenosquamous carcinoma of the bile duct. Inset: keratinised malignant cells.

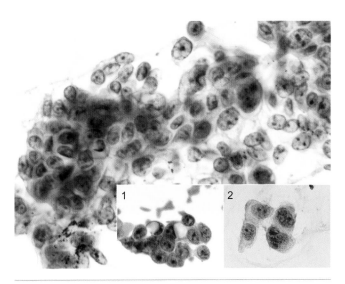

Fig. 10.66 Mucinous adenocarcinoma. Markedly enlarged nuclei of malignant cells, with dense cytoplasm showing focal mucin vacuolation (inset 1). Poorly differentiated bile duct adenocarcinoma has large pleomorphic cells (inset 2).

Pancreas

- Unlike other abdominal organs such as the liver and kidney, a Tru-Cut® needle biopsy (TNB) of the pancreas is associated with a significant risk of complications
- EUS, transgastric or transduodenal FNA of pancreatic masses (Fig. 10.70) has provided an alternative procedure for acquiring tissue to confirm the presence of pancreatic cancer and, in many centres, has entirely replaced CT-guided biopsies

Sensitivity of pancreas EUS-FNA is variable, averaging 80% but ranging from 60% to 100%. Sensitivity of the procedure can increase over time, reflecting increasing experience with this technique.

Normal cytology: pancreas

Cytological findings (Figs 10.67–10.69)

Acinar epithelium

- Polygonal cells with ample cytoplasm which is dense and blue-green with the standard Papanicolaou stain, and purple and more obviously granular with a Wright–Giemsa stain
- Arranged in tight, grape-like clusters or balls
- Often attached to tissue fragments with ill-defined fibrovascular stroma
- Individual acinar units, single cells and bare nuclei
- Nuclei are round with finely stippled chromatin
- Small and eccentric nucleoli are often easily identified

Ductal epithelium

- Ductal cells tend to be sparse in FNA smears from normal pancreas
- More noticeable in the presence of duct obstruction secondary to tumour or chronic pancreatitis
- Cuboidal to columnar cells
- Larger than acinar cells
- Often arranged as monolayer sheets or strips of cells with a luminal edge of non-mucinous cytoplasm
- Honeycomb appearance
- Uniform, geometric distribution of round, regular nuclei without crowding
- Well-defined cell borders
- Nuclei display evenly distributed finely granular chromatin
- Inconspicuous nucleoli, may become enlarged and prominent when reactive
- Cytoplasm varies in amount from scanty to moderate
- Dense and non-mucinous to the eye

Islet cells

- Not usually recognised on FNA with routine stains
- Require special stains to highlight the neurosecretory granules for identification

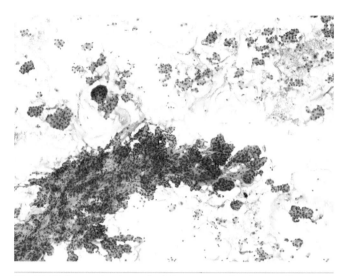

Fig. 10.67 Pancreatic acinar cells. Cohesive grape-like clusters of benign acinar cells are attached to a fibrovascular stroma and dispersed in the background.

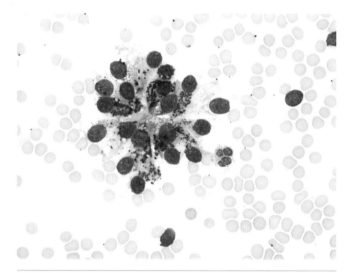

Fig. 10.68 Pancreatic acinar cell in acinar arrangement of polygonal cells with eccentric small round uniform nuclei, small nucleoli and abundant granular cytoplasm.

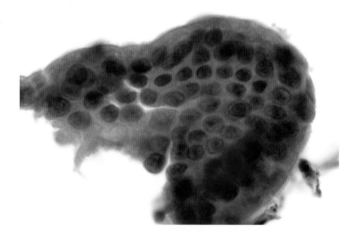

Fig. 10.69 Pancreatic ductal cells. Ductal cells most often appear as flat monolayered sheets of non-mucinous glandular cells with evenly distributed round uniform nuclei.

Differential diagnosis: Normal pancreatic epithelium

- Cellular aspirates in which acinar cells present a solid cellular smear pattern of monomorphic cells can be mistaken for a neoplasm
- Bare nuclei of acinar cells may be mistaken for lymphoid cells (nucleoli in acinar cells helpful)

Cytological findings: gastrointestinal cells in EUS-FNA of the pancreas (Figs 10.71–10.73 and Fig. 10.112 p. 348)

Duodenum

- Flat and cohesive monolayered sheet with a honeycomb pattern; occasionally papillary groups (intact villi, smaller groups and single cells)
- Sporadically placed goblet cells
- Non-mucinous glandular cells with brush border
- Lymphocytes ('sesame seeds') in the epithelium (variable)

Stomach

- Small sheets, strips and occasionally single cells and gastric pits
- Apical mucin cups in foveolar cells

Differential diagnosis: GI cells in FNA of the pancreas

- Pancreatic ductal cells leading to adequate interpretation of an inadequate sample
- Well-differentiated adenocarcinoma
- Mucinous cysts

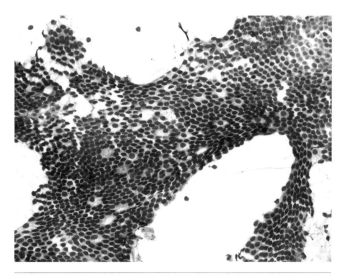

Fig. 10.71 Duodenal epithelium. Flat monolayered sheets of non-mucinous epithelium studded with goblet cells distinguish duodenal epithelium from pancreatic ductal cells or cyst lining epithelium.

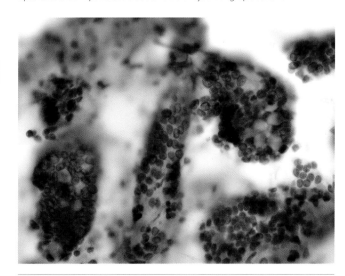

Fig. 10.72 Duodenal epithelium. Duodenal villi may be misinterpreted as carcinoma or papillae of IPMN. (see p. 347, Figs 10.105–10.107). Appreciation of goblet cells and intraepithelial lymphocytes will help identify the cells as duodenal in origin.

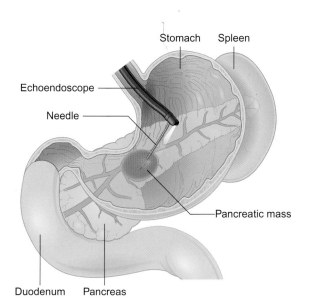

Fig. 10.70† The FNA needle is guided by the echoendoscope. Aspirates of masses in the pancreatic head are performed through the duodenum, and those in the body and tail of the gland via the stomach (see 'Cytological findings: gastrointestinal cells', Figs 10.71–10.73).

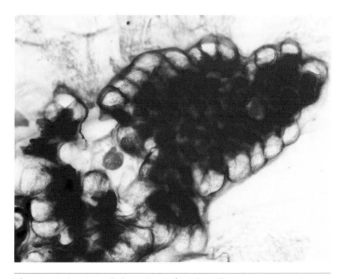

Fig. 10.73 Gastric epithelium. Gastric foveolar cells may appear mucinous and often demonstrate mucin in the upper third of the cytoplasmic compartment, forming an apical cup of mucin.

Pancreatitis

- The most important disease to be distinguished from chronic pancreatitis is pancreatic adenocarcinoma, which it can mimic clinically, on imaging, intraoperatively and on FNA
- Key cytological features to help distinguish benign reactive ducts from well-differentiated adenocarcinoma are:
  - cell group architecture, e.g. the arrangement of the cells within the groups
  - nuclear features

Acute pancreatitis

- Sudden onset, which may follow episodes of alcohol abuse, trauma or obstruction of the pancreatic duct by stones or tumour
- A relative contraindication for FNA as there is a slight risk of exacerbation of the pancreatitis

Cytological findings (Fig. 10.74)

- Acute inflammatory cells predominate
- Cellular debris
- Macrophages and fat necrosis
- Degenerated epithelial cells
- Granulation tissue including capillaries and reactive fibroblasts are seen in the healing phase

Chronic pancreatitis

- Result of repeated bouts of acute pancreatitis that lead to destruction of the acinar component
- Irreversible scarring of the parenchyma
- Causes: alcohol abuse, duct obstruction

Cytological findings (Figs 10.75–10.77)

- Scant cellularity
- Fragments of tissue composed of collagen and fibroblasts
- Scant chronic inflammatory cell component in the fibrotic tissue fragments
- Admixture with other pancreatic cells including acinar epithelium
- Ductal groups may be predominant cells on the smears
- Uniform distribution of cells in the group
- Minimal anisonucleosis
- Relatively even chromatin without parachromatin clearing
- Non-mucinous cytoplasm mostly
- Variable nuclear atypia

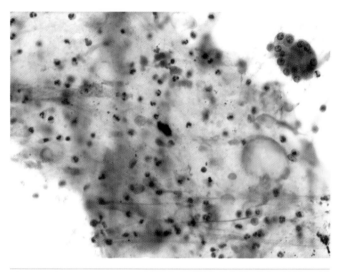

Fig. 10.74[†] Acute pancreatitis. Inflammatory debris, fat necrosis and benign pancreatic tissue support this interpretation. Note the single group of acinar cells (*upper right*).

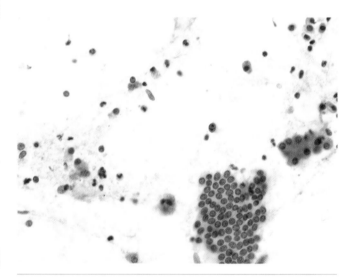

Fig. 10.75[†] Chronic pancreatitis. Mixed acinar and ductal cells with few inflammatory cells and histiocytes in the background.

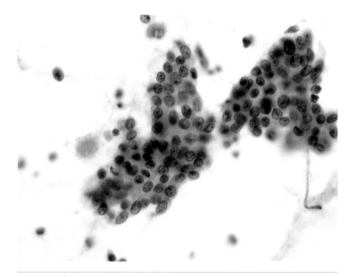

Fig. 10.76[†] Ductal cells with reactive atypia illustrated by slightly irregular nuclei, uneven spacing and nucleoli.

Autoimmune pancreatitis (AIP)

AIP is a sclerosing inflammatory, pancreatocentric autoimmune disease of the pancreas that frequently presents as a mass-forming lesion.

- Mimics pancreatic adenocarcinoma both clinically and radiologically
- Steroid-responsive disease
- Pancreatectomy is rarely justified
- Histology: periductal collar of lymphoplasmacytic inflammation, diffuse interlobular and/or lobular chronic inflammation, dense fibrosis and obliterative phlebitis (lymphoplasmacytic sclerosing pancreatitis)

Cytological findings: AIP (Figs 10.78, 10.79)

- Cytological features sufficient to diagnose the condition on FNA are present in less than one-third of cases
- FNA only occasionally provides a diagnosis of AIP
- Key cytological features:
    - presence of cellular stromal fragments
    - the cellularity due predominantly to embedded lymphocytes and plasma cells

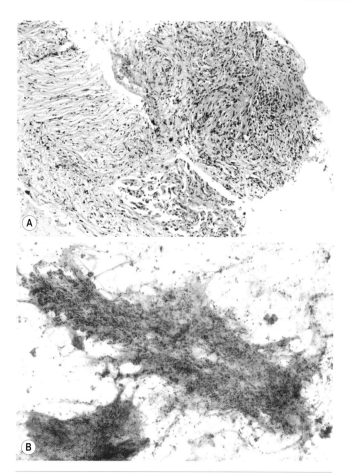

Fig. 10.78 Autoimmune pancreatitis. (A) Core biopsy or tissue fragments in cell block are very helpful in recognising the cellular stroma with embedded lymphocytes and plasma cells characteristic of this disease (H & E). (B) A clue to the diagnosis on FNA smears is recognising the characteristic cellular stroma with embedded lymphocytes and plasma cells. (From Hruban RH, Pitman MB, Klimstra DS. Tumors of the Pancreas. Atlas of Tumor Pathology, 4th series, fascicle 6. Washington, DC: American Registry of Pathology; Armed Forces Institutes of Pathology; 2007.)

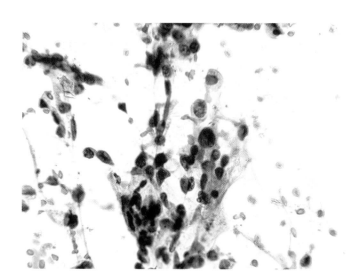

Fig. 10.77 Glandular cells with marked atypia in chronic pancreatitis is a pitfall for false-positive diagnosis. Ductal cells with atypia in the setting of chronic pancreatitis should be interpreted with caution.

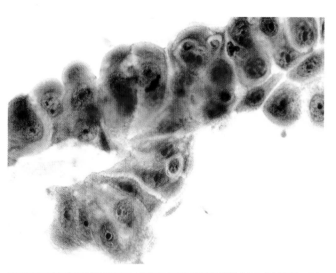

Fig. 10.79 Reactive changes may mimic malignancy. Note prominent nucleoli. Nuclear to cytoplasmic ratio and architecture are preserved. Inflammatory cells seen within the epithelium.

Ductal adenocarcinoma

- The vast majority (90%) of solid malignancies in the pancreas represent ductal adenocarcinoma or one its variants (See Box 10.2)
- Other solid malignancies of the pancreas encountered less commonly include:
  - pancreatic endocrine tumours
  - acinar cell carcinoma
  - pancreatoblastoma
  - metastatic neoplasms

Cytological findings (Figs 10.80–10.86 and Table 10.2, p. 343)

Well-differentiated ductal adenocarcinoma

- Nuclear contour irregularities
- Nuclear variation (>4 : 1) within a single group of cells
- Chromatin clearing and/or clumping
- 'Washed-out' nuclear chromatin (parachromatin clearing)
- Monolayer sheets with nuclear overlapping
- 'Drunken honeycomb' appearance
- Mitosis, necrosis and discohesion with single cells are useful but rarely present

Poorly-differentiated ductal adenocarcinoma

- Three-dimensional groups with nuclear crowding and overlap
- Easily identified intact malignant single cells
- Obvious nuclear membrane irregularities, hyperchromasia and coarse chromatin
- Mitosis and necrosis

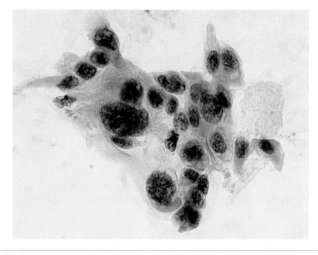

Fig. 10.80 Poorly differentiated ductal adenocarcinoma shows gross anisonucleosis, chromatin clearing and clumping and nuclear overlapping.

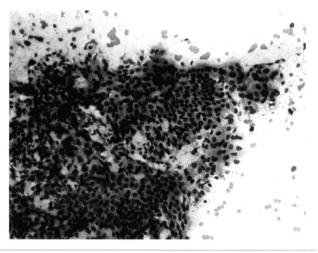

Fig. 10.81[†] Well-differentiated adenocarcinoma. Cohesive sheet of irregularly spaced nuclei in a 'drunken honeycomb' pattern.

Box 10.2   Histological classification of tumours of the pancreas

I. Epithelial neoplasms
  A. Exocrine neoplasms
   1. Serous cystic neoplasms
   2. Mucinous cystic neoplasms
     a. Mucinous cystadenoma
     b. Mucinous cystadenoma with moderate dysplasia
     c. Mucinous cystic neoplasm with carcinoma in situ
     d. Mucinous cystadenocarcinoma
   3. Intraductal papillary mucinous neoplasms (IPMN)
     e. IPMN-adenoma
     f. IPMN with moderate dysplasia
     g. IPMN with carcinoma in situ
     h. IPMN with an associated invasive carcinoma
     i. Intraductal oncocytic papillary neoplasm
   4. Invasive ductal adenocarcinoma and variants
   5. Acinar cell neoplasms
  B. Endocrine neoplasms
   1. Adenoma (0.5 cm)
   2. Well-differentiated pancreatic endocrine neoplasm of uncertain malignant potential

   3. Malignant well-differentiated pancreatic endocrine neoplasm
   4. Small cell carcinoma
  C. Epithelial neoplasms (of uncertain differentiation)
   1. Solid pseudopapillary neoplasm
   2. Pancreatoblastoma
  D. Miscellaneous
   1. Teratoma
   2. Lymphoepithelial cyst
II. Non-epithelial neoplasms
  A. Haemangioma
  B. Lymphangioma
  C. Leiomyosarcoma
  D. Malignant fibrous histiocytoma
  E. Lymphoma
  F. Paraganglioma
  G. Other
III. Secondary neoplasms (metastases to the pancreas)

(Modified from Hruban RH, Pitman MB, Klimstra DS. Tumors of the Pancreas. Atlas of Tumor Pathology, 4th Series, Fascicle 6. Washington, DC: American Registry of Pathology; Armed Forces Institutes of Pathology; 2007.)

Diagnostic pitfall

The underdiagnosis of well-differentiated adenocarcinoma as reactive epithelial changes is probably the greatest contributing factor for the relatively low sensitivity of FNA.

Further investigations: ductal adenocarcinoma

*   Oncogenes: K-ras mutations detected in more than 90% of pancreatic adenocarcinomas
*   Tumour suppressor genes: inactivation of p53, SMAD4 and p16
*   Mucin markers: over-expression of MUC1 and MUC4
*   Gene expression profiling studies: mesothelin, S100P and prostate stem cell antigen overexpression

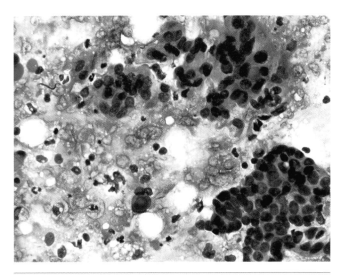

Fig. 10.84† Poorly differentiated adenocarcinoma. Epithelial cells with overtly malignant features including cellular clusters, large cells with high nuclear to cytoplasmic ratio, large irregular nuclei, single malignant cells and necrosis.

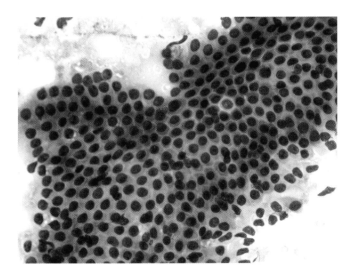

Fig. 10.82† Benign glandular epithelium. GI contamination and benign ductal cells appear as flat monolayered sheets of evenly spaced non-mucinous epithelium in contrast to the 'drunken honeycomb' pattern of adenocarcinoma illustrated in Fig. 10.81.

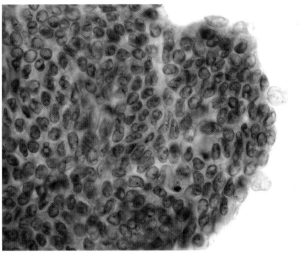

Fig. 10.85† Well-differentiated adenocarcinoma. Nuclear crowding and overlap, anisonucleosis of 4:1 in the same group and irregular nuclear membranes supports a malignant interpretation.

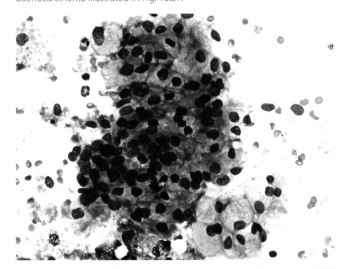

Fig. 10.83† Foamy gland pattern of adenocarcinoma. These deceptively malignant glandular cells demonstrate bland round nuclei but abnormally voluminous and visibly mucinous (foamy) cytoplasm.

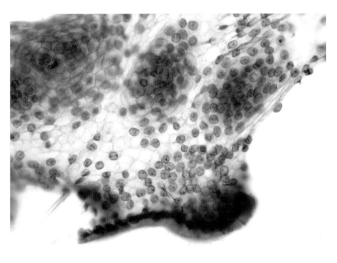

Fig. 10.86† Gastric epithelium. Uneven spacing can be seen due to normal gastric mucosal architecture. Note the islands of cells denoting gastric crypts.

Variants of pancreatic ductal adenocarcinoma

Undifferentiated carcinoma

Cytological findings: undifferentiated carcinoma (Fig. 10.87)

- Marked cellularity with prominent tumour diathesis
- Predominantly isolated and poorly cohesive cells with few cell clusters
- Bizarre pleomorphic single cells
- Scattered multinucleated giant cells with malignant nuclei
- Osteoclast-type giant cells are few
- Spindled cells
- Bizarre mitotic figures

- The identification of these variants is seldom of clinical relevance
- Clinically, these variants behave at least as aggressively as conventional tubular ductal adenocarcinoma
- Surgery remains the mainstay of treatment

Cytological findings: undifferentiated carcinoma with osteoclast-like giant cells (UCOGC) (Fig. 10.88)

- Dual cell population
- Spindle to polygonal epithelioid atypical mononuclear cells
- Bland multinucleated osteoclast-like giant cells
- Osteoid may be present

Differential diagnosis: undifferentiated carcinoma with osteoclast-like giant cells

- Undifferentiated (pleomorphic) carcinoma of the pancreas
- Other high-grade primary and metastatic malignant neoplasms with tumour giant cells
- Benign conditions with reactive stroma and giant cells

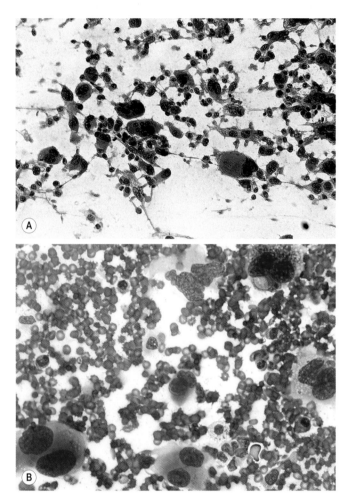

Fig. 10.87[†] Undifferentiated carcinoma. (A) This variant of adenocarcinoma is composed of large bizarre discohesive epithelioid to spindled giant malignant cells. A rare osteoclast-type giant cell may be noted (PAP). (B) The large bizarre malignant cells may be few and widely scattered.

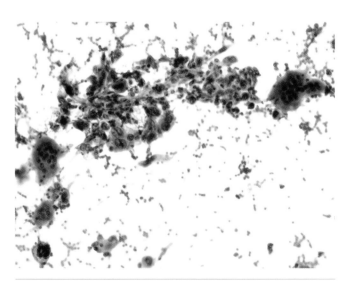

Fig. 10.88[†] Undifferentiated carcinoma with osteoclast-like giant cells. Malignant mononuclear cells are associated with usually readily apparent osteoclast-type giant cells.

Adenosquamous carcinoma and acinar cell carcinoma

Cytological findings: adenosquamous carcinoma (Fig. 10.89)

- Malignant glandular cells
- Malignant squamous cells; may not be keratinising

Cytological findings: acinar cell carcinoma (Fig. 10.90)

- Cellular smears, solid cellular smear pattern
- Loosely cohesive clusters and vague acini
- Single cells, including stripped naked nuclei
- Granular background of zymogen granules from stripped cytoplasm
- Monomorphic cells with round nuclei and prominent nucleoli
- Scant to moderate cytoplasm with granularity (best seen on air-dried smears)
- See Table 10.2 on p. 343

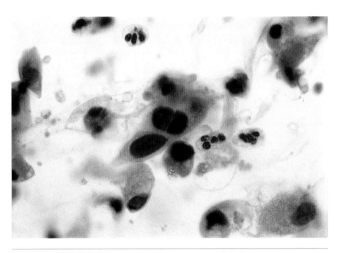

Fig. 10.89⁺ Adenosquamous carcinoma. Cluster of malignant squamous cells and neoplastic mucin-containing glandular cells.

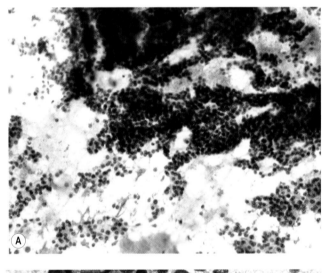

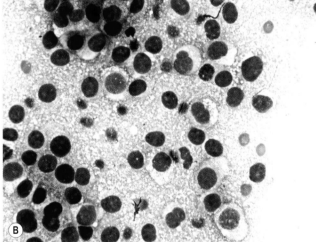

Fig. 10.90⁺ Acinar cell carcinoma. (A) Low-power smear pattern helps to distinguish malignant from benign acinar cells. Compare this cellular crowded sheet pattern to the organoid, grape-like pattern. (B) The characteristic granular cytoplasm of acinar cells may be dispersed in the background from stripped cells and is best noted on air-dried smears.

Solid pseudopapillary neoplasm of the pancreas (SPN)

- Occurs predominantly in adolescent girls and young women
- Radiologically, SPNs are well-circumscribed, generally large tumours often in the body and tail
- An indolent tumour of low-grade malignancy with metastases present in 10–15% of cases
- Long-term survival has been reported even in patients with metastases to the liver and peritoneum
- Complete resection of node-negative patients is considered curative
- See Table 10.2 on p. 343

Cytological findings (Figs 10.91, 10.92)

- Solid cellular smear pattern
- Papillary clusters with slender central fibrovascular cores with myxoid or collagenous stroma and loosely cohesive tumour cells
- Balls or globules of myxoid (metachromatic with Wright–Giemsa stain) stroma with or without a surrounding thick layer of neoplastic cells
- Monomorphically round to oval nuclei with nuclear grooves and indentations
- Finely granular chromatin and small to no nucleoli
- Cytoplasm is scanty and may contain perinuclear vacuoles and hyaline globules
- Foamy macrophages and necrosis (evidence of cystic change)

Differential diagnosis

- Pancreatic endocrine neoplasm (PEN)
- Acinar cell carcinoma
- Pancreatoblastoma

Further investigations

- SPNs are variably positive with cytokeratin and show nuclear reactivity with beta-catenin
- E-cadherin negative (while PENs show a membranous pattern of reactivity with both beta-catenin and E-cadherin)
- In conjunction with a chromogranin stain, this pattern of immunoreactivity can distinguish SPN from PEN

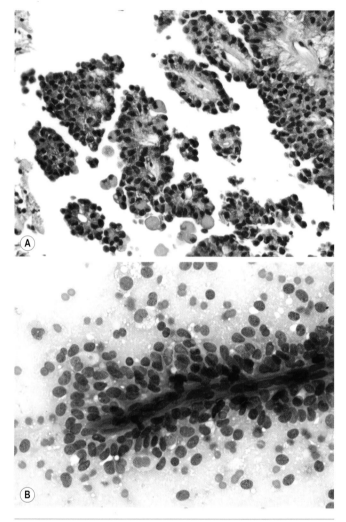

Fig. 10.91[†] Solid pseudopapillary neoplasm. (A) Papillary fragments with myxoid stromal cores are characteristic of this tumour (H & E). (B) Papillary fragments in an otherwise solid cellular smear pattern of monomorphic cells distinguishes SPN from its mimickers.

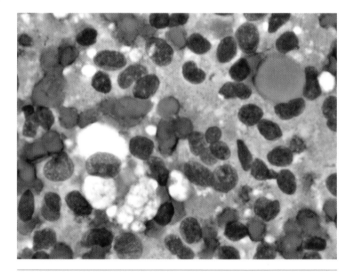

Fig. 10.92[†] Solid pseudopapillary neoplasm. Characteristic features of individual tumour cells include bland round to oval nuclei with nuclear grooves and indentations and occasional cytoplasmic perinuclear vacuoles and hyaline globules.

Pancreatic endocrine neoplasm (PEN)

- PENs are well-differentiated low-grade neoplasms of the endocrine cells with malignant potential
- The WHO recognises a three-tier classification (see Table 10.2, p. 343): well-differentiated endocrine neoplasms, well-differentiated endocrine carcinoma, and poorly differentiated endocrine carcinoma
- The most reliable feature of malignant behaviour in PENs is metastasis to regional lymph nodes or liver
- FNA samples are interpreted as 'pancreatic endocrine neoplasms' rather than carcinoma in most cases

Cytological findings: well-differentiated PEN (Fig. 10.93–10.98)

- Cellular smears, solid cellular smear pattern
- Predominantly single cells, some with stripped nuclei
- Loose, or more rarely, tightly cohesive clusters
- Blood vessels
- Rosette-like structures
- Monomorphic plasmacytoid population of small to medium-sized cells with occasional larger cells
- Round nuclei with finely stippled chromatin and smooth nuclear membranes, some binucleation
- Nucleoli small and inconspicuous, occasionally prominent
- Scant to moderate amounts of delicate cytoplasm (rarely vacuolated or oncocytic)
- Metachromatic cytoplasmic granules (on air-dried material)
- Mitoses, marked nuclear pleomorphism and necrosis absent or rare

Differential diagnosis: PEN

- Cystic degeneration
- Acinar cell carcinoma
- Solid pseudopapillary tumour
- Benign acinar cells
- Metastatic renal cell carcinoma

While in the past the majority of PENs were functional, non-functional tumours predominate today, and smaller, non-functioning neoplasms are increasingly incidental findings.

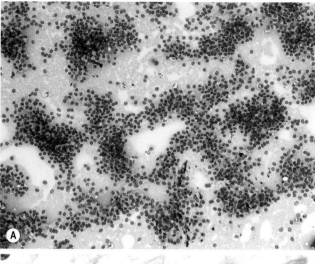

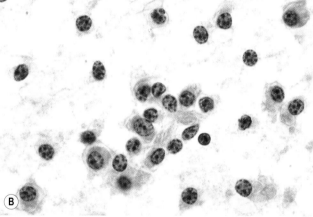

Fig. 10.93 Pancreatic endocrine neoplasm. (A) Monomorphic epithelial cells in a discohesive single cell smear pattern shared by the solid cellular neoplasms of the pancreas. (B) Monomorphic epithelial cells in loose clusters and singly. Cytoplasmic granules may be seen.

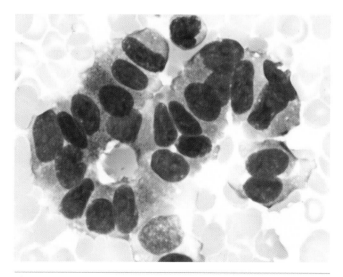

Fig. 10.94 Pancreatic endocrine neoplasm. Cells may be dispersed or arranged in small cords and acini. Note cytoplasmic granules.

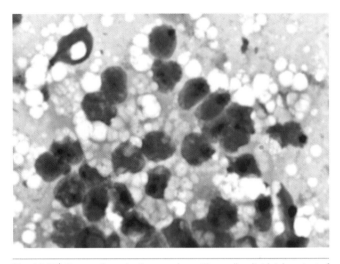

Fig. 10.95† Pancreatic endocrine neoplasm. Clear cell or lipid-rich variant of PEN must be distinguished from metastatic renal cell carcinoma

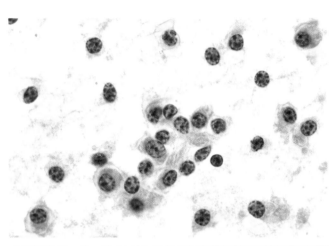

Fig. 10.97† Pancreatic endocrine tumour. A predominantly dispersed pattern of plasmacytoid tumour cells with eccentric nuclei, minor variation in nuclear size, stippled nuclear chromatin and dense and granular cytoplasm is typical.

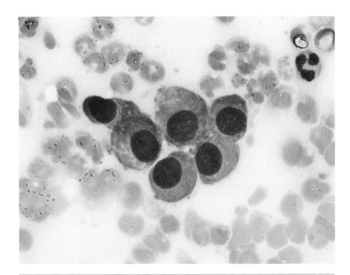

Fig. 10.96 Pancreatic endocrine neoplasm. Smears may be heavily bloodstained and relatively few dispersed cells resembling plasma cells should alert the observer to the possibility of PEN. Immunocytochemistry is helpful (see Fig. 10.97).

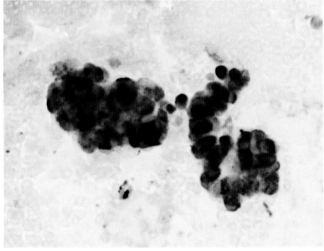

Fig. 10.98 Synaprophysin positivity in tumour cells confirms the diagnosis.

Poorly differentiated PEN (small cell carcinoma) (Fig. 10.99)

- Extremely rare and is readily distinguishable from well-differentiated endocrine neoplasm/carcinoma
- The histological features are indistinguishable from small cell carcinomas of the lung
- The cytological features are identical to small cell carcinomas of the lung (nuclear moulding, finely granular chromatin, inconspicuous nucleoli and scant cytoplasm)
- The differential diagnosis includes metastatic small cell carcinomas, especially from the lung

It is important to distinguish these poorly differentiated endocrine carcinomas from well-differentiated endocrine tumours as the survival in affected individuals is measured in months, unlike patients with even metastatic well-differentiated PENs, whose prognosis is considerably better.

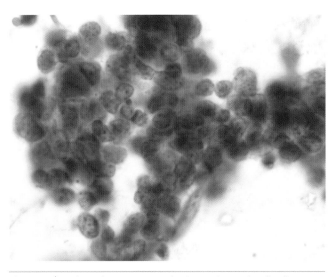

Fig. 10.99[†] High-grade pancreatic endocrine carcinoma (small cell carcinoma). Markedly irregular hyperchromatic cells with nuclear moulding are noted in this high-grade neuroendocrine carcinoma.

Table 10.2 Solid cellular neoplasms of the pancreas

	Pancreatic endocrine neoplasm	Acinar cell carcinoma	Solid pseudopapillary neoplasm	Pancreatoblastoma
Clinical features	40–60 years old M = F; 50% functional	Adults in their 60s >> children; M:F = 4:1; lipase hypersecretion syndrome in some	20–30 years old F >>> M	2–3 years old >> 40 years old M = F; 50% Asian
CT/EUS features	Round, generally small (1–2 cm) well-defined and circumscribed solid, occasionally cystic masses	Well-defined and circumscribed, often lobulated homogeneous solid, occasionally cystic masses, avg. 10 cm	Well-defined and circumscribed solid and cystic masses, avg. 10 cm; often in the tail	Well-defined and circumscribed masses, avg. 10 cm
Cytological features				
Smear background	Generally clean	Clean or granular from stripped cytoplasm	Clean or filled with haemorrhagic debris, foamy histiocytes and giant cells	Generally clean
Smear pattern	Dyscohesive, single cell pattern; few small clusters	Solid sheets and groups, acinar structures, single cells; loss of organoid grape-like clustering	Highly cellular with papillary fragments, loose clusters and single cells; fibrovascular cores with myxoid stroma	Cellular with clusters and single cells; stroma with vessels; recognising squamoid corpuscles requires cell block
Nuclei	Round to oval and eccentrically placed in the cell	Round and uniform with mild anisonucleosis	Uniform, oval with nuclear grooves and indentations	Tri-lineage epithelial differentiation with most cells demonstrating acinar features
Nuclear chromatin	Coarse, stippled, 'salt-and-pepper'	Coarse	Even and finely granular	Variable
Nucleoli	None or small but can be prominent	Usually prominent but may be absent	Absent to inconspicuous	Usually prominent
Mitoses	Variable but usually none or rare	None to rare	Absent	Variable
Cytoplasm	Dense to finely granular, rarely clear or oncocytic	Relatively abundant and granular	Scant to moderate with occasional perinuclear vacuole or hyaline globule	Generally granular
Immunohistochemical stains	Pan-keratin, chromogranin, synaptophysin, CD56, Leu7, NSE, variable hormonal markers	Trypsin, chymotrypsin, lipase and elastase, pan-keratin	Vimentin, alpha-1-antitrypsin, CD10, NSE, CD56; beta-catenin	Dependent on differentiation; squamoid corpuscles are usually not immunoreactive

(From Pitman MB, Deshpande V. Endoscopic ultrasound-guided fine needle aspiration cytology of the pancreas: a morphological and multimodal approach to the diagnosis of solid and cystic mass lesions. Cytopathology 2007; 18:331–347.)

Pancreatic cysts

Cysts of the pancreas constitute a broad spectrum of entities from benign to pre-malignant to malignant (see Table 10.3).

Although cyst cytology alone is often non-diagnostic, when evaluated in the context of the clinical history, radiological features, gross cyst fluid observations and ancillary tests (see Table 10.4), accuracy can be greatly improved. An educated and experienced cytopathologist is critical for accurate interpretation.

The purpose of preoperative investigations of a cystic lesion that will affect patient management is primarily to distinguish between:

- mucinous neoplasms
- pseudocysts
- serous cystadenomas

Table 10.3 Pancreatic cystic mass lesions

	Pseudocyst	Serous cystadenoma	Mucinous cystic neoplasm	Intraductal papillary mucinous neoplasm
Clinical features	Associated with pancreatitis and trauma; most pancreatitis related to alcohol	65 years old F > M	40–50 years old female	65 years old M > F
CT/EUS features	Most are single, unilocular, thin-walled cysts without septations	Large, mostly microcystic; some with central stellate scar with starburst calcifications; some with few and large cysts	Thick-walled, often calcified solitary, multiloculated, well-circumscribed cysts in the body or tail; no communication with the pancreatic duct	Main duct, branch duct and combined types. Cysts are single or multiple and connect to the main pancreatic duct; 70% in the head; thick wall, multiple septations and mural nodule correlate with high grade
Cytological features				
Smear background	Amorphous cyst debris	Clean to bloody	Variably thick mucin; mucin may be thin and clear	Variably thick mucin; mucin may be thin and clear
Smear pattern	Variably cellular without epithelial cell component	Hypocellular; frequently acellular	Acellular to hypocellular in low-grade neoplasms bland mucinous cells; variably atypical glandular cells in higher grade neoplasms	Acellular to hypocellular in low-grade neoplasms bland mucinous cells; variably atypical glandular cells in higher grade neoplasms; may see papillary structures
Nuclei	NA	Round and regular; bland	Bland to variably atypical	Bland to variably atypical
Nuclear chromatin	NA	Smooth and even	Variable	Variable
Nucleoli	NA	None	Absent to conspicuous	Absent to conspicuous
Mitoses	None	None	Generally absent	Generally absent
Cytoplasm	Histiocytes may have dense cytoplasm and mimic epithelial cells	Scant but visible and finely vacuolated	Mucinous, more obvious in low-grade neoplasms	Mucinous, more obvious in low-grade neoplasms
Cyst fluid analysis	High amylase in thousands U/L; low CEA > 200 ng/mL	Low amylase and low CEA, 200 ng/mL	Variable amylase, typically low; CEA usually 200 ng/mL	Amylase generally high; CEA usually 200 ng/mL

(From Pitman MB, Deshpande V. Endoscopic ultrasound-guided fine needle aspiration cytology of the pancreas: a morphological and multimodal approach to the diagnosis of solid and cystic mass lesions. Cytopathology 2007; 18:331–347).

Table 10.4 Biochemical cyst fluid parameters

	Pseudocyst	Serous cystadenoma	Mucinous Cystic Tumour	Mucinous cystadenoma
Ca 125	Low	Variable	Variable	Variable
CEA	Low	Low	High	High
CA 15-3	Low	Low	Low	High
CA 72-4	Low	Low	Low	High
CA 19-9	Low	Low	High	High
Amylase	High	Low	Variable	Variable

Non-neoplastic cysts of the pancreas

Pseudocyst

A pancreatic pseudocyst has no epithelial lining. It contains collections of pancreatic secretions, necrotic debris and blood following from damage to the pancreatic parenchyma secondary to the release and activation of pancreatic enzymes.

Cytological findings (Fig. 10.100)

- Histiocytes and neutrophils are invariably seen
- Background of granular and proteinaceous debris
- Scattered foamy and/or haemosiderin-laden macrophages
- Flecks of calcification
- Necrotic fat cells
- Inflammatory cells
- Absence of epithelial cells

Differential diagnosis

- Gastrointestinal contamination, epithelium and/or mucin
- Mistaking epithelioid histiocytes for serous or mucinous epithelial cells
- Mucoid fibrinous debris from complicated pseudocyst misinterpreted as mucin of a mucinous cyst

Lymphoepithelial cyst

Lymphoepithelial cyst is a rare benign squamous-lined cyst with subepithelial non-neoplastic lymphoid tissue.

Cytological findings (Figs 10.101, 10.102)

- Anucleate squames and abundant keratinous debris
- Mature superficial squamous cells
- Lymphocytes are usually present but amount is variable and may be quite scant
- Cholesterol clefts

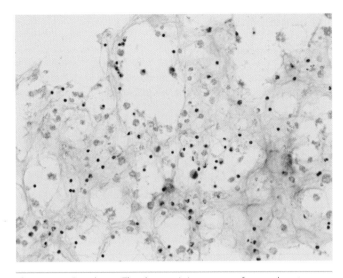

Fig. 10.100 Pseudocyst. The characteristic contents of a pseudocyst include proteinaceous debris and a variable number of inflammatory cells, which may be dominated by epithelioid histiocytes that must be distinguished from epithelial cells.

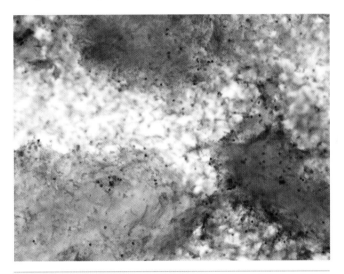

Fig. 10.101[†] Lymphoepithelial cyst. A background of anucleated squamous cells and keratinous debris are typical of the contents of a lymphoepithelial cyst. Note the sprinkling of lymphocytes in the background.

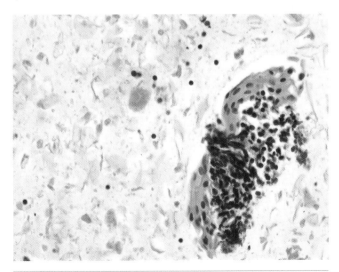

Fig. 10.102[†] Lymphoepithelial cyst. The presence of an intact cyst wall with squamous cell lining and subepithelial lymphoid tissue may occasionally be seen, as shown here in this cell block preparation.

Cystic neoplasms

Serous cystadenoma

Serous cystadenoma (microcystic or glycogen-rich cystadenoma) is a benign, typically microcystic, neoplasm that produces serous fluid.

Cytological findings (Fig. 10.103)

- Hypocellular
- Cuboidal non-mucinous epithelial cells
- Flat sheets with a honeycomb pattern, small flat clusters or single cells
- Bland, round or oval euchromatic nuclei without prominent nucleoli
- Clear, finely vacuolated cytoplasm
- Cytoplasmic glycogen demonstrated by PAS with and without diastase
- No intracellular or extracellular mucin
- Association with haemosiderin-laden macrophages in some cases

Differential diagnosis

- Acellular and hypocellular samples
- Epithelioid histiocytes
- Gastrointestinal contaminating epithelium

Intraductal papillary mucinous neoplasm (IPMN) (Figs 10.104–10.109)

IPMN is a slow-growing neoplasm with a good prognosis, which makes cytological diagnosis important for management (Fig. 10.104).

- Neoplasms of the pancreatic duct epithelium
- Intraductal papillary growth
- Thick mucin secretion
- Show varying degrees of dysplasia
  - range from adenoma to invasive carcinoma
  - dysplastic changes of borderline neoplasms and carcinoma in situ in between
- According to the site of involvement
  - main duct type
  - branch duct type
  - combined type

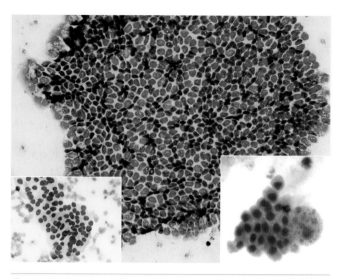

Fig. 10.103 Serous cystadenoma. The tumour cells are uniform cuboidal cells with bland central nuclei, smooth nuclear membranes and even chromatin. (*Inset left*) High-power view. (*Inset right*[1]) Non-mucinous cytoplasm and regularly spaced nuclei.

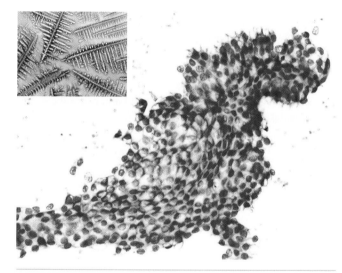

Fig. 10.104 Neoplastic mucinous cyst. Bland sheet of mucin secreting epithelium from an IPMN. (*Inset*) Thin mucin may define itself with a 'ferning' pattern, which distinguishes it from a proteinaceous background.

Cytological findings: intraductal papillary mucinous neoplasm with low-grade dysplasia (adenoma)

- Variable amounts of mucin, thin and thick
- Low cellularity
- Papillary fragments
- Mucinous glandular epithelium with mucin occupying more than one-third of the columnar cytoplasmic compartment
- Absence of nuclear atypia
- No background necrosis

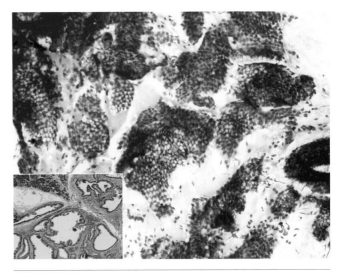

Fig. 10.107 IPMN. Papillary fragments and sheets of mucin-secreting epithelium. (*Inset*) Histology of IPMN.

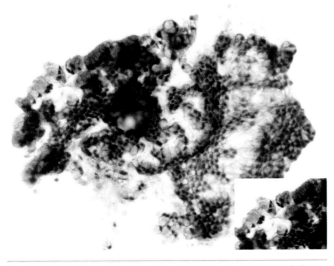

Fig. 10.105 IPMN – with low-grade dysplasia. Bland mucinous epithelium has round, regular nuclei, abundant mucinous cytoplasm and a low nuclear to cytoplasmic ratio (*inset*).

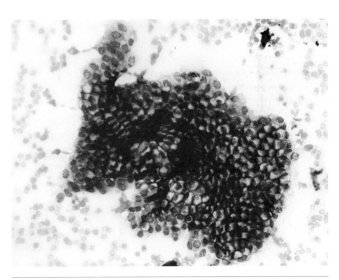

Fig. 10.108 IPMN. Absence of nuclear atypia makes differentiation from GI contaminants difficult.

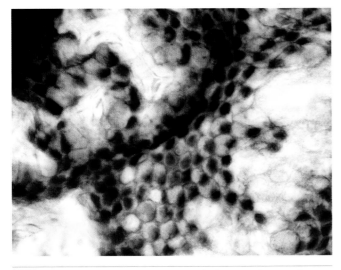

Fig. 10.106 IPMN – same case as Fig. 10.99, high-power view reveals mucinous secretion in every cell.

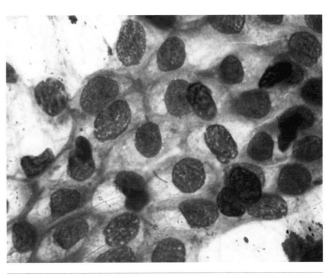

Fig. 10.109 IPMN. Mucinous glandular epithelium with mucin occupying more than one-third of the columnar cytoplasmic compartment

Cytological findings: intraductal papillary mucinous neoplasm with moderate dysplasia and higher (Figs 10.110–10.112)

In addition to the above findings for lesions with low-grade dysplasia:

- Increased cellularity relative to adenoma
- Recognisable cytological atypia with increased grade:
  - single intact cells
  - doublets
  - small cell clusters
  - cellular papillary groups
  - nuclear irregularity
  - increased nuclear: cytoplasmic ratio, decreased cytoplasmic mucin
  - irregular nuclear membranes
  - nucleoli
- Abundant background inflammation and necrosis support malignancy

CEA levels above 200 ng/mL are reported to distinguish non-mucinous from mucinous cysts, with very high levels of CEA correlating with malignancy.

Differential diagnosis: IPMN (Fig. 10.112)

- Scant and under-representative sample
- Thin or non-detectable mucin
- Obscuring inflammation, necrosis and debris
- GI contamination in EUS-guided aspirates
- Low CEA levels
- Peripancreatic cysts such as duplication cysts
- Secondarily cystic solid neoplasms

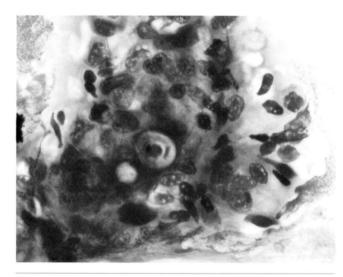

Fig. 10.111 IPMN with features of malignancy amounting to an adenocarcinoma. Architectural and cytological atypia contribute to the diagnosis.

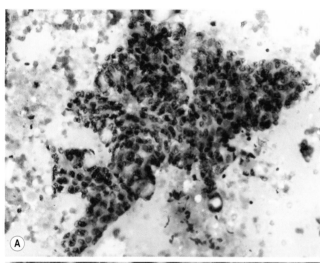

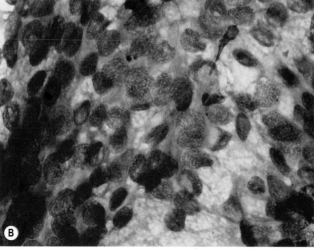

Fig. 10.110 IPMN with moderate to severe dysplasia. (A) Low-power view shows papillary clusters and disturbance of cell architecture. (B) High-power view shows overlapping and crowding, 'drunken' honeycomb pattern, but no frank evidence of malignancy.

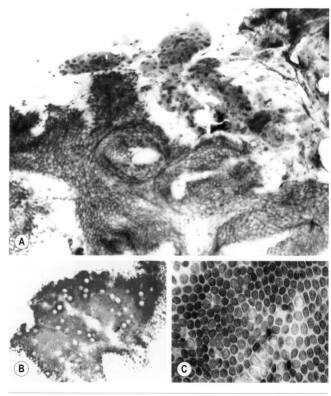

Fig. 10.112 (A) Stomach mucosa may present as sheets of bland mucin secreting epithelium (see also Fig. 10.73). (B) Intestinal contaminant has mucin-secreting goblet cells dispersed regularly resembling holes in the epithelium. (C) High-power view of duodenal epithelium shows no mucin secretion (compare with Fig. 10.109).

Mucinous cystic neoplasm (MCN) of the pancreas

MCN is a neoplastic mucin-producing cyst that, in almost all cases, occurs in females, does not communicate with the pancreatic ductal system, is lined by mucinous epithelial cells with varying degrees of atypia (Table 10.2, p. 343), and by definition contains subepithelial ovarian-type stroma.

Cytological findings (Figs 10.113–10.116)

- Thick, colloid-like mucin with or without mucinous epithelium
- Thin, watery mucin
- Often low cellularity due to typically low-grade neoplasms
- Mucinous epithelium with mucin filling cytoplasmic space (low-grade neoplasms)
- Variable nuclear atypia, background inflammation and necrosis

Differential diagnosis

- Thin or undetectable mucin
- GI contamination in EUS-guided aspirates
- Low CEA levels
- Peripancreatic cysts such as duplication cysts
- Secondary cystic solid neoplasms

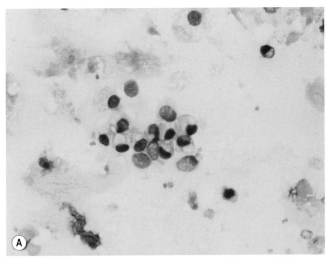

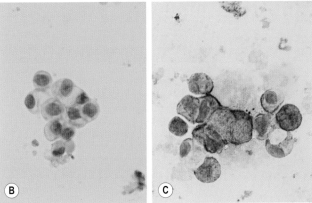

Fig. 10.113 Mucinous cystadenoma. (A) Low-grade epithelium displays small, round basal nuclei and cytoplasmic mucin that fills the cytoplasmic compartment. (B) PAP stain, same case. (C) BerEP4 epithelial marker positive. (D) Intracytoplasmic mucin positive (PAS-d).

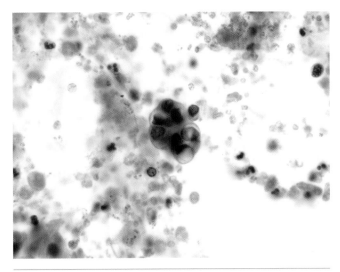

Fig. 10.114[†] Mucinous cystic neoplasm with invasive carcinoma (mucinous cystadenocarcinoma). Cluster of malignant cells with irregular nuclear membranes and residual mucin vacuoles in a background with coagulative necrosis supports the interpretation of malignancy.

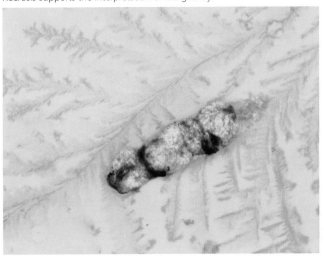

Fig. 10.115 Epithelial cells in a mucinous background. Nuclear detail often difficult to distinguish from macrophages; special stains and epithelial markers often helpful.

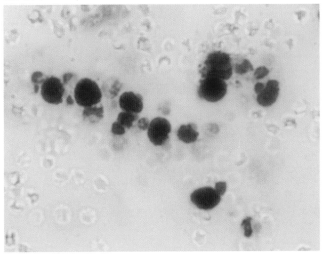

Fig. 10.116 MCN. Same case as in Fig. 10.114. Mucin stain (PAS-d) shows strong cytoplasmic positivity.

The role of FNA in management of pancreatic lesions

Management options for patients are broad and dependent on many factors including:

* patient age
* symptoms
* malignant potential of the lesion
* co-morbid conditions of the patient

Management of patients with neoplastic cysts is based on the preoperative distinction of:

* non-mucinous from
* mucinous cysts

Diagnostic accuracy with sufficiently high sensitivity and specificity depends on a multimodal team approach that combines the clinical and radiological patient information with the cytological impression and the results of ancillary studies (Fig. 10.117).

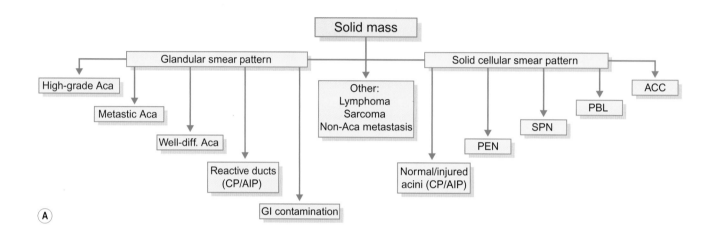

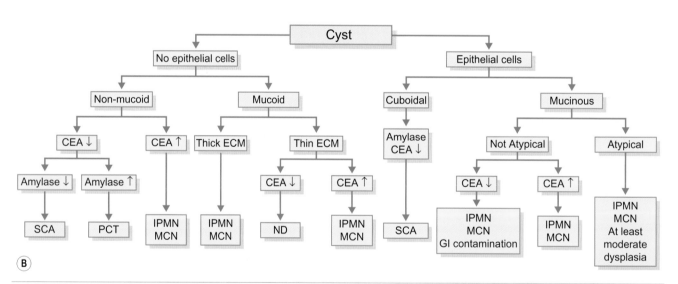

Fig. 10.117[†] A diagnostic algorithm for the cytopathologist is outlined. The diagnostic differential starts with the basic information from the radiological image: Is the lesion (A) solid or (B) cystic? (A) Aca, adenocarcinoma; CP, chronic pancreatitis; AIP, autoimmune pancreatitis; GI, gastrointestinal; PEN, pancreatic endocrine neoplasm; SPN, solid pseudopapillary neoplasm; PBL, pancreatoblastoma; ACC, acinar cell carcinoma. (B) CEA, carcinoembryonic antigen; ECM, extracellular mucin; SCA, serous cystadenoma; PCT, pseudocyst; IPMN, intraductal papillary mucinous neoplasm; MCN, mucinous cystic neoplasm; ND, non-diagnostic; SCA, serous cystadenoma.

CHAPTER 11

Childhood tumours

Contents

Introduction   351

Lymphoma   353

Neuroblastoma   354

Nephroblastoma   355

Rhabdomyosarcoma   357

Ewing's (sarcoma) family of tumours (pPNET)   358

Introduction

- Childhood tumours are rare, corresponding to less than 1% of all malignancies (one case of cancer is encountered annually among 10 000 children up to 15 years of age)
- More than half of malignancies in children are acute leukaemias and central nervous system tumours
- Hodgkin disease and germ cell tumours are more frequent in adolescents than in children
- Neuroblastoma, nephroblastoma and retinoblastoma are exceptional in adolescents
- The most common presenting symptoms of childhood tumours are listed in Box 11.1 and Table 11.1

Role of the cytopathologist

- The cytopathologist has a crucial role for the optimal therapy, diagnosis and management of childhood tumours. Definitive cell typing of small round cell tumours is mandatory for enrollment of patients in specific therapeutic protocols, which has led to a significant increase in disease-free survival rates. Immediate cytological assessment is a critical step that helps to establish the initial diagnostic impression and points to the need for obtaining additional tissue material for pertinent ancillary studies. In addition a complete history, physical examination, and radiological and laboratory evaluations are of critical importance in arriving at a definitive diagnosis (Table 11.1)

- Optimally, fine needle aspiration (FNA) of the lesion should be performed by, or at least in the presence of, a cytopathologist who will verify the quality and the quantity of the material obtained by rapid staining and process the specimen according to the first 'on-site' diagnosis
- The presence of the cytopathologist when obtaining the sample is crucial for:
  - checking sample adequacy
  - ensuring proper handling of the specimen
  - smearing and fixation
  - use of ancillary techniques
- It is essential that the cytopathologist is fully involved in the regular multidisciplinary team meetings for correlating the clinical, radiological, cytological and other laboratory findings

Box 11.1 Common tumours in the foetus and newborn

- Teratoma (usually benign)
- Vascular malformations
- Sarcomas
- Brain tumours
- Neuroblastoma
- Retinoblastoma
- Leukaemias

Obtaining a cytological sample from a child

- Palpable lesions: children are given local anaesthesia such as EMLA (APP Pharmaceuticals) cream which is applied over the area to be sampled 30 minutes to 1 hour prior to the procedure
- Babies are held down in order to ensure that they will not move during the procedure
- Older children who recognise the doctor and injections are asked to cooperate, and they usually do so perfectly
- If they are unable to cooperate, the sample is taken under sedation or light general anaesthesia
- In both cases, the cytopathologist performs the procedure
- Non-palpable lesions: usually ultrasound-guided FNA done either by the cytopathologist or the radiologist

The optimal needles used are 0.6–0.7 mm in diameter.

Main malignant small round cell tumours of childhood

1. Lymphomas
   - Burkitt's, lymphoblastic and centroblastic variant of Diffuse Large B cell lymphoma
   - Small cell type of Diffuse Large B cell lymphoma
2. Neuroblastoma (small and/or large cells)
3. Nephroblastoma (small and/or large cells)
4. Rhabdomyosarcoma of the alveolar type (small and/or large cells)
5. Germ cell tumours (large cells)
6. Other soft tissue sarcomas (small and/or large cells)
   - Malignant peripheral nerve sheath tumour
   - Liposarcoma
   - Malignant rhabdoid tumour
   - Desmoplastic small round cell tumour
7. Ewing's/pPNET family of tumours (small cells)
8. Liver tumours (small or large cells)

Table 11.1 Presenting symptoms and commonly associated suspected diagnoses

Usual presenting symptoms	Most frequent potential diagnoses
LYMPHADENOPATHY	
Localised	Infection (mononucleosis)
	Malignancy
Generalised	Systemic infection (mononucleosis)
	Autoimmune, storage or metabolic disease
	Drug-induced hyperplasia
THORACIC MASS	
Anterior mediastinum	Acute lymphoblastic leukaemia (T cell)
	Lymphoblastic lymphoma
Middle mediastinum	Lymphoma (Hodgkin)
	Metastases (from subdiaphragmatic tumours)
	Infections (tuberculosis, histoplasmosis)
Posterior mediastinum	Neuroblastoma
	Ganglioneuroma
	Neurofibroma
Chest wall	Ewing's/pPNET
	Alveolar soft part sarcoma
	Langerhans cell histiocytosis
BONE PAIN AND/OR MASS	
Localised	Osteomyelitis
	Ewing's/pPNET
	Osteosarcoma
	Langerhans cell histiocytosis
	Non-Hodgkin lymphoma
Diffuse	Acute leukaemia
	Metastases (Ewing's/pPNET, neuroblastoma)
Abdominal or pelvic mass	Congenital malformation (neonatal period)
	Nephroblastoma, neuroblastoma
	Lymphoma (Burkitt's)
	Hepatic, germ cell and ovarian tumours
	Inflammatory process (abscess)
LUMP OR SWELLING	
Extremities	Rhabdomyosarcoma
Orbit	Rhabdomyosarcoma, retinoblastoma
	Lymphoma, neuroblastoma
	Langerhans' cell histiocytosis
Sacrum	Sacrococcygeal teratoma

pPNET, peripheral primitive neuroectodermal tumour (included in the Ewing's family of tumours)

Lymphoma

About 10% of all childhood neoplasms are lymphomas and most of these are of the non-Hodgkin type.

- The most frequently encountered lymphoma types in childhood are summarised in Table 11.2
- More than 90% of NHL are high-grade lymphomas and include precursor and mature B-cell, T-cell or natural killer-cell neoplasms

Cytological findings: Burkitt's and Burkitt's-like lymphomas (Fig. 11.1)

- Relatively uniform population of isolated medium-sized tumour cells
- Rounded nuclei with a high mitotic rate
- Granular or speckled chromatin with multiple small but prominent nucleoli
- Thin rim of dense blue cytoplasm with small lipid vacuoles
- Tingible body macrophages (producing a 'starry sky' pattern on histological sections), often prominent apoptotic bodies in the background

Diagnostic pitfalls: BL and BLL

- B-cell lymphoblastic lymphoma
- Diffuse large B-cell lymphoma in BLL (atypical)
- Extramedullary myeloid malignancies (granulocytic or myeloid sarcoma)
- Other small round cell tumours (see p. 352 and Box 11.2, p. 356): CD45 may be absent in BL

For other lymphoma and leukaemia types refer to Chapter 7.

Further investigations

Please refer to Chapter 13, pp. 411–412.

Table 11.2 Most frequent non-Hodgkin lymphomas in children and adolescents

Lymphoma type	Frequency	Main sites involved	Immuno-phenotype
Burkitt (and Burkitt-like)	40%	Cervical lymph nodes, tonsil, jaw, abdomen, kidneys, ovaries, bone marrow, CNS	B cell
Lymphoblastic Precursor T	25%	Mediastinum, peripheral lymph nodes, liver, spleen, kidneys, retroperitoneum, testes, bone marrow, CNS	Pre-T cell
Precursor B	5%	Cervical lymph nodes, skin, bone	Pre-B cell
Diffuse large B cell (includes mediastinal)	20%	Peripheral lymph nodes, tonsil, bone, mediastinum, retroperitoneum, liver, bone marrow (rare), primary CNS	B cell
Anaplastic, large cell	10%	Skin, soft tissue, bone, peripheral lymph nodes, mediastinum, liver, bone marrow, CNS (rare)	T cell or null cell

CNS, central nervous system. (Adapted from Link MP, Weinstein HJ. Malignant non-Hodgkin lymphoma in children. In: Pizzo PA and Poplack DG (eds) Principles and Practice of Pediatric Oncology, 5th edn. Philadelphia: Lippincott Williams & Wilkins; 2006.)

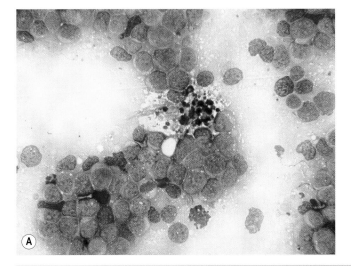

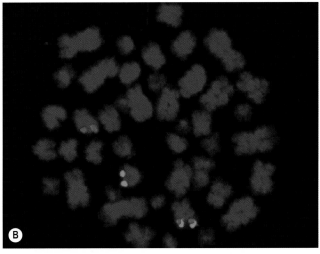

Fig. 11.1[†] (A) Burkitt's lymphoma. Medium-sized lymphoid cells with scanty blue cytoplasm showing lipid vacuoles. Note the dense chromatin and the presence of several mitoses and of a macrophage with tingible bodies (MGG).[†] (B) Burkitt's lymphoma. FISH on a metaphase with a *c-myc* 'break apart' probe showing a translocation of part of *c-myc* gene to chromosome 14 (*green spots*). Part of the gene is still visible on chromosome 8 (*red*). The second-normal *c-myc* gene is composed of two overlapping parts on normal chromosome 8.

Neuroblastoma

- The third most common childhood malignancy and follows leukaemia/lymphomas and tumours of the central nervous system
- Mean age at diagnosis is 2.5 years for both sexes
- May arise in the adrenal medulla or from any sympathetic ganglia within the retroperitoneum, posterior mediastinum, neck and sacral regions

Cytological findings

- In well-differentiated neuroblastoma: small round cells (Fig. 11.2)
- Variable number of Homer–Wright rosettes (Fig. 11.3A)
- Neurofibrillary background (neuropil) (Fig. 11.3B)
- Ganglion cells, which are large cells with one or more nuclei and prominent nucleoli are observed in ganglioneuroblastoma (Fig. 11.4)
- Ganglioneuroma shows only few mature ganglion cells admixed with spindled cells (Schwann cells) (Fig. 11.5). Neuroblasts and neurofibrillary background are lacking in these mature forms
- In poorly differentiated neuroblastoma: small round cells, nuclear moulding (Fig. 11.6A); rosettes and neuropil are rare or absent

Diagnostic pitfalls

- In contrast to the rosette-like structures sometimes observed in Ewing's/peripheral primitive neuroectodermal tumour (PNET), nephroblastoma, rhabdomyosarcoma, desmoplastic small round cell tumour, hepatoblastoma and melanotic progonoma, the Homer–Wright rosettes seen in well-differentiated neuroblastoma usually contain neuropil
- Ewing's/pPNET, monophasic blastemal nephroblastoma may be confused with poorly differentiated neuroblastoma (see list of 'Small round cell tumours', p. 352 and Box 11.2, p. 356)
- As these tumours are heterogeneous, the definite diagnosis of maturation into ganglioneuroma is not reliable on cytological specimens (a small neuroblastic component may not be sampled). This distinction requires extensive histopathological examination of the surgical specimen

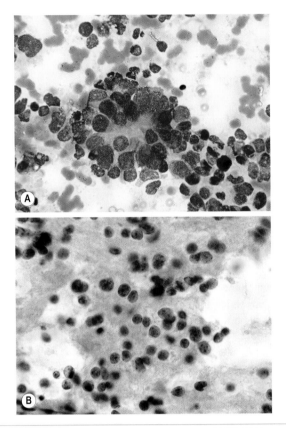

Fig. 11.3[†] (A) Neuroblastoma. Homer–Wright rosette (MGG). (B) Neuropil (neurofibrillary background) in a poorly differentiated neuroblastoma (PAP).

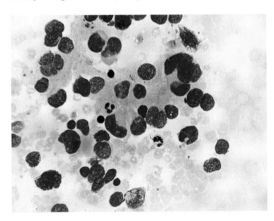

Fig. 11.4[†] Ganglioneuroblastoma. Note the presence of large differentiated neuroblasts and of neuropil.

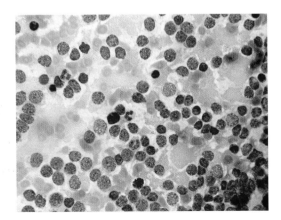

Fig. 11.2[†] Neuroblastoma. Immature neuroblasts (MGG).

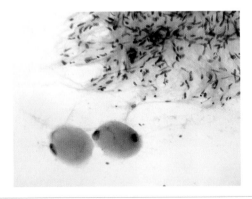

Fig. 11.5[†] Ganglioneuroma. Two mature ganglion cells and numerous spindle-shaped (Schwann) cells (PAP).

Further investigations

- Immunocytochemistry using an antibody against NB84 is positive in all well-differentiated neuroblastomas and in the majority of poorly differentiated tumours
- NB84 may also stain 25% of Ewing's/pPNET tumours and 50% of desmoplastic small round cell tumours
- Nephroblastomas are negative for NB84
- Prognosis is predicted by the combination of: patient age, clinical stage, DNA ploidy and presence of *MYCN* (2p24) oncogene amplification as detected by fluorescence in situ hybridisation (FISH) (see Chapter 13, p. 411, Fig. 13.50)
- Tumours which are near diploid or near tetraploid and which harbour a *MYCN* amplification (Fig. 11.6B) correlate with a poor outcome

Nephroblastoma (Figs 11.7, 11.8)

- Nephroblastoma is the fourth most common childhood malignancy
- Occurs during the neonatal period and is usually associated with congenital and chromosomal abnormalities

Cytological findings: nephroblastoma (Wilms' tumour) and other renal tumours

- Classic triphasic nephroblastoma:
  1. Epithelial elements: small round tumour cells with distinct cytoplasm, sometimes arranged in tubular structures (Fig. 11.7A)
  2. Mesenchymal or stromal elements: spindle-shaped tumour cells arranged in loose sheets intermixed with a myxoid or collagenous matrix (Fig. 11.7B)
  3. Undifferentiated blastemal elements: small and round tumour cells with little cytoplasm (Fig. 11.7C). Anaplastic foci may be detected (Fig. 11.8)
- Recognition may be difficult in biphasic or even monophasic variants of nephroblastoma

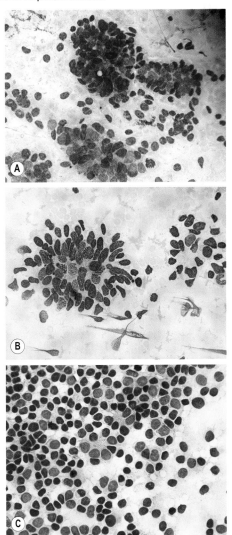

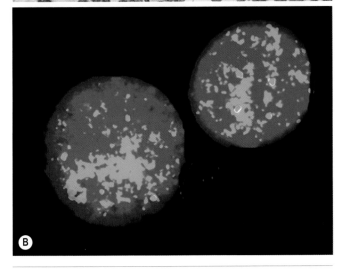

Fig. 11.6† (A) Neuroblastoma. Immature neuroblasts showing nuclear moulding (MGG). (B) FISH on interphase nuclei in neuroblastoma: amplification of the *MYCN* gene (*pink*) in malignant immature neuroblasts showing a multiple copies pattern. The control probe is chromosome 2 centromere (*green*).

Fig. 11.7† Nephroblastoma. (A) Epithelial component: small round or slightly irregular tumour cells arranged in tubular structures. (B) Stromal component: some spindle-shaped tumour cells arranged in loose sheets. (C) Blastomatous component: small round tumour cells without distinct cytoplasm.

Differential diagnosis: renal tumours of childhood

- **Clear cell sarcoma,** usually biphasic with round and spindle-shaped tumour cells (see Box 11.3)
- **Rhabdoid tumour of kidney** composed of large cells with abundant eosinophilic cytoplasm, irregular nuclei and prominent nucleoli
- **Congenital mesoblastic nephroma:**
  - classic type contains spindle cells without mitoses or necrosis reminiscent of infantile fibromatosis
  - cellular type contains round cells with mitoses and necrosis, reminiscent of infantile fibrosarcoma

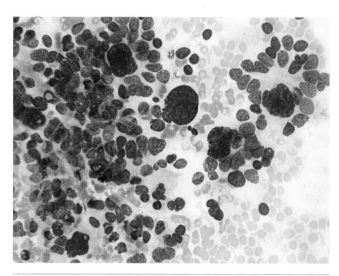

Fig. 11.8[†] Anaplastic nephroblastoma. Note the at least threefold enlarged hyperchromatic nuclei (MGG).

Diagnostic pitfalls: nephroblastoma (Wilms' tumour) and other renal tumours

- When epithelial cells predominate: multicystic nephroma, angiomyolipoma, renal cell carcinoma, clear cell sarcoma of the kidney, small round cell tumours
- When mesenchymal (stromal) elements predominate: congenital mesoblastic nephroma, soft tissue tumours (ancient schwannoma), clear cell sarcoma of the kidney, rhabdoid tumour and rhabdomyosarcoma (see Box 11.3)
- When blastemal cells predominate: nephrogenic rests, nephroblastomatosis, and small round cell tumours (see p. 352, Small round cell tumours)

Further investigations

- *Immunocytochemistry:*
  - WT1 positive in only 70% of nephroblastomas
  - staining of nuclei may also be seen in desmoplastic small cell tumours, lymphoblastic lymphoma and neuroblastoma, and cytoplasmic staining can be present in rhabdomyosarcoma
  - malignant rhabdoid tumour of the kidney: positive for various cytokeratins, epithelial-membrane antigen, desmin, and neurofilaments
- *Cytogenetics:*
  - no specific chromosomal translocation has been described in Wilms' tumour
  - rhabdoid tumour of the kidney: 22q11.12 deletion (hSNF5/INI1 gene)
  - cellular congenital mesoblastic nephroma consistently shows a translocation t(12;15)(p13;q25)
  - subtypes of renal cell carcinomas exhibit a Xp11.2 translocation

Box 11.2 Main malignant round and spindle cell tumours

1. Nephroblastoma (small and/or large cells)
2. Rhabdomyosarcoma (small and/or large cells)
3. Non-rhabdomyosarcoma soft tissue tumours (small and/or large cells)
   - Synovial sarcoma
   - Malignant peripheral nerve sheath tumour

Box 11.3 Main malignant spindle cell tumours

1. Nephroblastoma (small and/or large cells)
2. Rhabdomyosarcoma of embryonal type (small and/or large cells)
3. Non-rhabdomyosarcoma soft tissue tumours (small and/or large cells)
   - Synovial sarcoma
   - Malignant peripheral nerve sheath tumour
   - Fibrosarcoma
   - Leiomyosarcoma

Rhabdomyosarcoma

- Rhabdomyosarcoma is the fifth most common childhood tumour
- Represents half of all malignant soft tissue tumours in infants and children
- Median age at diagnosis is 5 years
- The most frequent sites of involvement are: head and neck (35%), genitourinary tract (22%), and extremities (18%)

Morphology and prognosis

Rhabdomyosarcomas of childhood are categorised with distinct prognostic significance into these morphological types:

- The *embryonal* type (65%):
  - stroma-rich, spindle cell appearance, no evidence of an alveolar pattern
  - has an intermediate prognosis
  - specific entities associated with a better prognosis
    - the botryoid variant (bladder, vagina or nasopharynx)
    - spindle cell or leiomyomatous variant (paratesticular region, orbit, extremities)
- The *alveolar* type (20%):
  - densely packed small round tumour cells lining septations
  - a solid variant is also recognised
  - generally has a bad prognosis
  - anaplastic foci may be present in embryonal and alveolar rhabdomyosarcoma – a poor prognostic sign

Cytological findings

- Embryonal and alveolar rhabdomyosarcomas may only be suggested cytologically in 80% of the cases
- Embryonal rhabdomyosarcoma: large and highly cellular tissue fragments, moderate or abundant stroma, a variable number of individual cells
- Tumour cells predominantly immature with uniform, slightly oval or round nuclei and small amounts of cytoplasm
- Rare cells mimicking rhabdomyoblasts with single or multiple nuclei and variable amounts of cytoplasm (Fig. 11.9)
- Alveolar rhabdomyosarcomas usually yield high-cellularity specimens. Individual tumour cells are small and round and the number of mature rhabdomyoblasts may vary from single to numerous (Fig. 11.10)

Further investigations

- *Immunocytochemistry*: muscle-specific (alpha smooth muscle antigen, desmin) and skeletal muscle (MyoD1, myogenin); however, desmin may be observed in some Ewing's/pPNET and myogenin may be difficult to detect on smears
- *Molecular genetic techniques*:
  - alveolar rhabdomyosarcomas: specific translocations between the FKHR gene located at 13q14 t(2;13)(q35;q14) translocation (PAX3-FKHR gene fusion), and the t(1;13) (p36;q14) translocation (PAX7-FKHR gene fusion)
  - embryonal rhabdomyosarcoma: loss of heterozygosity (LOH) at 11p15

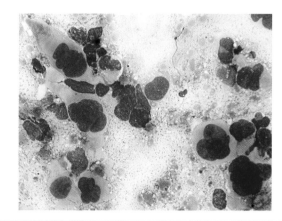

Fig. 11.9[†] Rhabdomyosarcoma. Nuclear pleomorphism and multinucleated tumour cells with elongated cytoplasm.

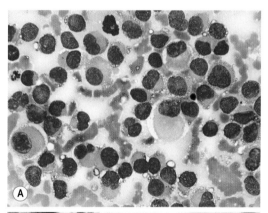

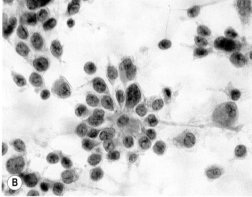

Fig. 11.10[†] (A) Alveolar rhabdomyosarcoma. Dissociated small round tumour cells and a few elements with eccentric nuclei (MGG). (B) Alveolar rhabdomyosarcoma (PAP).

Diagnostic pitfalls

- *Large and highly cellular fragments* in embryonal type should be differentiated from benign lesions such as:
  - infantile myofibromatosis
  - haemangioendothelioma
  - neurofibroma
- *Small round tumour cells*, mainly observed in the alveolar type; other small round cell tumours:
- Rhabdomyoblasts may mimic tumour cells observed in malignant rhabdoid tumours or in embryonal sarcoma (not otherwise specified)

Ewing's (sarcoma) family of tumours (pPNET)

- The Ewing's (sarcoma) family of tumours are peripheral primitive neuroectodermal tumours (pPNET) or peripheral neuroepitheliomas
  - previously known as: Ewing tumour (classic, atypical and peripheral neuroepithelioma), Askin's tumour (malignant small cell tumour of the thoracopulmonary region), malignant ectomesenchymoma, biphenotypic sarcoma, and olfactory neuroblastoma (esthesioneuroblastoma)
- These tumours commonly occur in bones but may also be seen in soft tissues
- The second most common malignant primary bone tumour in childhood, following osteosarcoma
- Mean age at diagnosis is 15 years

Cytological findings

- Cytological specimens are usually very cellular
- Clusters of loosely cohesive cells and single small round tumour cells
- Tumour cells are fragile (naked or stripped nuclei are often observed)
- Two cell subtypes:
  - one with hyperchromatic ('dark' cells) nuclei and scant cytoplasm corresponds probably to cells undergoing apoptosis
  - the other is composed of cells with larger amounts of cytoplasm containing glycogen vacuoles and round or ovoid nuclei with a finely granular chromatin and one to three small nucleoli ('light' cells) (Figs 11.11, 11.12)
- Rosettes may be seen (25%), but without detectable neuropil inside or outside the rosettes
- According to some authors, rosettes are never seen in the 'classic' Ewing's tumour

Diagnostic pitfalls

- Osteomyelitis
- Primary bone sarcomas (small cell osteosarcoma, mesenchymal chondrosarcoma)
- Langerhans cell histiocytosis/eosinophilic granuloma of bone
- Other small round cell tumours (from soft tissues and metastatic neuroblastoma)

Further investigations

- *Immunocytochemistry*
  - CD99 stains the vast majority (90–100%) of tumour cells, but also stains a significant number of cells from other tumours, lymphoblastic lymphoma, neuroblastoma, rhabdomyosarcoma, desmoplastic small round cell tumours
  - small round cell tumours and synovial sarcomas
  - cytokeratins detectable in 10% of Ewing's sarcomas
- *Molecular genetic techniques* (Fig. 11.13)
  - the t(11;22)(q24;q12) translocation (*EWS-FLI1* gene fusion) in 85% of cases
  - the t(21;22)(q22;q12) translocation (*EWS-ERG* gene fusion) in 10–15% of cases
  - the other types of gene fusions are very rare

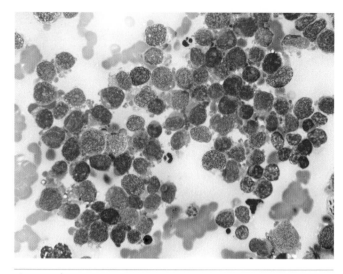

Fig. 11.11[†] Ewing's sarcoma. Loosely cohesive small round tumour cells with distinct cytoplasm. Some nuclei are smaller and hyperchromatic and correspond to apoptotic cells.

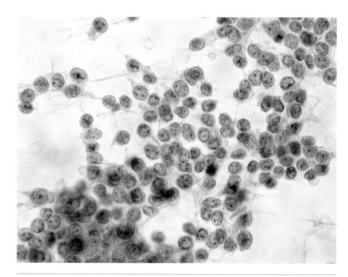

Fig. 11.12[†] Ewing's sarcoma. Tumour cells showing vacuolated cytoplasm and monomorphous nuclei with slightly nuclear molding sarcoma.

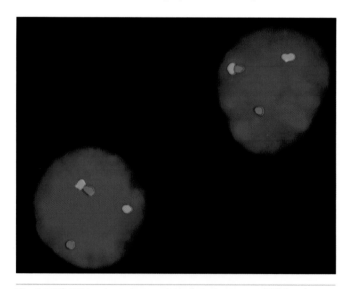

Fig. 11.13[†] FISH on interphase nuclei in Ewing's sarcoma: EWS 'break apart' probe which detects the split of EWS gene. Normal gene shows the double colour overlapping spots. The part of translocated gene (*red*) is on the other partner chromosome. This probe allows detection of the classic translocation t(11;22) but also all other translocation variants.

CHAPTER 12

Miscellaneous

Contents

Cerebrospinal fluid   360

Skin   366

Malignant tumours   369

Soft tissue and musculoskeletal system   372

Synovial fluid   387

Cytology laboratories throughout the world occasionally receive samples that are rare. The expertise in reading these is often lacking because of the low exposure to such material. Unless it is a specialised Central Nervous System unit, cerebrospinal fluid is received only occasionally, mainly for investigation of infections, staging of lymphoma and the detection of metastatic disease. Similarly, the skin cytology, scrapes and aspirates are performed only sporadically in any general hospital unit therefore a basic knowledge about the techniques of cell preparation and interpretation are valuable. Cytology is usually not a first line investigation for soft tissue lesions but, since these occur in all body sites, cytopathologists will in the course of their career get exposed to some unusual morphological presentations where the principles of malignant cytological diagnosis may not apply. Joint fluid investigation is usually a domain of specialised rheumathology units. However, occasionally,they find their way to the general cytopathologist who needs to be able to perform some elementary investigations and issue a meaningfull report.

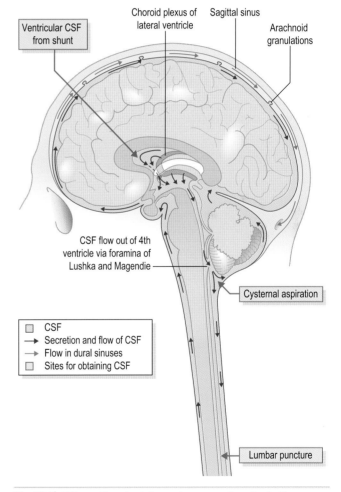

Fig. 12.1[†] CSF secretion, circulation and common sites of collection.

Cerebrospinal fluid

Cerebrospinal fluid (CSF) is secreted by the choroid plexus, circulates around the brain and spinal cord and within the ventricles and is reabsorbed into the venous system via arachnoid granulations (Fig. 12.1).

Samples of CSF are usually taken by lumbar puncture (LP), or from the cisterna or a ventricular shunt. The volume is limited and samples require special care, as other tests besides cytology may be needed.

Clinical indications for CSF cytology

* Clinical or radiological suspicion of involvement of subarachnoid space or ventricles by a cellular infiltrative process
* Raised CSF cell count or protein level
* Previous history of CNS or other tumour
* Unexplained headache and other neurological symptoms

Preparation methods for CSF cytology

* The laboratory procedures associated with receiving, preparing and reporting a CSF sample are shown in Fig. 12.2 and is described in Chapter 13

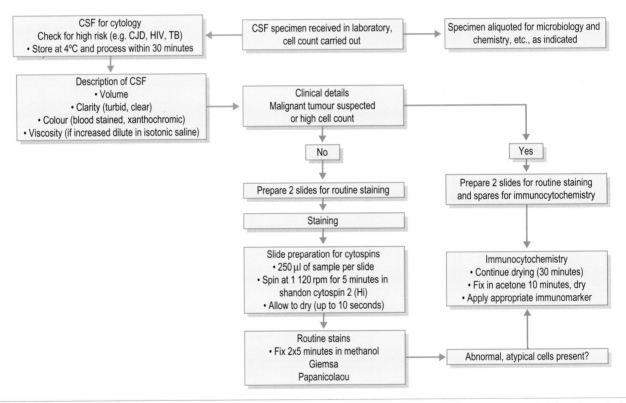

Fig. 12.2[†] Diagnostic approach to CSF in a cytology laboratory. Flow diagram of standard procedures for handling and processing of CSF specimens in the neurocytology laboratory.

Cytological findings: normal CSF (Fig. 12.3)

- Normally CSF is almost acellular
- Isolated macrophages, lymphocytes or neutrophil polymorphs may be seen and are of no pathological significance
- Introduction of chondrocytes either singly or in clusters into the CSF may occur during a lumbar puncture procedure
- Traumatic LP tap can introduce a few red blood cells into the CSF
- Normal cells shed from the choroid plexus or ventricular surface showing a benign cuboidal morphology may be seen in the CSF occasionally. Their preservation may vary
- Clusters of normal meningothelial cells are rarely seen in the CSF, often demonstrating a typical cell whorl formation
- Fragments of normal brain parenchyma may be introduced into the CSF during a ventriculostomy or shunt insertion for the treatment of hydrocephalus
- Large neuronal cells with prominent nucleoli, sometimes of a pyramidal shape, may be mistaken for atypical cells including germ cell tumours

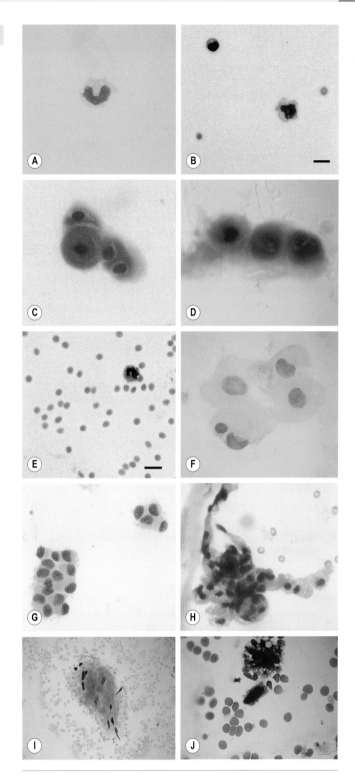

Fig. 12.3[†] Normal cells and contaminants in CSF. (A) Normal macrophage. (B) Normal lymphocytes. (C,D) Chondrocytes in small clusters. (E) Traumatic spinal tap leading to red blood cell contamination. (F,G) Choroid plexus cells. (H) Normal meningothelial cells with central whorl. (I) Fragment of normal brain parenchyma. (J) Large neuronal cells with prominent nucleoli.

Bacterial infections (Fig. 12.4A–D)

- **Pyogenic organisms** lead to cloudy CSF with a high polymorph count. Gram stain may show organisms
- **TB meningitis:** Florid lymphocytosis with lymphocytes numbering thousands/ml. ZN stain and microbiology investigations for TB are essential

Viral infections (Fig. 12.4E–G)

- **Aseptic:** Lymphocytosis but numbers fewer than TB, averaging less than a hundred/ml. Lymphocytes are mature, with predominance of T cells. Non-Hodgkin lymphoma is in the differential but this is usually morphologically high grade so rarely poses difficulty. Herpes simplex virus and Mollaret's recurrent meningitis
- **HIV:** recurrent infections at time of seroconversion, viral encephalitis or opportunistic infection

Fungal infections (Fig. 12.4H, I)

- ***Cryptococcus neoformans*** in immunosuppressed patients is the commonest; shows spherical yeasts 5–10 μm with thick mucoid capsule on MGG, PAP, Alcian blue or India ink. The organism may lie in macrophages. There is a paucity of lymphocytes in CSF of immunosuppressed patients

Other infectious causes

- **Lyme disease meningitis** (*Borrelia burgdorferi*) shows mild lymphocytosis, few polymorphs
- ***Acanthamoeba* spp.** and **toxoplasmosis:** mononuclear pleocytosis

Unknown causes of inflammation

- **Sarcoidosis, multiple sclerosis, autoimmune and vascular disorders** all cause variable lymphocytosis, and/or haemorrhage (Fig. 12.4J)

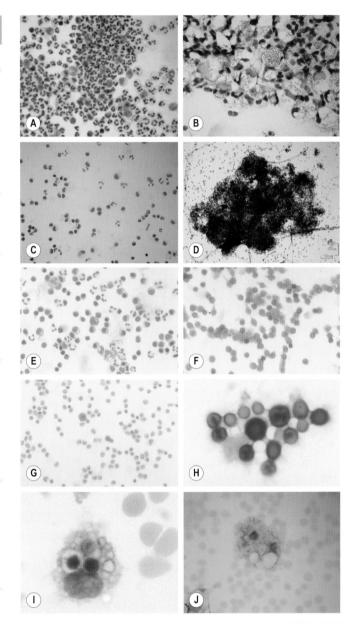

Fig. 12.4 Inflammatory and infectious CSF findings.

- (A) Acute bacterial meningitis with numerous polymorphs in the CSF. (B) Gram-negative bacteria are visible within macrophages, in a case of acute meningitis. (C) Pleocytosis of the CSF in tuberculous meningitis with both polymorphs and neutrophils present. (D) A cohesive mass of chronic inflammatory cells and epithelioid histiocytes in a CSF sample from a patient with tuberculous meningitis.
- (E) Mixed acute and chronic inflammatory cell infiltrates in acute viral aseptic meningitis. The lymphoid cells include small lymphocytes in addition to activated cells. (F) Viral meningitis: immunohistochemistry for CD3 confirms that a large number of the small lymphocytes, as well as some of the activated cells, are T cells. (G) Immunohistochemistry for CD20 shows occasional larger and small B cells.
- (H) *Cryptococcus* organisms in CSF as visualised with Alcian blue stain in a case of chronic meningitis. (I) *Cryptococcus* organisms present within macrophages in the CSF.
- (J) Siderophage (haemosiderin-laden macrophage) in CSF sample indicative of recent haemorrhage.

CSF in primary CNS tumours

- Only 10–20% of positive CSF samples are from primary CNS tumours
- For many diffuse tumours, biopsy is better than CSF cytology. LP is contraindicated if the CSF pressure is raised
- Gliomas, medulloblastomas, embryonal, pineal and germ cell tumours tend to spread through the CSF, shedding tumour cells directly into the subarachnoid space

Cytological findings (Figs 12.5–12.8)

- **Glioma cells** tend to be cohesive, so do not disseminate well in CSF and cell processes are not seen. The cells express GFAP
- **Malignant astrocytomas/glioblastoma multiforme** (GBM): cells and nuclei are pleomorphic with coarse chromatin. The cells show apoptosis, mitoses and multinucleation. Differential diagnosis: melanoma, sarcoma, PNET
- **Oligodendroglioma**: cells are larger than lymphocytes and show nuclear atypia; similar to other glial tumours
- **Ependymoma**: tightly packed groups, variable findings with grade of malignancy of the tumour
- **Leptomeningeal gliomatosis** (LG): due to extensive spread from a deeper glioma, CSF may show lymphocytes only
- **Medulloblastoma/PNET**: cerebellar tumour spreading to CSF in 25% of cases (commonest CNS primary seen in CSF). Small cells in clumps, nuclear moulding, high N:C ratio, mitoses, necrosis and inflammation. Distinguish from other small cell tumours. Synaptophysin positive on immunocytochemistry
- **Other primary CNS tumours**: germ cell tumour (biphasic, PLAP positive); choroid plexus tumour (papillary groups); pineal tumour (resemble PNET); meningioma (infrequent in CSF)

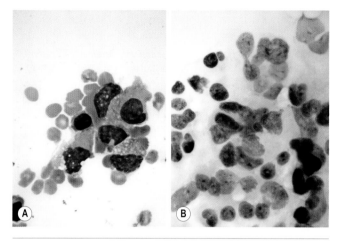

Fig. 12.6[†] (A) Oligodendroglioma: pleomorphic cells with fine chromatin. (B) Pleomorphic group of malignant cells from GBM.

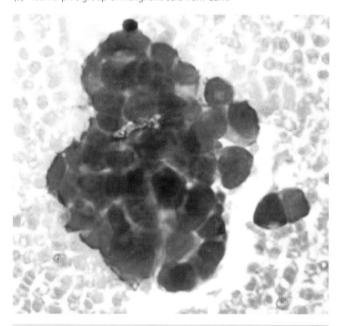

Fig. 12.7[†] Cluster of cohesive malignant cells from an anaplastic ependymoma.

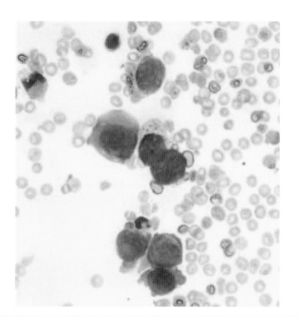

Fig. 12.5[†] Germinoma: large malignant cells with prominent nucleoli. Note small lymphocytes in background.

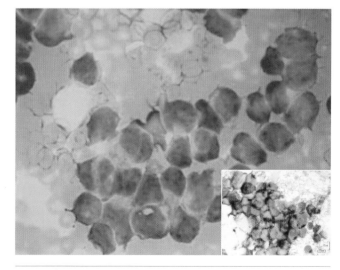

Fig. 12.8[†] PNET/medulloblastoma: pleomorphic cells with little cytoplasm, nuclear moulding. (Inset) Synaptophysin positivity.

CSF in secondary CNS tumours

- Metastatic malignancy in CSF usually occurs with a known primary, rarely the initial presentation
- Cells enter CSF via bloodstream, may circulate free in CSF without involving CNS tissues
- Breast and lung carcinoma are common primaries
- Most terminal melanoma cases have tumour cells in CSF
- Lymphoma, leukaemia frequently involve CNS/meninges (see p. 365)
- Carcinomatous meningitis has a poor prognosis especially in the elderly or with localizing CNS signs

Cytological findings: carcinomatous meningitis (Figs 12.9–12.11)

- Single or clustered large malignant cells with a few background lymphocytes. Breast cancer cells often single
- Adenocarcinoma: may see mucous vacuoles PASD positive
- Squamous carcinoma cells often numerous, may show keratinisaton, pleomorphic nuclei, coarse chromatin
- Melanoma: large dissociated cells, eccentric nuclei, large nucleoli, melanin pigment in cytoplasm and in melanophages

Differential diagnosis: carcinomatous meningitis

- Primary CNS tumour versus metastasis: clinical details are essential, immune stains may help
- Reactive lymphocytosis or lymphoma versus metastatic small cell carcinoma, e.g. single cell spread from breast, lung, gastric carcinoma: immunocytochemistry (as discussed in Chapters 4 and 13)
- Artefact: shunt sample may contain benign tissue fragments

Further investigation

- Full clinical, radiological and biochemical details are essential
- Histochemical stains: PASD or mucicarmine for mucin, Masson–Fontana for melanin
- Immunocytochemistry: valuable if enough CSF is available or may need further samples

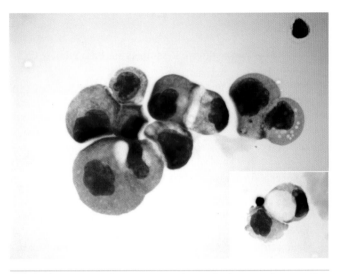

Fig. 12.9† Metastatic adenocarcinoma: cluster of cohesive malignant cells with mucinous vacuolation (inset).

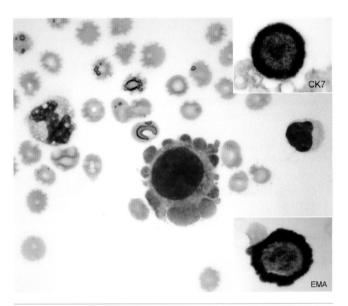

Fig. 12.10† Metastatic breast carcinoma: single malignant cells with ruffled borders. Insets positive for CK7 and EMA.

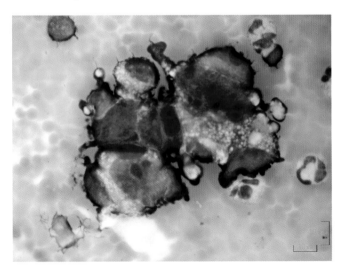

Fig. 12.11† Metastatic malignant melanoma: pleomorphic large malignant cells, prominent nucleoli, suggestion of pigment in cytoplasm.

CSF involvement in lymphomas and leukaemia

- Lymphoma/leukaemia frequently involve CNS; primary CNS lymphoma is rare
- LP useful for diagnosis and monitoring of treatment
- Presence of atypical lymphoid cells in CSF should prompt full investigation (bone marrow, lymph node sampling, HIV testing, neuroimaging)
- Childhood leukaemias usually do involve the CSF
- CSF is often drawn at the time of administering the prophylactic treatment

Cytological findings (Figs 12.12–12.15)

- **Acute lymphoblastic leukaemia:** high N:C ratio, smooth chromatin, prominent nucleoli, mitoses. Over 5 WBCs/mm³
- **Acute myeloid leukaemia:** mixed picture of immature and mature myeloid cells
- **Chronic lymphocytic lymphoma:** CNS spread not common, cells indistinguishable from small mature lymphocytes
- **Lymphomatous meningitis:** usually high-grade NHL types, rarely Hodgkin disease or low-grade NH lymphoma. Diagnostic if atypical lymphoid cells present

Differential diagnosis

- **Reactive lymphocytosis:** many causes; remember TB. Use immunocytochemistry and flow cytometry, repeat sampling
- **Metastatic small cell carcinoma** with single cell pattern: clinical details, immunocytochemistry

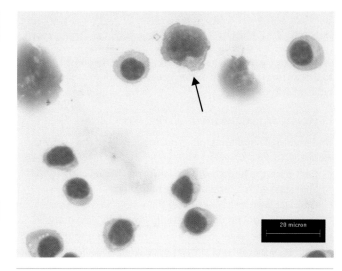

Fig. 12.13† Lymphoma. Cellular CSF with a mixed population of small lymphocytes and interspersed single large atypical lymphoid cells (*arrow*) (see Figs 12.14, 12.15).

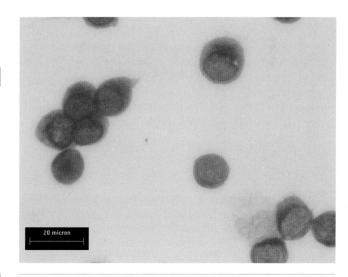

Fig. 12.14† Immunotyping of case in Fig. 12.13 showing frequent CD3-positive small T lymphocytes (see also Fig. 12.15).

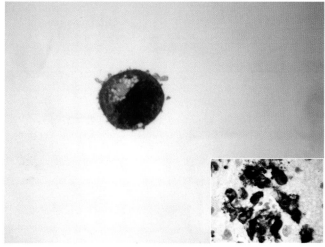

Fig. 12.12† Anaplastic large cell lymphoma in the CSF (Giemsa). (Inset) Histology was carried out of a region of cortex with abnormal imaging on MRI to confirm the CSF impression of lymphoma with atypical lymphoid cells which were CD30 positive in tissue section following cortical biopsy. Immunohistochemistry for ALK1 was also positive, confirming the diagnosis of anaplastic large cell lymphoma (primary CNS lymphoma).

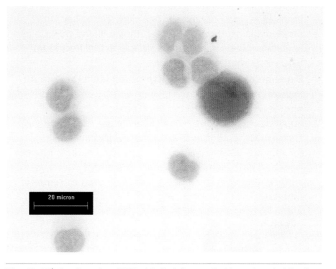

Fig. 12.15† B-cell marker CD79a labelled the atypical large lymphoid cells, confirming a diffuse large B-cell NHL involvement of CSF.

Skin

Skin cytology is a rapid, relatively non-invasive diagnostic technique. In many cases, it is sufficient for definitive diagnosis, and preferable to biopsy from areas such as the face to avoid or minimise scarring, particularly in conjunction with topical treatment modalities in some types of skin cancer.

Cytological features: normal skin (Figs 12.16, 12.17)

Under normal conditions, only squamous cells of the horny layer exfoliate.

- Cells from the horny layer are large, polyhedral and anuclear with a certain degree of folding
- Granular layer: cells are smaller than those in the horny layer; they contain deeply basophilic eratohyaline granules
- Squamous cell layer: cells vary in size according to their degree of maturity; in clusters of cells, intercellular bridges may be seen. Nuclei have well-defined, lacy chromatin
- Basal cell layer: this is composed of immature, germinative cells, seen histologically as a single row of small regular cells lying perpendicular to the underlying basement membrane, which anchors them (palisading). The nuclear:cytoplasmic ratio is high
- Melanocytes, conspicuous with their clear cytoplasm and small, dark nuclei, are scattered along the basal layer but are rarely seen in smears
- Langerhans cells, part of the immune system, are scarce and difficult to identify. A few inflammatory cells including lymphocytes, histiocytes and mast cells may also be seen in skin smears

Sampling techniques

- **Direct skin scrape**: A blunt or sharp curette, a double-ended elevator or a scalpel blade can be used. The skin should be cleansed before the procedure. The keratotic surface and any crusts must be removed completely to obtain a satisfactory representative smear. Four samples from superficial, crusted lesions should be taken from the periphery of the lesion, as the centre may be inflamed and necrotic
- **Touch imprint cytology**: This technique may be used successfully in ulcerating lesions and the cut surface of biopsies. A clean, dry microscope slide should be firmly pressed against the lesion after removal of any crusts. Slight abrasion of the surface exposes viable tissue, freeing up tissue fragments and individual cells
- **Fine needle sampling with aspiration (FNA) or without aspiration**: This technique may be employed to sample skin nodules and deeper lesions. Local anaesthetic is usually applied subcutaneously, particularly in the sensitive areas such as face, eyelids and lips. A narrow gauge needle, 0.7 mm (22–23G) in diameter is used. The needle is moved back and forth, sometimes almost tangentially to the skin surface, aiming at the raised edges of an ulcer or centre of a nodule. The needle contents are ejected and smeared in a thin layer on a glass slide (Fig. 12.18) (See Ch 13, FNA method)

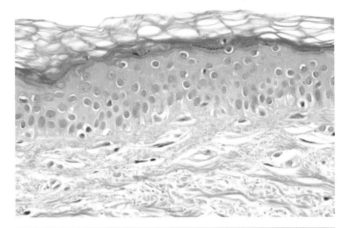

Fig. 12.16[†] Normal skin biopsy showing the epidermis and the upper dermis. The epidermis is composed of multilayered squamous cells (keratinocytes) and dendritic cells. Squamous cells, which form the bulk of cells in epidermis, possess intercellular bridges. The main dendritic cells found are Langerhans cells and melanocytes.

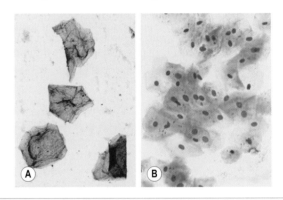

Fig. 12.17 Scrapes of the normal body surfaces. (A) skin scrape shows anuclear squamous cells (toluidine blue). (B) Scrape of the oral mucosa shows nucleated mature squamous cells (RAL 44).

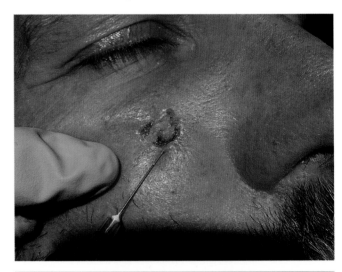

Fig. 12.18 Basal cell carcinoma, face. FNA capillary sampling without aspiration, allowing the material to enter the needle by capillary attraction, is particularly suitable for cellular nodules such as lymph nodes or melanoma metastases.

Skin infections

- **Leprosy**
- **Leishmaniasis**
- **Herpes virus**
- **Superficial fungal infections**

Cytological findings: leprosy (Fig. 12.19)

- Foamy macrophages containing bundles of acid-fast bacilli in Ziehl–Neelsen-stained preparations
- Loosely cohesive epithelioid cell granulomas, macrophages and varying amounts of lymphocytes

Differential diagnosis: leprosy

- The smear may sometimes resemble sarcoidosis
- The bacterial index may vary widely in mid-borderline leprosy and in many cases no bacteria are found

Cytological findings: leishmaniasis (Fig. 12.20)

- Macrophages containing intracytoplasmic amastigotes (Leishman bodies)
- Extracellular amastigotes in the background
- The amastigotes are spherical or ovoid, 2–3 μm in size. It may be possible to detect the nucleus and the rod-shaped kinetoplast in some of the amastigotes

Cytological findings: herpes virus (Fig. 12.21)

- Multinucleated cells measuring between 20 and 30 μm in diameter with up to 30 nuclei
- Nuclear moulding and margination of chromatin
- Pale, eosinophilic, ground glass-like intranuclear inclusion bodies
- Inflammatory cells

Differential diagnosis: herpes virus

- The large eosinophilic inclusions may be confused with nucleoli
- Multinucleated giant cells in pemphigus vulgaris lack nuclear inclusions and moulding and are accompanied by acantholytic cells

Cytological findings: superficial fungal infections (Fig. 12.22)

- Fungal spores, hyphae or pseudohyphae

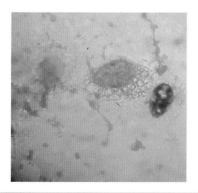

Fig. 12.19[†] Leprosy. Acid-fast bacilli in bundles in a foamy macrophage and scattered in the background (smear, Ziehl–Neelsen).

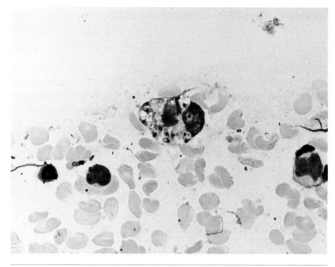

Fig. 12.20[†] Leishmaniasis. Macrophage with amastigotes in its cytoplasm. From an ulcerated lesion (smear).

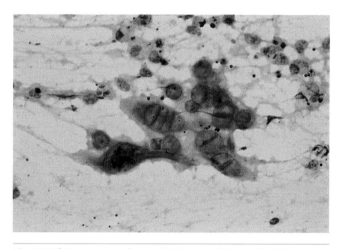

Fig. 12.21[†] Herpes virus infection. Multinucleated giant cells with ground-glass nuclei and nuclear moulding.

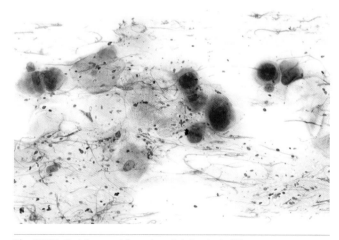

Fig. 12.22 Budding yeast forms in actinic keratosis. Skin scrape.

Seborrhoeic keratosis (Fig. 12.23)

Seborrhoeic keratosis is a common benign pigmented hyperplastic and keratotic skin lesion occurring as multiple oval brown to black plaques, mainly on the trunk in adults. Clinically they may be mistaken for malignant melanoma.

Cytological findings: pemphigus vulgaris (Fig. 12.24)

- Numerous single, rounded acantholytic cells with cyanophilic cytoplasm
- Large hyperchromatic nuclei with pronounced nucleoli and perinuclear halos
- Neutrophils, eosinophils and lymphocytes in the background

Differential diagnosis: pemphigus vulgaris

- Acantholytic cells may be misinterpreted as suspicious for malignancy

Cytological findings: actinic keratosis (Fig. 12.25)

- Cellular smears
- Single cells and groups of dyskaryotic keratinocytes with uneven or 'feathery' edges
- Intercellular bridges often seen
- Polyhedral or spindle-shaped cells
- Raised nuclear:cytoplasmic ratio
- Nuclei are enlarged and may have vesicular chromatin
- Nucleoli may be seen

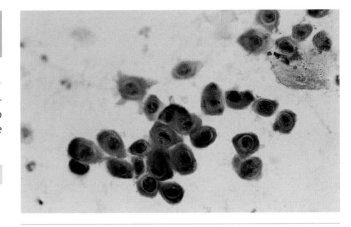

Fig. 12.24† Pemphigus. Rounded single cells with perinuclear halos (skin scrape).

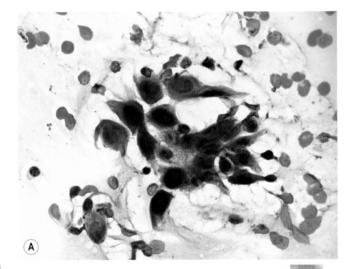

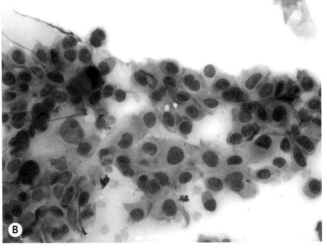

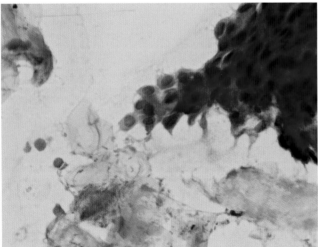

Fig. 12.23† Seborrhoeic keratosis. Sheets of basal and squamous cells and anucleate squames (skin scrape).

Fig. 12.25† Actinic keratosis. (A) Dysplastic squamous cells with intercellular bridges and enlarged nuclei. Clean background (skin scrape). (B) Dysplastic squamous cells with enlarged nuclei with nucleoli.

Malignant tumours

Basal cell carcinoma

- Basal cell carcinoma (BCC) is the most frequent of all cancers in fair-skinned populations
- Occurs most often on sun-exposed areas
- Malignant, locally aggressive epithelial tumour that very rarely metastasises
- Variable clinical appearance: superficial, nodular or morphoeic types
- Cytological diagnosis of either air-dried or alcohol-fixed scrapes or FNA smears is reliable if sufficient material is obtained (see Fig. 12.18)

Cytological findings (Figs 12.26–12.28)

- Cellular smear
- Tightly cohesive sheets of small uniform hyperchromatic cells with scanty cytoplasm and indistinct cell borders
- Well-defined, club-like groups of atypical cells
- Focal peripheral palisading in sheets and club-like structures
- Hyperchromatic round or oval nuclei with fine granular chromatin
- Little variation in nuclear size and shape
- Scattered tumour cells seldom seen

Differential diagnosis

- Metastatic small cell carcinoma
- The basaloid cell component of pilomatrixoma may resemble BCC. However, it differs in clinical presentation and contains 'ghost' cells and multinucleate giant cells
- The basosquamous type may be difficult to differentiate from keratoacanthoma and squamous cell carcinoma
- Basaloid cells in smears from sebaceous gland tumours may be difficult to distinguish from BCC
- Merkel cell carcinoma may pose problems but has greater cellular dissociation and lacks club-like structures

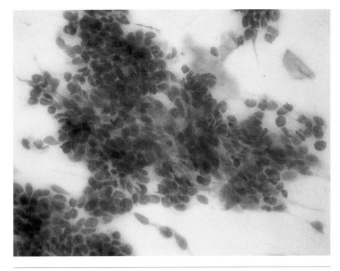

Fig. 12.27[†] Basal cell carcinoma. Groups of atypical basal cells with fragments of pink-staining basal membrane matrix.

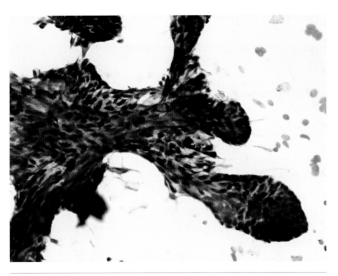

Fig. 12.28[†] Basal cell carcinoma. Smooth-edged, club-like fragments of atypical basal cell with peripheral palisading.

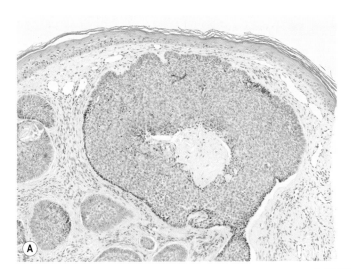

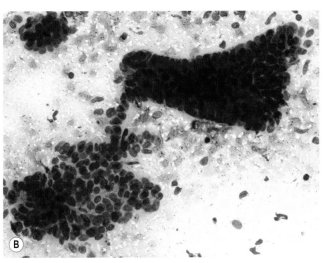

Fig. 12.26[†] (A) Basal cell carcinoma. Sheets of atypical basal cells with peripheral pallisading of the nuclei. Punch biopsy. (B) Basal cell carcinoma. Same case, FNA sample. Smooth-edged fragments and atypical basal cells with peripheral palisading.

Squamous cell carcinoma, malignant melanoma

Cytological findings: squamous cell carcinoma (Fig. 12.29)

- Single cells due to loss of cohesion
- Often highly orangeophilic cells due to abnormal keratinisation (PAP)
- Solid fragments of less-differentiated tumour cells
- Bizarre cell shapes, e.g. tadpole cells
- Large irregular nuclei with nucleoli
- Polymorphs and occasional eosinophils

Diagnostic pitfalls: squamous cell carcinoma (Fig. 12.29)

- Actinic (solar) keratosis and Bowen's disease lack the extremes of cytoplasmic and nuclear pleomorphism typical of SCC (see Fig. 12.25AB)
- Regenerative squamous epithelium at the edge of an ulcer shows hyperchromatic nuclei with nucleoli, mitoses and polymorphs. However, the squamous cells are cohesive and the nuclear:cytoplasmic ratio is low
- Scrapings from a keratoacanthoma may be difficult to differentiate from a highly differentiated SCC

Cytological findings: malignant melanoma (Figs 12.30, 12.31)

- Cellular smears
- Dissociated single cells with occasional loosely cohesive groups of cells
- Cells may vary considerably in size and shape
- Variable nuclear:cytoplasmic ratio
- Hyperchromatic eccentric nuclei
- Large nucleoli (often macronucleoli), often multiple
- Atypical mitoses
- Binucleate or multinucleated cells
- Cytoplasmic pigment may be seen
- Fine cytoplasmic vacuolation
- Peripheral condensation of the cytoplasm, often well defined

Differential diagnosis: malignant melanoma

- Cytological appearance of malignant melanoma is quite variable
- Some smears show large, undifferentiated cells
- The nuclei may vary greatly in size and shape and may contain macronucleoli
- Some have intranuclear vacuoles
- Others contain spindle-shaped cells, singly and in sheets, or round cells
- The amount of pigment is variable and may be in the cytoplasm or the background of the smear

FNA is not indicated in primary melanocytic lesions where an excision biopsy should be performed as a first-line investigation.

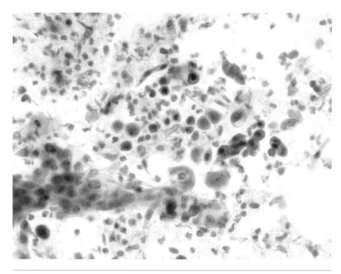

Fig. 12.29[†] Squamous cell carcinoma. Atypical keratinised cells, fragments of atypical cells with large nuclei and bizarre ('tadpole') cells.

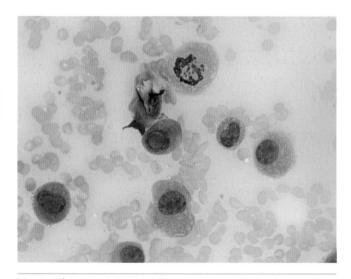

Fig. 12.30[†] Metastasis from a malignant melanoma. Single, pleomorphic cells with macronuclei and one cell in mitosis.

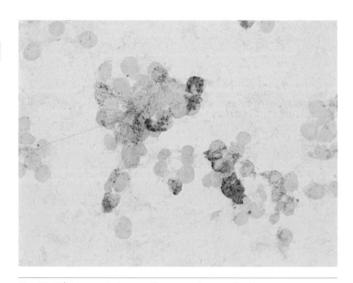

Fig. 12.31[†] Metastasis from malignant melanoma. Positive immunocytochemical staining for HMB-45 (FNA).

Other skin tumours

- **Pilomatryxoma**
- **Primary cutaneous lymphoma**
- **Merkel cell carcinoma**

Cytological findings: pilomatrixoma (Fig. 12.32)

- Clusters of basaloid cells with small to medium-sized, round nuclei with distinct nucleoli and peripheral condensation of the cytoplasm often well defined
- Nuclear moulding may be present among basaloid cells
- Sheets of squamous 'ghost' cells
- Calcium deposits
- Scattered naked nuclei from basal cells
- Fibrillary pink material enveloping basaloid cells
- Multinucleated giant cells

Fig. 12.32[†] Pilomatrixoma. Clusters of basaloid cells and squamous cells with ghost-like nuclei from nodule in the scalp.

Cytological findings: primary cutaneous lymphoma (Fig. 12.33)

- Primary cutaneous lymphomas are a heterogeneous group of diseases comprising clonal accumulations of lymphocytes originating in the skin
- Cutaneous lymphoma should always be considered in the presence of atypical lymphoid cells in smears from skin lesions
- Diagnosis is based on the clinical and cytological findings in addition to immunophenotyping and genotyping of the neoplastic lymphocytes (PCR gene rearrangement in T-cell lymphoma)

Apart from primary cutaneous lymphomas, systemic non-Hodgkin lymphomas may also involve the skin.

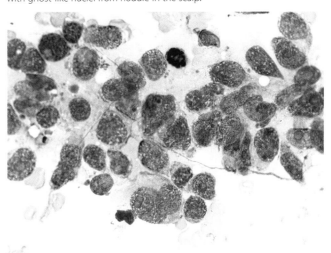

Fig. 12.33[†] Anaplastic large cell lymphoma, cutaneous type. Large anaplastic cells with pleomorphic nucleus. Some multinucleated cells may also present, resembling Reed–Sternberg cells. Reactive neutrophils and macrophages infiltrate the lymphomatous lesion. Unlike systemic CD30 ALCL, the expression of the ALK protein is not found in primary cutaneous tumours.

Cytological findings: Merkel cell carcinoma (Fig. 12.34)

- Cellular smears usually composed of small atypical non-cohesive cells
- Small clusters forming rosette-like structures may also be seen
- Fragile cells often resulting in crush artefact
- Numerous apoptotic bodies and occasional mitotic figures
- Nuclei relatively uniform in size, round or oval with minimal nuclear irregularities
- Nuclear chromatin finely dispersed, with an occasional visible nucleolus
- Lack of discernible cytoplasm (rare cells may show eccentric dense cytoplasm with a hyaline appearance indenting the nucleus, particularly evident in MGG staining)
- Cell-to-cell moulding and nuclear moulding
- Necrotic dirty background with occasional tingible body macrophages

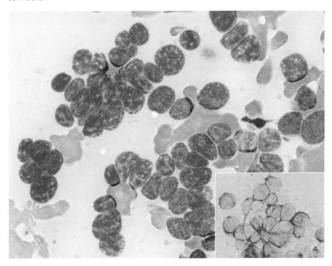

Fig. 12.34[†] Merkel cell carcinoma. FNA smear impression is that of a poorly differentiated small blue cell neoplasm resembling metastasis from a small cell carcinoma, lymphoma or BCC. (Inset) Merkel cell carcinoma stains positively with neuroendocrine markers and cytokeratins, as shown here, distinguishing it from lymphoma.

Soft tissue and musculoskeletal system

FNA as the diagnostic pre-treatment method for musculoskeletal tumours is accepted in many orthopaedic tumour centres, provided that the final cytological diagnosis is based on the combined evaluation of clinical data, radiographic findings and cytomorphology.

There are two main indications for fine needle aspiration (FNA) of soft tissue and bone lesions:

- the diagnosis before the definitive treatment
- the investigation of lesions clinically suspicious of tumour recurrence or metastasis

The role of FNA cytology in management of soft tissue and bone tumours

- The most important preoperative information for the orthopaedic surgeon is whether the lesion is a true soft tissue tumour, either benign or malignant
- In cases of benign soft tissue tumours, the cytopathologist must be able to differentiate correctly between benign lipomatous tumours, nerve sheath tumours, the so-called pseudosarcomas and fibrous tumours such as desmoid fibromatosis
- With bone lesions, FNA may also replace open biopsy in the primary diagnosis. It is the task of the cytopathologist to distinguish benign and malignant primary bone tumours from metastatic deposits and from the range of benign reactive and inflammatory conditions of bone

Table 12.1 Different preparation methods of fine needle aspirates for immunocytochemistry. Advantages and disadvantages

Preparation method	Advantages	Disadvantages
Direct smear	No preparation	Stripped nuclei and cytoplasmic background make evaluation of cytoplasmic antibodies difficult. No problem with nuclear antibodies
Cytospin preparation	For many years the most common method for immunocytochemistry	False negative results may happen when the expression of antibodies is focal
Cell block preparation	A cell block preparation is to compare with a histological 'mini-biopsy'. Easy to compare results with IC on histological samples and to perform controls	At times difficult to aspirate sufficient material for preparation
Liquid based cytology (ThinPrep)	Monolayer of cells. 'Clean' background. Material can be saved	All antibodies not yet tested and evaluated

Technical procedures (Table 12.1)

FNA of soft tissue tumours

- Performed in the same way as for epithelial tumours
- For deep-seated intramuscular or intermuscular tumours, a needle with a stylet is preferable to avoid sampling subcutaneous fat and other tissue surrounding the tumour
- The orthopaedic surgeon ought to decide the site of the insertion point, but if this is not possible, the vertex of the tumour is the best choice
- Tattooing of the skin area at the insertion point is valuable if the surgeon wishes to include the needle tract in the surgical specimen
- Core needle biopsy for immunohistochemistry can also be taken

FNA of bone

- It is not possible to penetrate intact cortical bone with thin needles
- Partly destroyed or eroded bone can usually be penetrated quite easily with a 22-gauge needle
- If the cortical bone is almost intact, an 18-gauge needle can be used, through which a 23-gauge needle may be inserted into the lesion and multiple aspirations performed
- Local anaesthetic must be used before aspiration

Ancillary methods

Immunocytochemistry

Immunocytochemistry is at present the most common ancillary method used. When aspirates are used for immunocytochemistry, different preparation methods have been tried and used (see Chapter 13 Immunocytochemistry).

Cytogenetics

Cytogenetics, especially molecular genetic techniques such as RT-PCR and FISH, have during recent years been important diagnostic aids. FNA preparations are suitable for both these techniques (see Table 12.6, p. 385).

Cytological findings in normal and reactive soft tissues

Cytological findings: normal soft tissues

Fibrous tissue

- Normal fibroblasts are spindle-shaped cells with slender contours. Cytoplasmic borders may be indistinct but unipolar or bipolar processes can usually be seen

Adipose tissue

- Normal adipose tissue cells are found in fragments or clusters in smears showing large fat cells with abundant univacuolated cytoplasm and small dark regular nuclei

Striated muscle

- Fragments of muscle fibres are pink or amphophilic on Papanicolaou staining, eosinophilic with H&E and deep blue in MGG-stained preparations

Cytological findings: reactive soft tissues

Fibroblasts (Fig. 12.35)

Reactive fibroblasts/myofibroblasts:

- Fusiform, rounded or triangular
- Abundant cytoplasm
- Nuclei vary in size and take on rounded, ovoid, spindly or irregular contours
- Chromatin is often irregularly distributed and nucleoli may be prominent
- Binucleated cells are common

Fat (Fig. 12.36)

Reactive adipose tissue fragments may show:

- Myxoid background
- Capillary network is often more prominent
- Fragments are more cellular than normal due to reactive increase in fibroblasts, endothelial cells and sometimes also due to the presence of histiocytes
- Adipocytes may show a multivacuolated cytoplasm
- Histiocytes with vacuolated or foamy cytoplasm are observed

Striated muscle (Fig. 12.37)

The principal reactive changes observed in striated muscle are regenerative in origin.

- Muscle fibres usually appear as large multinucleated cells
- Varying shapes including spindly, rounded and straplike forms. They are known as muscle giant cells (see Nodular fasciitis, p. 376)

Typical examples of reactive fibroblasts/myofibroblasts are present in smears from post-traumatic states and in the benign pseudo-sarcomatous soft tissue lesions.

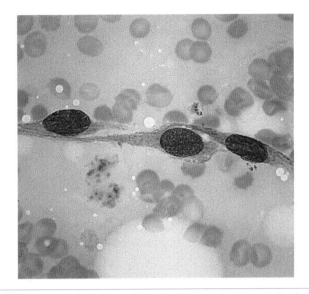

Fig. 12.35[†] Fibroblasts. The nuclei are ovoid, rounded or elongated with regular chromatin distribution and small or absent nucleoli. Stripped nuclei are a common finding.

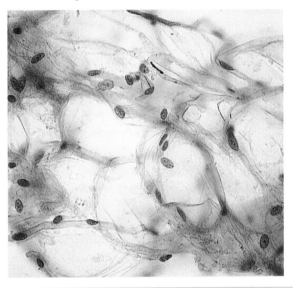

Fig. 12.36[†] Adipose tissue. Reactive adipose tissue is found in post-traumatic states and in adipose tissue surrounding non-adipose tumours.

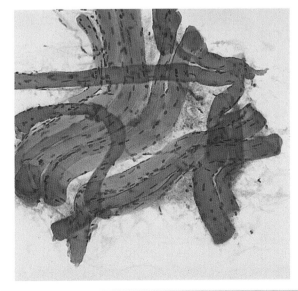

Fig. 12.37[†] Striated muscle. The peripherally placed nuclei are small, rounded and dark. Cross-striations may be observed.

Cytological findings in normal and reactive bone

Osteoblasts (Fig. 12.38)

- Arranged as single cells or small clusters or rows
- Uniform cells of rounded or triangular shape
- Abundant cytoplasm, which contains a characteristic clear area or 'Hof' adjacent to the nucleus or midway in the cytoplasm
- The nuclei are round with a central nucleolus
- Situated very close to the cytoplasmic membrane, almost protruding through it

Osteoclasts (Fig. 12.39)

- Scattered single large cells with abundant cytoplasm and multiple uniform rounded nuclei arranged closely together
- In MGG-stained smears, a characteristic cytoplasmic red granulation is seen

Chondrocytes (Fig. 12.40)

- Almost never seen as dissociated cells
- May be observed in lacunae in cartilaginous fragments composed of a hyaline matrix, which is reddish-blue to violet with MGG, or pink with H&E staining. In Papanicolaou-stained preparations the matrix has a pale grayish-red amphophilic fibrillary appearance

Cytological findings: reactive changes

- Proliferating fibroblasts/myofibroblasts
- Proliferating osteoblasts, often with reactive changes (Fig. 12.38)
- Osteoclastic giant cells (Fig. 12.39)
- Occasionally small calcifications

The characteristic findings are the mixture of proliferating fibroblasts/myofibroblasts, osteoblasts and osteoclastic giant cells.

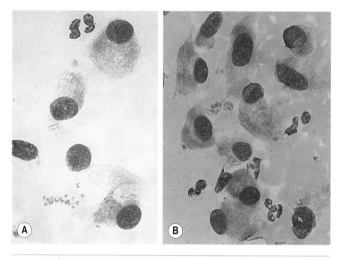

Fig. 12.38[†] Osteoblasts. (A) The typical osteoblast is rounded or triangular with a round eccentrically placed nucleus and a perinuclear clear 'Hof'. (B) Reactive osteoblasts vary in size and shape and anisocytosis may be marked.

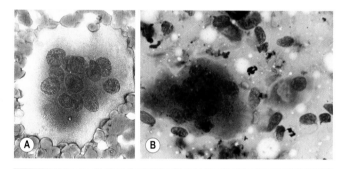

Fig. 12.39[†] Osteoclast. (A) A large cell with abundant cytoplasm showing red granules and multiple uniform nuclei (MGG). (B) An osteoclast-like giant cell and proliferating osteoblasts in myositis ossificans.

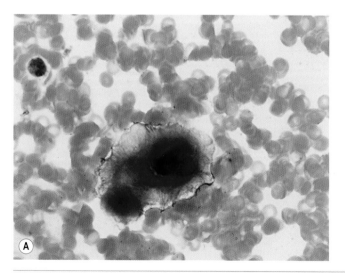

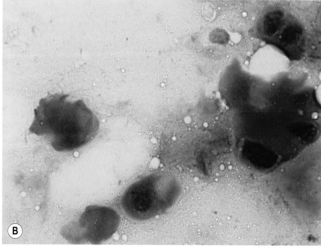

Fig. 12.40[†] (A,B) Chondrocytes. Small fragments of strongly stained hyaline matrix with chondrocytes.

Soft tissue tumours

Benign soft tissue tumours (Figs 12.41–12.44)

Benign soft tissue tumours are far more common than sarcomas. While most tumour types have benign and malignant counterparts, almost all sarcomas arise *de novo* rather than from malignant transformation of a benign tumour.

The main clinical problem is to differentiate the various benign variants from liposarcoma. The main clue to a benign diagnosis is the absence of atypical lipoblasts, but clinical details such as age, site and size are also of importance.

Benign adipocytic tumours (Table 12.2)

Cytological findings: lipoma (Fig. 12.41)

- Fatty tissue fragments
- Few dissociated adipocytes
- Fragments of striated muscle or regenerating muscle fibres ('muscle giant cells') in inter-intramuscular lipoma

Table 12.2 Various variants of benign lipomatous tumours and the main diagnostic pitfalls

Tumour type	Main pitfalls
Common lipoma	Normal adipose tissue
	Important to certify that the needle is within the target
	Well-differentiated liposarcoma
Lipoblastoma/ lipoblastomatosis	Common lipoma
	Myxoid liposarcoma (extremely rare in children)
Spindle cell lipoma	Neurilemmoma
	Myxoid liposarcoma
	Low-grade myxofibrosarcoma
Pleomorphic lipoma	Well-differentiated liposarcoma
Hibernoma	Common lipoma
	Granular cell tumour
	Adult rhabdomyoma
	Liposarcoma
Chondroid lipoma	Myxoid liposarcoma
	Extraskeletal myxoid chondrosarcoma

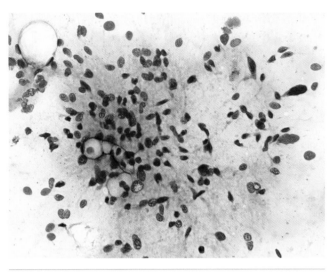

Fig. 12.42† Spindle cell lipoma. Smear from a tumour with abundant myxoid matrix, few fat cells and multiple uniform spindle cells (MGG).

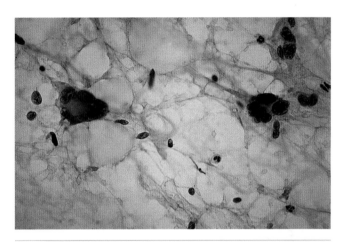

Fig. 12.43† Pleomorphic lipoma. Floret cells in FNA of pleomorphic lipoma. Large multinucleated cells with abundant cytoplasm and with overlapping nuclei along the cytoplasmic border.

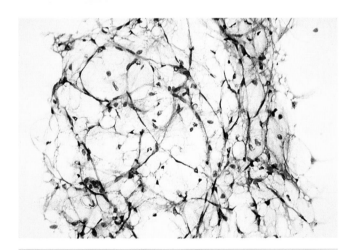

Fig. 12.41† Lipoma. Part of a fragment of adipose tissue. Large fat cells with small, dark nuclei. Thin capillary strands intersect the fragment.

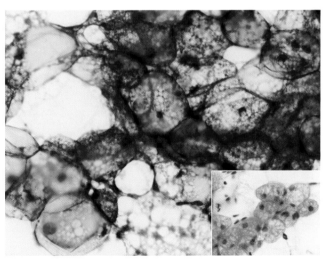

Fig. 12.44† Hibernoma. Small tumour fragments composed of vacuolated fat cells with small nuclei. (Inset) H&E appearance of hibernoma.

Benign fibroblastic/myofibroblastic and fibrohistiocytic tumours

Nodular fasciitis

Nodular fasciitis is the commonest of the so-called benign pseudosarcomatous lesions. It affects all age groups but is most common in young adults. It is usually subcutaneous and the predilection sites are the upper extremities, trunk, and the head and neck region.

Cytological findings: nodular fasciitis (Fig. 12.45)

- Cellular aspirates
- Myxoid background matrix
- Dispersed cells are mixed with clusters or closely packed sheets of cells
- More or less marked anisocytosis and anisokaryosis
- Cells resembling ganglion cells
- Admixture of leucocytes and histiocytes

Proliferative myositis/fasciitis (Fig. 12.46)

Proliferative myositis/fasciitis is another pseudosarcomatous lesion, usually involving the trunk.

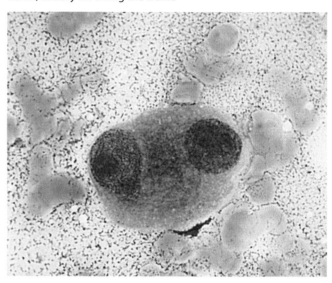

Fig. 12.46† Proliferative myositis/fasciitis: a characteristic cell; large, rounded and binucleate with abundant cytoplasm and nuclei opposite each other.

Desmoid fibromatosis

- A proliferation of fibroblasts, often in the shoulder region
- May recur locally

Cytological findings: desmoid fibromatosis (Fig. 12.47)

- Variable cell yield
- Cell clusters and dispersed cells
- Fragments of collagenised stroma
- The fibroblasts are spindle shaped with fusiform nuclei with moderate anisokaryosis
- Preserved cells show cytoplasmic processes
- Stripped nuclei common
- When smears originate from an infiltrative area of striated muscle, 'muscle giant cells' are found

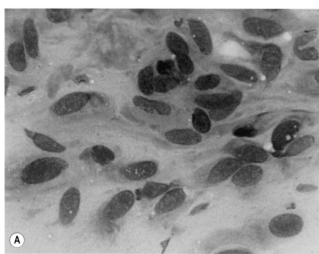

(A)

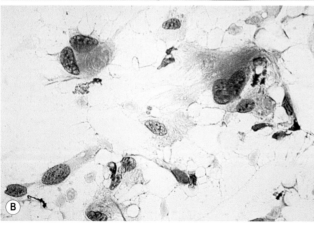

(B)

Fig. 12.45† Nodular fasciitis. (A) A myxoid background matrix with dispersed fibroblasts/myofibroblasts displaying moderate variation in shape and size. (B) Two binucleate cells, closely resembling ganglion cells, and one normal fibroblast.

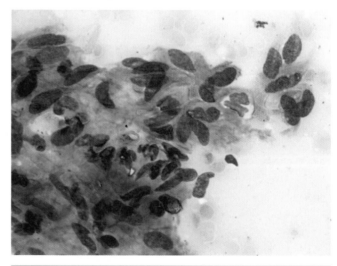

Fig. 12.47† Desmoid fibromatosis. A cluster of loosely attached fibroblast-like cells with ovoid nuclei and greyish-blue cytoplasm.

Tumours of peripheral nerves

Cytological findings: neurilemmoma (Figs 12.48, 12.49)

- Variable cellularity
- Tumour tissue fragments vary in size and cellularity
- Cohesive cells, rarely single tumour cells
- Occasional palisades of cells
- Indistinct cytoplasm, elongated nuclei, pointed ends
- Small rounded cells with rounded nuclei occasionally seen in moderate nuclear pleomorphism
- Myxoid background matrix occasionally
- Fragmented fibrillary background fragments

Cytological findings: granular cell tumour (Fig. 12.50)

- Dispersed cells and clusters
- Naked nuclei common
- Round nuclei, bland chromatin, prominent nucleoli
- Abundant granular cytoplasm, when preserved

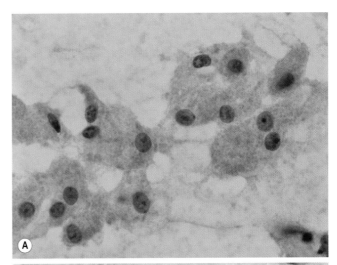

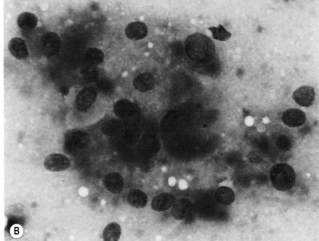

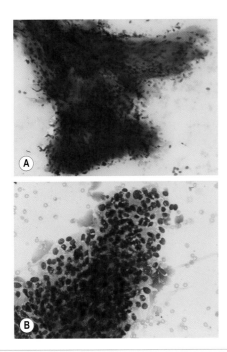

Fig. 12.48† Neurilemmoma. (A) A tumour tissue fragment with irregular borders with varying cellularity. (B) Small cells with rounded 'lymphocyte-like' nuclei are occasionally seen in the tumour fragments.

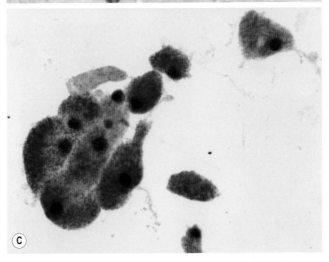

Fig. 12.49† Ancient neurilemmoma. The large cells with pleomorphic, hyperchromatic, sometimes bizarre nuclei typical of an ancient neurilemmoma are deceptively like sarcoma cells.

Fig. 12.50† (A,B) Granular cell tumour. The tumour cells have abundant granular cytoplasm and rounded bland nuclei with prominent nucleoli. (C) ThinPrep-preparation stained with S 100 protein.

Miscellaeneous soft tissue tumours
(Figs 12.51–12.54 and Table 12.3)

Table 12.3 Soft tissue tumours with a myxoid background matrix. Important cytological features in the differential diagnosis

Tumour	Cytological findings
Nodular fasciitis	Marked anisocytosis and anisokaryosis in proliferating fibroblasts/myofibroblasts. Single and binucleated cells resembling ganglion cells
Neurilemmoma	Mainly tissue fragments, dispersed cells uncommon. Fibrillary background in fragments. Nuclei with pointed ends, comma or fish-hook shaped. Nuclear palisading. Infrequently Verocay body structures
Neurofibroma	Mixture of dispersed cells and cell clusters. Cell morphology as neurilemmoma
Intramuscular myxoma	Abundant myxoid background. Rather poor cellularity. Slender tumour cells with long cytoplasmic processes and elongated nuclei. Occasional vessel fragments and 'muscle giant cells' in background
Ganglion	Abundant myxoid background. Poor cellularity. Scattered round cells with rounded nuclei
Myxofibrosarcoma	Abundant myxoid background. Tumour tissue fragments mixed with dispersed cells. Curvilinear vessel fragments in the myxoid matrix. Variable cellular and nuclear atypia
Low-grade fibromyxoid sarcoma	Variable pattern, often myxoid background. Dispersed cells mixed with cell clusters. Spindle cells with slight to moderate atypia. Occasionally curvilinear vessel fragments in the myxoid matrix
Myxoid liposarcoma	Abundant myxoid background. Tumour tissue fragments with myxoid matrix and a distinct branching capillary network. Slight to moderately atypical lipoblasts
Extraskeletal myxoid chondrosarcoma	Varying amount of myxoid matrix. Cell clusters, cell balls and branching cells mixed with dispersed cells. Rounded, elongated cells. Rounded, ovoid or spindly nuclei. Slight to moderate atypia

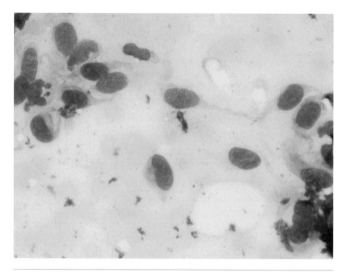

Fig. 12.52[†] Soft tissue leiomyoma. The tumour cells have faintly stained grey-blue cytoplasm and blunt-ended uniform nuclei.

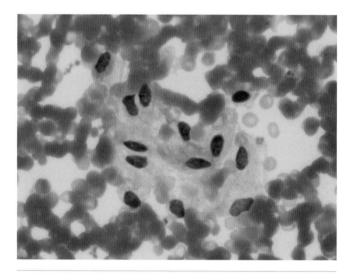

Fig. 12.53[†] Haemangioma. A small cluster of spindle-shaped cells with ovoid nuclei in a haemorrhagic background.

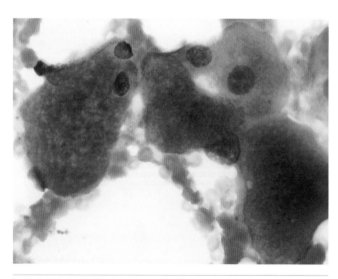

Fig. 12.51[†] Adult rhabdomyoma. Large cells with abundant granulated cytoplasm and rounded nuclei with prominent nucleoli.

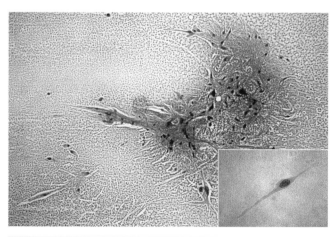

Fig. 12.54[†] Intramuscular myxoma. Overview: an abundant myxoid background matrix and myxoid tumour fragment containing spindle cells with bipolar cytoplasm. (Inset) The typical myxoma cell has very long, thin cytoplasmic processes.

Liposarcoma (Figs 12.55–12.57)

Malignant tumours of adipose tissue according to the WHO classification of soft tissue tumours

- Atypical lipomatous tumour/well-differentiated liposarcoma
  - lipoma-like
  - sclerosing
  - inflammatory
  - spindle cell
- Dedifferentiated liposarcoma
- Myxoid liposarcoma
- Hypercellular (round cell liposarcoma)
- Pleomorphic liposarcoma

Cytological findings: myxoid liposarcoma (Fig. 12.56)

- Abundant myxoid background substance
- Vacuolated tumour tissue fragments with myxoid matrix and branching capillary network
- Almost no dispersed cells
- Uni- or multivacuolated slightly atypical lipoblasts, often alongside the capillary fragments
- Spindly or rounded uniform mesenchymal cells other than lipoblasts
- No mitoses
- Cytogenetics: see Table 12.6, p. 385

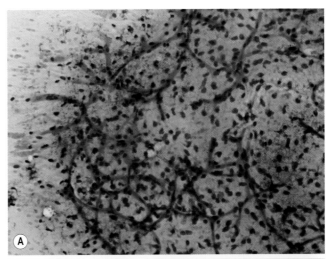

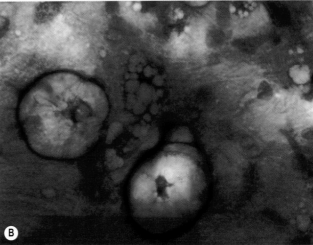

Fig. 12.56[†] Myxoid liposarcoma. (A) A moderately cellular tissue fragment with a myxoid background matrix and a network of branching capillaries. A few univacuolated lipoblasts are seen (MGG). (B) Detail from the tumour fragment in (A). Multivacuolated lipoblasts with scalloped nuclei.

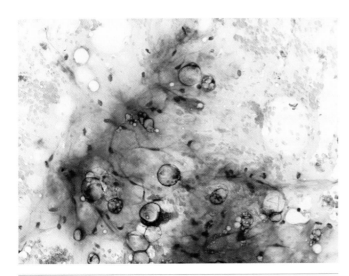

Fig. 12.55[†] Atypical lipomatous tumour/well-differentiated liposarcoma. In this case, slightly to moderately atypical, uni- and multivacuolated lipoblasts predominate.

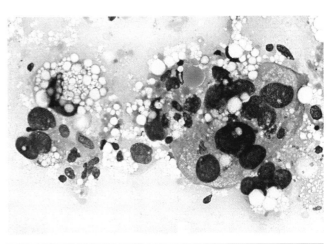

Fig. 12.57[†] Pleomorphic liposarcoma. Highly atypical lipoblasts, some of which are multinucleated.

Cytological findings: pleomorphic sarcoma of MFH type (Fig. 12.58)

- Often highly cellular yield
- Tissue fragments, cell clusters, dispersed tumour cells
- Spindle-shaped fibroblast-like cells
- Pleomorphic, histiocyte-like tumour cells
- Tumour cells of indeterminate origin
- Large multinucleated tumour cells
- Often marked nuclear pleomorphism and atypia. Large irregular nucleoli
- Mitotic figures, often atypical

Cytological findings: malignant peripheral nerve sheath tumour (Fig. 12.59)

- Cellular smears
- A mixture of fascicles of tightly packed sarcoma cells
- Dispersed cells
- Stripped nuclei
- Indistinct cytoplasm
- Elongated nuclei, often with pointed ends or wavy configuration
- Often embedded in a fibrillary background substance similar to the background in neurilemmoma aspirates

Cytological findings: leiomyosarcoma (Fig. 12.60)

- Very variable cell yield
- Cohesive clusters, tissue fragments or large fascicular tumour fragments
- Rather few dissociated cells
- Blue or magenta background matrix in clusters and fascicles
- Abundant cell cytoplasm with indistinct borders
- Degenerate bare nuclei
- Blunt-ended or cigar-shaped elliptic nuclei, sometimes segmented or with nuclear vacuoles

Differential diagnosis: pleomorphic sarcomas

- Pleomorphic liposarcoma
- High-grade pleomorphic leiomyosarcoma
- Pleomorphic MPNST
- Anaplastic large cell lymphoma
- Anaplastic carcinoma
- Sarcoma-like malignant melanoma

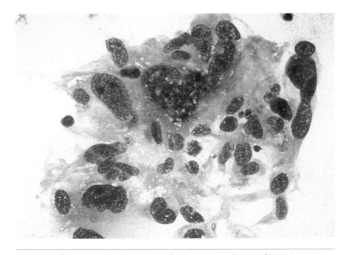

Fig. 12.58[†] Pleomorphic sarcoma of MFH type. A cluster of loosely attached pleomorphic cells with marked anisokaryosis.

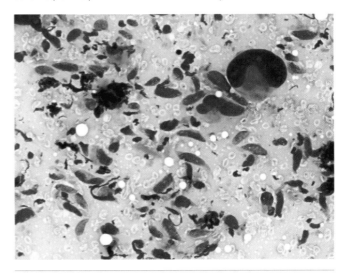

Fig. 12.59[†] Malignant peripheral nerve sheath tumour. Atypical spindle cells in a fibrillary background matrix. Note the nuclei with pointed ends. Atypical spindle cells with fibrillary cytoplasm; nuclei have coarse chromatin and prominent nucleoli and marked cellular pleomorphism.

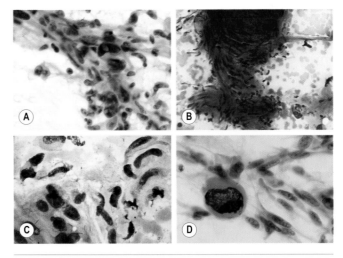

Fig. 12.60[†] Leiomyosarcoma. (A) A fascicle of cohesive tumour cells mixed with few dispersed cells. (B) The cells in the fragments are often embedded in a dense matrix. (C) Part of a fascicle of elongated cells with blunt-ended nuclei. (D) In high-grade tumours, mitotic figures may be found.

Rhabdomyosarcoma

Rhabdomyosarcoma is an aggressive tumour predominantly of young adults and children, widely distributed anatomically, but found principally in the head and neck region, the genitourinary tract and retroperitoneum, and in the extremities. The classic main histological types in order of frequency are

- Embryonal (Fig. 12.61, Table 12.4)
- Alveolar (Fig. 12.62)
- Pleomorphic (Fig. 12.63)

Further investigations: rhabdomyosarcoma

The immunocytochemical hallmarks of the various subtypes of rhabdomyosarcoma are the positive staining with muscle-specific actin, desmin and the specific markers for striated muscle, myogenin and Myo-D1 (Fig. 12.62). Myoglobin is occasionally present in more differentiated myoblasts. Almost all cases of alveolar rhabdomyosarcoma present with the chromosomal aberration t(2;13)(q35;q14), resulting in a fusion transcript between the PAX3 and FKHR genes (see Ch 11 p. 357 and Table 12.6, p. 385).

Table 12.4 Important cytological findings in the differential diagnosis of small cell malignant tumours in childhood and adolescence

Tumour	Cytology
Embryonal rhabdomyosarcoma	Occasionally myxoid background matrix. Often marked anisocytosis and anisokaryosis. Fusiform, strap-shaped, ribbon-like, triangular or rounded myoblast-like cells. Predominance of fusiform cells in the spindle cell type
Alveolar rhabdomyosarcoma	Predominantly small cell pattern. Rounded or pear-shaped primitive myoblast-like cells with eccentric nuclei. Cytoplasm eosinophilic in H&E and grey-blue in MGG. Cytoplasmic vacuolation. Occasionally multinucleated giant cells with small nuclei
Neuroblastoma	Small cell pattern. Occasionally large cells resembling ganglion cells. Mixture of dispersed cells and cell clusters of loosely attached cells. Moulded cell clusters. Neutrophil background. Occasional rosettes. Dark rounded or irregular nuclei. In preserved cells, often long thin cytoplasmic processes connecting one cell to another
Classic, conventional Ewing's sarcoma	Mixture of dispersed cells and groups of cells. Often stripped nuclei and cytoplasmic background Double cell population. Large light cells with rounded nuclei and abundant thin cytoplasm with vacuoles or clear spaces. Small dark cells with scanty cytoplasm and irregular hyperchromatic nuclei. Bland nuclear morphology. Inconspicuous nucleoli
Atypical Ewing's sarcoma/PNET	Variable anisocytosis and anisokaryosis. Double cell population less evident. Often rosettes. Rounded or spindly cells with small cytoplasmic processes. In PNET often marked nuclear pleomorphism (rhabdomyoblast-like cells, cells with rhabdoid morphology)
Desmoplastic small round cell tumour	Mixture of dispersed cells and clusters of loosely attached cells. Rounded or ovoid cells with scant cytoplasm and rounded, ovoid nuclei with finely granular chromatin and small nucleoli

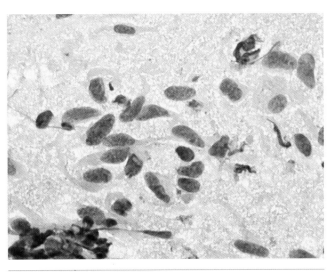

Fig. 12.61[†] Embryonal rhabdomyosarcoma, spindle cell variant. Moderately pleomorphic spindly cells with fusiform nuclei with alternating pointed or blunt ends.

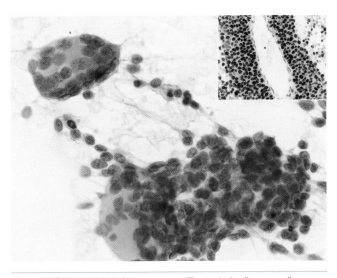

Fig. 12.62[†] Alveolar rhabdomyosarcoma. The typical cells are small, rhabdomyoblast-like with eosinophilic cytoplasm and rounded paracentral nuclei with prominent nucleoli. The small cell population is often mixed with multinucleated tumour cells. (Inset) Nuclear positivity for Myo-D1.

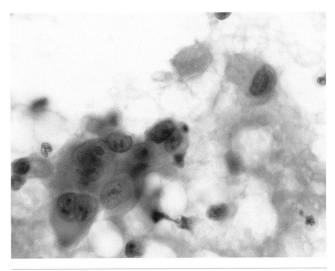

Fig. 12.63[†] Pleomorphic rhabdomyosarcoma. One clue to the diagnosis is the presence of highly atypical myoblast-like cells with eosinophilic cytoplasm and eccentric atypical nuclei.

Synovial sarcoma

Synovial sarcoma may present in the vicinity of joints but most often occurs in the extremities without any connection to joints, and is also found at other sites such as trunk wall, the abdominal wall and pharyngeal region.

Cytological findings (Figs 12.64, 12.65)

- Cellular aspirates
- Dispersed cells and tissue fragments
- Stripped nuclei
- Branching capillaries with attached tumour cells
- Spindly or ovoid bland nuclei
- In biphasic tumours, occasionally small acinar-like structures
- Mitotic figures common in the tissue fragments
- The presence of mast cells in many aspirates
- Immunocytochemistry: EMA, CK7, CK19, BCL2, CD99, S100 +/−
- Cytogenetics, see Table 12.6, p. 385

Differential diagnosis

- Synovial sarcoma may be very difficult to distinguish from the other spindle cell tumours such as solitary fibrous tumour and spindle cell sarcomas such as fibrosarcoma, MPNST and malignant haemangiopericytoma

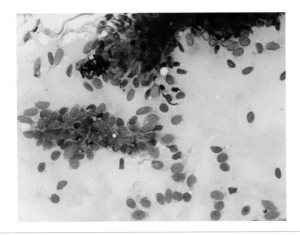

Fig. 12.64† Synovial sarcoma. The typical smear is composed of a mixture of fragments of tightly packed cells and dispersed cells of which stripped nuclei are common.

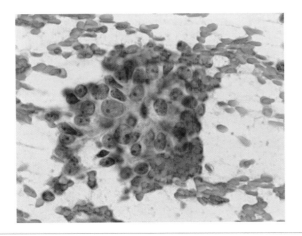

Fig. 12.65† Synovial sarcoma. In biphasic tumours, glandular-like structures may be present.

Alveolar soft part sarcoma (Fig. 12.66)

This rare sarcoma, occurring mainly in young adults and adolescents, develops in the deep soft tissues of the lower extremities or in soft tissues internally.

Cytological findings: Alveolar soft part sarcoma

- single and small groups of polyhedral malignant cells
- granular cytoplasm
- anisokaryosis and prominent nucleoli
- many bare nuclei
- characteristic crystals observed in PAP-stained smears within the cytoplasm and in the background near the tumor cells
- Immunocytochemistry: Desmin pos, Actin pos
- Cytogenetics, see Table 12.6, p. 385

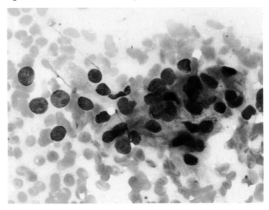

Fig. 12.66† Alveolar soft part sarcoma. Often a mixture of clustered and dispersed cells. Stripped nuclei with prominent nucleoli is a common finding.

Clear cell sarcoma (Fig. 12.67)

Clear cell sarcoma or malignant melanoma of soft parts is prone to occur in relation to tendons and aponeuroses in young adults.

Immunocytochemically, most clear cell sarcomas stain positively for S-100 and HMB-45. Metastatic melanoma is the most important diagnostic pitfall with cytological and immunocytochemical findings the same as clear cell sarcoma. However, characteristic translocation (t12;22) is seen only in clear cell sarcoma (see Table 12.6, p. 385).

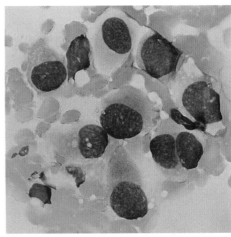

Fig. 12.67† Clear cell sarcoma. A group of cells of epithelial appearance with sharp cytoplasmic borders and rounded nuclei of sarcoma cells. Cells are mostly dissociated, but small clusters of loosely attached cells are also present. The cells are spindle shaped or polygonal with abundant pale cytoplasm and rounded or ovoid large nuclei.

Definition of the cytological criteria for interpreting FNA samples from primary bone tumours is at present largely confined to malignant neoplasms, since FNA findings in very few benign tumours have been thoroughly documented (Table 12.5).

Table 12.5 Primary bone tumours/lesions with clearly defined cytological features enabling a specific diagnosis to be made

Benign	Malignant
Giant cell tumour	Osteosarcoma
Osteoblastoma	Chondrosarcoma
Chondroblastoma	Ewing's family of tumours
Langerhans cell histiocytosis	Chordoma

Chondroma

Occur at all ages and may be multiple.

Cytological findings: chondroma (Fig. 12.68)

- Cartilaginous fragments with cells in lacunar spaces
- Cells with small regular nuclei
- Cellular pleomorphism not uncommon

Chondroblastoma

Chondroblastomas occur most often in young people, especially in the second decade, but are commoner in males, and are often painful. The most usual site is the epiphysis of the long bones, but they may also be found in small tubular and flat bones.

Cytological findings: chondroblastoma (Fig. 12.69)

- Mononuclear cells, well-formed cytoplasm, round nuclei
- Multinucleated osteoclast-like cells
- Fragments of chondroid matrix

Chondrosarcoma

This group of tumours occurs in adults, in the fourth to seventh decades. Predominant sites are the bones of the trunk and upper ends of femur and humerus, and a few are extraskeletal.

Cytological features: chondrosarcoma (Fig. 12.70)

- Fragments of hyaline cartilage
- Myxoid background matrix
- Mononuclear and binucleated tumour cells often in lacunae
- Large rounded individual cells with well-defined cytoplasm
- Nuclei rounded or irregular and lobulated
- Cytogenetics: see Table 12.6, p. 385

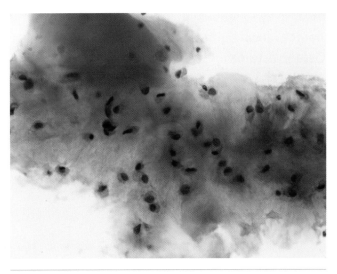

Fig. 12.68[†] Chondroma. A cartilaginous fragment, strongly blue-violet with irregularly distributed small cells with bland nuclei.

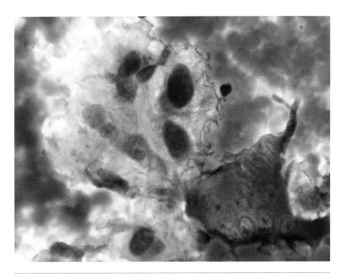

Fig. 12.69[†] Chondroblastoma. A small group of chondroblast-like cells embedded in a red-blue chondroid matrix. One osteoclast-like cell (*bottom right corner*).

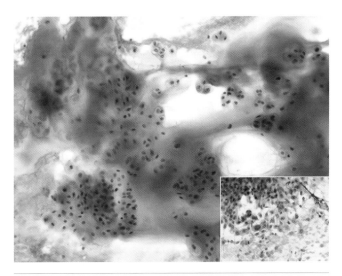

Fig. 12.70[†] Chondrosarcoma. Low-grade malignant chondrosarcoma. Cartilaginous fragments with irregularly dispersed uniform cells. Note the variable cellularity (MGG). (Inset) High-grade malignant chondrosarcoma. A highly cellular tumour fragment exhibiting marked nuclear atypia.

Osteogenic tumours

Osteoblastoma

This benign bone-forming tumour has a definitive predilection for males in the first three decades of life and may be difficult to diagnose on FNA.

Cytological findings: osteoblastoma (Fig. 12.71)

- Cells of osteoblastic type, mononuclear and binucleated
- Clusters of spindle cells
- Osteoclastic cells

Osteosarcoma

Osteosarcoma is the commonest of all primary malignant bone tumours. The majority of patients are in the second and third decades of life, but osteosarcoma has been reported in children less than 10 years of age and in middle-aged or elderly patients. Histologically, there are several types of osteosarcoma: osteoblastic, chondroblastic, fibroblastic, telangiectatic and small cell type.

Cytological findings: osteosarcoma (Fig. 12.72)

- Mixture of cell clusters and dispersed cells
- Pleomorphic pattern of obviously malignant cells
- Relatively frequent mitoses, including atypical forms
- Intercellular tumour matrix of osteoid within clusters
- Benign osteoclastic giant cells
- Epithelioid tumour cells, which may be of osteoblastic type or resemble chondroblasts in osteoblastic or chondroblastic variants, respectively
- Atypical spindle-shaped fibroblast-like cells in fibroblastic types

Differential diagnosis: osteosarcoma in FNA

- Benign tumours/lesions
- Reactive osteoblastic proliferations (pseudomalignant myositis ossificans)
- Fracture callus
- Aggressive osteoblastoma
- Giant cell tumour
- Malignant tumours
- Primary pleomorphic sarcoma of bone (MFH-like)
- High-grade malignant chondrosarcoma
- Dedifferentiated chondrosarcoma
- Metastatic anaplastic carcinoma
- Anaplastic large cell lymphoma
- Ewing's family of tumours (small cell osteosarcoma)

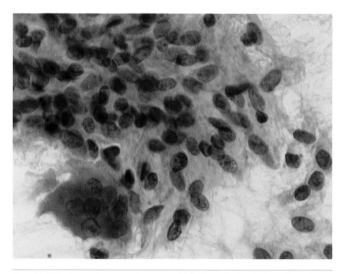

Fig. 12.71[†] Osteoblastoma. A group of tightly packed spindly cells and osteoblast-like cells and one osteoclast-like cell.

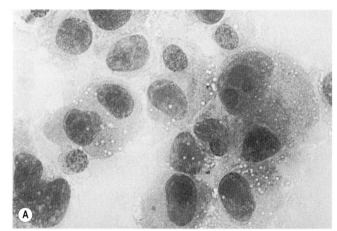

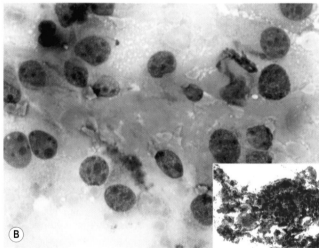

Fig. 12.72[†] Osteoblastic osteosarcoma. (A) Mostly rounded tumour cells with eccentric nuclei and abundant cytoplasm (MGG). (B) Thin strands of tumour osteoid encircling a group of tumour cells. (Inset) Osteoblastic osteosarcoma. Strong cytoplasmic staining for alkaline phosphatase.

Bone: miscellaneous lesions

Langerhans cell histiocytosis (Fig. 12.73)

Langerhans cell histiocytosis, when localised in the bone also known as eosinophilic granuloma, is a lesion characterised by proliferation of histiocytic cells of Langerhans type, with a variable number of eosinophils, neutrophils, lymphocytes and plasma cells.

Ewing's family of tumours (ES/PNET)

ES/PNET comprises a number of tumours of presumed neuroectodermal origin, involving extraskeletal and skeletal sites. ES/PNET includes classic Ewing's sarcoma, atypical Ewing's sarcoma, the so-called Askin tumour and peripheral neuroepithelioma (see also Ch 11 and Table 12.6 on this page).

Cytological findings: classic ES (Fig. 12.74)

- As a rule, cellular smears
- A mixture of dissociated cells and cell clusters and groups
- Naked nuclei and a cytoplasmic background common
- A double cell population; large cells with abundant cytoplasm with vacuoles or clear spaces (dissolved glycogen) and rounded bland nuclei with finely granular chromatin
- Small nucleoli (large light cells) and smaller cells with scanty cytoplasm and irregular dark nuclei (small, dark cells)
- The dark cells often in moulded groups within the cell clusters

Diagnostic pitfalls: Ewing's sarcoma

- Osteomyelitis
- Primary bone sarcomas (small cell osteosarcoma, mesenchymal chondrosarcoma)
- Langerhans' cell histiocytosis/eosinophilic granuloma of bone
- Other small round cell tumours (from soft tissues and metastatic neuroblastoma)

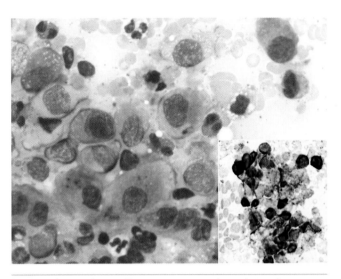

Fig. 12.73[†] Langerhans cell histiocytosis. A mixed population of Langerhans histiocytes, eosinophils and neutrophils. The typical nuclear morphology, irregular nuclei with folded nuclear membrane, the so-called 'coffee-bean' nuclei. Inset: CD1 positivity confirms the diagnosis.

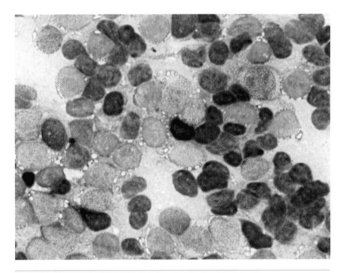

Fig. 12.74[†] Classic Ewing's sarcoma. Typical double cell population with large light cells featuring vacuolated cytoplasm and small dark cells with irregular dark nuclei.

Table 12.6 Cytogenetic investigations in some of the common sarcoma types

Tumour type	Cytogenetic abnormality
Alveolar soft part sarcoma	t(X;17)(p11;q25)
Clear cell sarcoma	t(12;22) and t(2;22)
Extraskeletal myxoid chondrosarcoma	t(9;22)(q22;q12)
Ewing sarcoma/PNET	t(11;22)(q24;q12)
Liposarcoma, myxoid and round cell	t(12;16((q13;p11)
Liposarcoma, well differentiated	Ring chromosome 12
Rhabdomyosarcoma, alveolar	t(2;13)(q35;q14)
Rhabdomyosarcoma, embryonal	Loss of 11p15
Synovial sarcoma	t(X;18;p11;q11)

Bone: metastatic tumours and reporting of FNA in bone and soft tissue lesions

Metastatic lesions are the malignant tumours most commonly encountered in bone. Carcinomatous metastases in the skeleton are mainly derived from the breast, kidney, lung, prostate, thyroid, liver and cutaneous and extracutaneous malignant melanoma. See Table 12.7 for the main immunostains used for identifying the primary tumour.

Table 12.7 Important antibodies to apply to suggest the primary site when a bone metastasis is the first sign of the tumour

Primary site	Antibody	Comment
Kidney	CK8/18; CK7/20; CD10,RCC	CK8/18+; CD10+; CK7/20–
Lung	Squamous cell carcinoma: CK5/6; CK7	CK5/6+; CK7 +/–
	Adenocarcinoma: CK7/20; TTF-1	CK7+; TTF-1+; CK20–
	Small cell carcinoma: CK7/20; TTF-1, synaptophysin, CD 56	TTF-1+; CK7/20–
Breast	CK7/20; ER; PGR, G6PD-15, mammoglobin	CK7+; CK20–
Thyroid	Thyroglobulin; TTF-1, calcitonin	TTF-1+; calc–
Prostate	CK8/18; CK7/20; PSA	CK8/18+; CK7/20–
Liver	Hepar-1; pCEA; CK7/20	CK7/20–
Malignant melanoma	S-100 protein; HMB45; Melan A	S-100+; HMB45+; Melan A+

Table 12.8 Soft tissue tumours/lesions with definitive cytological features making diagnosis of tumour type possible

Benign	Malignant
Nodular fasciitis	Leiomyosarcoma
Proliferative fasciitis/myositis	Liposarcoma
Myositis ossificans	Synovial sarcoma
Lipoma	Rhabdomyosarcoma
Neurilemmoma	Ewing's family of tumours
Desmoid fibromatosis	Neuroblastoma
Elastofibroma	Low-grade fibromyxoid sarcoma
Solitary fibrous tumour	Myxofibrosarcoma
Intramuscular myxoma	Angiosarcoma
	Malignant peripheral nerve sheath tumour (MPNST)
	Extraskeletal myxoid chondrosarcoma
	Epithelioid sarcoma

The cytological report

On the basis of clinical data and radiological findings alone, it may be difficult even for experienced orthopaedic surgeons and radiologists to decide whether a soft tissue tumour is benign or malignant or even if the lesion is a true soft tissue tumour.

The cytological diagnosis becomes the most important parameter in determining further management. See Tables 12.8 and 12.9 for the main tumour types and categories.

To avoid misleading diagnoses and misinterpretation of reports, FNA diagnoses of soft tissue and bone tumours can be issued, subject to prior discussion with the orthopedic surgeons and radiologists, as follows:

- sarcoma, including highly suspicious for sarcoma
- malignant tumour other than sarcoma
- benign
- non-diagnostic, including insufficient material for diagnosis and inconclusive findings with regard to benignity or malignancy

Table 12.9 Soft tissue sarcoma classification and grading based on predominant cytomorphological phenotypes

Small round cell sarcomas	Spindle cell sarcomas
Ewing's sarcoma/primitive neuroectodermal tumour (PNET)	Fibrosarcoma
Rhabdomyosarcoma (childhood types)	Leiomyosarcoma
Neuroblastoma	Synovial sarcoma
Mesenchymal chondrosarcoma	Malignant peripheral nerve sheath tumour
Desmoplastic small round cell tumour	Gastrointestinal stromal tumour (GIST)
Pleomorphic sarcomas	Epithelioid/polygonal cell sarcomas
Pleomorphic malignant fibrous histiocytoma (MFH)	Epithelioid sarcoma
	Clear cell sarcoma (melanoma of soft parts)
Pleomorphic liposarcoma	Alveolar soft part sarcoma
Extraskeletal osteosarcoma	Malignant schwannoma
Pleomorphic rhabdomyosarcoma	Malignant granular cell tumour
Pleomorphic leiomyosarcoma	
Angiosarcoma	
Myxoid sarcoma	
Myxoid liposarcoma	
Myxofibrosarcoma (myxoid MFH)	
Low-grade fibromyxoid sarcoma	
Extraskeletal myxoid chondrosarcoma	

(Modified from Singh HK, Kilpatrick SE, Silverman JF. Fine needle aspiration biopsy of soft tissue sarcomas: utility and diagnostic challenges. Adv Anat Pathol 2004; 11:24–37.)

Synovial fluid

- Synovial fluid is a transudate of plasma with added saccharide-rich molecules, notably hyaluronic acid and lubricin, produced by synoviocytes lining the cartilage covering the bone ends of certain joints, with no underlying basement membrane
- The fluid allows multidirectional movement of the bones forming the joint
- Synovial fluid cytology is used mainly for diagnosis of inflammatory and degenerative joint diseases

Basic approach to synovial fluid microscopy

- Combines examination of cells with recognition of non-cellular particulate material (crystals, etc.)
- Quantification of cell types is important in assessing abnormal joint fluid
- A four-step sequential analysis is used:
  - Gross analysis: colour, clarity and viscosity
  - The nucleated cell count performed on an unstained saline suspension, expressed per unit volume
  - The 'wet prep': a coverslipped drop is examined with part-closed condenser and polarised light for crystals, and particulate material (see Figs 12.75–12.78)
  - The cytocentrifuged preparation (see page 388)

The 'wet prep': crystal identification (Figs 12.75–12.78)

- Monosodium urate: 5–30 μm needle-shaped crystals, negatively birefringent. Diagnostic of gout
- Calcium pyrophosphate dehydrate: short rectangles, found with increasing age
- Hydroxyapatite: tiny with polarised light, seen better when stained with Alizarin red and polarised: present in destructive arthropathies
- Lipids: vary in shape and type, e.g. cholesterol, cholesterol esters, found in inflammatory conditions, haemorrhage, trauma
- Steroids: from intra-articular injection, lasting up to 10 weeks

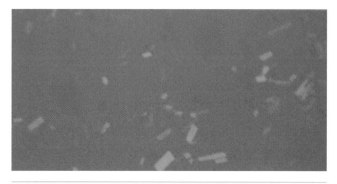

Fig. 12.76[†] Polarised light 'wet prep': note the weakly birefringent crystals of calcium pyrophosphate.

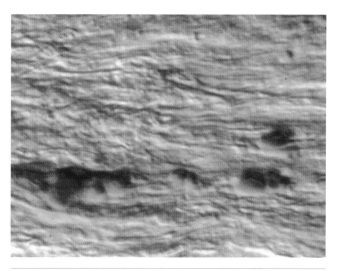

Fig. 12.77[†] Hydroxyapatite crystalloids in a fibrin clot stained with Alizarin red.

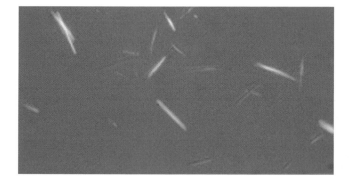

Fig. 12.75[†] Unstained synovial fluid 'wet prep' viewed between crossed polarisers with an interference plate in the light path, giving the magenta background. Note the highly birefringent needle-shaped urate crystals.

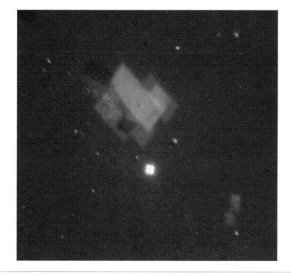

Fig. 12.78[†] Large flat notched plate-like cholesterol crystal with small bright lipid liquid crystal below showing Maltese cross pattern.

The 'wet prep': other particulate material (Fig. 12.79)

- Cartilage fragments: surface sheen with clusters of chondrocytes, seen in osteoarthritis, bone necrosis
- Collagen/fibrocollagenous fragments
- Debris from prostheses can mimic crystals
- Extraneous material: usually iatrogenic
- Ragocytes: cells found in the joints in rheumatoid arthritis; RA cell. Such cells are produced when polymorphonuclear leucocytes ingest aggregated IgG immunoglobulin, rheumatoid factor, fibrin and complement

The cytocentrifuge preparation (Figs 12.80–12.82)

- Fluid usually diluted to standardise, and stained with modified Giemsa and Gram stain for organisms in septic arthritis
- Polymorphs predominate in inflammatory arthropathies (gout, septic and rheumatoid arthritis); lymphocytes, macrophages and synoviocytes in non-inflammatory (osteoarthritis, trauma)
- Rieder cells: 15 μm diameter with large lobed nuclei, a feature of rheumatoid disease due to toxic effects
- Macrophages common in all arthritic types and may ingest apoptotic bodies
- Other cells: eosinophils (haemorrhage), LE cells (ingested nuclear material in lymphocytes suggest LE), mast cells (non-specific)

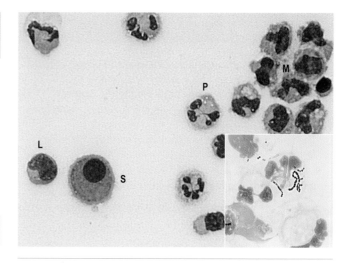

Fig. 12.80† Main cell types in synovial fluid: P, polymorph; L, lymphocyte; M, macrophage; S, synoviocyte. (Inset) Gram-positive cocci in a cytocentrifuge preparation.

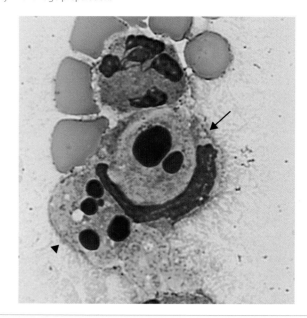

Fig. 12.81† Cytophagocytic mononuclear cell containing an apoptotic cell (*arrow*) with a similar cell at lower left border (*arrowhead*).

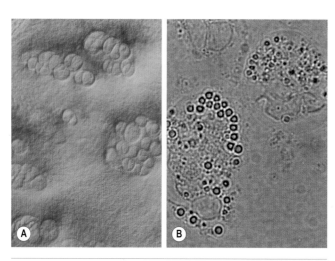

Fig. 12.79† 'Wet preps' showing (A) cartilage fragment with attached clustered chondrocytes, (B) ragocyte with cytoplasmic granules.

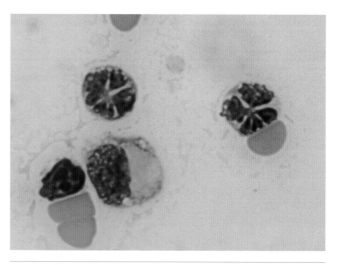

Fig. 12.82† Rieder cells. Note lobulated nuclei with central pale area.

Management of synovial fluid cytology

Figures 12.83–12.85 show algorithms to follow for the diagnostic management of synovial fluid samples.

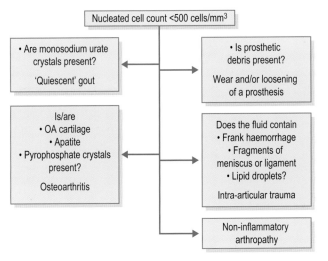

Fig. 12.83† Diagnostic algorithm for a 'low cell count' fluid.

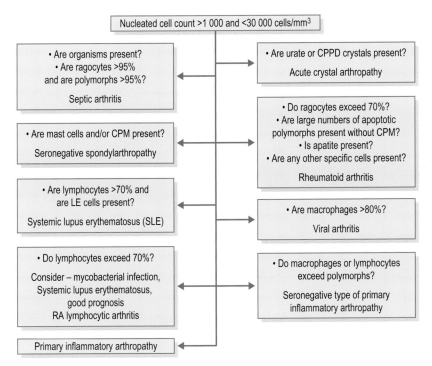

Fig. 12.84† Diagnostic algorithm for a 'conventional inflammatory arthropathy'.

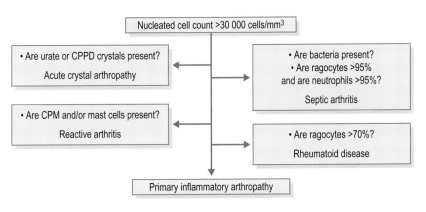

Fig. 12.85† Diagnostic algorithm for a 'high cell count' fluid. There are four main causes of very high cell counts: acute crystal arthritis, septic arthritis, reactive arthritis and an acute rheumatoid flare. However, the last is extremely rare nowadays because of the changing nature of rheumatoid disease and the availability of over-the-counter medications.

CHAPTER 13

Techniques

Contents

Routine procedures – John E. McGloin   392

Immunocytochemistry – Nataša Nolde   398

Polymerase chain reaction – Tim Diss   404

In situ hybridisation (ISH) – Alexander Valent   410

Routine procedures

Exfoliative cytology

The exfoliative material most commonly received in cytology laboratory is from the cervix:

- Cervical, vaginal, endocervical, endometrial
- Brushings – bronchial, biliary, oesophageal, gastrointestinal
- Fluids – urine, body cavity fluid (pleural, peritoneal, pericardial effusions, hydrocele), cerebrospinal (CSF), cystic (breast, thyroid, renal, ovarian), washings
- Secretions – sputum, discharge
- Skin scrape

Collection and transport of cytological material

- Cervical samples are performed by suitably trained sample takers and taken as either alcohol-fixed direct smears or placed in a liquid-based medium for subsequent preparation (Fig. 13.1)
- Fluids are best transported in sterile containers and prepared as fresh as possible. The optimal amount of effusion for cytological investigation is 25 mL but if special investigations or cell blocks are required, then a larger volume will be needed (Figs 13.2, 13.3)
- Washings consist of cells suspended in normal saline and the cells are well preserved. Samples should be free of excessive blood or mucin
- Brushings can be taken as either alcohol-fixed smears or, where the technology is available, in a liquid-based medium. The brush should be rinsed in normal saline to maximise cell yield (Figs 13.4A, B)
- CSF samples are small-volume samples, typically around 1 mL and they deteriorate quickly. They should be transported and processed as soon as possible
- The entire contents of a cyst should be sent to the laboratory, up to 25 mL in volume
- Urine samples should consist of a 2 to 3 hour whole output specimen and not the first of the day or 24 hour collection. Urothelial cells deteriorate with time but the addition of 50 mL industrial methylated spirit (IMS) will act as a preservative
- Sputum samples can be taken first thing in the morning to capture overnight secretions but before teeth brushing or breakfast
- Scrapings from skin and other surfaces should be spread onto glass slides and fixed as appropriate for the staining method

General points

- If immediate transport of samples is not possible, refrigerate at 4°C
- Liquid-based cytology samples are viable for 6 weeks
- Clots can be removed from samples, fixed in formalin and processed in histology to produce sections

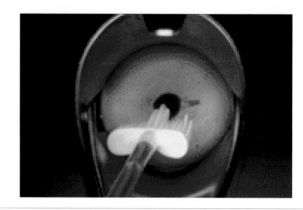

Fig. 13.1 Exfoliative cytology. Cells are removed from the surface of the cervix using a brush.

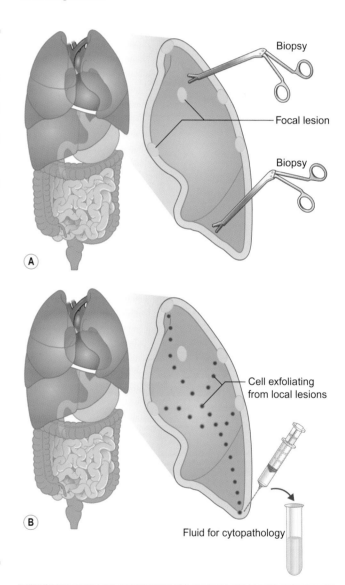

Fig. 13.2 Sampling of pleural lesions: biopsy (A) versus effusion cytology (B). Focal lesions may be missed by biopsy. However, cells exfoliated from any of these focal lesions are pooled in the fluid and should be present in a related effusion or washing. (From Shidham VB, Atkinson BF. Cytopathologic Diagnosis of Serous Fluids. 1st edn. London: Elsevier; 2007)

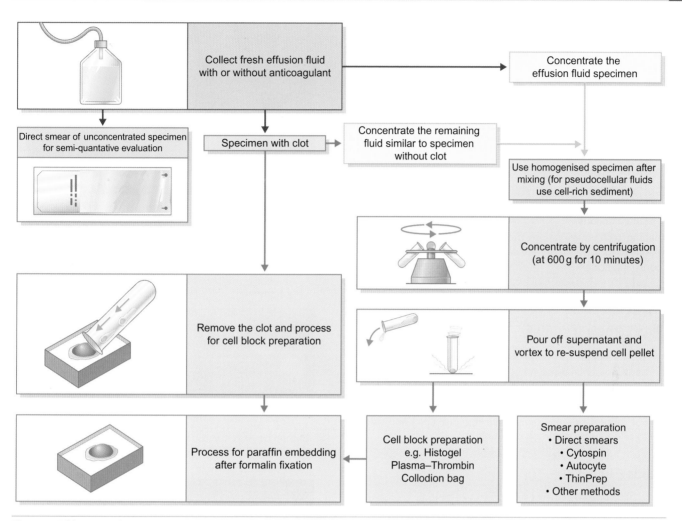

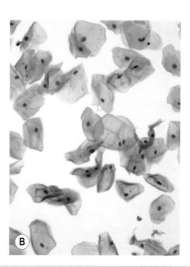

Fig. 13.3 Exfoliative cytology. Treatment pathway for handling serous fluid to produce slides or a cell block. (From Shidham VB, Atkinson BF. Cytopathologic Diagnosis of Serous Fluids. 1st edn. London: Elsevier; 2007)

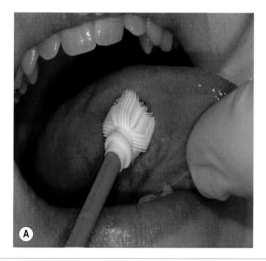

Fig. 13.4A Cells are taken by brushing the oral mucosa. Cells from the brush can either be brushed directly onto a glass slide and fixed or transferred into a liquid medium to be processed later.

Fig. 13.4B Microscopic view of squamous cells taken by oral brushing, smeared directly onto a slide and stained with Papanicolaou stain.

Fine needle aspiration cytology (FNAC)

FNAC is different from exfoliative cytology in that a thin needle is used to obtain cells from a superficial or deep masses. It is a less invasive procedure than biopsy (see Chapter 7, p. 173, Fig. 7.1).

In the outpatient clinic, FNAC is commonly used, with or without ultrasound, to sample superficial lumps (Fig. 13.5) such as:

- Lymph node
- Salivary gland
- Thyroid
- Breast
- Subcutaneous

Imaging techniques can be used, in conjunction with a longer needle, to locate and aspirate deeper-seated masses in the head, thorax and abdomen.

Cytological preparations

Direct smear (Fig. 13.6)

- Spread sample by using one glass slide on top of another, applying gentle pressure:
    - if too thin, results in poor cellularity and distortion of cells
    - if too thick, difficult to visualise cells
- For sputum, examine sample in a Petri dish ('pick and smear') to select suitable portion of sample

Fluids (Fig. 13.7)

A cytocentrifuge is used if a fluid is of small volume or poorly cellular, yielding a small deposit after centrifugation

Fluid samples are centrifuged in order to:

- Concentrate the cells
- Assess the amount and nature of the deposit
- Allow multiple preparations to be made

Prewashing the sample in tissue culture medium or normal saline reduces cell debris and background staining

If a sizable deposit is obtained, cell preparations can be made by direct smears (Fig. 13.6).

Cell block (Fig. 13.8)

Cell blocks allow cytology samples to be converted into tissue blocks that can be sectioned (Fig. 13.8 and 13.9B). To prepare a cell block:

- A substantial centrifuged deposit is required
- Deposit is converted into a pellet by using:
    - fibrin to produce a clot
    - embedding in agar
    - using a commercial kit
- The pellet is fixed in formalin and embedded in paraffin wax from which sections can be cut

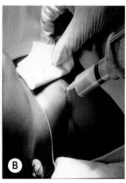
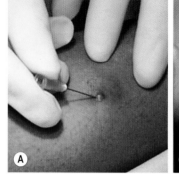

Fig. 13.5 (A) FNA can be taken using a needle only (capillary method). The needle tip is moved in and out of the lesion until blood is seen in the hub of the needle. Material is expelled from the needle onto a slide using a syringe. (B) The needle is attached to a syringe and syringe holder in order to use suction to obtain a specimen. This is often used to drain cystic lesions and the fluid expelled into a container to be processed in the laboratory.

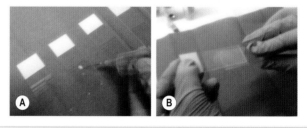

Fig. 13.6 (A) Expelling material from the needle onto the slide. (B) Gentle spreading of the sample between the two adhering glass slides.

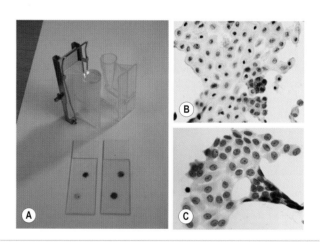

Fig. 13.7 (A) Cytocentrifuge apparatus showing cuvettes and resulting cytospin preparations. (B) PAP-stained cytospins show mesothelial cells in a monolayer distribution. (C) MGG, same case.

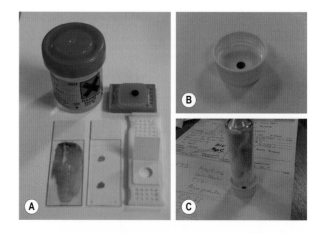

Fig. 13.8 (A) Cell block apparatus showing (clockwise from upper left): formalin-fixed sample, paraffin cell block, slide for cell block preparation, haematoxylin and eosin-stained slide and MGG-stained cytology slide. (B, C) A 'poor man's cell block' method.

- Sufficient cellular material is needed to produce a pellet of cells for processing
  - a 'poor man's cell block' method involves ejecting the contents of a needle into the lid of a universal container. A gauze soaked with 10% formalin is inserted into the container, which is then closed upside down. Formalin vapours fix the material within 6 hr. After this, a sample is fixed and can be removed with a scalpel blade or forceps.

Cell imprints (Fig. 13.9)

Imprints can be obtained from fresh tissue specimens, such as lymph nodes. The application of a glass slide with firm, gentle pressure to a freshly cut surface of a lymph node or tumour surface allows a monolayer of cells to be taken from the surface of the sample (Fig. 13.9).

This approach is suited to using a rapid staining method (see p. 397).

Liquid-based cytology (LBC)

- The LBC technologies rely on processing machines and can be used for both cervical and non-cervical cytological samples
- LBC reduces bloodstaining, disperses mucin, and produces a monolayer of cells that is representative of the whole sample. It can be used for ancillary techniques

Fixation

- The correct fixation is vital in order to best demonstrate the cellular material in samples
- Papanicolaou (PAP) staining requires cytological material to be fixed immediately in 95% alcohol (see Fig. 13.13)
- May Grunwald Giemsa (MGG) staining requires cytological material to be air-dried prior to fixation in methanol (see Fig. 13.14) (Fig. 13.10A, B, see p. 396)

Most common pitfalls (Fig. 13.10)

- FNAC: failure to release the suction in the syringe to allow pressure to equalise before removal of the fine needle from the lump will result in cells sucked into the barrel of the syringe rather than the needle. The syringe can be washed out with saline but some material may be lost
- Direct smears: if excessive pressure is applied when spreading, cells can be distorted or broken up ('smearing artefact'). Smears that are too thin show more smearing artefact while smears that are too thick may show poor staining
- Blood: excessive blood can dilute cell populations and cause poor staining due to the thickness of the smear. Use of density media can separate a layer of epithelial cells ('buffy coat') from red blood cells to give a cellular preparation

Heavily bloodstained samples can be treated with 10% glacial acetic acid to lyse the blood, and then washed with normal saline.

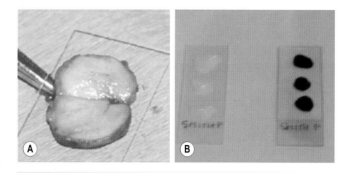

Fig. 13.9 (A) Touch preparation made by pressing a clean glass slide against a dissected lymph node. (B) Unstained and stained slides derived from lymph node touch preparation.

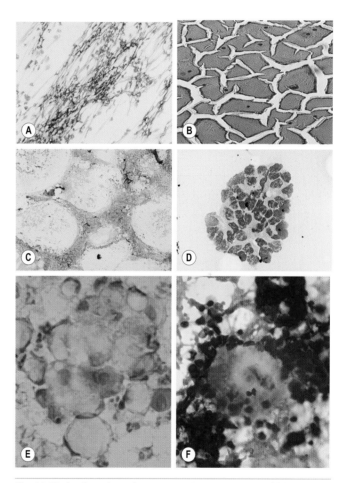

Fig. 13.10 Artefacts due to improper specimen preparation. (A) Smearing artefact due to excessive pressure. (B) Excessive blood present, diluting out cell content. The blood forms thick, cracked patches. (C) Holes in the sample due to spraying fixative being used too close to the slide. (D) Slow air drying in a closed container may cause air-drying artefact. (E) Air-dried preparation stained by Papanicolaou method. Incorrect fixation causes cells to be poorly defined. Nuclear detail is poor, showing grey-blue nuclei with fuzzy chromatin. Cytoplasmic staining is weak and shows a limited colour range. (F) Alcohol-fixed MGG preparation. Incorrect fixation causes nuclei to be overstained and definition is lost. Cells are clumped, cytoplasmic staining is heavier and red blood cells stain brown.

Staining methods

Two routine staining methods are in routine use in cytology, each requiring a different type of fixation prior to the staining (see flow-charts, p. 397):

- Papanicolaou stain (PAP) is used for samples immediately fixed in 95% alcohol ('wet-fixed') preparations
- May Grunwald Giemsa stain (MGG) is used for air-dried preparations

Incorrect fixation introduces artefacts that make visualisation of cells difficult (see Fig. 13.10E, F).

Papanicolaou stain (Fig. 13.11)

Papanicolaou staining is a polychrome method which depends on the degree of cell maturity and cellular metabolic activity. The three main advantages of this staining procedure are:

- Good definition of nuclear detail
- Cytoplasmic transparency
- Indication of cellular differentiation of squamous epithelium

The haematoxylin nuclear stain demonstrates chromatinic patterns of normal and abnormal cells. The counterstains, Orange-G and EA (eosin-azure) have a high alcoholic concentration which provides cytoplasmic transparency (see p. 397). This enables clear visualisation through areas of overlapping cells, mucus and debris.

May Grunwald Giemsa stain (Fig. 13.12)

May Grunwald Giemsa was originally a haematological stain that facilitated the differentiation of blood cell types. It was used primarily to stain peripheral blood smears and bone marrow aspirates.

Nuclei stain dark red to purple, while cytoplasm stains varying shades of grey/blue, with keratin showing a bright turquoise blue colour. Thick sheets and clusters do not stain well as the stain penetrates poorly. Thin smears or monolayers show optimal staining. Mucin shows metachromasia with pink/magenta colouration but can mask cellular detail if excessive. Blood stains a pale grey/gold colour.

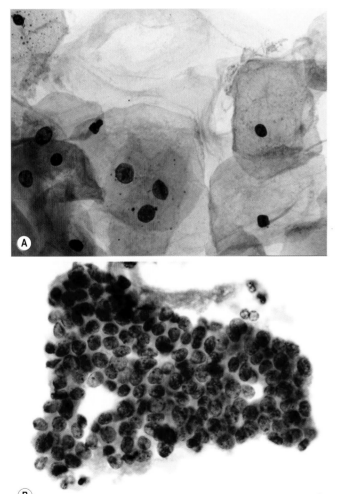

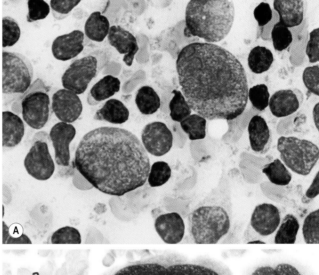

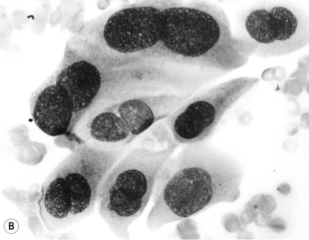

Fig. 13.11 Examples of PAP staining. (A) Cervical squamous epithelium shows the nuclear detail well, differential counterstaining and cytoplasmic transparency. (B) A crisp nuclear detail is essential for diagnosis and enables the diagnosis of endocervical glandular neoplasia in the case shown here.

Fig. 13.12 May Grunwald Giemsa staining. (A) FNA of lymph node shows good nuclear and cytoplasmic detail. (B) FNA of salivary gland with clean morphological detail, binucleation, anisonucleosis, coarse chromatin, prominent nucleoli and well-defined cytoplasm containing granules.

Papanicolaou staining method flowchart

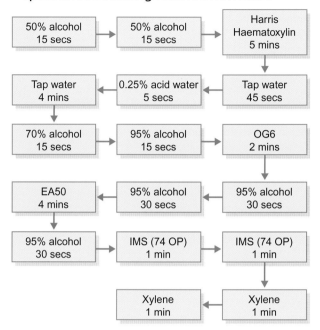

```
50% alcohol     →   50% alcohol     →   Harris
15 secs             15 secs             Haematoxylin
                                        5 mins
                                          ↓
Tap water       ←   0.25% acid water ←   Tap water
4 mins              5 secs              45 secs
  ↓
70% alcohol     →   95% alcohol     →   OG6
15 secs             15 secs             2 mins
                                          ↓
EA50            ←   95% alcohol     ←   95% alcohol
4 mins              30 secs             30 secs
  ↓
95% alcohol     →   IMS (74 OP)     →   IMS (74 OP)
30 secs             1 min               1 min
                                          ↓
                    Xylene          ←   Xylene
                    1 min               1 min
```

MGG staining method flowchart

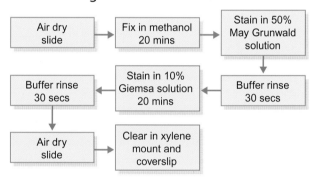

```
Air dry         →   Fix in methanol  →   Stain in 50%
slide               20 mins              May Grunwald
                                         solution
                                           ↓
Buffer rinse    ←   Stain in 10%     ←   Buffer rinse
30 secs             Giemsa solution      30 secs
  ↓                 20 mins
Air dry         →   Clear in xylene
slide               mount and
                    coverslip
```

Diagnostic pitfalls: PAP staining

- Varying thickness of material on slide
- Type of fixative used
- Inadequate filtering of stain solutions
- Age of staining solution
- Degree of usage of staining solutions
- Use of chlorinated tap water
- pH of water can effect nuclear staining
- Temperature of water
- Insufficient rinsing after acid
- Air drying of slides between solutions
- Improper draining of slides during staining

Rapid staining method (Fig. 13.13)

- Stain is similar to a Romanowsky-type stain
- Staining time is a few minutes
- Single cells are well demonstrated
- Thick clusters are less well demonstrated
- Slides can subsequently be stained with MGG stain

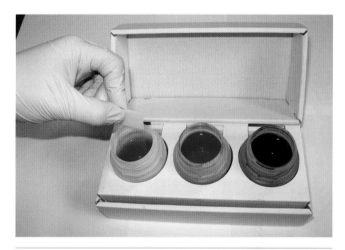

Fig. 13.13 Rapid staining kit can be used in the cases where a diagnosis is required instantly. The procedure takes only a few minutes.

The most commonly used histochemical stains on cytological preparations are

- Periodic acid–Schiff (PAS) ± diastase
  - glycogen, mucin (persists after diastase digestion)
- Grocott
  - fungi – Aspergillus, Candida, Pneumocystis spp.
- Ziehl–Neelsen
  - Tuberculosis bacilli

Other special stains that can be performed include:

- Periodic acid–Schiff (PAS) ± diastase
  - glycogen, mucin (persists after diastase digestion)
- Oil Red O
  - lipids
- Southgate's mucicarmine
  - neutral mucin, *Cryptococcus* spp.
- Carbol chromotrope
  - eosinophils
- Gram
  - Gram-positive bacteria
- Perls
  - iron deposits
- Masson–Fontana
  - melanin pigment

Immunocytochemistry

Introduction

Immunocytochemistry (ICC) has emerged as a powerful investigative tool that can provide supplemental information to routine morphological assessment of cytological samples. The use of ICC to study cellular markers that define specific phenotypes has provided important diagnostic, prognostic, and predictive information relative to disease status.

Main applications of ICC

- Sample types
  - fine needle aspiration (FNA)
  - exfoliative cytology (body fluids, urine, cerebrospinal fluid, gynaecological material)
- Indications
  - supplemental information in cancer diagnostics
  - assessment of predictive markers (ER, PR, HER2)
  - prognostic information (Ki 67)

Sample preparation

- Smear (Fig. 13.14A)
- Liquid based cytology (LBC) slides (Fig. 13.14B)
- Cytospin (Fig. 13.14C)
- Cell block sections

Fixation

- Must be done immediately
- Prior or after slide preparation
- For at least 30 min!
- In most cases at 4°C
- Type of fixative depends on antigen (Ag) investigated

Fixatives

- Methanol
- Ethanol
- LBC fixatives
- Commercial sprays containing polyethylene glycol and alcohol; must be removed prior to staining
- Combination of fixatives (e.g. Delaunay's fixative)
- Acetone (as a component in combination of fixatives or as a step in fixation procedure)
- Air drying followed by rehydration

Antigen retrieval (AR) in ICC

Increases cell membrane permeability.

Provides access to previously masked Ag.

In ICC, majority of Ag can be demonstrated without AR.

In some situations AR is required: Ki-67, cyclin D1, hormone receptors.

- (A) Heat-mediated AR
  - usually performed in an aqueous medium, with pH about 2.0, 7.0 or 10.0
  - most frequent methods use citrate buffer, pH 6.0 or TRIS/EDTA buffer, pH 9.0
  - optimal temperature: near the boiling point of water (it can be reached using a microwave oven, an autoclave, a water bath or a pressure cooker)
  - length of exposure to heat varies with regard to Ag investigated
  - exposure to heat is followed by cooling
- (B) Enzyme-mediated AR
- (C) Combination of heat-mediated and enzyme-mediated AR

Each laboratory must determine the best method of AR for their particular circumstances.

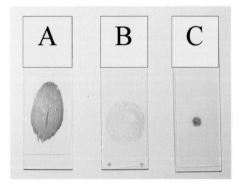

Fig. 13.14 Examples of appropriate sample preparation for ICC staining: smear (A), LBC slide (B), cytospin (C).

Manually/automated

Direct/indirect methods (Fig. 13.15)

- • (A) Direct method
  - – one-step staining method
  - – involves a labelled antibody (Ab), reacting directly with Ag in the cell
  - – Ab can be labelled with a fluorescent dye or with an enzyme (horseradish peroxidase (HRP) or alkaline phosphatase (AP)), which is activated by substrate addition
  - – detection: light (enzyme) or fluorescent (fluorophore) microscope
  - – simple and quick
  - – less sensitive (inadequate signal amplification)
- • (B) Indirect method
  - – an unlabeled primary Ab reacts with cell Ag
  - – a labelled secondary Ab reacts with primary Ab
  - – signal amplification and sensitivity are better when compared to direct method
  - – second Ab can be labelled with a fluorescent dye or with an enzyme
  - – most frequently used methods: peroxidase anti-peroxidase (**PAP**) method, avidin-biotin complex (**ABC**) method and labelled streptavidin biotin (**LSAB**) method
  - – above mentioned methods involve three layers: (1) unlabeled **primary Ab**, (2) **biotinylated secondary Ab** which binds to primary Ab and (3) **a third layer**, which is specific for each particular method and binds to labelled secondary Ab

PAP method (Fig. 13.16)

- • The third layer is a rabbit Ab linked to peroxidase, making a stable PAP complex
- • Excellent sensitivity; due to PAP complex the level of amplification upon substrate activation is 100 to 1000 times greater than just secondary Ab amplification
- • Lower quantities of primary Ab are required per slide

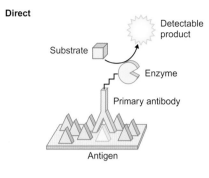

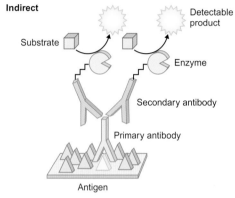

Fig. 13.15 Schematic presentation of direct and indirect ICC methods.

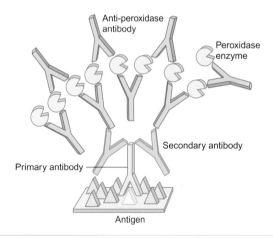

Fig. 13.16 PAP method.

ABC method (Fig. 13.17)

- The third layer is a complex of avidin-biotin peroxidase
- After addition of diaminobenzidine (DAB) or other chromogen substrate, the complex produces a coloured end product visible in light microscopy

LSAB method (Fig. 13.18)

- Similar to ABC, avidin-biotin peroxidase in the third layer is replaced by an enzyme streptavidin complex
- Streptavidin-biotin-enzyme complexes are smaller than avidin-biotin complexes in ABC method, thus epitopes on antigens in LSAB method are more easily tagged compared to ABC method. LSAB method is therefore 5 to 10 times more sensitive compared to ABC method
- Compared to avidin, which has an isoelectric point of 10 and has therefore tendency for electrostatic binding to the cells, streptavidin is uncharged. Also, in contrast to avidin, streptavidin does not contain carbohydrate groups which might bind to cell lectins. Both characteristics of avidin result in more prominent background staining in ABC method compared to LSAB method

Polymeric methods (Fig. 13.19)

- One of the latest in ICC
- Polymeric technology increases sensitivity, reduces the number of assay steps and minimises non-specific background staining that could appear in ABC/LSAB methods due to binding of avidin/streptavidin on endogenous cell biotin
- Application of primary Ab is followed by addition of enzyme labelled polymer that, following addition of substrate chromogen, gives a coloured end product visible in light microscopy

ICC staining

- Nuclear (Figs 13.20–13.22)
- Cytoplasmic (Figs 13.23, 13.24 and 13.28)
- Membranous (Figs 13.25–13.28)

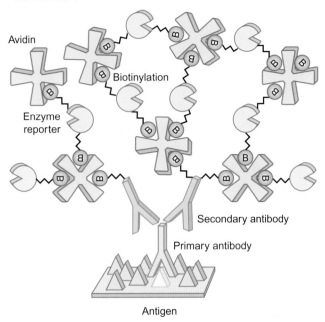

Fig. 13.17 ABC method.

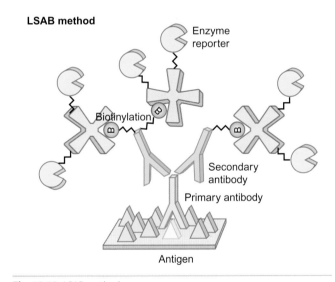

Fig. 13.18 LSAB method.

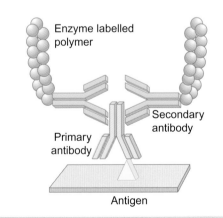

Fig. 13.19 Polymeric method.

Internal quality control

Use of positive and negative controls is essential in every staining run to ensure the correct result.

Positive control (PC)

- ICC reaction of PC must be positive in order to establish the proper performance of the staining reagents and methods
- The most appropriate PC: cytological samples or cell lines, containing cells with known antigens or cells with known levels of Ag expression (e.g. PC for HER2)
- PC must be fixed in the same manner as diagnostic samples
- PC can be stored from 1 month to a few years, depending on type of antigen and fixative used
- PC can be stored (1) in methanol at 4°C, (2) at room temperature following methanol fixation and 10% polyethylene glycol, coating, (3) as LBC slides, (4) as cell blocks, (5) as permanent preparations

Negative control (NC)

- The purpose of addition of NC in each ICC staining run is to evaluate non-specific ICC staining due to non-specific background staining or lack of Ab specificity
- NC is one of the regularly prepared samples for ICC on which only the antibody dilution reagent is applied, the primary Ab is withheld
- Negative ICC reaction is mandatory
- If positive staining occurs in NC, test specimen results must be considered invalid

External quality control

Participation in one of the immunocytochemical quality control schemes, for example, UK NEQAS http://www.ukneqas.org.uk, is recommended.

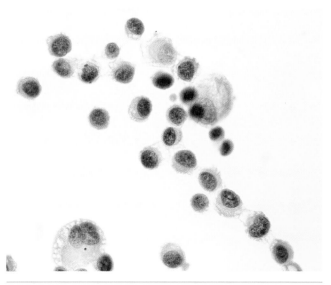

Fig. 13.20 Nuclear ICC reaction for oestrogen receptor (ER) on cytospin prepared from MCF 7 cell line (PC for ER) and fixed in methanol.

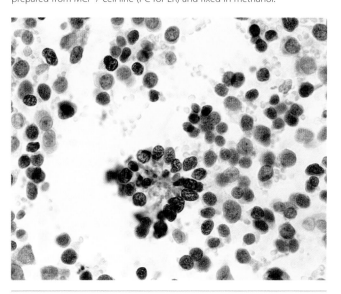

Fig. 13.21 Nuclear ICC reaction for progesterone receptor (PR) on cytospin prepared from FNA of breast carcinoma and fixed in methanol.

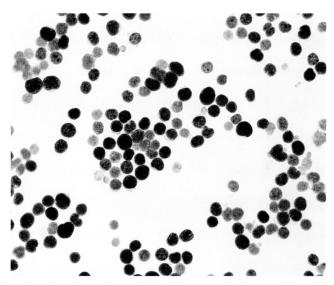

Fig. 13.22 Nuclear ICC reaction for Ki-67 (MIB-1) on cytospin prepared from FNA of T-cell lymphoblastic lymphoma and fixed in methanol. Heat-mediated antigen retrieval was used prior to ICC staining.

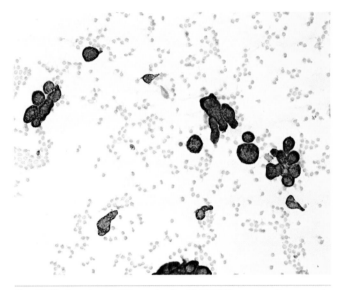

Fig. 13.23 Cytoplasmic ICC reaction for CK AE1/AE3 on cytospin prepared from FNA of breast carcinoma, fixed in methanol and 10% PEG.

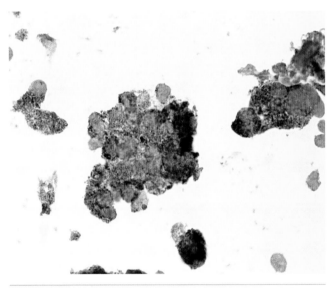

Fig. 13.24 Cytoplasmic ICC reaction for PSA on cytospin prepared from FNA of prostatic carcinoma metastasis, fixed in Delaunay and stained after Papanicolaou staining prior to ICC staining.

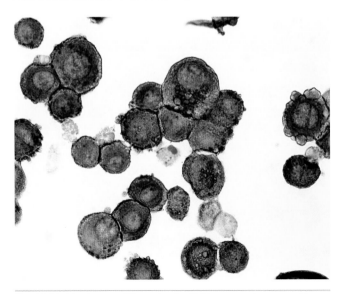

Fig. 13.25 Membranous ICC reaction for HER2 on cytospin prepared from SKBR3 cell line (3+ PC for HER2), and fixed in methanol.

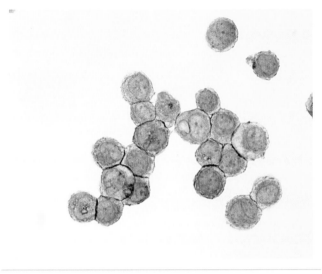

Fig. 13.26 Membranous ICC reaction for HER2 on cytospin prepared from MDA MB 453 cell line (2+ PC for HER2), and fixed in methanol.

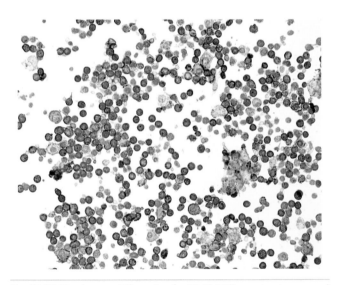

Fig. 13.27 Membranous ICC reaction for CD 45 (LCA) on cytospin prepared from FNA of chronic lymphadenitis and fixed in methanol.

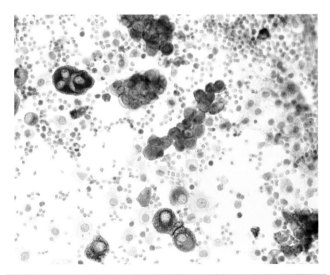

Fig. 13.28 Double ICC staining on cytospin (methanol fixation) prepared from pleural effusion of peritoneal adenocarcinoma shows calretinin-positive *mesothelial cells* (brown cytoplasmic ICC reaction: DAB chromogen, HRP) and Moc-positive *malignant cells* (red membranous ICC reaction: fast red chromogen AP).

Pitfalls – weak reaction/no reaction

- Inadequate fixation (Fig. 13.29)
- Inadequate dilution of primary Ab (Fig. 13.30) or failure to add Ab
- Inappropriate incubation time or temperature of incubation of primary Ab
- Inadequate antigen retrieval (Fig. 13.31)
- Primary Ab diluted in inappropriate buffer. *Solution:* use PBS or TBS as Ab diluent
- Inappropriate counterstaining
- Instrument malfunction
- Other

Pitfalls – background staining and unspecific bindage

- Inadequate or delayed fixation
- Contamination of polyclonal Ab
- Unspecific binding of Ab due to hydrophobic or electrostatic forces or endogenous peroxidase activity when using DAB chromogen. *Solution*: pre-treatment with H_2O_2 prior to incubation of primary Ab
- Unspecific binding due to activity of endogenous AP in cells when using AP as a label. *Solution*: pre-treatment with levamisole
- Avidin binding to endogenous biotin present in liver, kidney or hepatopancreatic cells when ABC/LSAB method is used. *Solution*: pre-treatment of unconjugated avidin with biotin saturation (Fig. 13.32)
- Sample is too concentrated
- Inadequate rinsing
- Excessive incubation in chromogen substrate
- Instrument malfunction
- Other

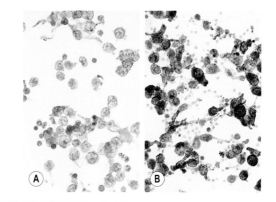

Fig. 13.30 Weak ICC reaction for HMB-45 at Ab dilution 1:1500 (A) and adequate ICC reaction at Ab dilution 1:100 (B).

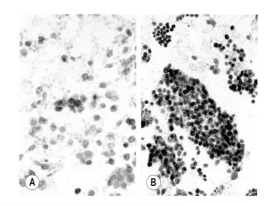

Fig. 13.31 Weak ICC reaction for ER where antigen retrieval was not used (A) and appropriate ICC reaction after heat-mediated antigen retrieval in TRIS/EDTA (B).

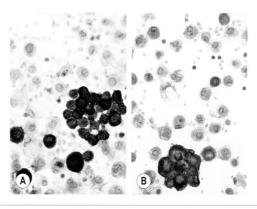

Fig. 13.32 ICC reaction for calretinin with (A) and without (B) avidin-biotin blockade. An unspecific staining of histiocyte cytoplasm is present when avidin-biotin blockade is not used.

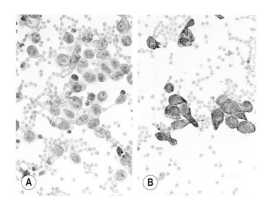

Fig. 13.29 Weak ICC reaction for CK7 in the centre (A) and adequate ICC reaction on the edge (B) on the same cytospin.

Polymerase chain reaction

Introduction

Polymerase chain reaction (PCR) permits amplification and simplified analysis of any known nucleic acid target. Suitable DNA or RNA can be extracted from cytological preparations. PCR can be used for the analysis of clonality of lymphocyte populations, translocations and mutations. The results can be correlated with cytology (Fig. 13.33) to aid diagnosis, prognosis and prediction of response to therapy.

Rationale

- PCR works by using a DNA polymerase enzyme to copy chosen short stretches of DNA in vitro
- The selected regions are targeted using two specific single-stranded DNA oligonucleotides ('primers') which define the limits of the amplified region (Fig. 13.34)
- By repeating this process many times, large amounts of the desired fragment are generated, which makes it easy to study in the absence of the remainder of the genome
- The presence or absence of the region can be assessed as well as its length and nucleotide sequence, using electrophoresis, sequencing or other methods (Fig. 13.35)

Sample types

Most cytological samples can be used as a source of DNA for PCR analysis, including:

- Fluids
- Direct smears
- Cytospin preparations
- Cell blocks

Nucleic acid extraction

Nucleic acids tend to be well preserved in cytological specimens compared to histological samples which have been subjected to formaldehyde fixation and processing. Commercial kits can be employed to simply, reliably and cost-effectively extract DNA or RNA, depending on the analysis required.

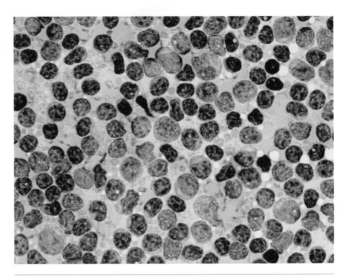

Fig. 13.33 Molecular genetic information can aid diagnosis when cytology and immunophenotyping are inconclusive, such as in this case of a population of small lymphocytes.

One cycle of PCR

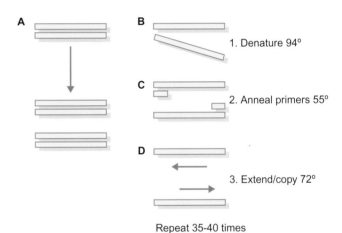

1. Denature 94°
2. Anneal primers 55°
3. Extend/copy 72°

Repeat 35-40 times

Fig. 13.34 (A) One cycle of polymerase chain reaction (PCR) doubles target DNA numbers by (B) denaturing target DNA, (C) annealing primers and (D) primer extension.

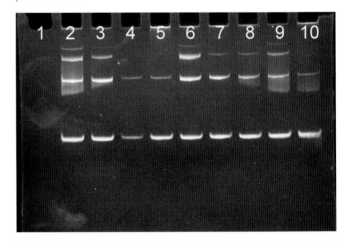

Fig. 13.35 Polyacrylamide gel electrophoresis of PCR products. Quality of DNA extracts can be tested by PCR amplification of fragments of 100, 200, 300 and 400 base pairs. In degraded samples, larger fragments cannot be amplified (such as lanes 4, 5 and 10).

Techniques

- DNA extraction
- End-point PCR (Fig. 13.36). DNA amplification followed by gel electrophoresis. Standard methodology. Amplification followed by fluorescent fragment analysis. More precise – requires dedicated instrument and fluorescent labelling of primers
- Real-time PCR (when quantification or improved specificity and sensitivity are required) (Fig. 13.37). Non-specific fluorescent dyes that bind to double-stranded DNA or labelled probes that bind specifically to PCR products
- Interpretation

Applications

- Lymphoma
- Sarcoma
- Infectious agents
- Identity of individual (disputed sample origin)
- Predictive mutation (e.g. lung cancer)

Nucleic acid targets

- Lymphomas
  - Immunoglobulin genes (e.g. heavy chain)
  - T-cell receptor genes (e.g. TCR-gamma) T(14;18)
- Sarcomas
  - T(11;22) (EWS-FLI1)
  - T(X;18) (SYT-SSX)
- Lung cancer
  - EGFR mutation
  - KRAS mutation
  - BRAF mutation
- Infectious agents
  - HPV
  - TB

Pitfalls

- Poor DNA quantity/quality
- Sampling error – lack of target cells in selected material
- Normal cells masking tumour
- Cross-contamination causing false positives
- Non-specific amplification leading to difficulties in interpretation

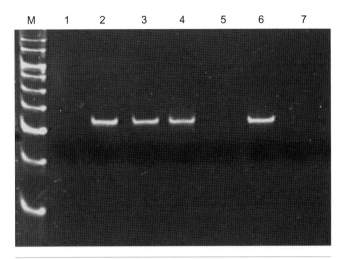

Fig. 13.36 End-point PCR. T(X;18) has been amplified and PCR products run on an 8% polyacrylamide gel and stained with ethidium bromide. M, size markers; 1, negative control; 2, positive control; 3–7, test cases. Positive cases carrying the translocation are indicated by the presence of a band of the expected size.

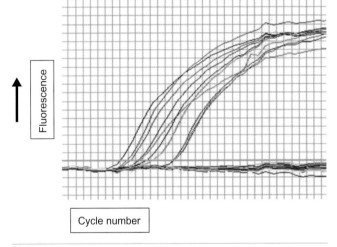

Fig. 13.37 Real-time PCR. T(X;18) has been amplified using a real-time PCR machine. The amplification of specific product has been monitored cycle by cycle (*X-axis*) by measuring fluorescence (*Y-axis*). Positive cases are indicated by exponential increase in fluorescence whereas negative cases show no increase in fluorescence (*horizontal plots*).

Clonality analysis

- Lymphoproliferative disorders are often difficult to resolve cytologically and immunocytochemically. Clonality analysis can help confirm monoclonality of B cells or T cells by PCR amplification of antigen receptor genes
- In B-cell proliferations: immunoglobulin heavy and light chain genes are amplified
- In T-cell proliferations: T-cell receptor genes are amplified (Figs 13.38, 13.39)

Method of cell preparation in suspected lymphoma

- DNA extracted from residual FNA sample
- Control gene amplification to confirm that adequate DNA has been extracted
- In suspected T-cell lymphoma:
  - T-cell receptor beta or gamma chain genes are targeted
- In suspected B-cell lymphoma:
  - Immunoglobulin heavy chain and kappa light chain genes are targeted

PCR product analysis (Figs 13.39, 13.40)

- PCR products are run on polyacrylamide gels and stained with ethidium bromide
- Polyclonal products appear as a smear or ladder (suggests a reactive process)
- Monoclonal products appear as dominant bands (suggests a neoplastic process)
- This analysis can also be carried out using capillary electrophoresis with fluorescently labelled primers

Pitfalls

- False-negative results due to failure of primer binding. This can result from variation in target sequence and somatic mutations
- False-positive results due to poor resolution of products

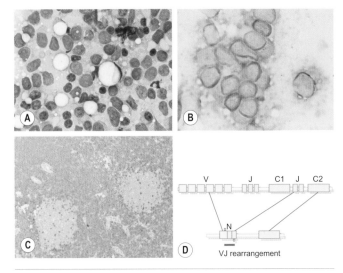

Fig. 13.38 (A) T-cell lymphoma, (B) CD3, (C) CD3, (D) TCR-gamma chain gene rearrangement – PCR primers target the V and J regions and amplify the variable junctions.

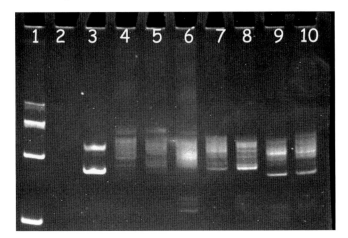

Fig. 13.39 Polyacrylamide gel of T-cell receptor gamma chain gene PCR products. Lane 1, control gene amplification confirms presence of adequate DNA; 2, negative control; 3, positive control (dominant band); 4–6 polyclonal cases (smears); 7–8 and 9–10 (T cell lymphoma from Fig. 13.38) two monoclonal test cases in duplicate (dominant bands).

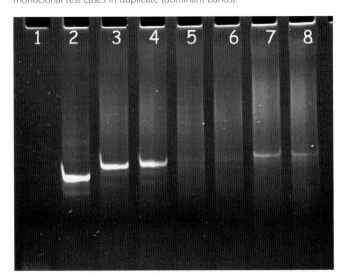

Fig. 13.40 Polyacrylamide gel of immunoglobulin heavy chain PCR products. Lanes: 1, negative control; 2, monoclononal control: B cell lymphoma (dominant band); 3 and 4, monoclonal case in duplicate (dominant band); 5 and 6 polyclonal case in duplicate (smears); 7 and 8, monoclonal case in duplicate (dominant band).

Diagnosis of lymphomas

Certain chromosome translocations are characteristic of specific lymphoma types. These can be used as diagnostic markers in difficult cases. Examples include:

- Detection of t(14;18) in follicular lymphoma (Fig. 13.41)
- T(11;14) in mantle cell lymphoma

Diagnosis of sarcomas

Many sarcomas also have hallmark translocations. Diagnosis can be helped by detection of:

- T(11;22) in Ewing's sarcoma
- T(X;18) in synovial sarcoma
- T(12;22) in clear cell sarcoma (Fig. 13.42)

Method: Lymphomas

- Genomic DNA is amplified using primers spanning the translocation breakpoints
- Products are run on polyacrylamide or agarose gels
- Products, which are variable in length due to variation in breakpoints, are only seen in the presence of the translocation (Fig. 13.43)

Method: Sarcomas

- RNA is extracted and converted to cDNA using reverse transcription
- This is amplified using PCR primers that span the exon boundaries of fusion transcripts
- Products are run on polyacrylamide or agarose gels
- Products (also variable in length) are only seen in the presence of the translocation
- Translocations can also be detected using real-time PCR (Fig. 13.43)

Pitfalls

- False negatives due to breakpoint variability
- Degradation of DNA or RNA

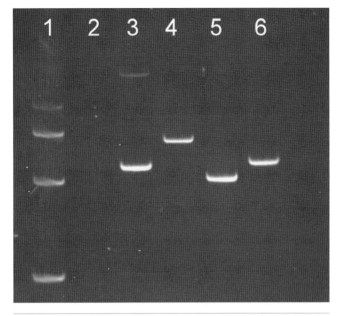

Fig. 13.41 PCR detection of t(14;18) in follicular lymphoma. Lane 1, size markers; 2, negative control; 3, positive control; 4–6 test cases (all positive).

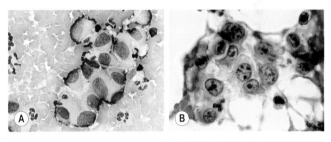

Fig. 13.42 Clear cell sarcoma – pleural fluid. Large cells with eccentric nuclei and prominent nucleoli. Epithelial markers were negative. PCR detected T(12;22) confirming a diagnosis of clear cell sarcoma (see Ch 12, Fig. 12.67).

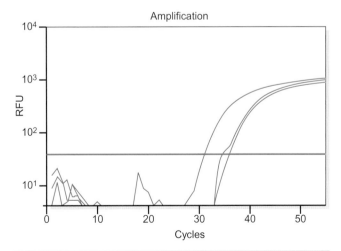

Fig. 13.43 RT-PCR detection of t(12;22) EWS/ATF1. The traces with an exponential shape indicate positivity, whereas traces from negative samples remain below the horizontal bar.

Epidermal growth factor receptor (EGFR)

- Patients with non-small cell lung carcinoma harbouring specific activating mutations in the EGFR gene have been shown to respond better to tyrosine kinase inhibitors than those with other EGFR mutations or no mutations (Figs 13.44, 13.45)
- Cytological specimens are frequently used as a source of DNA for this analysis
- Mutations include exon 19 deletions, L858R, L861Q and exon 20 insertions

Selection of first-line therapy in non small cell lung carcinoma (NSCLC)

- Extract DNA from FNA or other sample
- Check quality of extract
- Detect the most common mutations in EGFR gene using real-time PCR. This is highly sensitive; 1% mutant cells can be detected in a wild-type background
- Other techniques such as fragment analysis and Sanger sequencing can be used to detect other variants
- First-line therapy:
    - mutation-positive: TKI inhibitors
    - mutation-negative: chemotherapy

Pitfalls

- Not all mutations detected
- Some cell preparation procedures such as cell blocks may degrade DNA

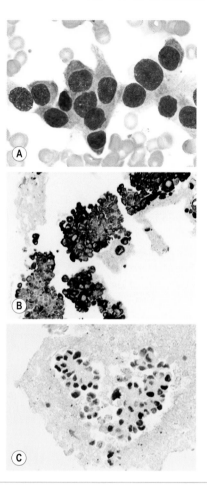

Fig. 13.44 Lung adenocarcinoma stained with (A) MGG, (B) CK7, (C) TTF1.

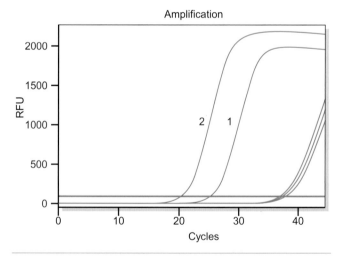

Fig. 13.45 Real-time PCR detection of EGFR exon 19 deletion. Positive trace for the deletion (*blue 1*) emerges within 12 cycles of the control trace (*blue 2*) in this patient. The additional traces shown in green represent amplification of a control reaction present in all wells and indicate a lack of PCR inhibitors in these samples.

- Human papillomavirus
- Tuberculosis
- *Pneumocystis carinii*
- *Toxoplasma* spp.
- *Candida albicans*

Mycobacterial infection (Fig. 13.46)

Primers target the IS6110 insertion sequence, which is a repetitive mobile sequence present at high copy numbers (1–24) in Mtb complex (*M. tuberculosis*, *M. bovis*, *M. bovis* BCG, *M. africanum*, *M. microti*).

Pitfalls in detection of infectious agents

- Target DNA present in the absence of active bacterium, for example, after treatment
- False positives due to cross-contamination between tissue samples during cut-up/processing/sectioning
- False negatives due to poor DNA quality or rare target sequence
- Poor extraction efficiency due to bacterial cell wall

Pneumocystis carinii (Fig. 13.47)

- Cannot be cultured
- PCR important in cases where morphology is inconclusive

Future developments in molecular diagnostics

Other targets:

- Diagnostically useful cancer-related mutations and translocations
- More targeted therapy related to specific mutations (for example, B-RAF, PI3KC2)
- High-throughput expression arrays and next-generation sequencing
- Mutation screening techniques such as high-resolution melt analysis (HRM)

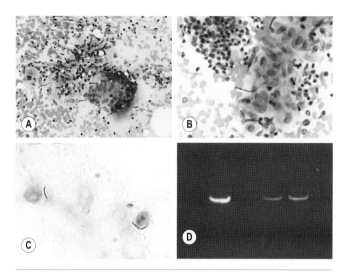

Fig. 13.46 TB infection. (A) MGG, (B) MGG, (C) ZN, (D) PCR amplification of TB DNA showing 100bp product from positive samples.

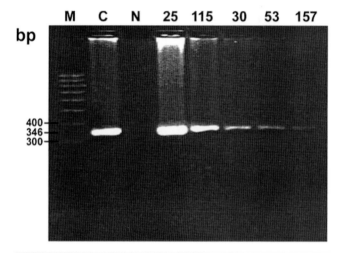

Fig. 13.47 PCR detection of *Pneumocystis carinii* in bronchoalveolar lavages and sputa. A 346bp product is seen in positive cases (25, 115, 30, 53 and 157). (Reproduced from Pinlaor et al. PCR diagnosis of *Pneumocystis carinii* on sputum and bronchoalveolar lavage samples in immuno-compromised patients. Parasitol Res (2004) 94: 213–218.)

In situ hybridisation (ISH) (Figs 13.48, 13.49)

In situ hybridisation allows a visual assessment of structural or numerical genetic aberrations such as:

- Translocations, inversions
- Low gene copy number abnormalities (gains or deletions of chromosome arms including one or several genes)
- High gene copy number aberrations (amplifications)

The principle

- DNA probe complementary to the gene or a sequence of interest is produced and labelled. Labelled probe is hybridised to the target gene in nuclei
- Three different ISH methods are actually available:
  - **FISH** (**F**luorescent in situ hybridisation)
  - **CISH** (**C**hromogenic in situ hybridisation)
  - **SISH** (**S**ilver in situ hybridisation)
- FISH uses the fluorescent labelled probe and the fluorescent microscope is needed for analysis
- CISH uses the indirectly labelled probe and enzymatic reaction is used to develop a chromogenic reaction, or the fluorescent probe is hybridised and the fluorochrome-directed antibodies will develop the chromogenic signal. Microscopic analysis of results is done in bright-field microscope
- SISH is a fully automated technique to detect chromogenic signals with silver nanoparticles which are deposited at the side of the target hybridised probe. The bright field microscope is used

DNA probes

(1) DNA repeat probes
  (A) Centromeric probes
  (B) Subtelomeric probes
(2) Gene-specific probes
  (A) Split (break-apart) probes
  (B) Fusion/double fusion probes
  (C) Gene probes detecting amplifications or deletions

The largest majority of specific gene probes are available for FISH; the choice is limited for CISH and SISH.

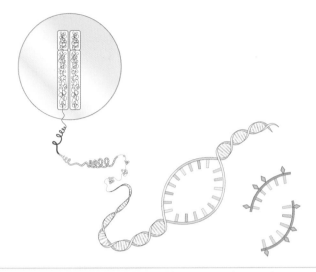

Fig. 13.48 DNA in nuclei as well as the fluorescent probe must be denatured to the single DNA strand at high temperature.

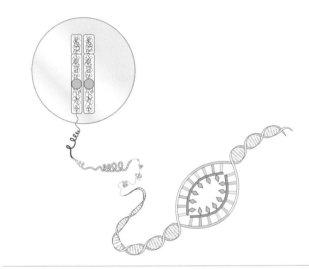

Fig. 13.49 Complementary probe single strands will hybridise to nuclei DNA single strands and detect a genetic rearrangement.

Types of preparation

* Smears
* Cytospins
* Cell blocks

FISH protocol flow chart

Slide preparation (let dry 2–12h)

↓

Fixation of material on the slide (methanol: acetic acid 9:1) 5-20 minutes at room temperature; time depends on cell density

↓

Enzymatic pretreatment (pepsin at 37°C/5–15 min, depends on cell density)

↓

Apply the probe on the slide, cover by coverslip

↓

Denaturation of the probe and the target together (co-denaturation) in hybridiser (temperature depends on used probes)

↓

Hybridisation overnight (37°C–44°C)

↓

Stringency wash (37°–65°–72°C)

↓

Slide mounting with DAPI and antifade medium

↓

Microscopy (analysis, photo documentation)

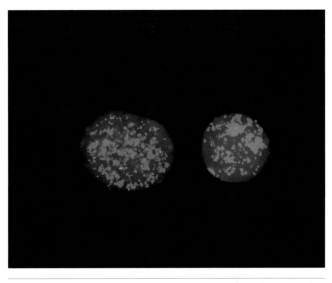

Fig. 13.50 Paediatric tumour: neuroblastoma. FISH with *MYCN* gene probe showing gene amplification (*red spots*). Control green probe is the chromosome 2 centromere.

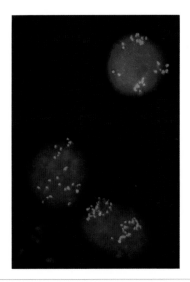

Fig. 13.51 Adult carcinoma: breast invasive duct carcinoma. FISH with *FGFR1* gene (*green*) showing gene amplification. Control probe (*red*) is the chromosome 8 centromere.

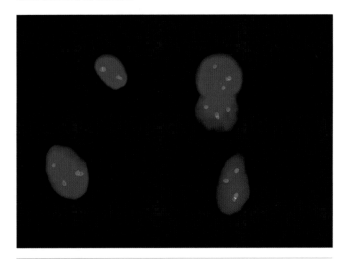

Fig. 13.52 Paediatric tumour: Ewing's sarcoma. One *EWS* gene is normal (*two spots together*) and the second is dissociated (*red and green*) due to a translocation. Lymphocyte shows two normal *EWS* genes (*red and green together*).

Fluorescence in situ hybridization in lymphomas: gene translocation (Figs 13.53–13.56)

In lymphomas, the more frequently used probes are the double fusion probes (in some cases the split probes are of interest).

The principle of the double fusion probe is the detection of two different chimeric genes created by the translocation between two different chromosomes. The probes are usually large and cover not only the gene but also the region flanking the gene of interest (for easy signal detection).

Differential diagnosis

- **Burkitt's lymphoma:** translocation t(8;14) between genes c-MYC and IGH
- **Large B-cell lymphoma:** translocation t(3;14) between genes BCL6/IGH or split of genes BCL6 or IGH (with other translocation partners)

Other translocations and genes detected by FISH in lymphomas

- Mantle cell lymphomas:
    - translocation t(11;14)
    - genes CCND1/IGH
- Follicular lymphomas:
    - translocation t(14;18)
    - genes IGH/BCL2
- MALT lymphomas:
    - translocations involving the gene MALT1 and other genes such as API2, IGH or BCL6

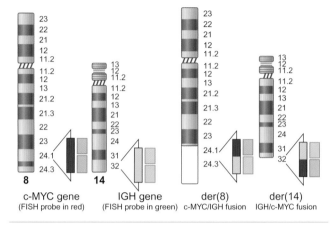

c-MYC gene (FISH probe in red)   IGH gene (FISH probe in green)   der(8) c-MYC/IGH fusion   der(14) IGH/c-MYC fusion

Fig. 13.54 Translocation t(8;14) will create two fusion genes, one on chromosome 8 and one on chromosome 14.

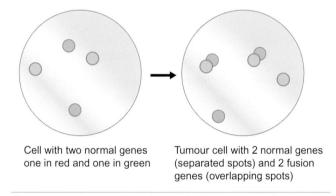

Cell with two normal genes one in red and one in green   Tumour cell with 2 normal genes (separated spots) and 2 fusion genes (overlapping spots)

Fig. 13.55 Interphasic nuclei with normal and two rearranged genes in Burkitt's lymphoma.

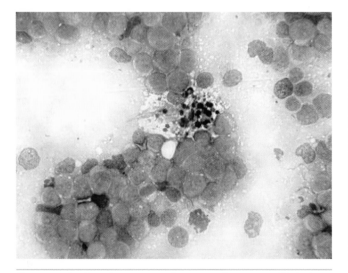

Fig. 13.53 Cytological preparation of a smear with suspicion of Burkitt's lymphoma.

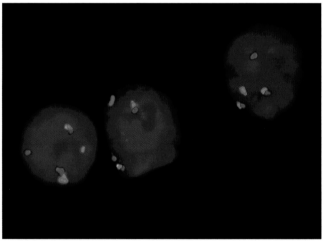

Fig. 13.56 FISH in Burkitt's lymphoma with double fusion probe, as illustrated by Figures 13.54 and 13.55.

Fluorescence in situ hybridisation in solid tumours: detection of gene amplification (Figs 13.57–13.61)

Gene amplification is an important increase of the gene copy number in a nucleus which is followed by a raise of protein level. The best known example is the amplification of the ERBB2 (HER2) gene in invasive breast carcinoma. Determination of HER2 status is done by: (A) immunohistochemistry (protein level), (B) FISH (gene copy number, used if IHC 2+).

The identification of HER2-positive cases is needed to include patients for targeted therapy trials.

The ERBB2 (HER2) gene status can be detected by all three methods: FISH, CISH, SISH.

Other solid tumours (different types), and the genes which are frequently amplified

- Neuroblastoma: MYCN
- Medulloblastoma: MYCN and c-MYC
- Liposarcoma: MDM2
- Non-small round cell lung carcinoma: EGFR

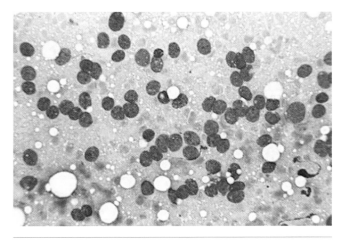

Fig. 13.57 FNA of invasive breast carcinoma.

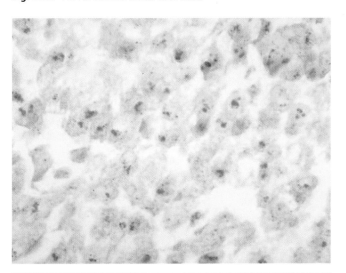

Fig. 13.58 CISH with HER2 probe in invasive breast cancer interphasic nuclei showing ERBB2 (HER2) amplification.

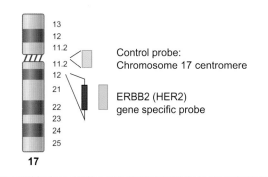

Control probe:
Chromosome 17 centromere

ERBB2 (HER2)
gene specific probe

Fig. 13.59 Chromosome view of the ERBB2 (HER2) gene in red and a control centromeric probe in green.

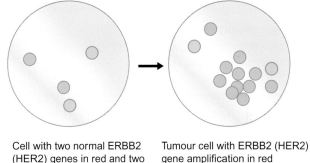

Cell with two normal ERBB2 (HER2) genes in red and two controls in green (chromosome 17 centromeric region)

Tumour cell with ERBB2 (HER2) gene amplification in red (multiple copies) and two control centromeric spots in green

Fig. 13.60 Interphasic nuclei showing normal nucleus and HER2 gene amplified nucleus.

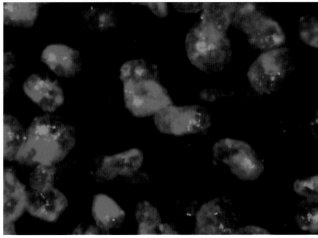

Fig. 13.61 FISH with ERBB2 (HER2) probe and 17 centromeric probe showing a gene amplification.

In mesenchymal tumours, the most frequently used probe is a split probe (in some cases a simple fusion probe can replace a split probe).

The principle of the split probe is the detection of the gene responsible for the tumour phenotype which is covered by a two-colour probe. In the case of translocation, the gene is split into two parts and the FISH probe will show the separate red and green signals. The split (or break-apart) probe is useful in the evaluation of genes which have two or more translocation partners.

Differential diagnosis of small round cell tumours

- Ewing's sarcoma (gene EWRS1)
- Alveolar rhabdomyosarcoma (gene FKHR)
- Lymphomas (gene c-MYC)

Other mesenchymal solid tumours and genes involved in their pathogenesis detected by FISH

- Round cell/myxoid liposarcoma: CHOP, FUS
- Synovial sarcoma: SYT
- Chondrosarcomas myxoid: EWSR1, CHN
- Fibrosarcoma: gain of whole chromosomes (can be detected by centromeric probes)

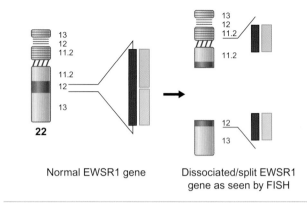

Normal EWSR1 gene   Dissociated/split EWSR1 gene as seen by FISH

Fig. 13.63 Schematic chromosome view of normal and split EWSR1 gene. This gene can be translocated to at least two different chromosome partners (not shown).

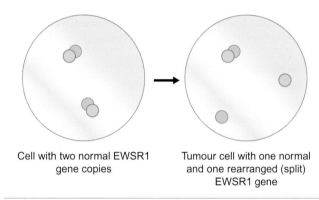

Cell with two normal EWSR1 gene copies   Tumour cell with one normal and one rearranged (split) EWSR1 gene

Fig. 13.64 In normal interphasic nuclei the probes are fused (either they appear close or they overlap and appear as yellow signal). In the case of Ewing's sarcoma due to a translocation, the spots are split and appear distant from each other.

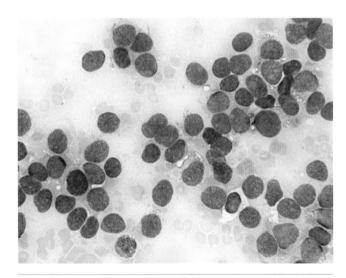

Fig. 13.62 FNA of small round cell tumour: Ewing's sarcoma.

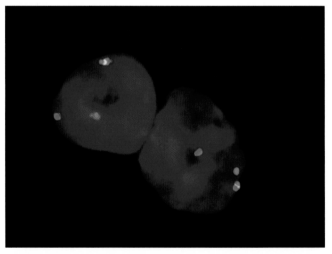

Fig. 13.65 FISH on interphasic nuclei showing a split (separation) of one EWSR1 gene, with the normal second gene.

CHAPTER 14

Self-assessment questions

Cytopathology, like the other academic disciplines, does not have a prescribed beginning and an end. The users of this book are therefore not expected to read it from cover to cover. Instead, they are more likely to find themselves wandering through the pages, looking at the pictures, starting to recognise the familiar conditions and then venturing to the less common. The prerequisite of appreciating the topics is a sound knowledge of basic histopathology. After this has been acquired, cytopathology becomes a visual treat, a puzzle: expecting the eye to see that bit further and engaging the imagination in how to construct a whole from the sum of its parts. And, as in any other puzzle, this process takes time and patience. To start with, a pressing clinical situation will urge the reader to compare the images from the book to those under the microscope, only to realise that different conditions may share some similar features. In these cases, the multidisciplinary meetings will reveal the clinical background and/or results of other investigations and highlight the fact that, as clinical cytopathologists, we are not alone in the diagnostic process. With time, through the important feedback from such meetings and the discussions around the teaching microscope as well as the organized tutorials and workshops, the accumulated knowledge will start replacing the imagination with facts (Figs 14.1–14.3).

The self-assessment chapter has been designed by the authors, all of whom have acquired knowledge and experience through the above process, with a wandering reader in mind. The cases presented here are taken from the main body of the book and have been chosen to put them in a clinical context. Therefore, go ahead, test your knowledge and see how much more there is to learn.

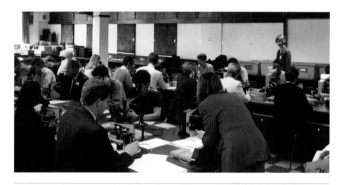

Fig. 14.2 Tutorials and workshops. Formal workshops, such as the one shown here, are a way of learning, expanding and sharing the knowledge of cytopathology.

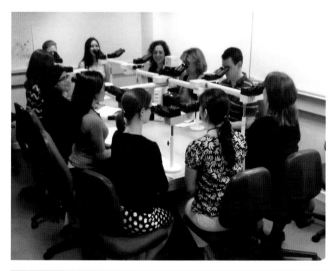

Fig. 14.1 Teaching microscope. A weekly discussion of interesting cases around a teaching microscope is one of the ways of gaining experience in cytopathology.

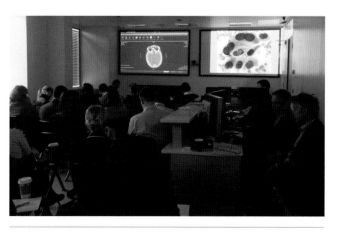

Fig 14.3 Multidisciplinary meetings (MDM). These are weekly gatherings of specialists involved in a particular discipline. The image shows a Head and Neck (HN) MDM where radiologists, histopathologists, cytopathologists, surgeons, oncologists and specialist nurses discuss new cases and follow up investigations of HN cancer patients.

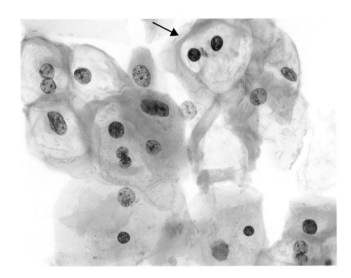

Case 1

Routine cervical cytology sample from a 32-year-old woman

- Describe the cells present.
- What is your diagnosis?
- What differential diagnoses would you consider?
- What additional investigations would you perform?
- What management would you recommend?

Answer: see Fig 2.60, and pp. 18 & 46.

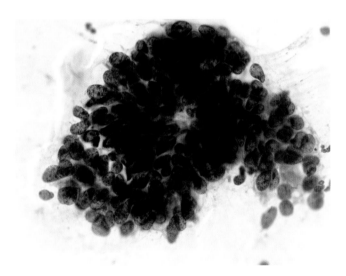

Case 2

Routine cervical cytology sample from a 48-year-old woman

- Describe the cells present.
- What is your diagnosis?
- What differential diagnoses would you consider?
- What is the management?

Answer: see Fig. 2.144, and pp. 41, 44 & 46.

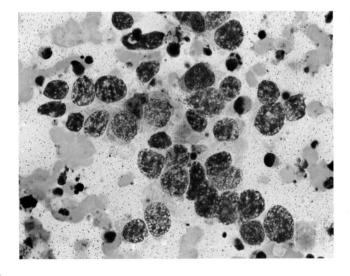

Case 3

EBUS-FNA lung from male aged 43 years

- Describe the cells present.
- What is the likely diagnosis?
- What is your differential diagnosis?
- What further investigations might help?
- What additional symptoms could the patient have?

Answer: see Fig. 3.45, and p. 70.

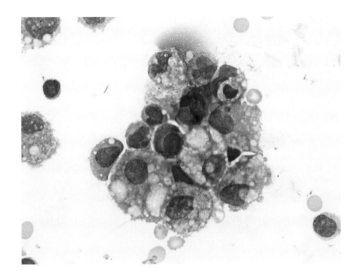

Case 4

Pleural fluid from female aged 79 years with bilateral effusions

- Describe the cells present.
- What is the differential diagnosis?
- What is the likely diagnosis?
- What further clinical information would support the diagnosis?
- Would it be worth examining a further sample?

Answer: see Fig. 4.16, and p. 108.

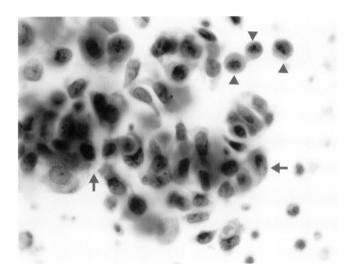

Case 5

Ascitic fluid from male aged 80 years

- Describe the cells present.
- What is the differential diagnosis?
- What is the likely diagnosis?
- What investigations would be helpful?

Answer: see Fig. 4.62, and p. 119.

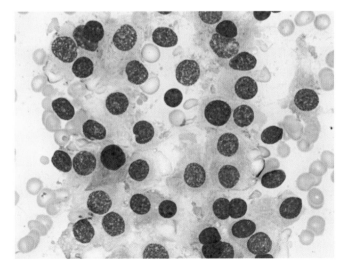

Case 6

FNA of thyroid from female aged 35 years with enlarged nodule in the left lobe

- Describe the cells present.
- What is the main feature of interest here?
- What is the likely diagnosis?
- How would you grade this FNA?
- What other investigations would you suggest to the clinician?

Answer: see Fig. 6.41, and p. 156.

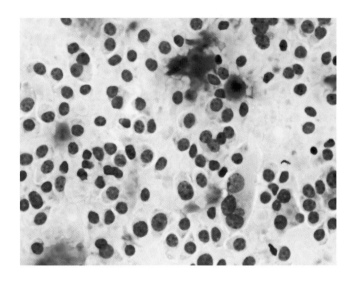

Case 7

FNA of thyroid from male aged 73 years with diffuse swelling of the thyroid

• Describe the cellularity of the smear.
• Describe the background of the smear.
• What is your differential diagnosis?
• What additional tests would you do?
• Would you discuss this case at the MDT?

Answer: see Fig. 6.90, and p. 167.

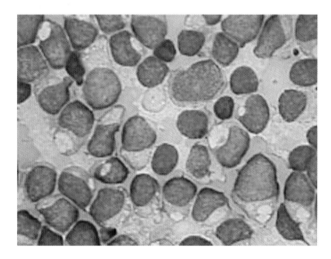

Case 8

Female aged 25 years with osteolytic lesion in the spine, isolated finding

• Describe the cells present.
• Is this a malignant lesion?
• What is the differential diagnosis?
• What additional tests would you perform?

Answer: see Fig. 7.126A, and p. 241.

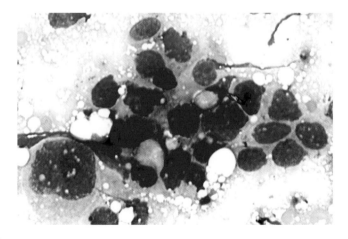

Case 9

FNA of breast lump from female aged 65 years

• Describe the cells present.
• What is the likely diagnosis?
• What is the differential diagnosis?
• How would you grade this lesion?

Answer: see Fig. 8.70, and p. 267.

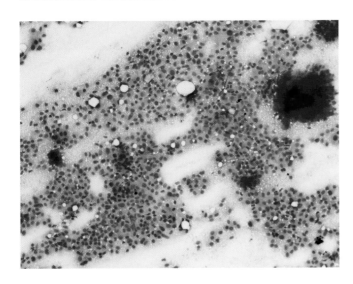

Case 10

FNA of salivary gland from male aged 53 years, on ultrasound a well-defined mass

- Describe the cellularity of the sample.
- Describe the background of the smear.
- What is a helpful feature here?
- What is your diagnosis?

Answer: see Fig. 9.13A, and p. 283.

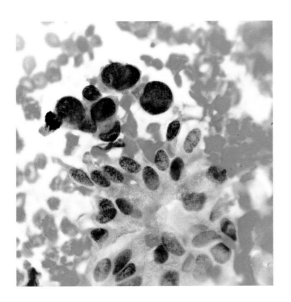

Case 11

Billiary brushings from male aged 69 years with common bile duct obstruction

- Describe the types of cells present.
- What is your diagnosis?

Answer: see Fig. 10.63, and p. 330.

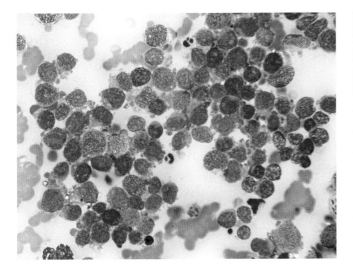

Case 12

FNA of mandible from male aged 15 years with diffuse swelling

- Describe the cellularity of the sample.
- Describe individual cells.
- What is the differential diagnosis?
- What immunocytochemistry marker(s) would you request?
- What molecular genetic tests would you perform?

Answer: see Fig. 11.11, and p. 358.

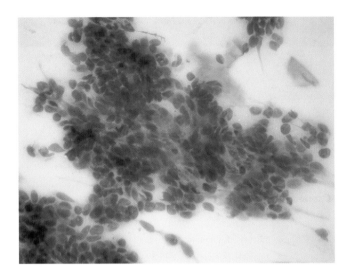

Case 13

FNA of skin from male aged 67 years, with itching

• Describe the cells in the smear.

• Describe the background of the smear.

• What is your diagnosis?

Answer: see Fig. 12.27, and p. 369.

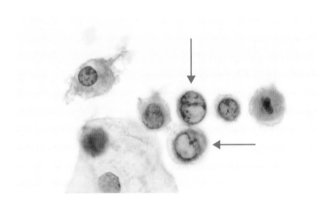

Case 14

Routine cervical cytology sample from a 39-year-old woman

• Describe the cells present.

• What is your diagnosis?

• What differential diagnoses would you consider?

• What is the management?

Answer: see Fig. 2.77, and pp. 25, 33 & 46.

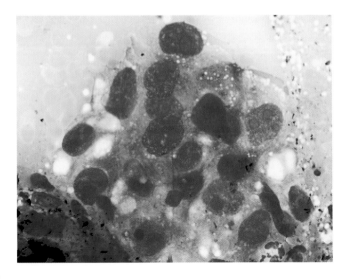

Case 15

EBUS-FNA of peripheral lung nodule from female aged 58 years

• Describe the cells present.

• What is the likely diagnosis?

• What is the differential diagnosis?

• What further clinical details should be checked?

• What investigations would help with the diagnosis?

Answer: see Fig. 3.51, and p. 72.

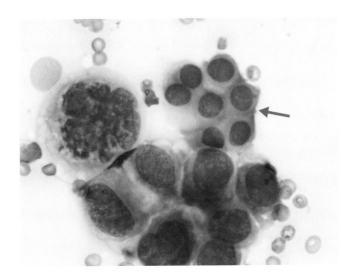

Case 16

Pleural fluid from male aged 59 years

- Describe the cells present.
- What is the differential diagnosis?
- What is the likely diagnosis?
- What further investigations on this sample would help to confirm the diagnosis?
- What is the prognosis for this patient?

Answer: see Fig. 4.46, and p. 116.

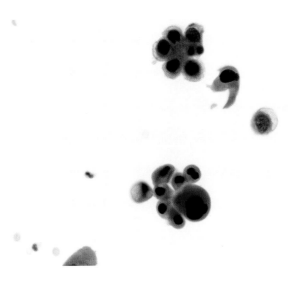

Case 17

Urine from male aged 62 years

- Describe the cells present.
- What is the likely diagnosis?
- What is the differential diagnosis?
- How would you grade this abnormality?
- What symptoms are likely to have been recorded?

Answer: see Fig. 5.21, and p. 139.

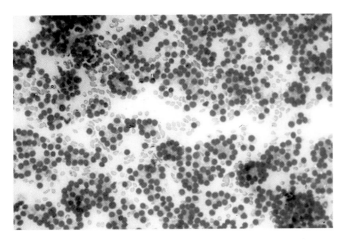

Case 18

FNA of thyroid from male aged 67 years with nodule in the right lobe, detected on ultrasound

- Describe the cellularity of the smear.
- Describe the cell arrangement.
- Describe the background of the smear.
- What is the likely diagnosis?
- How would you grade this smear in the cytology report?
- What is the differential diagnosis?

Answer: see Fig. 6.50, and p. 158.

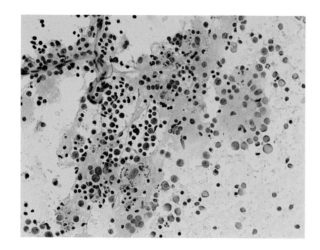

Case 19

• Describe the cells present.

• What is the likely diagnosis?

• What is the differential diagnosis?

• What additional investigation would you perform?

• Can cytology give a definitive answer in this case?

Answer: see Fig. 7.4D, and p. 177.

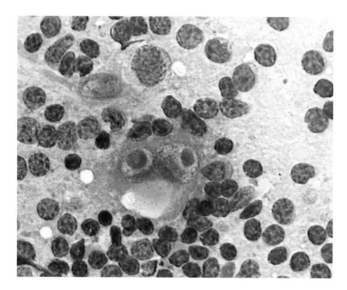

Case 20

FNA of cervical lymph node from 25-year-old male with history of night sweats and malaise

• Describe the diagnostic features in this smear.

• What is the differential diagnosis?

• What additional tests would you do?

• Does this patient need excision biopsy?

Answer: see Fig. 7.61B, and p. 204.

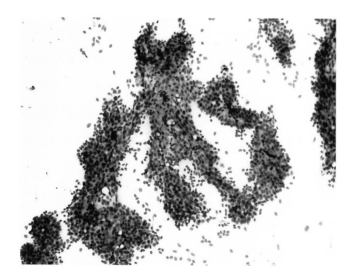

Case 21

FNA of breast lump from female aged 28 years

• Describe the cells present.

• What is the likely diagnosis?

• What is the differential diagnosis?

• What is the prognosis for this patient?

• What clinical features might have been found on examining the breast lump?

Answer: see Fig. 8.33, and p. 255.

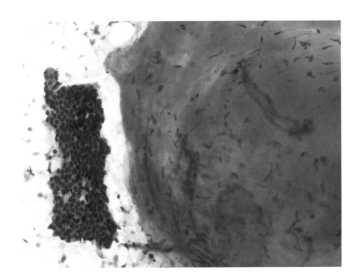

Case 22

FNA of breast lump from female aged 45 years

- Describe the cells present and other findings.
- What is the likely diagnosis?
- What is the differential diagnosis?
- On the findings, is it possible to say if this is benign or malignant?

Answer: see Fig. 8.45, and p. 257.

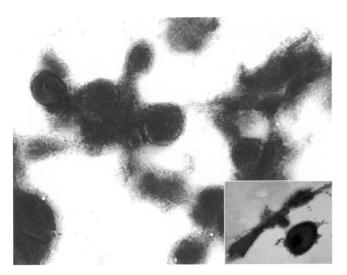

Case 23

FNA of submandibular gland from female aged 41 years with swelling of six months' duration

- Describe the cell arrangement.
- What is the prominent feature?
- What is the differential diagnosis of salivary gland lesions containing hyaline globules?
- What is the likely diagnosis here?

Answer: see Fig. 9.48, and p. 292.

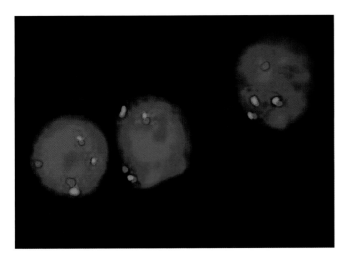

Case 24

Molecular investigation in a child with a mandibular mass

- What is the name of the investigation?
- What are the principles?
- What do red dots represent?
- Give an example of at least two conditions that can be diagnosed in this way.

Answer: see Fig. 13.56, and p. 412.

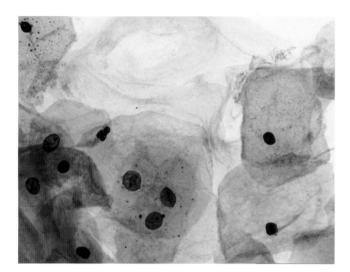

Case 25

Cervical smear from female aged 25 years

- What type of staining is this?
- What are the advantages of this stain?
- How was the specimen fixed?

Answer: see Fig. 13.11A, and p. 396.

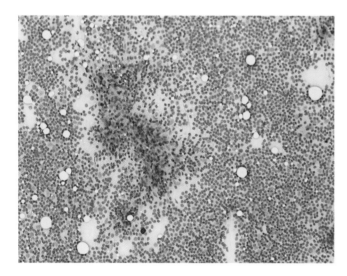

Case 26

FNA of parotid gland from male aged 69 years with diffuse swelling of left parotid gland

- Describe the cellularity of the smear.
- What is the prominent cell type?
- What is the differential diagnosis?
- What further tests would you do to establish a diagnosis?

Answer: see Fig. 9.93, and p. 304.

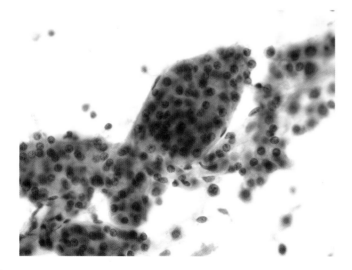

Case 27

FNA of liver from female aged 65 years, jaundiced

- Describe the cellularity of the sample.
- Describe the cell arrangement.
- What is the differential diagnosis?
- What additional tests would you perform?

Answer: see Fig. 10.28A, and p. 318.

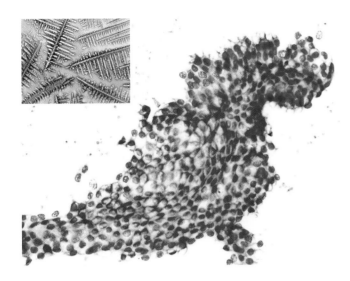

Case 28

FNA of pancreas from female aged 63 years.
Mucoid material obtained on FNA

• Describe the cells in the main image.

• Describe the background (inset).

• What is the main morphological feature of the cells?

• What is your diagnosis?

• Would you discuss this patient at the MDT?

Answer: see Fig. 10.104, and p. 346.

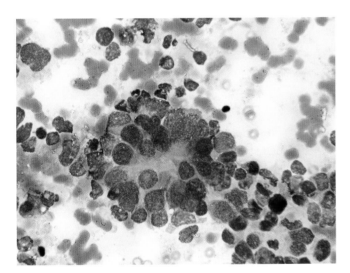

Case 29

FNA of lymph node from two-year-old female
with anaemia and malaise

• Describe the arrangement of the cells in the smear.

• What is the differential diagnosis?

• What is the likely diagnosis?

• What additional tests would you perform in this case?

Answer: see Fig. 11.3A, and p. 354.

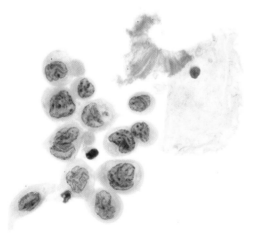

Case 30

Routine cervical cytology sample from a
27-year-old woman

• Describe the cells present.

• What is your diagnosis?

• What differential diagnoses would you consider?

• What is the management?

Answer: see Fig. 2.108, and pp. 33 & 46.

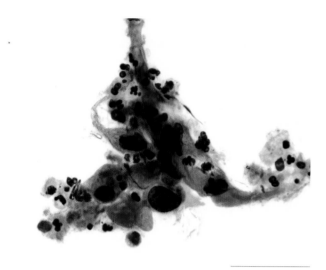

Case 31

FNA of lung mass from male aged 68 years, ex-smoker

- Describe the cell types present.
- What is the likely diagnosis?
- What is your differential diagnosis?
- What further investigations on this sample would help?
- What is the most likely site in the chest for this lung mass?

Answer: see Fig. 3.26, and p. 66.

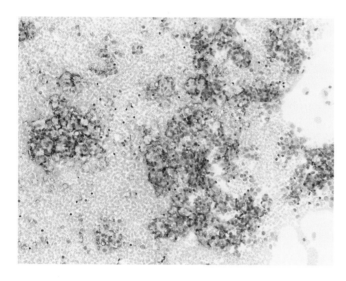

Case 32

Left ovarian aspirate from a 34-year-old woman. Ovary contains a 2cm smooth-walled cyst

- Describe the cells present.
- What is your diagnosis?
- What possible differential diagnoses would you consider?
- What is your management?

Answer: see Fig. 2.188A, and p. 53.

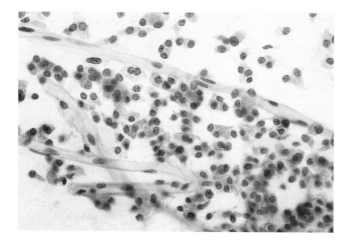

Case 33

Bronchial brushing from male aged 40 years with nodule in right main bronchus

- Describe the two cell types present.
- What is your diagnosis?
- What is the differential diagnosis?
- What investigations would confirm your diagnosis?
- What is the likely prognosis for this patient?

Answer: see Fig. 3.75, and p. 77.

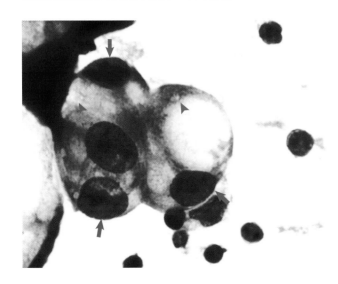

Case 34

Pleural fluid from female aged 53 years

- Describe the cells present.
- What is the differential diagnosis?
- What is the likely diagnosis?
- What clinical details could be relevant?
- What further investigations would you perform on this sample?

Answer: see Fig. 4.36, and p. 114.

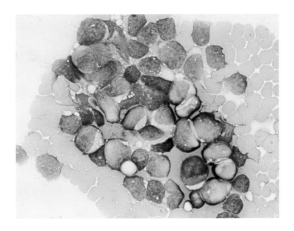

Case 35

Pleural fluid from male aged 46 years

- Describe the cells present.
- What is the differential diagnosis?
- What is the likely diagnosis?
- What further investigations on this sample would be helpful?
- What treatment is this patient likely to have had when first diagnosed with this tumour?

Answer: see Fig. 4.91A, and p. 131.

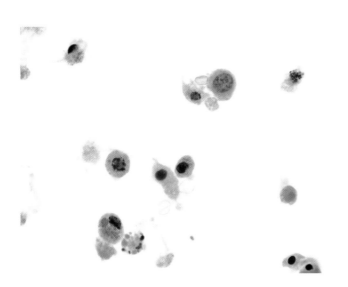

Case 36

Urine from male aged 40 years

- Describe the cells present.
- What is the likely diagnosis?
- What is the differential diagnosis?
- How would you grade this abnormality?

Answer: see Fig. 5.28, and p. 141.

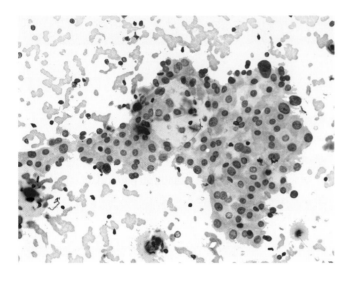

Case 37

FNA of thyroid from female aged 65 years with diffuse enlargement of the thyroid

• Describe the cells.

• Describe the background of the smear.

• Describe the cell arrangement.

• What is the likely diagnosis?

• What additional tests would you suggest to the clinician?

Answer: see Fig. 6.26, and p. 153.

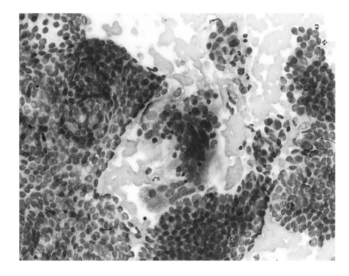

Case 38

FNA of thyroid from female aged 17 years with enlarged right lobe

• Describe the cellularity of the smear.

• Describe the cell arrangement.

• What is your diagnosis?

• How would you grade this smear for the cytology report?

• Is this case appropriate for the MDT discussion?

Answer: see Fig. 6.69, and p. 163.

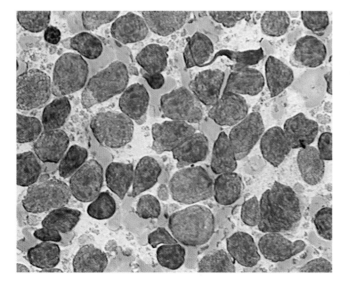

Case 39

FNA of lymph node from female aged 45 years with a several-week history of malaise

• Describe the cells present.

• What is the likely diagnosis?

• What is the differential diagnosis?

• What additional investigations would you perform?

Answer: see Fig. 7.37A, and p. 194.

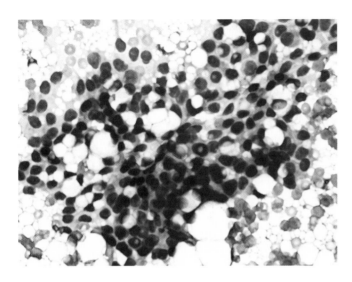

Case 40

FNA of breast lump from female aged 35 years

- Describe the cells present.
- What is the likely diagnosis?
- What is the differential diagnosis?
- What clinical details might be relevant in assessing these findings?

Answer: see Fig. 8.8, and p. 247.

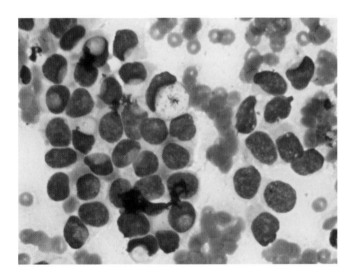

Case 41

FNA of abnormal area on mammography from female aged 52 years

- Describe the cells present.
- What is the likely diagnosis?
- What is the differential diagnosis?
- Would any special stains be helpful?

Answer: see Fig. 8.82, and p. 269.

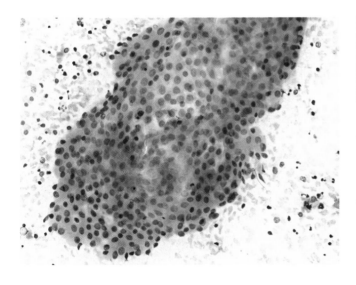

Case 42

FNA of parotid gland from male aged 75 years with swelling at the angle of the mandible

- Describe the predominant cell type in this smear.
- Describe the background of the smear.
- What is your diagnosis?
- What is your differential diagnosis?

Answer: see Fig. 9.21, and pp. 285 & 307.

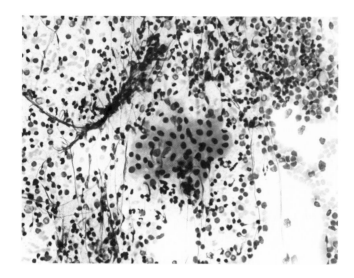

Case 43

FNA of submandibular gland from male aged 70 years, smoker

• Describe the cells in this smear.

• What is your diagnosis?

• What is the differential diagnosis?

Answer: see Fig. 9.54, and p. 294.

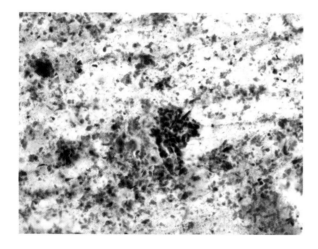

Case 44

FNA of liver from male aged 75 years with multiple liver lesions on ultrasound

• Describe the cellularity of the sample.

• Describe the background.

• What is the likely diagnosis?

• What additional tests would you perform?

• What clinical information would you require?

Answer: see Fig. 10.51, and p. 325.

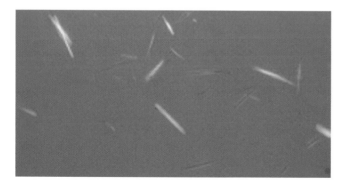

Case 45

Synovial fluid from male aged 79 years with joint pain

• What is this investigation?

• What does it show?

• What type of cell preparation would you use?

• In which cases would you use it?

Answer: see Fig. 12.75, and p. 387.

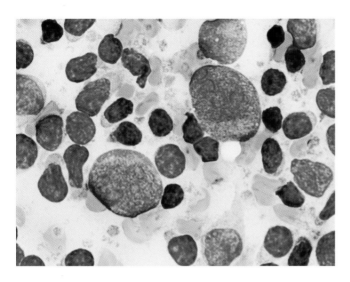

Case 46

FNA of lymph node from male aged 27 years

- What is the stain used in this smear?
- What are the advantages of this staining?
- How was the specimen fixed?

Answer: see Fig. 13.12A, and p. 396.

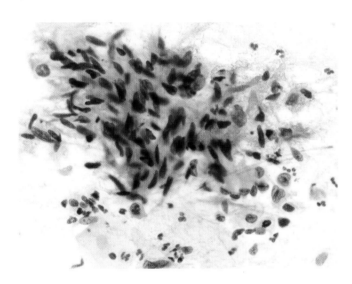

Case 47

Routine cervical cytology sample from a 44-year-old woman with irregular bleeding

- Describe the cells present.
- What is your diagnosis?
- What differential diagnoses would you consider?
- What is your management?

Answer: see Fig. 2.117, and pp. 35, 37 & 46.

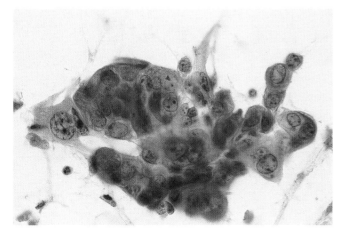

Case 48

Bronchoalveolar lavage from young male, post-infective episode

- Describe this group of cells.
- What change has occurred in these cells?
- Which features favour a benign process?
- What are the long-term risks with these changes?
- Would any follow-up be necessary at this stage?

Answer: see Fig. 3.14, and p. 62.

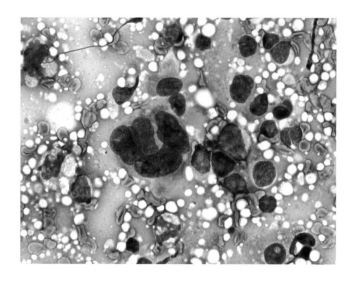

Case 49

Touch prep from mediastinal mass, male aged 26 years

• Describe the cells present.

• What is the likely diagnosis?

• What is the differential diagnosis?

• How can the diagnosis be confirmed cytologically?

• How would this tumour be graded?

Answer: see Fig. 3.113, and p. 87 and Chapter 7.

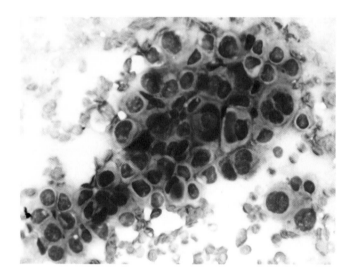

Case 50

FNA of solitary lung mass from female aged 75 years

• Describe the cells present.

• What is your diagnosis?

• What is the differential diagnosis?

• What further clinical information is necessary?

• What stain has been used for this sample?

Answer: see Fig. 3.35, and p. 68.

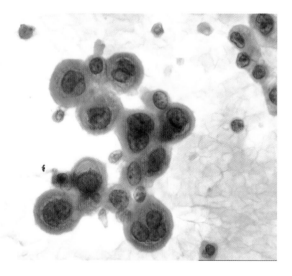

Case 51

Pleural fluid from male aged 78 years, previous dockyard worker

• Describe the cells present.

• What is the differential diagnosis?

• What is the likely diagnosis?

• What further investigations should be used to confirm the diagnosis?

• What is the prognosis and the medicolegal significance of the likely diagnosis?

Answer: see Fig. 4.73, and p. 124.

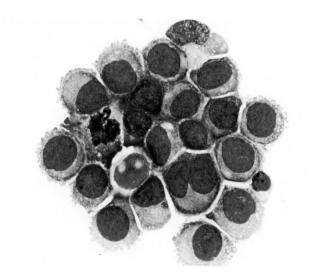

Case 52

Ascitic fluid from male aged 70 years with weight loss and anaemia

• Describe the cells present.

• What is the differential diagnosis?

• What is the likely diagnosis?

• What immunostains would be helpful diagnostically?

• Would any histological stains be helpful on this sample?

Answer: see Fig. 4.95B, and p. 133.

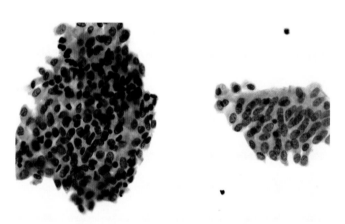

Case 53

Urine from male aged 50 years

• Describe the cells present.

• What type of cell is seen?

• What pathology, if any, do the findings suggest?

• What further information would you seek to confirm your opinion?

Answer: see Fig. 5.15, and p. 138.

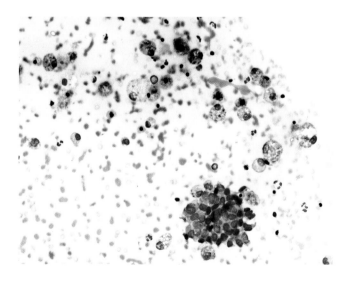

Case 54

FNA of thyroid from female aged 27 years

• Describe the cells and the background.

• Are the appearances typical of a lymph node aspirate?

• What would you need to find out from the clinical and radiological assessments?

• What additional tests would you perform?

• What is the likely diagnosis?

Answer: see Fig. 6.21A, and p. 151.

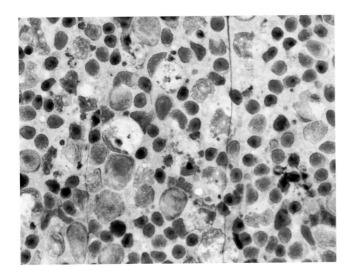

Case 55

FNA of lymph node from female aged 37 years with enlarged left cervical node, and three-week history of fever and malaise

• What are the diagnostic features in this smear?

• What is the likely diagnosis?

• What is the differential diagnosis?

• Does this patient need an excision biopsy?

Answer: see Fig. 7.9, and p. 179.

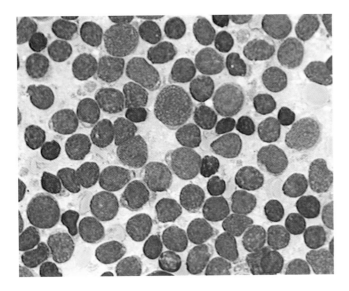

Case 56

FNA of mediastinal lymph nodes from male aged 15 years with a history of shortness of breath

• Describe the cells present.

• What is the likely diagnosis?

• What is the differential diagnosis?

• What additional tests would you perform?

• Can FNA deliver a conclusive diagnosis is this case?

Answer: see Fig. 7.19, and p. 184.

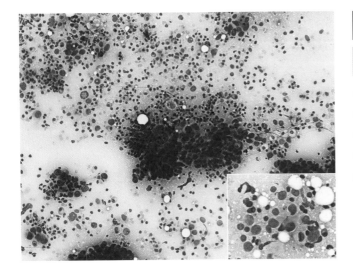

Case 57

FNA of breast lump from female aged 40 years

• Describe the cells present.

• What is the likely diagnosis?

• What is the differential diagnosis?

• What is the significance of the mixed cell types in the aspirate?

Answer: see Fig. 8.86, and p. 270.

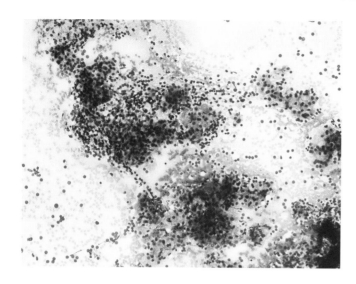

Case 58

FNA of parotid gland from female aged 43 years with a mass in the parotid gland

• Describe the cellularity of the sample.

• Describe the background of the smear.

• What is the differential diagnosis?

• What is the likely diagnosis?

Answer: see Fig. 9.35, and p. 289.

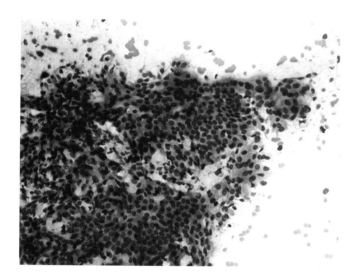

Case 59

FNA of pancreas from female aged 82 years, jaundiced

• Describe the cellularity of the sample.

• Describe the cell arrangement.

• What is the differential diagnosis?

• What is your diagnosis?

Answer: see Fig. 10.81, and p. 336.

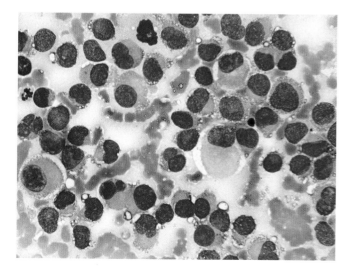

Case 60

FNA of lymph node from male aged 5 years with scrotal swelling

• Describe the cells in the smear.

• Describe the cell arrangement.

• What is differential diagnosis?

• What additional tests would you perform?

Answer: see Fig. 11.10A, and p. 357.

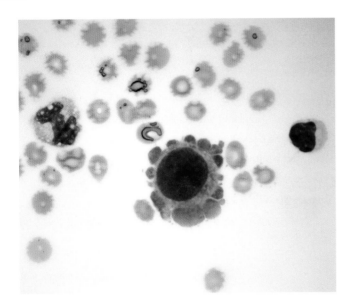

Case 61

CSF from female aged 53 years, with headache

- Describe the cells in the smear.
- What is the likely diagnosis?
- How would you confirm it?
- What additional clinical information would you seek?

Answer: see Fig. 12.10, and p. 364.

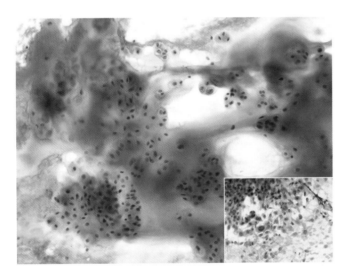

Case 62

FNA of upper end of femur mass from male aged 67 years

- Describe the background of this smear.
- What is the likely differential diagnosis?
- What other tests would you perform?
- Which other investigation is essential to compare with the FNA?

Answer: see Fig. 12.70, and p. 383.

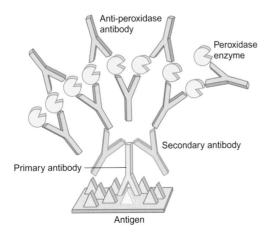

PAP method

Case 63

Principles of immunocytochemistry

- What does PAP stand for?
- How many layers does this method involve?
- What constitutes each layer?

Answer: see Fig. 13.16, and p. 399.

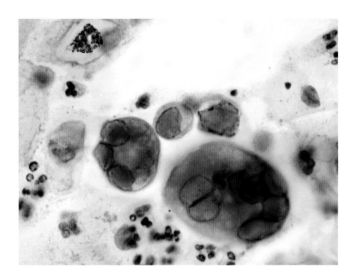

Case 64

Sputum from female aged 29 years with history of severe weight loss and cough

- Describe the cells present.
- What is the likely diagnosis?
- What is the differential diagnosis?
- How could the diagnosis be confirmed?
- What other clinical details could be relevant in this case?

Answer: see Fig. 3.128, and p. 90.

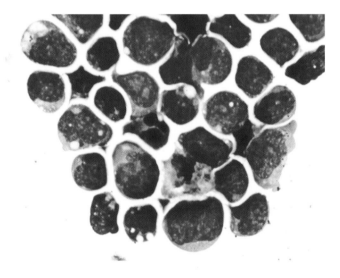

Case 65

Pleural fluid, milky coloured sample, from male aged 65 years

- Describe the cells present.
- What is the differential diagnosis?
- What is the likely diagnosis?
- What further investigations should be performed on this sample?
- What is the significance of the gross appearance of the fluid?

Answer: see Fig. 4.68 inset, and p. 121.

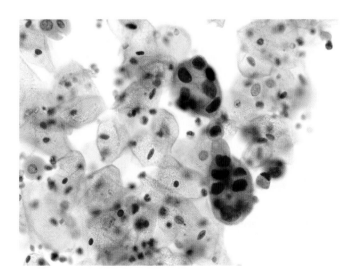

Case 66

Urine from female aged 59 years

- Describe the cells present.
- What is the likely diagnosis?
- What is your differential diagnosis?
- What further clinical details could be relevant?

Answer: see Fig. 5.33, and p. 142.

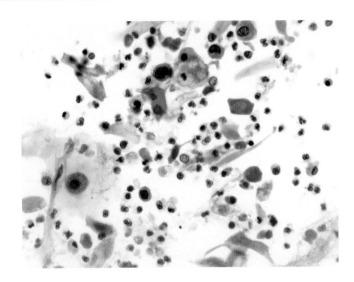

Case 67

Urine from female aged 75 years

- Describe the cells present.
- What is the likely diagnosis?
- What is the differential diagnosis?
- What is the significance, if any, of the keratinised cells seen?

Answer: see Fig. 5.30, and p. 141.

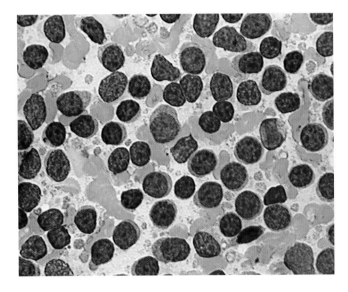

Case 68

FNA of lymph node from 64-year-old male with anaemia

- Describe the cells present.
- What is the likely diagnosis?
- What is the differential diagnosis?
- What additional investigations would you perform?
- Can cytology give a definitive answer in this case?

Answer: see Fig. 7.21, and p. 186.

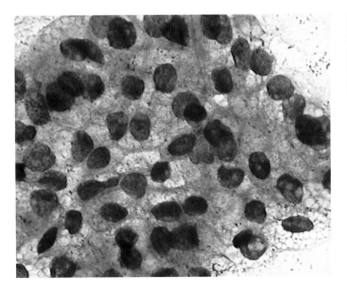

Case 69

FNA of supraclavicular lymph node from male aged 53 years

- Describe the diagnostic features.
- What is the likely diagnosis?
- How would you confirm it?
- What clinical history would you expect in this case?

Answer: see Fig. 7.70, and p. 207.

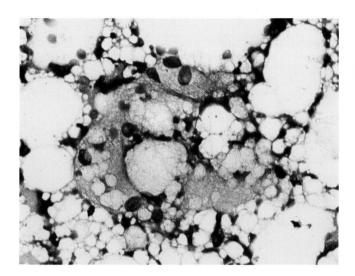

Case 70

FNA of breast lump from female aged 39 years

- Describe the cells present.
- What is the likely diagnosis?
- What is the differential diagnosis?
- What clinical details could be relevant to the diagnosis?

Answer: see Fig. 8.12, and p. 249.

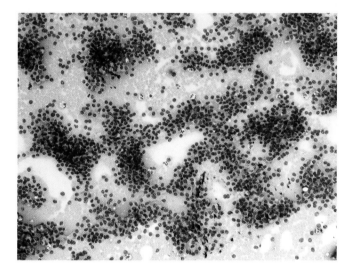

Case 71

FNA of pancreas from male aged 55 years with obstructive jaundice

- Describe the cellularity of the smear.
- Describe the cell arrangement.
- What is the differential diagnosis?
- What additional tests would you perform?
- What other clinical information may you require?

Answer: see Fig. 10.93A, p. 341 and Table 10.2, p. 343.

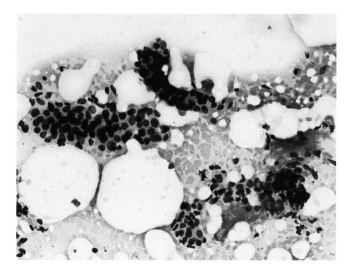

Case 72

FNA of breast lump from female aged 46 years

- Describe the cells present.
- What is the likely diagnosis?
- What is the differential diagnosis?
- What grade would you give to these findings?

Answer: see Fig. 8.76, and p. 268.

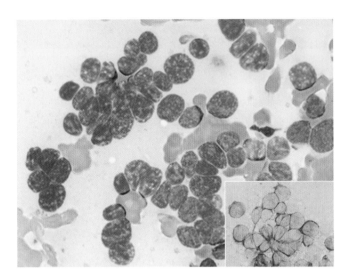

Case 73

FNA of skin nodule from male aged 85 years with history of bluish skin nodule for some months

- Describe the cells in the smear.
- What is the differential diagnosis?
- What additional tests would you perform?
- What is the marker used in the inset photograph

Answer: see Fig. 12.34, and p. 371.

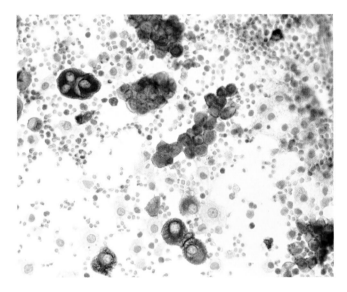

Case 74

Pleural effusion from a patient with peritoneal carcinoma

- Describe the findings.
- What is the purpose of double immunocytochemistry staining?
- What do the antibodies highlight?
- If one of these is an epithelial marker, what is your diagnosis?

Answer: see Fig. 13.28, and p. 402.

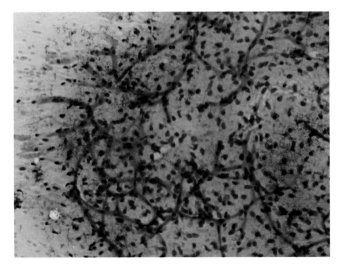

Case 75

FNA of retroperitoneal mass from female aged 67 years with abdominal discomfort

- Describe the cellularity of the sample.
- What is the main feature of this smear?
- What additional stains would you perform?
- What is your differential diagnosis?

Answer: see Fig. 12.56A, and p. 379.

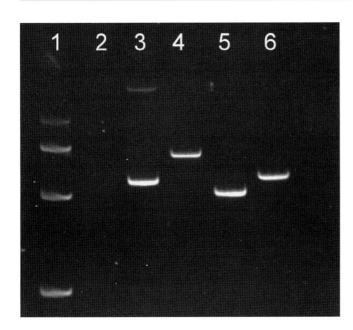

Case 76

A test to detect t(14;18) has been performed on FNA of lymph nodes with suspicion of lymphoma. (Lanes: 1, size markers; 2, negative control; 3, positive markers; 4–6, test cases).

• Describe the method used

• Describe the findings in test cases (lanes 4, 5 & 6)

• What is the diagnosis?

• What other DNA sequences can be targeted by this method?

Answer: see Fig. 13.41, and p. 407.

Subject Index

Note: vs denotes differential diagnosis, or comparisons

A

Abrikossov (granular cell) tumour, breast 259, 259f
abscess
    amoebic, of liver 312
    breast 252, 252f
    liver 312
    pyogenic, of liver 312
    subareolar 250, 250f
acid fast bacilli 88, 89f
acinar cell(s), pancreatic *see* pancreatic acinar cells
acinar cell carcinoma (pancreas) 339, 339f, 343t
    lymph node metastases 207f
acinar epithelium
    pancreatic 332
    salivary gland 280f
acinic cell carcinoma (salivary gland) 280, 288, 288f–289f, 307f
    cystic variant 289f
    differential diagnosis 288, 289f
actinic (solar) keratosis 368, 368f
Actinomyces 20f, 95f, 312
actinomycotic bacteria, lung infection 88f
acute basophilic leukaemia 238, 238f
acute erythroid leukaemia 236, 236f
acute leukaemia
    of ambiguous lineage 240, 240f
    not otherwise specified 238, 238f
acute lymphoblastic leukaemia 184f, 365
acute megakaryoblastic leukaemia 237, 237f
acute monoblastic and monocytic leukaemia 235, 235f
acute monoblastic leukaemia 235, 235f
acute monocytic leukaemia 235, 235f
acute myeloid leukaemia (AML) 196f, 209t, 227–241
    CSF in 365
    cytological findings 196f, 227–228, 227f
    with myelodysplastic-related changes 230, 230f
    not otherwise specified
        acute erythroid leukaemia 236, 236f
        acute megakaryoblastic leukaemia 237, 237f
        acute monoblastic and monocytic leukaemia 235, 235f
        acute myelomonocytic leukaemia 234, 234f
        acute panmyelosis with myelofibrosis 239, 239f
        with maturation 233, 233f
        without maturation 232, 232f, 237
        minimal differentiation 231, 231f
    with recurrent genetic abnormalities
        acute promyelocytic leukaemia 228, 228f
        inv(16) or t(16;16) 229, 229f
        t(8;21) 227, 227f
acute myelomonocytic leukaemia 234, 234f
acute panmyelosis with myelofibrosis 239, 239f
acute promyelocytic leukaemia (PML) 228, 228f
adenocarcinoma
    bile ducts *see* cholangiocarcinoma
    bladder 139
    cervical *see under* cervical carcinoma
    colonic *see* colonic carcinoma
    duodenal, metastatic cells in serous effusions 118f
    endometrial *see* endometrial carcinoma
    endometrioid 57f
    gastric, metastatic cells in effusions 118f
    lung *see under* lung tumours
    mesothelioma *vs* 115, 127t
    metastatic 114f
        CSF in 364, 364f
        serous effusions 112f, 118f
    ovarian 57f, 117f
    pancreatic *see* pancreatic ductal adenocarcinoma
    polymorphous, salivary gland 296, 296f, 306f
    respiratory tract reactive changes *vs* 62
    salivary duct 297, 297f
    urinary tract *see* urinary tract malignancy
adenocarcinoma cells, mesothelioma *vs* 124, 127t
adenoid cystic carcinoma
    lung *see under* lung tumours
    salivary gland 281f, 283f, 292, 292f–293f, 306f
        differential diagnosis 286, 292
        histology 292
adenolymphoma *see* Warthin's tumour
adenoma
    bile duct (extrahepatic) 331
    bile duct (intrahepatic) 313, 313f
    breast *see under* breast
    hepatocellular 316
    nipple 262–263
    oncocytic *see* oncocytic adenoma
    pleomorphic *see under* salivary gland tumours
    thyroid *see* thyroid gland neoplasms
    tubular 258, 258f
    villous, bile ducts 331
adenoma/carcinoma sequence 137
adenomyoepithelioma, breast 266b, 260f
adenosquamous carcinoma
    bile ducts (extrahepatic) 331, 331f
    lung 72f
    pancreas 339, 339f

adipose tissue
    benign tumours 375, 375f, 375t
    malignant tumours 379–380
        see also liposarcoma
    normal cytology 373, 373f
    reactive changes 373, 373f
ALK protein 371f
alkaline phosphatase 212f, 384f
allergic bronchopulmonary aspergillosis 97, 97f
allergic bronchopulmonary disease 97, 97f
    differential diagnosis 97
alpha-fetoprotein (AFP) 317t, 320, 322
Alternaria 61f
alveolar casts 93
    amphophilic 93, 93f
alveolar proteinosis, pulmonary 101, 101f
alveolar rhabdomyosarcoma *see* rhabdomyosarcoma, alveolar type
alveolar soft part sarcoma 382, 382f
alveolitis, fibrosing *see* fibrosing alveolitis
amphophilic material, pulmonary alveolar proteinosis 101, 101f
amphophilic plaque, amyloidosis 101f
amylase crystals, sialadenitis 301f
amyloid deposits
    liver 314, 314f
    medullary carcinoma of thyroid 166f–167f
    plasma cells with 190f
amyloidosis 189, 190f
    liver 314, 314f
    lung 101, 101f
anaemia, refractory
    with excess blasts (RAEB) 223, 223f
    refractory cytopenia with unilineage dysplasia 220, 220f
    with ring sideroblasts 221, 221f
anaplastic large cell lymphoma (ALCL) 202, 203f
    ALK-ALCL 202
    ALK+ALCL 202, 202f–203f
    childhood 353t
    CSF 365f
    histiocytic sarcoma *vs* 242f
    primary cutaneous (C-ALCL) 202, 203f, 371f
anaplastic lymphoma kinase (ALK1) 202, 202f
'anchovy paste', echinococcal cyst of liver 312f
angiofollicular lymph node hyperplasia 181, 181f
angioimmunoblastic T-cell lymphoma (AITL) 201, 201f
angiomyolipoma, liver 315, 315f
angiosarcoma
    liver 324, 324f
    post-irradiation, breast 275f
anisocytosis, anaplastic large cell lymphoma 203f

anisonucleosis 38f, 154f, 156f, 161f, 203f
anisopilocytosis 213f
antigen retrieval, immunocytochemistry 398, 403f
anucleate squames
    cervical transformation zone 6, 7f
    epidermoid cyst (breast) and 259f
    lymphoepithelial cyst (pancreas) 345, 345f
    ovarian cystic teratoma 56
    skin 368f
    vulval 47f
apocrine carcinoma of breast 254f, 272, 272f
apocrine cells (breast) 253, 254f
    anisonucleosis 263f
    apocrine carcinoma 254f
    atypical 254f
    hyperplasia with atypia and 263f
    metaplastic 259
apocrine metaplasia, breast 253f
Arias–Stella changes 44
artefacts 395f
    air drying 395f
    cervical smears 11, 12f
    fibroadenoma, atypia 256f
    P. jirovecii differential diagnosis 93
    smearing 395, 395f
arthritis, diagnostic algorithm 389f
arthropathy, inflammatory, diagnostic algorithm 389f
asbestos, mesothelioma and 123
asbestos body 99, 99f
asbestosis 99
ascitic fluid/ascites 110f
    acute myeloid leukaemia blast cells 196f
    Burkitt's lymphoma in 195f
    gastric carcinoma 115f
    malignant epithelial cells 196f
    metastatic breast carcinoma 116f
    metastatic duodenal carcinoma 118f
    metastatic ovarian carcinoma 117f
    ovarian serous papillary carcinoma 114f
    rhabdomyosarcoma 196f
Askin's tumour *see* Ewing's (sarcoma) family of tumours
aspergillosis, allergic bronchopulmonary 97, 97f
Aspergillus infection 92f
    allergic bronchopulmonary aspergillosis 97, 97f
    lung 92, 92f, 97
asthma 97, 97f
    adenocarcinoma *vs* 72f
astrocytoma, CSF in 363
Auer rods 224, 227–228, 227f–228f, 232f
Australian Modified Bethesda System (AMBS), cervical intraepithelial neoplasia 27t
autoimmune pancreatitis (AIP) 335, 335f
avidin-biotin complex (ABC) method 399–400, 400f, 403f

B

bacterial infections
    cerebrospinal fluid (CSF) in 362, 362f
    cervical/vaginal 15f–16f, 16
    lung *see* lung infections
Bartonella henselae, infection (cat-scratch disease) 179, 179f

basal cell(s), skin 366
    in basal cell carcinoma of skin 369f
basal cell adenocarcinoma, salivary gland 299f
basal cell adenoma, salivary gland 306f
basal cell carcinoma of skin 366f, 369, 369f
    differential diagnosis 369
basaloid cells
    adenoid cystic carcinoma (salivary gland) 292f–293f
    pilomatrixoma 371, 371f
    salivary gland FNA 306
    sebaceous gland tumours 369
basophil(s), acute basophilic leukaemia 238, 238f
basophilic cytoplasm, lymphoblasts 183f
B-cell lymphoma 182t
    in chronic lymphocytic leukaemia 205
    diffuse large cell *see* diffuse large B-cell lymphoma (DLBCL)
    high-grade, primary effusion *see* primary effusion lymphoma
    PCR product analysis 406f
    see also B-lymphocytes
BCG treatment, urine cytology after 144, 144f
BCL2-positive cells, follicular lymphoma 192f
BCR-ABL1 fusion gene 210
benign pseudosarcomatous lesions 376
beryllium, lymphadenopathy 180
Bethesda System, reporting
    cervical glandular abnormalities 40t
    cervical smears 24, 27t
    thyroid cytopathology 170, 170t
bile 311, 311f, 327
    malignant epithelial cells producing 319f
    sampling 326
bile duct(s) (extrahepatic) 326–331
    adenocarcinoma 330, 330f–331f
    adenosquamous carcinoma 331, 331f
    anatomy 309f
    brush/catheter samples 326
        see also bile duct brushings
    carcinoma 326
    cystadenocarcinoma, mucinous 331, 331f
    cystadenoma 331
    cystic mucinous neoplasms 331, 331f
    dysplasia of epithelium 329, 329f–330f
        high-grade 329, 329f
        low-grade 329, 329f
    fine-needle aspiration samples 326–327
    inflammatory processes 328, 328f
    intraductal papillary tumour 330, 330f
    liquid-based cytology (LBC) 326
    neoplasms 326b, 330–331
    normal cytology 327, 327f
        bile duct brushings 327, 327f
        FNA samples 327
    papillary carcinoma, well-differentiated 331
    parasitic infection 328, 328f
    premalignant lesions 326
    reactive changes 328, 328f
    sampling for cytology 326
    villous adenoma 331
bile duct(s) (intrahepatic) 316f
    adenocarcinoma *see* cholangiocarcinoma
    adenoma 313, 313f
    hamartoma 313, 313f

bile duct brushings 326
    adenocarcinoma 330, 330f
    cholangiocarcinoma differential diagnosis 323, 323f
    cystadenoma/cystadenocarcinoma *vs* 331
    inflammatory and reactive processes 328f
    malignancy types, sensitivity for 331
    normal cytology 327, 327f
bile duct epithelium 316f
    in adenocarcinoma 330f
    dysplasia 329, 329f
        see also under bile duct(s) (extrahepatic)
    normal 310, 327f
    reactive changes 328f
    regenerative and degenerative changes 328
bile pigment 311, 311f
bile plugs, canalicular 311f
biliary papillomatosis 330, 330f
biliary tree
    sampling for cytology 326
    see also bile duct(s) (extrahepatic); gallbladder
BK virus 143, 143f
bladder, HPV infection 144, 145f
bladder carcinoma 139
    adenocarcinoma 139
    metastatic serous effusions 119f
    transitional cell (urothelial) *see* transitional cell carcinoma
blastoma, pulmonary 81, 82f
Blastomyces dermatitidis, lung infection 94, 94f
blood, in specimens 395, 395f
'blue blobs', cervical smears/samples 11, 13f
B-lymphoblastic leukaemia/lymphoma 183, 183f–184f
B-lymphocytes
    mature, neoplasms 182t, 185–197
        see also specific tumours
    monocytoid, cat-scratch disease 179, 179f
    precursors, neoplasms 183
        lymphoblastic leukaemia/lymphoma 183, 183f–184f
    see also B-cell lymphoma
bone 372
    cytogenetics 372
    immunocytochemistry 372
    Langerhans cell histiocytosis 385, 385f
    mass, childhood tumours 352t
    normal cytology 374, 374f
    pain, childhood tumours 352t
    reactive changes 374, 374f
    tumours *see* bone tumours
bone marrow aspiration 174, 174f
    complications 174
bone marrow disorders 175
    see also specific leukaemias/tumours
bone tumours 383
    benign 383t
        chondroblastoma 383, 383f
        osteoblastoma 384, 384f
    childhood 352t
    cytological report 386
    FNA cytology for management 372
    malignant 383t
        see also chondrosarcoma; Ewing's sarcoma (classic); osteosarcoma
    metastatic 386, 386t

Borrelia burgdorferi infection 362
Bowen's disease 370
branchial cleft cyst 303, 303f
breast 245–277
   abscess 252, 252f
   adenomyoepithelioma 266b, 260f
   apocrine cells *see* apocrine cells (breast)
   apocrine metaplasia 253f
   benign changes 253, 266b
     apocrine cells 254f
     lactational changes 258, 258f
   benign fibrocystic change 253, 253f–254f
   benign tumours/tumour-like lesions 255–
     260, 265t, 266b
   borderline epithelial lesions 263–264
     cellular (florid) papillary lesions 264
     columnar cell lesions 263
     lobular intraepithelial neoplasia 264
   carcinoma *see* breast carcinoma
   cellular (florid) papillary lesions 264
   columnar cell lesions 263, 263f
   complex sclerosing lesions 262–263, 262f
   cysts 253
     apocrine cells in fluid 254f
     foamy macrophages 253, 253f
   duct ectasia 250, 250f, 259, 260f
   ductal cells 246f, 248f
   enlargement, male *see* gynaecomastia
   epidermoid cyst 259, 259f
   epithelial cells 245f–246f, 261f
     reactive atypia 250f
     sclerosing lymphocytic lobulitis 252f
   epithelial hyperplasia *see* breast,
     hyperplasia
   fat necrosis 249, 249f
     differential diagnosis 249, 249f
   fibroadenoma *see* fibroadenoma (breast)
   fibroblasts 247f
   fibrocystic change, gynaecomastia *vs* 248
   fibrocystic lesions 262–263
   fibroepithelial neoplasms 246, 266b
   fine-needle aspiration (FNA) 245–246, 247f
     capillary technique 247
     multidisciplinary team role 277
     palpable lesions 247
     reporting 277, 277t
     role in management 277
   galactocele 248
   granular cell tumour 259, 259f
   granulomatous mastitis *see* mastitis,
     granulomatous
   gynaecomastia 248, 248f
   hamartoma 258
   hyperplasia 261, 261f
     carcinoma *vs* 253, 254f, 263
     florid, gynaecomastia *vs* 248
   hyperplasia with atypia 263
   hyperplasia without atypia 261
   inflammatory conditions 249–252
   intramammary lymph node 259, 259f
   lactating adenoma 258, 258f
   lactation pattern 247f
   lactational changes 258, 258f
   lobular intraepithelial neoplasia 264, 264f
   lobules, normal histology 245f
   lymphoma (primary) 275, 275f
     mantle cell 276f
   male, tumours, WHO classification 266b

malignant tumours 265–270, 265t, 266b
   carcinosarcoma 274
   epithelial *see* breast carcinoma
   myoepithelioma 274, 274f
   phyllodes tumour 275, 275f
   post-irradiation angiosarcoma 275f
   precursor lesions 266b
   sarcoma 275
   uncommon 275
mesenchymal tumours, WHO classification
   266b
metastatic tumours (extramammary
   primary) to 266b, 275, 276f
   lymphomas 276f
microglandular adenosis 261
mucocele-like lesions 264, 264f
myoepithelial cells 247f–248f
myoepithelial lesions 266b
normal 245–248, 245–246, 245f
nucleoli 247f
papilloma (benign) 262–263, 262f
periductal mastitis *see* mastitis, periductal
pregnancy-related changes 246
radial sclerosing lesions 262
sclerosing lymphocytic lobulitis 252, 252f
subareolar abscess 250, 250f
subareolar papillomatosis 262–263
terminal duct lobular units (TDLU),
   dilatation 263
tubular adenoma 258, 258f
tumour-like lesions 255–261
   see also breast, benign tumours
vacuolation 247f
breast carcinoma 113, 265–270
   apocrine 254f, 272, 272f
   clear cell (glycogen rich) 273, 273f
   colloid (mucinous) 271, 271f
   differential diagnosis
     columnar cell changes 263
     epithelial hyperplasia 253, 254f, 263
     fibroadenoma 255
     hyperplasia with atypia 263
   ductal 265, 267
     FISH with *FGR1* gene 411f
     high-grade 267f–268f
     intermediate-grade 268f
     invasive 267
     low-grade 267f–268f
     metastatic 142f
   ductal carcinoma in situ 268f
   false-positive, fibroadenoma 255
   glycogen rich 273, 273f
   HER2 gene amplification 413, 413f
   immunocytochemistry, cytoplasmic
     reaction 402f
   inflammatory 252, 252f
   invasive 266b, 413f
     ductal 267
     fat necrosis *vs* 249, 249f
     FISH, gene amplification 413, 413f
     lobular 269–270
   lipid-rich 273, 273f
   lobular 265, 269–270, 269f
     differential diagnosis 270
     intracytoplasmic vacuoles 269f
     invasive 269–270
     metastatic 43f, 116f
     pleomorphic type 269f, 270

medullary, with lymphoid stroma 270,
   270f
metaplastic 274, 274f
   CSF in 364, 364f
   differential diagnosis 274
metastatic
   adenocarcinoma cells in effusions 116f
   cells in serous effusions 112f–116f,
     113–119
   dual cell population 115f
   dual immunostaining 134f
   ductal, urine cytology 142f
   lobular 43f
   in lung 80f
   mesothelioma *vs* (pleural fluid) 126f
   small cell carcinoma of lung *vs* 70f
   mucinous (colloid) 271, 271f
   neuroendocrine 271, 271f
     diagnostic pitfalls 271
   osteoclast-like giant cells 251f, 273, 273f
   papillary 272, 272f
   progesterone receptor 401f
   tubular 270, 270f
     differential diagnosis 270
breast clinic, 'one stop' 277, 277f
bridges, intercellular, actinic keratosis 368, 368f
British Association of Cytopathology (BAC) 27t,
   40t
bronchial brushing 64
   bronchial carcinoid 77f
   large cell carcinoma 75f
   normal cytology 60f–61f
   pulmonary blastoma 82f
   reactive changes 63f, 74f
   squamous cell carcinoma differential
     diagnosis 68f
     dysplasia *vs* 67f
bronchial epithelium
   cilia 60f–61f
   hyperplasia 62, 63f
   normal 60, 60f–61f, 74f
   reactive changes 62, 63f
     drug toxicity causing 63
   squamous metaplasia 62, 62f
bronchial lining 59f
bronchial tumours 64f
bronchiectasis 96, 96f
bronchiolar cells, hyperplastic 72f
bronchitis, chronic 64
bronchoalveolar cell carcinoma (BAC) *see* lung
   tumours, adenocarcinoma - lepidic
   predominant
bronchoalveolar lavage (BAL)
   adenocarcinoma with lepidic growth
     pattern 73f
   bacterial infections 88f
   fibrosing alveolitis 74f
   fungal infections 94f
   hyperplastic bronchiolar cells 72f
   normal cytology 60
   P. jirovecii infection 93f
   pulmonary alveolar proteinosis 101, 101f
   reactive changes 62f–63f
   Strongyloides infection 95, 95f
   viral infections 91f
bronchogenic carcinoma 64
bronchopneumonia 88
bronchopulmonary fistula 109f

bronchoscope, flexible, with ultrasound probe (EBUS-TBNFA) 64f
brushings 392
   bile duct *see* bile duct brushings
   bronchial *see* bronchial brushing
   oral mucosa 393f
buffered balanced salt (BBS) solution 175
Burkitt's leukaemia 197
Burkitt's lymphoma (BL) 197, 353t
   in ascitic effusion 195f
   chromosomal translocation 197, 197f
     FISH 412, 412f
   cytological findings 197, 197f, 353, 353f
   diagnostic pitfalls 353
   differential diagnosis 197
   immunomarkers 130f, 197
Burkitt's-like lymphoma (BLL) 353, 353t

C

calcium pyrophosphate dihydrate crystals 387, 387f
calretinin staining 131f, 403f
Candida infections
   cervical/vaginal 16, 17f, 40
   lung 94
cannonballs 122t
carcinoid tumours
   lung *see* lung tumours, carcinoid
   lymph node metastases 207f
carcinoma *see individual carcinomas*
carcinoma cells, in serous effusions *see* serous effusions
carcinomatous meningitis 364
carcinosarcoma
   breast 274
   pulmonary 81
Castleman's disease 181, 181f
cat-scratch disease 179, 179f
CD3
   reactive follicular hyperplasia 175f
   T-cell lymphomas 199f, 365f, 406f
   T-lymphoblastic leukaemia 184f
   viral meningitis 362, 362f
CD5, reactive follicular hyperplasia 175f
CD10-positive cells 175f, 183f–184f
CD15, Reed–Sternberg-like cell in small lymphocytic lymphoma 186f
CD19, reactive follicular hyperplasia 175f
CD20 362, 362f
   diffuse large B-cell lymphoma 193f–194f, 205f–206f
   follicular lymphoma 192f
   mantle cell lymphoma 191f
   post-transplant lymphoproliferative disease 206f
   primary effusion lymphoma 195f
   small lymphocytic lymphoma 186f
CD30
   anaplastic large cell lymphoma 202, 202f–203f
   diffuse large B-cell lymphoma 194f
   Hodgkin's lymphoma 204t
CD34, sinusoids in hepatocellular carcinoma 320, 320f
CD45, immunochemistry staining 402f
CD68-positive cells 242f, 244f
   macrophages 178f, 218f

CD79a marker 365f
cell block preparations 394–395, 394f
cell cannibalism 51f
cell imprints 395, 395f
central nervous system (CNS) tumours
   primary, CSF in 363, 363f
   secondary 364
     CSF in 364, 364f
     differential diagnosis 364
centroblasts
   follicular lymphoma 192, 192f
   non-specific lymph node hyperplasia 177, 177f
   normal lymph node 176, 176f
centrocytes
   follicular lymphoma 192, 192f
   non-specific lymph node hyperplasia 177, 177f
   normal lymph node 176, 176f
'cercariform' cells 68f
cerebrospinal fluid (CSF) 359–365
   bacterial infections 362, 362f
   diagnostic approach 360f
   fungal infections 362, 362f
   indications for cytology 360
   inflammatory diseases 362, 362f
     unknown aetiology 362
   lymphoma and leukaemia 365, 365f
   normal cells and contaminants 361f
   primary CNS tumours 363, 363f
   processing of specimens 360f
   sampling 360, 392
   secondary CNS tumours 364, 364f
   secretion, circulation and collection sites 359f, 360
   viral infections 362, 362f
cervical carcinoma
   adenocarcinoma (primary) 40, 40f–41f
     diagnostic pitfalls 44
     rosette formation 41f
   adenocarcinoma in-situ 40
   precancerous changes 3, 25
     see also cervical intraepithelial neoplasia (CIN)
   radiotherapy, vaginal smear changes after 22, 22f
   squamous cell (invasive) 25, 35
     diagnostic pitfalls 37, 37f
     FIGO staging 35
     macronuclei 35, 36f
     poorly differentiated 36f
     repair/regeneration *vs* 23, 36f–37f, 37
     spindle cells 35f–36f
     tadpole cell 35, 36f
     tumour bud, invasive 35f
     tumour diathesis 35f
cervical epithelium, Papanicolaou staining 396f
cervical glandular intraepithelial neoplasia (CGIN) 41f
   cell clusters, characteristics 44t
   cytology 40
   diagnostic pitfalls/differential diagnosis 21, 21f, 44
     endometrial polyps 44, 45f
     endometrial pseudostratified epithelium 44, 44f
     reserve cell hyperplasia 44, 45f
     tuboendometrioid metaplasia 44, 45f

high-grade 41f
   management 46
   pseudostratification 40, 41f
cervical infections 16
   bacterial 15f–16f, 16
   fungal 16, 17f
   protozoa 16, 17f
   viral 18–19, 18f
     diagnostic pitfalls 18
     HPV 18, 18f
     HSV 19, 19f
cervical intraepithelial neoplasia (CIN) 25–37
   abnormal chromatin pattern 25, 25f, 29f
     moderate/severe dyskaryosis 30, 30f–31f
   cell clusters, characteristics 44t
   CIN I (mild dyskaryosis) 26f, 28, 28f
     differential diagnosis 28
   CIN II (moderate dyskaryosis) 26f, 30, 30f
   CIN III (severe dyskaryosis) 26f, 30, 30f
     keratinising 30, 37, 37f
     necrosis with 37f
     see also dyskaryosis (cervical), severe
   glandular *see* cervical glandular intraepithelial neoplasia (CGIN)
   grades 25, 26f
   low-grade, 'test of cure' 46, 46f
   management 46
   see also dyskaryosis (cervical, squamous)
cervical screening 1
cervical smears/cytology 3–4
   abnormal, management 46
     follow-up after and HPV testing 46
     glandular dyskaryosis 46
     squamous dyskaryosis 46
   anucleate squames 6, 7f
   artefacts in processing 11, 12f
   atrophic 13f
   Bethesda System 24, 27t
   borderline nuclear changes 38, 38f
     HPV testing and association 38, 38f
     management 38
     regenerative atypia 39f
   CIN *see* cervical intraepithelial neoplasia (CIN)
   contaminants (external/atmospheric) 11, 12f
   conventional/direct smears 24, 24f
   endocervical cells *see* endocervical cells
   endometrial carcinoma cells 42
   endometrial cells *see* endometrial cells
   epithelial pearl 6, 6f
   epithelium, Papanicolaou staining 396f
   glandular neoplasms 40–44
     see also cervical carcinoma
   granulation tissue (immature) 23f
   histiocytes 9f
   hyperchromatic crowded group 21f
   hyperkeratosis 6, 7f
   iatrogenic changes 20–22
     diagnostic pitfalls 20
     hormonal therapy 20
     intrauterine devices 20, 20f
     radiation 22, 22f
     surgery 21, 21f
   infections *see* cervical infections
   infestations 11, 11f–12f
   inflammatory cells 10, 10f
   liquid based cytology samples 24, 24f

metaplastic cells 6, 7f, 14f
navicular cells 13f, 28
normal 6–11, 6f
  endocervical cells 8, 8f–9f
  endometrial cells 8, 9f
  inflammatory cells 10, 10f
  intermediate cells 6f–7f
  metaplastic cells 6, 7f
  reserve cells 10, 10f
  squamous cells 6, 6f
Papanicolaou staining 396f
parabasal cells 11, 13f
  in atrophic cervicitis 14
  atrophic/degenerate 13f, 15f
postmenopausal changes 11
  atrophic cervicitis, parabasal cells 15f
  'blue blobs' 11, 13f
  continued oestrogenization 11
  parabasal cells 11, 13f
precancerous changes 3, 25
  see also cervical intraepithelial neoplasia
    (CIN)
pregnancy and post-partum 11, 13f
reactive/inflammatory changes, mild
  dyskaryosis vs 28
repair and regeneration 23, 23f
  extreme regenerative atypia 39f
  squamous cell carcinoma vs 23, 36f–37f, 37
  stromal cells 23, 23f
reserve cells 10, 10f
  hyperplasia 10, 10f
sample adequacy 24, 24f
  reasons for inadequacy 24
sampling method 392
spermatozoa 11, 11f
squamous carcinoma see cervical carcinoma
squamous cells 6, 6f–7f
  in acute cervicitis 11, 14f
  borderline 38
  carcinoma see cervical carcinoma
  degenerative karyolysis 15f
  immature, borderline nuclear changes 39f
  intermediate cells 6, 6f–7f
  parakeratotic 6, 6f
  'pearl' and 'raft' formation 6, 6f
  repair changes 23, 23f
  'skewering', candida pseudohyphae 17f
  superficial cells 6, 6f
  Trichomonas vaginalis infection 17f
squamous metaplasia 4
  complete/incomplete 5f
  high-grade dyskaryosis vs 32f–33f
  immature 32f–33f, 33, 37, 39f
transformation zone cytology see cervical
  transformation zone
tubo-endometrioid metaplasia 21, 21f
'two cell population' 22
vacuolation of cytoplasm,
  radiotherapy-induced 22f
cervical transformation zone 4, 4f–5f
  normal cell cytology 6–11
  see also specific cell types under cervical
    smears/cytology
cervicitis 14
  atrophic 14, 15f
  follicular 14, 15f, 16, 34f
    high-grade dyskaryosis vs 33, 34f
  non-specific changes 14, 14f–15f

cervix
  exfoliative material 392, 392f
    method of sampling 392
  normal anatomy 3–4, 3f
  normal cytology see cervical smears/
    cytology
  normal histology 4f, 8f
  repair and regeneration 23, 23f
  squamocolumnar junction 5f
    after puberty 4, 5f
    'original' 4, 4f–5f
    post-menopause 4, 4f
    before puberty 4, 5f
  transformation zone see cervical
    transformation zone
CGIN see cervical glandular intraepithelial
  neoplasia (CGIN)
Charcot–Leyden crystals 97, 97f
chemotherapy effect
  respiratory system 63f, 68f
  urine cytology 144
childhood myelodysplastic syndrome 226f
childhood tumours 351–358
  common tumours and incidence 351–352,
    352t
    foetus and newborn 351b
  cytopathologist's role 351
  Ewing's family of tumours see Ewing's
    (sarcoma) family of tumours
  juvenile myelomonocytic leukaemia 218,
    218f
  lymphoma see lymphoma
  nephroblastoma see nephroblastoma
  neuroblastoma see neuroblastoma
  obtaining cytological samples 352
  osteosarcoma see osteosarcoma
  presenting symptoms and diagnoses 352t
  rhabdomyosarcoma see rhabdomyosarcoma
  round and spindle cell tumours 356b
  small round cell tumours 352
  spindle cell tumours 356b
cholangiocarcinoma 313, 323
  cytological findings 323, 323f
  metastatic serous effusions 119f
cholesterol crystals 152f, 301f
chondroblastoma 383, 383f
chondrocytes 374, 374f
  in CSF 361, 361f
  in synovial fluid 'wet prep' 388f
chondroid hamartoma 81, 81f
chondroid lipoma 375t
chondroma 383, 383f
chondrosarcoma 383, 383f
  myxoid (extraskeletal) 378t
choroid plexus, cells shed from 361, 361f
chromosomal translocation 412f
  acute myeloid leukaemia
    t(8;21) 227, 227f
    t(16;16) 229, 229f
  Burkitt's lymphoma 412, 412f
  clear cell sarcoma 407, 407f
  detection pitfalls 407
  Ewing's sarcoma 407, 407f
  FISH 412
  follicular lymphoma 412
  large B-cell lymphoma 412
  MALT lymphoma 412
  mantle cell lymphoma 412

PCR 407
  sarcoma 407
  synovial sarcoma 407
chronic eosinophilic leukaemia not otherwise
  specified (CEL-NOS) 215, 215f
chronic lymphocytic leukaemia (CLL) 185,
  185f–186f
  atypical/variants 185
  B-cell lymphoma development 205
  CSF in 365
  differential diagnosis 186f
  serous effusions 120, 120f
chronic myeloid leukaemia (CML) 210,
  210f–211f
  BCR-ABL1 positive 210
chronic myelomonocytic leukaemia (MDS/
  MPN-CMML) 217, 217f
chronic obstructive airways disease (COAD) 96,
  96f
chylous effusions 104t, 120
ciclosporin toxicity 63f
cilia, bronchial epithelium 60f–61f
ciliary tufts, detached, serous effusions 108,
  109f
cirrhosis of liver 316
  reactive mesothelial cells in effusions 110,
    110f
CK7, immunocytochemistry staining 403f
clear cell carcinoma
  breast 273, 273f
  endometrial 43f, 52f
  ovarian 43f, 57f
  renal, breast metastasis 276f
clear cell sarcoma 382, 382f
  chromosomal translocation detection 407,
    407f
  metastatic melanoma vs 382
  pleural fluid 407f
  renal, in children 356
clonality analysis 406, 406f
  cell preparation method 406
  PCR product analysis 406, 406f
  pitfalls 406
  T-cell receptor 406f
c-myc gene 353f
coccoid overgrowth, cervical 16f
'coffee-bean' nucleus 385f
collagen balls, serous effusions 108, 109f
'collagenous spherulosis' 260f
colloid
  'chewing-gum' 162
  thyroglossal cyst 152f
  thyroid gland 147f–149f, 165f
colloid carcinoma, breast 271, 271f
colloid goitre 148, 148f–149f
colloid nodules (thyroid) 147, 148f–149f
colonic carcinoma
  adenocarcinoma, metastatic
    to liver 325, 325f
    to lung 80f
    to lymph nodes 207f
    to ovary 57f
  immunomarkers 131f
colorectal tumours
  adenocarcinoma, pseudostratified glandular
    cluster 142f
  urinary tract adenocarcinoma vs 141,
    142f

colposcopy 46
columnar epithelium, bronchi 59f
condyloma, flat, koilocytosis 18f
congenital mesoblastic nephroma 356
congestive cardiac failure 107
connective tissue tumours, secondary, of lung
    65t
contaminants
    cervical smears 11, 12f
    P. jirovecii differential diagnosis 94f
    respiratory tract samples 61f, 68f
cornflake artefacts, cervical smears 11, 12f
corpus amylaceum 135f
corpus luteum cyst 54f
cotton fibres, cervical smear 12f
Creola body 72f, 97, 97f
Cryptococcus neoformans
    in CSF 362, 362f
    lung infection 94, 94f
crystal arthropathies, diagnostic algorithm
    389f
CSF *see* cerebrospinal fluid (CSF)
Curschmann's spiral 96f, 97
cyclophosphamide 63
cyst(s)
    branchial cleft 303, 303f
    breast *see* breast, cysts
    corpus luteum 54f
    cytological material collection 392
    echinococcal, of liver 312, 312f
    epidermoid, breast 259, 259f
    lymphoepithelial *see* lymphoepithelial cyst
    ovarian *see* ovarian cysts
    pancreatic *see* pancreas, cysts
    paraovarian 55
    retention, salivary gland 301f
    thyroglossal *see* thyroglossal cyst
    thyroid *see* thyroid cysts
cystadenocarcinoma
    bile ducts, extrahepatic 331, 331f
    mucinous *see* mucinous
        cystadenocarcinoma
    serous, of ovary 56f
cystadenoma
    bile ducts, extrahepatic 331
    hepatobiliary 315, 315f
    mucinous *see* mucinous cystadenoma
    serous *see* serous cystadenoma
cystic teratoma, mature, ovarian 56, 57f
cytocentrifuge 394, 394f
cytodiagnosis 1
cytogenetics
    bone and soft tissue 372
    nephroblastoma 356
cytomegalovirus (CMV)
    inclusion bodies, lung infection 91f
    urine cytology 144, 145f
cytopathic effects, viral infections of lung 90
cytopathology 1
cytopenia, refractory *see entries beginning
    refractory cytopenia*
cytophagocytic mononuclear cell 388f
cytoplasm, Papanicolaou staining 396
cytospin preparations
    for immunocytochemistry 394–395, 398f
    lymph node/bone marrow conditions 175
cytotoxic therapy effect *see* chemotherapy
    effect

D

dacryocytes, primary myelofibrosis 213, 213f
'decoy' cells, inclusional, human polyomavirus
    143, 143f
dendritic cell(s), follicular 176f
dendritic cell neoplasms 242–243
desmin, malignant cells positive for 196f
desmoid fibromatosis 376, 376f
desmoplastic small round cell tumour 381t
diabetic mastopathy 252, 252f
diffuse large B-cell lymphoma (DLBCL) 193
    anablastic type 193
    angioimmunoblastic T-cell lymphoma
        change to 201f
    breast metastasis 276f
    centroblastic type 193, 194f
    childhood 353t
    CSF in 365f
    cytological findings 193, 193f
    differential diagnosis 193
    FISH, chromosomal translocation 412
    immunoblastic type 193, 193f
        in HIV infection 205, 205f
    immunophenotype 193
    pleomorphic type 194f
    pleural effusions 121f
    post-transplant lymphoproliferative disease
        206f
    Richter's syndrome and 185
    salivary gland 299f
    T-cell rich 193, 194f
direct skin scrape 366
direct smears 394, 394f
    artefacts and pitfalls 395, 395f
    cervical cytology 24, 24f
    for immunocytochemistry 398f
DNA probes 410
Doderlein bacilli 6, 7f, 16, 16f
drug toxicity, pulmonary 100t
    reactive changes 63, 63f
duct ectasia 259, 260f
ductal adenocarcinoma, pancreatic *see*
    pancreatic ductal adenocarcinoma
ductal carcinoma *see* breast carcinoma, ductal
ductal cells
    breast *see* breast
    pancreatic *see* pancreatic ductal cells
    salivary gland 280
ductal epithelium
    pancreatic 332
    salivary gland 280f, 300f
duodenal aspirates, normal bile duct cytology
    327
duodenal carcinoma
    adenocarcinoma, metastatic, serous effusion
        118f
    metastatic, serous effusion 118f
duodenal epithelial cells, in EUS-FNA of
    pancreas 333, 333f
duodenal villi 333f
dyserythropoiesis
    acute myeloid leukaemia with
        myelodysplastic-related changes 230,
        230f
    refractory cytopenia of childhood 226, 226f
    refractory cytopenia with unilineage
        dysplasia 220, 220f

dysgranulopoiesis, acute myeloid
    leukaemia 230, 230f
dyskaryosis (cervical, glandular) 46
    see also cervical glandular intraepithelial
        neoplasia (CGIN)
dyskaryosis (cervical, squamous) 15f, 25
    abnormal chromatin pattern 25, 25f
    cellular features 25
    characteristics 25
    chromasia variations 26f
    grading 25, 26f, 27t
    HPV and/vs 29f
    hyperchromatic 25, 25f, 28f–29f
    hypochromatic (pale cell) 25, 25f, 29f–30f
    intrauterine device effect 20f
    management 46
    mild/low-grade (CIN I) 26f, 28, 28f–29f
        differential diagnosis 28
    moderate (CIN II) 26f, 30, 30f, 33f
        differential diagnosis 32f–33f, 33
        repair/regeneration vs 23
    severe/high-grade (CIN III) 26f, 30, 30f–32f
        bland cell variant 30, 32f
        differential diagnosis 33
        endometrial cells *vs* 33, 33f
        follicular cervicitis *vs* 33, 34f
        histiocytes *vs* 32f–33f, 33
        immature squamous metaplasia
            vs 32f–33f, 33
        irregular nuclear membrane 30f
        keratinisation 31f–32f
        necrosis with 37f
    terminology system comparison 27t
    see also cervical intraepithelial neoplasia
        (CIN)
dyskaryosis (vulval) 48f
dyskaryosis (vulvovaginal), urine cytology 136f
dysplastic nodule, hepatic *see under* liver
dysthrombocytopoiesis 230, 230f

E

Echinococcus, cyst in liver 312, 312f
echoendoscope, FNA, pancreatic material 332,
    333f
ectocervix, hyperkeratosis 6, 7f
ECTP terminology, cervical intraepithelial
    neoplasia 27t
ectopion, cervical 4, 5f
effusions *see* pleural effusions; serous effusions
embryonal carcinoma, mediastinal 86, 87f
embryonal sarcoma 324, 324f
emperipolesis 51f, 178f
    essential thrombocythaemia 214, 214f
emphysema 64
endocervical canal, normal 8f
endocervical cells 8, 8f–9f
    acute inflammation involving 39f
    borderline 38, 39f
    dyskaryotic, in cervical adenocarcinoma 40f
    honeycomb arrangement of cells 8, 8f
    mucus 8f
    multinucleate 10f
    normal ciliated 9f
    nuclear size variations 9f
    picket-fence arrangement of cells 8, 8f–9f,
        14f
endocervical polyps 44

endocervicitis 44
endometrial carcinoma 42
  adenocarcinoma 42, 42f–43f
  atypical cells 42f
  clear cell 43f, 52f
  papillary serous 43f, 51f
  serous 51f–52f
    psammoma bodies 43f, 52f
endometrial cells
  in cervical smears 8, 9f, 20
    severe dyskaryosis vs 33, 33f–34f
  tubular 50f
  uterine cytology 50, 50f
endometrial cluster 42f–43f, 136f
endometrial cytology
  cell cannibalism 51f
  hyperplasia 51
  malignancy 51
  non-neoplastic conditions 50
  normal 50–51, 50f
  papillary aggregate 51f
endometrial epithelial cells 9f
endometrial polyps, CGIN diagnostic pitfall and 44, 45f
endometrial pseudostratified epithelium, CGIN vs 44, 44f
endometrial sarcoma, stromal, metastasis to breast 276f
endometrioid adenocarcinoma, ovarian 57f
endometriosis 54f, 109f
endoscopic retrograde pancreatography (ERCP) 309f
endoscopic ultrasound, FNA see under fine-needle aspiration (FNA)
endothelial cells
  hepatocellular carcinoma 318, 318f–319f
  spindle-shaped hyperchromatic nuclei 324, 324f
Entamoeba gingivalis, lung infection 95, 95f
Entamoeba histolytica, liver abscess 312
Enterobius vermicularis 11, 11f
eosinophil(s)
  abnormal, acute myeloid leukaemia with inv(16) or t(16;16) 229, 229f
  basophilic 229, 229f
  chronic eosinophilic leukaemia 215
  in sputum sample 97, 97f
eosinophilic effusions 111f
eosinophilic granuloma 243, 385, 385f
  see also Langerhans cell histiocytosis (LCH)
ependymoma 363, 363f
epidermal growth factor receptor (EGFR) 408, 408f
epidermoid cyst, breast 259, 259f
epithelial cells
  breast see breast
  gastric see gastric epithelial cells
  hepatoblastoma 322
  intestinal exfoliated, ileal conduit sample 138f
  malignant, in pleural effusion 196f
  see also epithelium
epithelial granuloma, urine cytology 144f
epithelioid cells
  cat-scratch disease 179, 179f
  fat necrosis of breast 249
  subacute thyroiditis 154f

epithelioid granuloma
  subacute thyroiditis 154f
  tuberculous lymphadenitis 178, 178f
epithelium
  acinar see acinar epithelium
  bile duct see bile duct epithelium
  bronchial see bronchial epithelium
  cervical, Papanicolaou staining 396f
  columnar, respiratory system 59f
  ductal see ductal epithelium
  endometrial pseudostratified 44, 44f
  mucin-secreting see mucin-secreting epithelium
  oncocytic see oncocytic epithelium
  squamous, regenerative 370
  thyroid see thyroid epithelium
  see also epithelial cells
Epstein–Barr virus (EBV), primary effusion lymphoma and 195
ERBB2 (HER2) gene, amplification 413, 413f
erythroblasts 223f–224f
erythroid precursors
  nests, primary myelofibrosis 213, 213f
  refractory anaemia with ring sideroblasts 221, 221f
  unclassifiable myelodysplastic neoplasms 219f
erythroleukaemia 236, 236f
essential thrombocythaemia (ET) 214, 214f
European Commission Training Programme (ECTP) 27t
Ewing's (sarcoma) family of tumours 358, 385
  cytological findings 358, 358f, 381t
  'dark' and 'light' cells 358
  diagnostic pitfalls, and investigations 358
  differential diagnosis 354–355
  immunocytochemistry 358
  molecular genetic techniques 358, 358f
Ewing's sarcoma (classic) 381t
  chromosomal translocation detection 407, 407f
  cytological findings 385f, 414f
  FISH, EWS gene 411f, 414f
EWS gene 411f
EWSR1 gene 414f
exfoliative cytology 392
  collection/transport of material 392, 393f
  sites and samples 392, 392f
extramedullary haemopoiesis, liver 314, 314f
exudates 104t

F

'faggot cells' 228, 228f
fallopian tube carcinoma 42
fasciitis
  nodular 376, 376f, 378t
  proliferative 376, 376f
fat necrosis, breast see under breast
female genital tract 3–56
  Müllerian-type epithelium 42
  normal anatomy 3–4, 3f
  see also cervix; entries beginning cervical, endometrial, ovarian
FGFR1 gene, FISH, breast carcinoma 411f

fibroadenoma (breast) 255
  cytological findings 255, 255f–256f
    naked nuclei 256f
    stromal fragment 256f
  differential diagnosis 255
    low-grade ductal carcinoma 267f–268f
  juvenile 257f
  in lactation 258, 258f
fibroblast(s) 247f, 373
  reactive 373, 373f
fibroblastic reticular cell tumour 244, 244f
fibroblastic tumours, benign 376
fibrohistiocytic tumours, benign 376
fibromatosis, desmoid 376, 376f
fibromyxoid sarcoma 378t
fibrosing alveolitis 98f–99f
  adenocarcinoma vs 72f, 74f
fibrous tissue 373
  reactive 373, 373f
fibrous tumour, solitary, lung/pleura 81, 81f–82f
fine-needle aspiration (FNA) 1, 394
  bone 368, 372
  breast see breast
  EUS-FNA (endoscopic ultrasound) 309f, 326, 333
    pancreas 332
  increasing use 1
  lymph nodes see lymph node(s)
  ovary 53, 53f
  respiratory tract see respiratory system
  salivary glands see salivary gland
  skin samples 366
  soft tissue tumours see soft tissue tumours
  thyroid gland see thyroid gland
  thyroid nodules 148
fine-needle aspiration cytology (FNAC)
  techniques 394
  capillary method 247, 394f
  cell block preparations 394–395, 394f
  cell imprints 395, 395f
  common pitfalls 395, 395f
  direct smears 394, 394f
  fixation 395
  fluid preparation 394, 394f
  for lymph nodes 173, 173f
  sample preparation 394–395
  sample sites 394
fine-needle sampling without aspiration, skin samples 366
fixation 395
  artefacts and incorrect method 395f
flow cytometry, FNA aspirate from lymph node 175, 175f
fluorescence in situ hybridisation (FISH) 411
  Burkitt's lymphoma 353f
  double fusion probe 412, 412f
  Ewing's family of tumours 358, 358f
  gene amplification detection 413
  gene translocation (solid tumours) 414
  lymph node samples 175
  lymphomas 412
  neuroblastoma 355f
  preparation types 411
  probes 410
  protocol flowchart 411
  split probe 414
focal nodular hyperplasia 316, 316f–317f

foetus, common tumours 351b
follicle centre lymphoma,
    immunocytochemistry 191t
follicular carcinoma, thyroid *see* thyroid
    carcinoma, follicular
follicular dendritic cells 176f
follicular lesions, thyroid *see* thyroid gland
follicular lymphoma 192
    cytological findings 192, 192f
    FISH and chromosomal translocation 412
    grades 192, 192f
    PCR detection 407f
    serous effusions 121f
foreign body giant cell reaction, chronic
    sialadenitis 301f
fungal infections
    cervical/vaginal 16, 17f
    CSF in 362, 362f
    lung *see* lung infections, fungal

G

galactocele 248
gallbladder 326–331
    anatomy 309f
    FNA samples 326
    primary tumours 326b
ganglion 378t
ganglion cells 354f
    ganglioneuroblastoma 354, 354f
ganglioneuroblastoma, ganglion cells 354,
    354f
ganglioneuroma 354, 354f
gastric carcinoma
    ascites 115f
    metastatic, serous effusion 118f
    signet ring cell 118f, 122t
gastric crypts 337f
gastric epithelial cells 337f
    in EUS-FNA of pancreas 333, 333f
gastric foveolar cells 333f
gastrointestinal tract carcinomas, effusions 118,
    118f
gene amplification
    breast carcinoma (HER2) 413, 413f
    detection, FISH 413
    other solid tumour 413
genetics, molecular 404f
    Ewing's family of tumours 358, 358f
    rhabdomyosarcoma 357, 381
    see also cytogenetics; polymerase chain
        reaction (PCR)
germ cell tumours, mediastinal *see* mediastinal
    tumours
germinal centres 177, 177f
germinoma, CSF in 363f
giant cells
    cervical transformation zone 10, 10f
    Kimura's disease 180, 180f
    Langerhans cell histiocytosis 180, 180f
    measles virus pneumonia 91f
    multinucleated
        fat necrosis of breast 249f
        herpes virus infection of skin 367, 367f
        histiocytic, subareolar abscess 250f
        sarcoidosis 179, 179f
        subacute thyroiditis 154f
        tuberculous lymphadenitis 178f

muscle 373
    osteoclast-like *see* osteoclast-like giant
        cells
    tumour cells, in serous effusions 122t
    Warthin–Finkeldey 180, 180f
Giemsa–Romanowsky stain, bile pigments
    311
glioblastoma multiforme, CSF in 363, 363f
glioma, CSF in 363
glove powder, cervical smears 12f
glycogen, cytoplasmic, koilocytes *vs* 18
glypican-3 (GPC3), hepatocellular
    carcinoma 320, 320f
goblet cells 59f, 96f, 333f
goitre 148
    colloid 148, 148f–149f
    multinodular 148, 150, 163f
    simple non-toxic 148
    toxic 148
Goodpasture's syndrome 100, 100f
granular cell tumour 377, 377f
    breast 259, 259f
    bronchial 81, 81f–82f
granular layer of skin, normal 366
granulation tissue cells 180, 180f
granulocytic precursors, hypolobulation/
    hypogranulation 222f
granuloma
    eosinophilic 243, 385, 385f
    epithelial in urine after BCG 144f
    epithelioid *see* epithelioid granuloma
    hepatic 312, 312f
    non-caseating, sarcoidosis 179, 179f
    pulmonary 98f, 98t
    silicone 251f
    suture, differential diagnosis 180, 180f
    talc 101, 101f
    tuberculosis 89f
granulomatous disease, pulmonary fibrosis due
    to 99t
granulomatous inflammation, liver 312
granulomatous lymphadenopathy 178
granulomatous mastitis *see* mastitis,
    granulomatous
Grave's disease 157f
Grocott's methenamine silver stain 93, 93f
ground-glass nuclear appearance 19f, 90f
gynaecomastia 248, 248f

H

haemangioma
    hepatic 315, 315f
    sclerosing (pneumocytoma) 81, 81f
    soft tissue 378f
haematolymphoid malignancies 182–207
    serous effusions 120, 120f–121f
    see also leukaemia; lymphoma
haematoxyphil body 111f
haematuria, urinary tract malignancy 139
haemopoiesis, extramedullary, liver 314, 314f
haemopoietic system 173–244
    see also bone marrow; lymph node(s);
        spleen
haemosiderin 311
    in liver 311, 311f, 319f
    macrophage with *see* macrophage(s)
    staining 311, 311f

halo, perinuclear *see* perinuclear halo
hamartoma
    bile duct 313, 313f
    chondroid 81, 81f
    lymphoid (Castleman's disease) 181, 181f
    mammary (breast) 258
    mesenchymal, hepatic 313, 313f
Hand–Schüller–Christian disease 243
Hashimoto's thyroiditis 153
hepatic haemangioma 315, 315f
hepatic splenosis 314, 314f
hepatitis, granulomatous 312, 312f
hepatobiliary cystadenoma 315, 315f
hepatobiliary ducts, carcinoma 313
hepatobiliary tract cytology 309
    see also bile duct(s) (extrahepatic); liver
hepatoblastoma 322, 322f
    differential diagnosis 322
    embryonal 322f
    fetal 322, 322f
hepatocellular adenoma 316, 317f
    differential diagnosis 317t
hepatocellular carcinoma 318–320
    acinar cell variant 321, 321f
    bile pigment in cells 311
    binucleated cell decrease 316, 318
    clear cell variant 321, 321f
    differential diagnosis 317t, 324f
        metastatic neuroendocrine carcinoma
            325f
    fibrolamellar variant 321, 321f
    immunocytochemistry 318, 321
    lymph node metastases 207f
    metastatic, immunocytochemistry 320
    moderately-poorly differentiated (high-
        grade), cytological findings 318, 319f
    variants 321
    well-differentiated (low-grade) 318,
        318f–319f
        benign hepatic nodules *vs* 317t
        capillarised endothelial cells of
            sinusoids 318f, 320, 320f
        reticulin stain 318, 320f
hepatocyte(s) 310, 310f
    bile pigment from 311
    fatty change 311, 311f
    macroregenerative nodule 316f
    malignant 318, 318f, 320f
        intracytoplasmic pale bodies 321f
        intranuclear pseudoinclusion 321f
        iron retention loss 311
        oxyphilic cytoplasm 321f
    monoclonal, benign neoplasm (adenoma)
        316
    neoplastic 318f
    pleomorphism 316
    reactive 316f–317f
hepatoma *see* hepatocellular carcinoma
hepatosplenic T-cell lymphoma 198, 198f
    differential diagnosis 198
Hep-Par-1 antibody (anti-hepatocyte) 320,
    320f
HER2
    gene amplification in breast carcinoma 413,
        413f
    immunochemistry staining 402f
herpes genitalis 19
herpes labialis 19

herpes simplex virus (HSV)
  cervical infection 19, 19f
  lung infection 90f
herpes virus, skin infection 367, 367f
hibernoma 375f, 375t
histiocyte(s) 33f
  CD1-positive 180f
  cervical transformation zone 9f
  epithelioid 98f
    granulomatous hepatitis 312f
    tuberculous lymphadenitis 178f
  foamy
    hepatobiliary cystadenoma 315f
    inflammatory pseudotumour of liver
      313f
  Rosai–Dorfmann disease 178
  severely dyskaryotic cells vs 32f–33f, 33
histiocytic neoplasms 242–243
histiocytic sarcoma (HS) 242, 242f
histiocytosis, Langerhans cell see Langerhans
  cell histiocytosis (LCH)
Histoplasma, lung infection 94, 94f
history, cytopathology 1
HIV infection, lymphoma associated 205, 205f
  diffuse large cell lymphoma 205, 205f
  Hodgkin's lymphoma 205, 205f
  primary effusion lymphoma 195, 205, 205f
HMB-45, immunocytochemistry staining 403f
Hodgkin's lymphoma 83, 182t, 204
  classical (CHL) 204, 204f
    subtypes 204
  differential diagnosis 204
    primary effusion lymphoma 196f
  in HIV infection 205, 205f
  immunocytochemistry 204t
  immunomarkers 134f
  lung involvement 83f
  mediastinal 87f
  nodular lymphocyte predominant 204
  post-transplant lymphoproliferative
    disease 206
  sarcoidosis vs 179
'Hof' perinuclear clear area, osteoblasts 374,
  374f
Homer–Wright rosettes 354, 354f
hormonal therapy, cervical cytology changes
  20
hormone replacement therapy (HRT), cervical
  cytology 20
'horseshoe' cells 202
human papillomavirus (HPV)
  bladder infection 145f
  cervical infections 18, 18f
    borderline nuclear changes and 38,
      38f
    mild dyskaryosis vs 29f
  testing, after CIN treatment 46, 46f
  urine cytology 144, 145f
  vulval hyperkeratosis and 48f
human polyomavirus infection, urothelial
  malignancy vs 143, 143f
Hürthle cell(s) 169f
Hürthle cell neoplasms 160, 161f
hyaline deposits, focal, Castleman's disease 181,
  181f
hyaline globules, salivary gland FNA 306
  adenoid cystic carcinoma 292f–293f, 306f
  basal cell adenoma 286, 286f

pleomorphic adenoma 306f
  polymorphous low-grade adenocarcinoma
    296f, 306f
  salivary tumours with 292
hyaline matrix, chondrocytes with 374, 374f
hyaluronic acid 124f
hydroxyapatite crystals 387, 387f
hyperkeratosis
  ectocervix 6, 7f
  vulval 47f–48f
hyperthyroidism 156

I

idiopathic hypereosinophilic syndrome 215
ileal conduit samples, urine cytology 137,
  138f
immune disorders, pulmonary fibrosis due to
  99t
immunoblasts 176, 176f
  angioimmunoblastic T-cell lymphoma 201,
    201f
  diffuse large B-cell lymphoma 193, 193f
immunocytochemistry (ICC) 398–403
  antigen retrieval 398
  applications 398
  bone and soft tissue 372
  Ewing's (sarcoma) family of tumours
    358
  fixation 398
  fixatives 398
  haemolymphoid malignant cells in effusions
    120, 122t
  hepatocellular carcinoma 318, 321
  lymphoma differential diagnosis 191t
  medullary carcinoma of thyroid 167f
  nephroblastoma 356
  neuroblastoma 355
  polymeric methods 400, 400f
  primary vs metastatic lung tumours 79t
  pulmonary lymphomas 83
  quality control see quality control
  rhabdomyosarcoma 357
  sample preparation 398, 398f
  sample types 398
  serous effusions see serous effusions
  staining 399–400
    background staining pitfall 403, 403f
    cytoplasmic 402f
    double 402f
    membranous 402f
    nuclear 401f
    unspecific staining pitfall 403, 403f
    weak reaction/no reaction pitfalls 403,
      403f
  staining methods 400
    ABC method 399–400, 400f, 403f
    direct 399, 399f
    indirect 399, 399f
    labelled streptavidin biotin method
      399–400, 400f
    PAP method 399, 399f
immunodeficiency-associated
  lymphoproliferative disorders 205
immunohistochemistry
  anaplastic carcinoma of thyroid 168t
  lung adenocarcinoma vs squamous cell
    carcinoma 71f

immunomarkers
  Burkitt's lymphoma 130f
  Hodgkin's lymphoma 134f
  linitis plastica gastric carcinoma 133f
  lung tumours 132f
  mesothelial cell 128t
  metastatic adenocarcinoma 130f
  metastatic breast carcinoma 130f, 134f
  metastatic melanoma 133f
  non-mesothelial cell 128t
  ovarian carcinoma 130f
  primary peritoneal carcinoma 134f
  rhabdomyosarcoma 134f, 381
  serous effusions 129t, 130f
  small cell carcinoma of lung 131f
immunosuppressed patients, pulmonary
  dysfunction 91t
in situ hybridisation (ISH) 410–414
  chromogenic (CISH) 410
  DNA probes 410, 410f
  FISH see fluorescence in situ hybridisation
    (FISH)
  principle 410, 410f
  silver (SISH) 410
Indian file arrangement, lobular breast
  carcinoma 269, 269f
  metastatic 116f, 122t
infections see specific infections and organs
infectious agents, detection 409
infestations, cervical smears 11, 11f–12f
inflammatory arthropathy, diagnostic algorithm
  389f
inflammatory cells
  cervical transformation zone 10, 10f
  respiratory tract aspiration sample 60
  serous effusions 108, 108f–109f
inflammatory changes, respiratory system
  62
inflammatory diseases, CSF in 362, 362f
inflammatory myofibroblastic tumour 81, 82f
inflammatory pseudotumour, liver 313, 313f
inguinal hernia sac 103f
inhibin, follicular cells 53f
intestinal epithelial cells, exfoliated,
  degeneration 138f
intracytoplasmic vacuoles 119t, 269f
intraduct papilloma, salivary gland 287,
  287f
intraductal papillary mucinous neoplasm (IPMN)
  (pancreatic) 336b, 344t, 346–348
  biochemisty/cyst fluid 344t
  cytological findings 346, 346f–347f, 347
  differential diagnosis 348, 348f
  low-grade dysplasia with 347, 347f
  moderate/severe dysplasia with 348f
intramammary lymph node 259, 259f
intramuscular myxoma 378f, 378t
intrauterine devices (IUDs), cervical cytology
  changes 20, 20f
iron pigment deposition, lung parenchyma 100,
  100f
islet cells, normal 332

J

juvenile myelomonocytic leukaemia (JMML)
  218, 218f
juvenile papillomatosis 79

K

keratin, orangeophilia
  cervical dyskaryosis 29f
  laryngeal keratosis 68f
keratinisation, malignant squamous cells in
  effusions 116f
keratinocytes 366f
keratoacanthoma 370
  basal cell carcinoma vs 369
Kikuchi–Fujimoto disease 179, 179f
Kimura's disease 180, 180f
koilocyte(s)
  borderline nuclear changes 38f
  cytoplasmic glycogen vs 18
  diagnostic pitfalls 18
  in HPV infections 18f, 38f
koilocytosis 18, 29f
K-ras mutations 337
Kuttner tumour 300

L

labelled streptavidin biotin (LSAB) method 399–
  400, 400f
lactation pattern, breast 247f
lactational changes, breast see breast
lactobacilli, cervical/vaginal 16, 16f
Langerhans cell(s), normal 366
Langerhans cell histiocytosis (LCH) 180, 180f,
  243, 243f, 385, 385f
  differential diagnosis 243
    Kimura's disease vs 180, 180f
Langhans giant cell 178f, 179
LE cells 111f, 388
leiomyoma, soft tissue 378f
leiomyosarcoma 380, 380f
  lymph node metastases 208f
Leishman bodies 367, 367f
leishmaniasis 367, 367f
leprosy 367, 367f
leptomeningeal gliomatosis, CSF in 363
leptothrix, cervical/vaginal 16, 16f
Letterer–Siwe disease 243
leukaemia
  acute see entries beginning acute
  Burkitt's 197
  chronic eosinophilic, not otherwise specified
    215, 215f
  chronic lymphocytic see chronic
    lymphocytic leukaemia (CLL)
  chronic myeloid see chronic myeloid
    leukaemia (CML)
  chronic myelomonocytic 217, 217f
  CSF in see cerebrospinal fluid (CSF)
  juvenile myelomonocytic 218, 218f
  plasma cell 189
  pulmonary involvement 83
  pure erythroid 236, 236f
  T-cell prolymphocytic 200f
  T-lymphoblastic see T-lymphoblastic
    leukaemia (T-ALL)
linitis plastica gastric carcinoma,
  immunomarkers 133f
lipids, in synovial fluid 387, 387f
lipoblast(s) 379f
lipoblastoma 375t
lipoblastomatosis 375t

lipofuscin 311
lipoid pneumonitis 100, 100f
lipoma 375, 375f
  chondroid 375t
  diagnostic pitfalls 375t
  liposarcoma vs 375t
  pleomorphic 375f, 375t
  spindle cell 375f, 375t
liposarcoma 379–380
  lipoma vs 375t
  myxoid 378t, 379, 379f
  pleomorphic 379f–380f, 380
  well-differentiated 379f
liquid-based cytology (LBC) 395
  biliary tree samples 326
  cervical samples 24, 24f
  for immunocytochemistry 398f
lithiasis, urine cytology 144, 145f
liver 309–325
  abscess 312
    actinomyces 312
    amoebic 312
    pyogenic 312
  adenoma (hepatocellular) 313, 313f, 317f
    differential diagnosis 317t
  amyloidosis 314, 314f
  anatomy 309f
  angiomyolipoma 315, 315f
  benign lesions 314
  benign neoplasms 315
  benign nodules 316, 317t
    cytological features 316
    hepatocellular carcinoma vs 317t
  bile duct hamartoma 313, 313f
  carcinoma see hepatocellular carcinoma
  cirrhosis see cirrhosis of liver
  cytological analysis methods 309
  dysplastic nodule 316, 316f
    differential diagnosis 317t
  echinococcal cyst 312, 312f
  extramedullary haemopoiesis 314, 314f
  fatty change 311, 311f
  fine-needle aspiration (FNA) 309
    abscess drainage 312
    complications 310
    contraindications 310
    management role 325
    safety, cytology specificity 309
  focal nodular hyperplasia 316, 316f
    differential diagnosis 317t
  granulomata (non-infectious) 312, 312f
  granulomatous inflammation 312
  haemangioma 315, 315f
  hepatobiliary cystadenoma 315, 315f
  infections 312
  inflammatory conditions 312
  inflammatory myofibroblastic tumour 313,
    313f
  inflammatory pseudotumour 313, 313f
  lesions mimicking neoplasms 313
  macroregenerative nodule 316, 316f
  malignant neoplasms 318–325
    embryonal sarcoma 324, 324f
    primary sarcoma 324, 324f
    see also angiosarcoma;
      cholangiocarcinoma; hepatoblastoma;
      hepatocellular carcinoma
  mesenchymal hamartoma 313, 313f

metastatic tumours in 320, 325
  colonic adenocarcinoma 325, 325f
  neuroendocrine carcinoma 325, 325f
  renal cell carcinoma 325, 325f
normal cytology 310–311, 310f
pigments 311, 311f
  bile pigment 311, 311f
  haemosiderin 311f, 319f
  lipofuscin 311
reactive conditions 312
small cell dysplasia 316
splenosis 314, 314f
xanthogranulomatous reaction 313f
lower uterine segment
  CGIN diagnostic pitfalls and 44, 45f
  iatrogenic changes 21, 21f
    differential diagnosis 21
  sampling 21
lumbar puncture 360–361, 361f
lung see entries beginning pulmonary; respiratory
  system
lung cancer see lung tumours
lung disorders 96–101
  allergic see allergic bronchopulmonary
    disease
  alveolar proteinosis 101, 101f
  amyloidosis 101, 101f
  bronchiectasis 96, 96f
  COAD 96, 96f
  diffuse parenchymal disease 99, 99f
  drug-associated toxicity 100t
  iatrogenic or idiopathic
    granulomata due to 98t
    pulmonary fibrosis due to 99t
  iron pigment deposition 100
  occupational see occupational diseases
  sarcoidosis 98
  talc granuloma 101, 101f
lung infections 88–95
  bacterial 88, 98t
    acute or chronic 88
    differential diagnosis 88
    in immunosuppressed patients 91t
    tuberculosis 88
  fungal 92, 98t
    Aspergillus 92, 92f
    in immunosuppressed patients 91t
    other fungi 94, 94f
    P. jirovecii see Pneumocystis jirovecii
      (P. carinii) infection
  granulomata due to 98t
  in immunosuppressed 91t
  parasitic 95, 95f
    differential diagnosis 95
  viral 90
    CMV 91f
    differential diagnosis and investigations
      90
    HSV 90f
    in immunosuppressed patients 91t
    measles 91f
lung tumours 59, 64–75
  adenocarcinoma 64–75
    cytological findings 71, 71f–72f
    differential diagnosis 71, 72f
    further investigations 71, 408f
    immunohistochemical algorithm 71f
    mesothelioma vs 115, 127t

metastatic 71
 poorly differentiated, serous effusions
  114f
 reactive changes *vs* 62
 vacuolation 71f–72f
adenocarcinoma - lepidic predominant
 73
 cytological findings 73, 73f–74f
 differential diagnosis 73, 74f, 78f
 further investigations 73
 mucinous 74f
adenoid cystic carcinoma 79, 79f
 differential diagnosis 79
adenosquamous carcinoma 72f
carcinoid 77, 77f
 cytological findings 77, 77f–78f
 differential diagnosis 69, 77, 78f
 spindle cell 78f
carcinoma, classification 65t
carcinoma in situ 68f
 differential diagnosis 66, 67f
diagnosis and management 64
diagnosis by cytology 64
epidermal growth factor receptor (EGFR)
 408
giant cell carcinoma 76f
immunocytochemical markers 79t, 132f
in immunosuppressed patients 91t
juvenile papillomatosis 79
large cell carcinoma 64–75
 case study 76
 cytological findings 75, 75f–76f
 differential diagnosis 75, 76f
leukaemia 83
lymphomas 78f, 83
 see also non-Hodgkin's lymphoma
lymphoproliferative disease 65t
mesenchymal 81–83
metastatic carcinoma 79
 differential diagnosis 79
 immunocytochemical markers 79t
 lymphoepithelial thymoma 85f
mucinous adenocarcinoma 74f
mucoepidermoid carcinoma 79
necrotic 64f
non-small cell 408
 first-line therapy selection 408
papillomas 79
polymerase chain reaction (PCR) 405
primary epithelial 65t
primitive neuroectodermal tumour
 (PNET) 78f
secondary 65t
serous effusion 132f
small cell *see* small cell carcinoma of lung
spread 64
squamous cell carcinoma 64–75
 cytological findings 66, 66f–67f
 differential diagnosis 66, 67f–68f
 further investigations 66
 immunohistochemical algorithm 71f
 keratinised 66, 66f–67f
 metastatic *vs* primary 68f
 non-keratinised 66, 66f–67f
 poorly differentiated 67f
 sputum sample 66f
 tadpole cells 66f
 well-differentiated 66f–67f

therapy selection, mutation detection for
 408
Lyme disease meningitis 362
lymph node(s)
 enlarged 173
 fine-needle aspiration (FNA) 173, 173f
  cytospin preparations 175
  flow cytometry 175, 175f
  lymphadenopathy management 174, 174f
  method 173, 173f
  molecular techniques 175
  Richter's syndrome 186f
  ultrasound guidance 173, 174f
  see also individual lymphomas
 hyperplasia, giant/angiofollicular
  (Castleman's disease) 181, 181f
 intramammary 259, 259f
 intraparotid 285f
 metastatic disease *see* lymph node
  metastases
 MGG staining 396f
 neoplastic lesions *see* lymphoid neoplasms;
  lymphoma
 non-specific hyperplasia 177, 177f
 normal 176–177, 176f
 primary tumours 182
  see also lymphoma
 reactive *see* lymphadenopathy, reactive
 residual follicle centres 177f
lymph node metastases 182, 207
 acinar cell carcinoma of pancreas 207f
 adenocarcinoma of colon 207f
 carcinoid tumours 207f
 differential diagnosis 180
 fine needle aspiration 207
 hepatocellular carcinoma 207f
 leiomyosarcoma 208f
 malignant peripheral nerve sheath tumour
  208f
 melanoma 208f
 renal cell carcinoma 208f
 small cell carcinoma of lung 207f
lymphadenitis
 chronic 402f
 granulomatous 178, 178f
 histiocytic necrotising (Kikuchi–Fujimoto
  disease) 179, 179f
 tuberculous 178, 178f
lymphadenopathy
 childhood tumours 352t
 chronic, children/adolescents 179
 diagnosis 173, 174f
  ancillary techniques 175
  cytospin preparations 175
 diagnostic algorithm 173, 174f
 granulomatous 178
 management, FNA role 174, 174f
 massive, sinus histiocytosis with 178, 178f
 reactive 174f, 178–181
  Castleman's disease 181, 181f
  cat-scratch disease 179, 179f
  granulomatous lymphadenopathy 178
  Kikuchi–Fujimoto disease 179, 179f
  Kimura's disease 180, 180f
  sarcoidosis 178–179, 179f
  sinus histiocytosis 178, 178f
  tuberculous lymphadenitis 178, 178f
 reactive follicular hyperplasia 175f

lymphoblastic leukaemia/lymphoma 183
 B-lymphoblastic leukaemia/lymphoma 183,
  183f–184f
 cytological findings 183, 183f–184f
 T-lymphoblastic leukaemia 183, 184f
lymphoblasts 183f–184f
 'hand mirror-like' 184f
 neoplasms 183
lymphocytes 176
 cervicitis 15f
 in CSF 361f
 synovial fluid 388f
 see also B-lymphocytes; lymphoid cells;
  T-lymphocytes
lymphocytic mastopathy 252, 252f
lymphocytic thyroiditis 153, 153f
lymphocytosis
 pleural fluid 110f
 reactive, CSF 364–365
lymphoepithelial cyst
 pancreas 345, 345f
 salivary gland 294f, 302f–303f, 303
lymphoepithelial lesion, salivary gland 305f
lymphoepithelial thymoma, metastatic
 carcinoma to lung 85f
lymphoglandular bodies 173
lymphoid cells
 giant, Castleman's disease 181, 181f
 lymphocytic thyroiditis 153, 153f
 lymphoepithelial cyst 303f
 lymphoma of thyroid 169f
 see also lymphocytes
lymphoid neoplasms 182, 182t
 histiocytic and dendritic cell 182t
 mature B-cell 182t, 185–197
  see also under B-lymphocytes
 mature T-cell/NK-cell 182t
  see also under T-lymphocytes
 precursor neoplasms 182t, 183
  see also lymphoblastic leukaemia/
   lymphoma; leukaemia; lymphoma
lymphoma 182–207
 anaplastic large cell *see* anaplastic large cell
  lymphoma (ALCL)
 B-cell *see* B-cell lymphoma
 breast 275, 275f
  metastases 276f
 Burkitt's *see* Burkitt's lymphoma
 CD20-positive cells 305f
 children and adolescents 352–353
 chromosomal translocations 407, 412
 clonality analysis for diagnosis 406
 CSF in *see* cerebrospinal fluid (CSF)
 diagnosis, FNA cytology 173
 diffuse large B-cell *see* diffuse large B-cell
  lymphoma (DLBCL)
 extranodal, hepatosplenic *see* hepatosplenic
  T-cell lymphoma
 extranodal marginal zone B-cell 304
 FISH 412
 follicle centre, immunocytochemistry
  191t
 follicular *see* follicular lymphoma
 hepatosplenic T-cell *see* hepatosplenic T-cell
  lymphoma
 HIV infection-associated *see* HIV infection,
  lymphoma associated
 Hodgkin's *see* Hodgkin's lymphoma

lymphoblastic
  childhood 353t
  of thymus 85f
  see also lymphoblastic leukaemia/
    lymphoma
lymphoplasmacytic, breast metastasis 276f
malignant cells in serous effusions 112,
  112f
MALT-lymphoma see MALT-lymphoma
mantle cell see mantle cell lymphoma
  (MCL)
marginal zone see marginal zone lymphoma
  (MZL)
mediastinal 87f
myeloid sarcoma vs 241
non-Hodgkin's see non-Hodgkin's
  lymphoma
polymerase chain reaction 405, 406f
primary cutaneous see primary cutaneous
  lymphoma
primary effusion see primary effusion
  lymphoma
recurrence, diagnosis by FNA 173
serous effusions 120, 120f
  algorithm for evaluation 128, 128f
small lymphocytic see small lymphocytic
  lymphoma (SLL)
T-cell see T-cell lymphoma
thyroid 168, 169f
lymphomatous meningitis, CSF in 365
lymphoplasmacytoid cells 188f
lymphoproliferative disease 182t
  immunodeficiency-associated 205
  post-transplant see post-transplant
    lymphoproliferative disease (PTLD)

M

macronucleoli, hepatocellular carcinoma 319f
macrophage(s)
  aspiration of respiratory tract sample 60,
    61f
  carbon pigment laden 60f
  CD68 positivity 178f
  cervical transformation zone 10, 10f
  in CSF 361f
  degenerative changes 108f, 111f
  foamy 89f
    breast cysts 253, 253f
    fat necrosis of breast 249f
    leprosy 367, 367f
  haemosiderin-laden 54f, 150f, 152f
    in CSF 362, 362f
  iron-laden 99f–100f, 100
  lipoid pneumonitis 100f
  lymph nodes (normal) 176, 176f
  mucocele 302f
  multinucleated see giant cells
  normal 176, 176f
  Rosai–Dorfmann disease 178, 178f
  serous effusions 108, 108f–109f
  sputum sample 60, 60f
  'starry sky' pattern, Burkitt's lymphoma 197
  synovial fluid 388, 388f
  thyroglossal cyst and 152f
  thyroid cyst and 150f
  tingible body 34f, 176f, 353, 353f

malignant melanoma see melanoma, malignant
malignant peripheral nerve sheath tumour see
  peripheral nerve sheath tumours
MALT-lymphoma 187, 188f, 304, 305f
  FISH and chromosomal translocation 412
mantle cell lymphoma (MCL) 191, 191f
  blastoid variant 191, 191f
  of breast 276f
  classical (typical) 191, 191f
  differential diagnosis 191, 191t
  FISH and chromosomal translocation 412
  immunocytochemistry 191t
  pleomorphic variant 191, 191f
marginal zone lymphoma (MZL) 187
  cytological findings 187, 187f–188f
  nodal 187, 188f
  splenic 187, 187f–188f
mast cells
  mastocytosis 216, 216f
  Warthin's tumour and 285f
mastitis
  acute 252, 252f
  granulomatous 251, 251f
    differential diagnosis 251
  periductal 250, 250f
    differential diagnosis 250
  tuberculous 251f
mastocytosis 216, 216f
mastopathy, diabetic/lymphocytic 252, 252f
'matchstick cells', biliary epithelium 327f
May Grünwald Giemsa (MGG) stain 396–397,
  396f
  method flowchart 397f
measles virus pneumonia 91f
mediastinal tumours 84–86
  germ cell tumours 86
    cystic seminoma 86f
    embryonal carcinoma 86, 87f
    malignant teratoma 86, 87f
    mature cystic teratoma 86, 87f
    seminoma 86f
  location 84f
  lymphoma 87f
  thymic carcinoma 84, 85f
  thymoma see thymoma
medulloblastoma, CSF in 363, 363f
megakaryoblasts, acute megakaryoblastic
  leukaemia 237, 237f
megakaryocytes 221f
  acute panmyelosis with myelofibrosis 239f
  binucleated 222f
  chronic myeloid leukaemia 210, 210f
  essential thrombocythaemia 214, 214f
  extramedullary haemopoiesis 314, 314f
  multinucleated 225f
  myelodysplastic syndrome with isolate
    del(5q) 224f
  polycythaemia vera 212f
  refractory cytopenia with unilineage
    dysplasia 220f
melanocytes, normal 366
melanoma, malignant 370
  amelanotic, lymph node metastases 208f
  differential diagnosis 370, 370f
  metastases 370f
    breast 276f
    clear cell sarcoma vs 382

CSF in 364, 364f
immunomarkers 133f, 370f
lung 76f
lymph node 208f
lymphoma pattern in effusions vs 120
serous effusions, carcinoma vs 115
of soft parts 382
vulval and vaginal 49, 49f
meningitis
  acute bacterial 362, 362f
  acute viral aseptic 362, 362f
  carcinomatous 364
  chronic 362, 362f
  Lyme disease 362
  lymphomatous, CSF in 365
  tuberculous 362, 362f
meningothelial cells, in CSF 361, 361f
Merkel cell carcinoma 371, 371f
  basal cell carcinoma vs 369
mesenchymal cells, hepatoblastoma 322
mesenchymal hamartoma, hepatic 313, 313f
mesenchymal tumours
  FISH 414
  respiratory system 81–83
mesothelial cell(s) 105
  adenocarcinoma cells vs 106f
  atypical 107, 107f, 110
    mesothelioma 125f
  ball (collagen ball) 109f
  calretinin staining 131f
  carcinoma cell group 106f
  degenerative changes 105, 106f
  dual cell approach to malignancy 107,
    112–113, 115f, 126f
    algorithm 113f
  as facultative macrophage 108
  immunocytochemistry staining 402f
  intercellular windows 105f–106f
  markers 128t
  mesothelioma 107f, 124f
  metastatic carcinoma 113, 113f
  morphology 105, 105f
  negative staining properties 128
  normal cytology 103f, 105, 105f
  nuclei 105, 105f–106f, 122t
  pleomorphic 106f–107f
  pleural effusion 402f
  reactive 104–105, 106f–107f
    active cirrhosis 110f
    carcinoma vs 115
    diagnostic pitfalls 107, 107f
    knobbly contours 106f
    malignant cells with 112
    mesothelioma cells vs 123–124, 125f–
      126f, 127t
    non-specific 107, 107f, 111f
    overdiagnosis of malignancy 107
  serous lining 103f
  washing process dislodging 106f–107f
  see also serous effusions
mesothelioma 123–124
  adenocarcinoma cells vs 124, 127t
  asbestos association 123
  carcinoma vs 115, 127t
  clinical details 123–124
  cytology 124
    diagnostic clues 124

deciduoid 125f
effusions 112, 124
hypercellular 126f
mesothelial cells 107f
metastases 123
metastatic breast carcinoma vs 126f
nuclear pleomorphism 126f
pathology 123f
peritoneal deciduoid 125f
pleural 123, 123f–125f
reactive mesothelial cells vs 123–124,
    125f–126f, 127t
sarcomatoid type 123
variants 123t, 124
working classification 123t
metaplastic cells, cervical transformation zone
    6, 7f
metastases see specific tumours, and organs
MGC staining, air-drying before fixation 395,
    395f
micromegakaryocyte 223f, 230f
molecular genetics see genetics, molecular
molecular techniques 410–414
    lymph node FNA samples 175
monocytosis 217f–218f
mononuclear cell, cytophagocytic 388f
monosodium urate crystals 387, 387f
Mott' cell 206f
mucicarmine stain 119f
mucin
    ferning 330f, 346f
    gastric epithelium and 333f
    staining 115
mucin vacuoles
    breast cancer 114f
    cholangiocarcinoma 323f
    metastatic adenocarcinoma, CSF sample
        364f
    mucinous adenocarcinoma, bile ducts
        331f
mucinous adenocarcinoma
    bile ducts 331f
    lung 74f
mucinous carcinoma, breast see breast
    carcinoma
mucinous cystadenocarcinoma
    bile ducts (extrahepatic) 331, 331f
    ovary 57f
    pancreatic 349f
mucinous cystadenoma
    ovary 55, 55f
    pancreas 349f
    see also pancreatic tumours, mucinous
        cystic neoplasm
mucinous cystic neoplasm, pancreas see under
    pancreas
mucinous tumour, intraductal papillary see
    intraductal papillary mucinous neoplasm
    (IPMN) (pancreatic)
mucin-secreting epithelium
    gastric mucosa 333f, 348f
    intraductal papillary mucinous
        neoplasm 346f–347f
    mucinous cystic neoplasm of pancreas 349,
        349f
mucocele, salivary gland see under salivary
    gland

mucocele-like lesions, breast 264, 264f
mucoepidermoid carcinoma
    lung see under lung tumours
    salivary gland see under salivary gland
        tumours
Mucor, lung infection 94, 94f
mucous cells
    mucoepidermoid carcinoma (salivary gland)
        120, 290, 290f–291f
    vacuolation 114, 120, 290f–291f
mucus, ferning 330f, 346f
mucus cells, respiratory tract aspiration sample
    60
multiple myelomatosis, serous effusions 120,
    120f
muscle, striated see striated muscle
muscle giant cells 373
musculoskeletal system 372–386
    tumours, FNA as diagnostic pre-treatment
        method 372
mycetoma, lung 92, 92f
MYCN gene probe 411f
mycobacterial infections, PCR detection 409,
    409f
Mycobacterium avium-intracellulare 89f, 178f
Mycobacterium tuberculosis 409, 409f
    see also tuberculosis
mycosis fungoides 200, 200f
myeloblasts 196f
    acute myeloid leukaemia without
        maturation 232f
    chronic myeloid leukaemia 210
myelodysplastic syndromes 209t, 220–226,
    220f
    childhood 226f
    with isolated del(5q) 224, 224f
    refractory anaemia with excess blasts (RAEB)
        223, 223f
    refractory cytopenia with multilineage
        dysplasia (RCMD) 222, 222f
    refractory cytopenia with unilineage
        dysplasia (RCUD) 220, 220f
    unclassifiable (MDS-U) 225, 225f
myelodysplastic/myeloproliferative neoplasms
    209t, 217–218
    chronic myelomonocytic leukaemia 217,
        217f
    juvenile myelomonocytic leukaemia 218,
        218f
    refractory anaemia with ring sideroblasts
        221, 221f
    unclassifiable myelodysplastic neoplasms
        219, 219f
myelofibrosis
    acute panmyelosis with 239, 239f
    phase in polycythaemia vera 212
    primary 213, 213f
myeloid neoplasms 209–244, 209t
myeloid sarcoma 241, 241f
myeloma
    non-secretory 189
    plasma cell see plasma cell myeloma
myeloproliferative neoplasms 209t, 210–216
    chronic eosinophilic leukaemia not
        otherwise specified 215, 215f
    chronic myeloid leukaemia see chronic
        myeloid leukaemia (CML)

essential thrombocythaemia 214, 214f
    mastocytosis 216, 216f
    polycythaemia vera 212, 212f
    primary myelofibrosis 213, 213f
myoepithelial carcinoma, salivary gland 299f
myoepithelial cells
    adenoid cystic carcinoma 292f
    breast 247f–248f
myoepithelial sialadenitis see sialadenitis
myoepithelioma
    benign, salivary gland 286, 286f
    malignant, breast 274, 274f
    salivary gland 286, 286f, 299f
myofibroblast(s) 373, 373f
myofibroblastic tumours, benign 376
myoglobin 381
myositis, proliferative 376, 376f
myxofibrosarcoma 378t
myxoid chondrosarcoma 378t
myxoid liposarcoma 378t, 379, 379f
myxoma, intramuscular 378f, 378t

N

Nabothian follicles 4f
natural killer (NK) cells, mature, neoplasms 182t,
    198–204
navicular cells, cervical smear 13f, 28
NB84 355
necrosis, tuberculous lymphadenitis 178, 178f
negative control (NC) 401
nephroblastoma (Wilms' tumour) 355–356
    anaplastic 356f
    ancillary technique value 356
    cytogenetics 356
    cytological findings 355, 355f
    diagnostic pitfalls 356
    differential diagnosis 356
    immunocytochemistry 356
    triphasic, features 355, 355f
nerve sheath tumour, salivary gland 299f
neurilemmoma 377, 377f, 378t
    ancient 377f
neuroblast(s) 354f–355f
neuroblastoma 354–355, 354f–355f, 381t
    diagnostic pitfalls 354
    FISH, MYCN probe 411f
    poorly differentiated 354, 355f
neuroendocrine carcinoma
    metastatic, to liver 325, 325f
    small cell carcinoma of lung vs 70f
neurofibroma 378t
neuropil 354, 354f
neutropenia, refractory cytopenia with
    unilineage dysplasia 220, 220f
neutrophil(s)
    ascitic fluid 110f
    cat-scratch disease 179, 179f
    cervicitis 11, 14f
    dysplastic, refractory cytopenia with
        unilineage dysplasia 220, 220f
    engulfed, endometrial carcinoma 42f
    inflammatory cells 10
    'pince-nez' appearance 220f, 227f
    see also polymorphonuclear cells
neutrophilic emperipolesis 51f
newborn, common tumours 351b

nipple
  adenoma 262–263
  discharge 250
  erosive adenosis 262–263
  Paget's disease 273, 273f
  retraction 250
  tumours, WHO classification 266b
nipple ducts, papilloma 262–263
NK cell neoplasms, WHO classification 182t
Nocardia asteroides 88f
nodular fasciitis 376, 376f, 378t
non-Hodgkin's lymphoma
  children and adolescents 353
  follicular *see* follicular lymphoma
  low-grade 169f, 192
  of lung 78f, 83, 83f
    differential diagnosis 83
    lung carcinoid *vs* 78f
    small cell carcinoma of lung *vs* 70f
  lymphoepithelial cyst *vs* 303f
  lymphoplasmacytic, differential diagnosis 186f
  mediastinal 87f
  T-cell type, of lung 83f
  thyroid gland 168, 169f
  see also lymphoma; *specific types of lymphoma*
nuclear inclusion bodies, HSV infection of cervical epithelial cells 19f
nuclear moulding, small cell carcinoma 69, 69f–70f, 78f
nuclei
  eccentric, medullary thyroid carcinoma 167f
  ground-glass 19f, 90f
  macronuclei 35, 36f
  mesothelial cells 105, 105f–106f, 122t
  naked, fibroadenoma (breast) 256f
  urothelial cells 138f, 144f–145f
nucleic acid, extraction 404–405
nucleoli
  breast 247f
  macronucleoli, hepatocellular carcinoma 319f

O

occupational diseases, lung 99
  granulomata due to 98t
  pulmonary fibrosis due to 99t
oestrogen receptor (ER), nuclear immunocytochemistry reaction 401f
oligodendroglioma, CSF in 363, 363f
oncocytic adenoma 161f
  oncocytic papillary carcinoma *vs* 165f
  salivary gland 287, 287f, 307f
oncocytic carcinoma, salivary gland 307f
oncocytic cell(s) 161f
  acinic cell carcinoma 307f
  mucoepidermoid carcinoma 307f
  salivary gland 307
  Warthin's tumour differential diagnosis 284, 307f
oncocytic epithelium
  lymphocytic thyroiditis 153, 153f
  oncocytic adenoma (salivary gland) 287f
  Warthin's tumour 284f–285f

oncocytic neoplasms
  salivary gland 307f
  thyroid gland 160, 161f
oral contraceptives, cervical cytology changes 20
oral mucosa, brushings 392, 393f
orangeophilia
  keratin *see* keratin
  mucoepidermoid carcinoma 294f
organ ischaemia, non-specific effusion 107
osteoblast(s) 374, 374f
osteoblastoma 384, 384f
osteoclast(s) 374, 374f
osteoclast-like giant cells
  breast carcinoma 251f, 273, 273f
  undifferentiated pancreatic carcinoma 338, 338f
osteogenic tumours 384
osteosarcoma 384, 384f
  children 358
  differential diagnosis (FNA) 384
ovarian cysts 53
  corpus luteum cyst 54f
  endometriotic 53, 54f
  functional 53, 53f
  luteinised follicular 53f
  regressing follicular 55
  serosal inclusion 55
  simple 55
ovarian neoplasms 42, 55
  benign 55
    mature cystic teratoma 56, 57f
    mucinous cystadenoma 55, 55f
    serous cystadenoma 55, 55f
  borderline epithelial 56, 56f
  malignant 56
    adenocarcinoma, effusions 117f
    clear cell carcinoma 43f, 57f
    endometrioid adenocarcinoma 57f
    mucinous cystadenocarcinoma 57f
    papillary carcinoma, effusions 117f
    serous cystadenocarcinoma 56f
    serous papillary carcinoma 114f
  metastatic
    ascitic fluid 114f, 117f
    from colonic adenocarcinoma 57f
    dual cell population 117f
    malignant cells in serous effusions 117f, 130f
    secretory vacuoles in cells 117f
ovary
  cytology 53–56, 53f
  endometriosis 54f
  fine-needle aspiration 53, 53f
owl's eye appearance, CMV inclusions 91f
oxalate crystals, thyroid cyst and 151f

P

Paget's cells 49f
Paget's disease of nipple 273, 273f
Paget's disease of vulva 49, 49f
palisading columnar cells 207f
pancreas 332–349
  acinar cells *see* pancreatic acinar cells
  acinar epithelium 332
  anatomy 309f, 333f
  biopsy, complication risk 333

cysts 344–349, 344t
  fluid biochemistry 344t
  non-neoplastic 345
  see also pancreatic pseudocyst
diagnostic algorithm 350f
ductal cells *see* pancreatic ductal cells
ductal epithelium 332
fine-needle aspiration 333f
  contraindication 334
  diagnostic algorithm 350f
  EUS-FNA 332, 333
  management of lesions 350
gastrointestinal cells in EUS-FNA 333, 333f
glandular epithelium 337f
lymphoepithelial cyst 345, 345f
normal cytology 332–333, 332f
  differential diagnosis 333
pseudocyst *see* pancreatic pseudocyst
reactive changes 335f
tumours *see* pancreatic tumours
pancreatic acinar cells 332
  acute pancreatitis 334f
  carcinoma *see* acinar cell carcinoma (pancreas)
  chronic pancreatitis 334f
  normal 332, 332f
pancreatic ductal adenocarcinoma 336–337, 336b
  ancillary studies 337
  autoimmune pancreatitis *vs* 335
  chronic pancreatitis *vs* 334
  diagnostic pitfalls 337
  foamy gland pattern 337f
  pleomorphic cells in serous effusions 118f
  poorly-differentiated 336, 336f–337f
  reactive changes *vs* 335f
  undifferentiated 338, 338f
    with osteoclast-like giant cells 338, 338f
  variants 338
  well-differentiated 336–337, 336f–337f
pancreatic ductal cells 332, 332f
  chronic pancreatitis 334f–335f
pancreatic endocrine neoplasms (PEN) 336b, 341–343, 343t
  classification 336b
  clear cell or lipid-rich variant 342f
  differential diagnosis 341
  metastatic, to liver 325, 325f
  poorly differentiated (small cell carcinoma) 343, 343f
  well-differentiated, cytology 341, 341f–342f
pancreatic islet cells, normal 332
pancreatic pseudocyst 344t, 345, 345f
  biochemical cyst fluid parameters 344t
  differential diagnosis 345
pancreatic tumours
  acinar cell carcinoma *see* acinar cell carcinoma (pancreas)
  adenocarcinoma *see* pancreatic ductal adenocarcinoma
  adenosquamous carcinoma 339, 339f
  cystic neoplasms 344t, 346–349
    see also intraductal papillary mucinous neoplasm (IPMN); serous cystadenoma
  endocrine neoplasms *see* pancreatic endocrine neoplasms (PEN)
  epithelial neoplasms 336b

histological classification 336b
intraductal papillary mucinous see
    intraductal papillary mucinous neoplasm
    (IPMN)
mucinous cystic neoplasm (MCN) 336b,
    344t, 346f–347f
    biochemical cyst fluid parameters 344t
    cytological findings 349, 349f
    differential diagnosis 349
non-epithelial neoplasms 336b
pleomorphic cells in serous effusions 118f
serous cystadenoma see serous
    cystadenoma
solid malignant neoplasms 336–343, 343t
    types 336
    see also pancreatic ductal adenocarcinoma
solid pseudopapillary neoplasm (SPN) 340,
    340f, 343t
undifferentiated (pleomorphic) 338
pancreatitis 334–335
    acute 334, 334f
    autoimmune (AIP) 335, 335f
    chronic 334
        cytological findings 334, 334f–335f
        pancreatic adenocarcinoma vs 334
pancreatoblastoma, summary of features 343t
Papanicolaou (PAP) smears see cervical smears/
    cytology
Papanicolaou (PAP) staining 396, 396f
    cervical epithelium 396f
    liver pigments 311, 326
    method flowchart 397f
papillary adenocarcinoma, breast 272, 272f
papilloma
    biliary 330, 330f
    breast 262–263, 262f
    intraduct, salivary gland 287, 287f
    lung 79
    nipple ducts 262–263
papova virus 143, 143f
Pappenheimer bodies 222
parabasal cells, cervical see cervical smears/
    cytology
paracoccidioidomycosis 94f
paraimmunoblasts 186f
parakeratotic cells, urine cytology 145f
paraovarian cysts 55
parasitic infections
    extrahepatic bile ducts 328, 328f
    lung see lung infections
paravacuolar granules, thyroid hyperplasia
    156f
parenchymal lung disease, diffuse 99, 99f
parotid gland 279f
    lymph node in 285f
    pleomorphic adenoma 282
pathology services, rationalisation 1
Pelger–Hüet anomalies 227, 227f
pemphigus vulgaris 368, 368f
periductal mastitis see mastitis, periductal
perinuclear halo
    inflammatory, in cervicitis 15f
    koilocytes vs 18
    pemphigus vulgaris 368, 368f
peripheral nerve sheath tumours, malignant
    380, 380f
    lymph node metastases 208f
peripheral nerve tumours 377–378

peripheral neuroepitheliomas see Ewing's
    (sarcoma) family of tumours
peripheral primitive neuroectodermal tumours
    (pPNET) see Ewing's (sarcoma) family of
    tumours
peripheral T-cell lymphoma 199
    cytological findings 199, 199f
peritoneal carcinoma, primary,
    immunomarkers 134f
peritoneal fluid
    macrophage 108
    metastatic ovarian carcinoma 117f
    reactive mesothelial cells 106f
    see also serous effusions
Perl's stain 100
peroxidase anti-peroxidase (PAP) method 399,
    399f
Philadelphia chromosome 210
phyllodes tumour
    benign 255, 257
        cytological findings 257, 257f
        mucinous, differential diagnosis 255
    malignant 275, 275f
pilomatrixoma 371, 371f
    basal cell carcinoma of skin vs 369
plant particle, cervical smears 12f
plasma cell(s), normal lymph node 176
plasma cell leukaemia 189
plasma cell myeloma 189, 190f
    asymptomatic (smouldering) 189
    clinical variants 189
    differential diagnosis 189
    further investigations 189
plasma cell neoplasms 190f
plasmacytoma, solitary, of bone 190f
pleomorphic adenoma see under salivary gland
    tumours
pleomorphic diffuse large B-cell lymphoma
    (DLBCL) 194f
pleomorphic lipoma 375f, 375t
pleomorphic liposarcoma 379f–380f, 380
pleomorphic mantle cell lymphoma (MCL) 191,
    191f
pleomorphic rhabdomyosarcoma 381f
pleomorphic sarcoma, differential diagnosis
    380
pleural effusions/fluid 103, 120
    adenocarcinoma 106f
    cell types 109f
    clear cell sarcoma 407f
    diffuse large B-cell lymphoma 121f
    endometriosis 109f
    haematoxyphil body 111f
    immunocytochemistry staining 402f
    lymphocytosis 110f
    metastatic cells 113f
        breast carcinoma 113f, 115f–116f
    primary effusion lymphoma 195, 195f
    Reed–Sternberg cell in 196f
    see also serous effusions
pleural lesions, biopsy 392f
Pneumocystis jirovecii (P. carinii) infection 93
    cytological findings 93, 93f
    differential diagnosis 93
    further investigations 93, 409, 409f
pneumocytoma (sclerosing haemangioma) 81,
    81f
pneumonia, measles virus 91f

pneumonitis, lipoid 100, 100f
polycythaemia vera (PV) 212, 212f
    phases 212
polymerase chain reaction (PCR) 404–409
    applications 405
    chromosomal translocation detection
        407
    electrophoresis of products 404f, 406f
    end-point 405, 405f
    future developments 409
    infectious agent detection 409
    lymphoma detection 406, 407f
    mutation detection for therapy selection
        408
    nucleic acid extraction 404–405
    nucleic acid targets 405
    pitfalls 405–409
    rationale 404, 404f
    real-time 405, 405f, 407, 407f–408f
    sample types 404
    techniques 405
polymeric technology,
    immunocytochemistry 400, 400f
polymorphonuclear cells
    in cytoplasm of tumour cells 51f
    exudate, lung infections 88, 88f
    synovial fluid 388f
    see also eosinophil(s); neutrophil(s)
polymorphous low-grade adenocarcinoma
    (PLGA) 296, 296f, 306f
popcorn cells 204, 204f
positive control (PC) 401
postmenopausal changes, cervical samples see
    cervical smears
post-partum cervical smears 11, 13f
post-transplant lymphoproliferative disease
    (PTLD) 182t, 206
    cytological findings 206, 206f
    early lesion 206, 206f
    monomorphic 206, 206f
    polymorphic 206, 206f
pregnancy
    breast changes 246
    cervical smears 11, 13f
primary cutaneous lymphoma 200, 200f, 371,
    371f
    Merkel cell carcinoma vs 371f
primary effusion lymphoma (PEL) 121f, 195
    cytological findings 195, 195f
    differential diagnosis 195, 196f
    in HIV infection 195, 205, 205f
    plasmablastic variant 205, 205f
primary myelofibrosis (PM) 213, 213f
primary sclerosing cholangitis 328, 328f
primitive neuroectodermal tumour (PNET)
    CSF in 363, 363f
    Ewing's/peripheral see Ewing's (sarcoma)
        family of tumours
    lung 81, 82f
    lung carcinoid vs 78f
    neuroblastoma vs 354
progesterone receptor, breast carcinoma 401f
prolymphocytes 186f
prostatic carcinoma
    adenocarcinoma 141
    immunocytochemistry, cytoplasmic reaction
        402f
    metastatic, in lung 80f

metastatic serous effusions 119f
urine cytology 142f
protozoa
cervical infections 16, 17f
vaginal infections 16
psammoma bodies 20, 20f
endometrial carcinoma 43f
ovarian serous cystadenocarcinoma 56f
ovarian serous papillary carcinoma 114, 114f
serous effusions 108, 109f, 114, 122t
serous endometrial carcinoma 52f
thyroid disorders with 162, 163f
thyroid papillary carcinoma 162, 163f, 164
pseudo-Chediak–Higashi granules 227, 227f
pseudocyst see pancreatic pseudocyst
pseudo-Gaucher cell 211f
pseudomyxoma peritonei 122t
pseudo-Pelger anomaly 220f
pseudo-Pelger–Hüet anomaly 230, 230f
pseudopod formation, blasts, acute
megakaryoblastic leukaemia 237, 237f
pseudosarcomatous lesions, proliferative
myositis/fasciitis 376f
pseudostratification, cervical glandular
intraepithelial neoplasia 40, 41f
pulmonary alveolar proteinosis 101, 101f
pulmonary blastoma 81, 82f
pulmonary disorders see lung disorders
pulmonary embolism, reactive mesothelial cells 110
pulmonary fibrosis, conditions associated 99t
pulmonary granuloma 98f, 98t
pulmonary infarction, reactive mesothelial cells 110
pulmonary infections see lung infections
pulmonary toxicity, drugs associated 100t
pure erythroid leukaemia 236, 236f

Q

quality control 401
external 401–403
internal 401
negative (NC) 401
positive (PC) 401

R

radiation, cervical cytology changes due to 22, 22f
radiotherapy effect, urine cytology 144
ragocyte, in synovial fluid 'wet prep' 388f
rapid staining method 397, 397f
reactive follicular hyperplasia 175f
reactive lymphadenopathy see
lymphadenopathy, reactive
Reed–Sternberg cells 83, 83f, 87f, 134f, 196f, 204
in Hodgkin's disease in HIV infection 205f
in Richter's syndrome 185
types 204f
Reed–Sternberg-like cell, small lymphocytic
lymphoma 186f
refractory anaemia with excess blasts (RAEB) 223, 223f
refractory anaemia with ring sideroblasts (RARS) 221, 221f

refractory cytopenia of childhood (RCC) 226, 226f
refractory cytopenia with multilineage dysplasia (RCMD) 222, 222f
refractory cytopenia with unilineage dysplasia (RCUD) 220, 220f
renal carcinoma, metastatic
clear cell carcinoma, to breast 276f
to liver 325, 325f
to lymph nodes 208f
serous effusions 119f
renal tumours, childhood 356
nephroblastoma see nephroblastoma
reserve cells
cervical transformation zone 10, 10f
hyperplasia 10, 10f
CGIN diagnostic pitfalls and 44, 45f
respiratory tract aspiration sample 60, 62
respiratory system 59–101
diagrammatic representation 59f
disorders see lung disorders
dysplasia, squamous cell carcinoma vs 67f
exfoliative samples 59
fine-needle aspiration (FNA) 59–60, 64
EBUS-FNA 59, 64, 70f
large cell carcinoma 75f–76f
lung tumours 64
normal 60, 60f–61f
small cell carcinoma 69f–70f
squamous cell carcinoma 67f–68f
hyperplasia 62
infections 62
see also lung infections
lung tumours see lung tumours
mesenchymal tumours 81–83
normal cytology 59f, 60
aspiration sample 60, 61f
bronchial brushing 60f–61f
bronchoalveolar lavage 60
contaminants 61f
differential diagnosis 60
exfoliative sample 60, 60f–61f
FNA samples 60, 60f–61f
sample type 60
sputum sample 60, 60f
sputum sample (inadequate) 61f
reactive changes 62
adenocarcinoma - lepidic pattern vs 74f
atypical squamous metaplasia vs 62
basal cell hyperplasia 63f
case study 63
cytotoxic therapy effect 63f
degenerative inflammatory 62
differential diagnosis 62
drug toxicity causing 63, 63f
enlarged bronchial epithelial cells 63f
hyperplasia 62, 63f
squamous cell carcinoma vs 62
squamous metaplastic cells 62, 62f
squamous cell carcinoma see squamous cell
carcinoma (SCC)
squamous metaplasia 62, 62f
atypia in, squamous cell carcinoma vs 66, 67f
tumours see lung tumours
retention cyst, salivary gland 301f
reticular cell tumour, fibroblastic 244, 244f
rhabdoid tumour of kidney 356

rhabdomyoblasts 357
rhabdomyoma 378f
rhabdomyosarcoma 357, 357f, 381
alveolar type 357, 357f, 381f, 381t
chromosomal aberration 357, 381
diagnostic pitfalls 357
in ascitic fluid, primary effusion lymphoma
vs 196f
diagnostic pitfalls 357
embryonal type 357, 381f, 381t
diagnostic pitfalls 357
spindle cell variant 381f
further investigations 381
immunomarkers 134f, 381
morphology and prognosis 357
pleomorphic 381f
rheumatoid arthritis, reactive mesothelial cells in
effusions 110, 111f
Richter's syndrome 185, 186f
Rider cells 388, 388f
Riedel's thyroiditis (Riedel's struma) 155, 155f
ring sideroblasts 219f, 221f, 225f
refractory anaemia with 221, 221f
Rosai–Dorfmann disease 178, 178f
rosette formation, cervical glandular
intraepithelial neoplasia 40

S

salivary duct carcinoma 297, 297f
salivary gland 279–308
acinar atrophy 300f
acinar cells 280, 300f
acinar epithelium 280f
anatomy 279f
basaloid cells 306
chronic sialadenitis 285f, 294f
cystic changes, metastatic squamous cell
carcinoma vs 295
cystic degeneration 284
cysts 302–307
mucous see salivary gland, mucocele
diagnostic algorithm 308f
ductal cells 280
ductal epithelium 280f, 300f
fine-needle aspiration (FNA) 282, 306
algorithm 308f
common diagnoses 308t
hyaline globules see hyaline globules
image-guided FNA 279f
lymphoepithelial cyst 294f, 302f–303f, 303
lymphoepithelial lesion 305f
lymphoid infiltration 305f
mucocele 302, 302f
differential diagnosis 302, 302f
mucoepidermoid carcinoma vs 291f, 302f
myoepithelial sialadenitis see sialadenitis,
myoepithelial
neoplastic conditions see salivary gland
tumours
non-neoplastic conditions 300, 308t
pathogenesis, clinical findings 300
normal 280, 280f
differential diagnosis 280
histology 279f
oncocytic cells 307
Warthin's tumour vs 284
retention cyst 301f

sarcoidosis 301f
sialadenitis *see* sialadenitis
sialosis 287f
squamous cells in aspirates 294–295
squamous metaplasia 284, 285f, 294f
   Warthin's tumour 294f
salivary gland tumours 281–298, 308t
   acinic cell carcinoma *see* acinic cell
     carcinoma
   adenocarcinoma, mucoepidermoid
     carcinoma *vs* 290
   adenoid cystic carcinoma *see* adenoid cystic
     carcinoma
   adenolymphoma (Warthin's tumour) *see*
     Warthin's tumour (adenolymphoma)
   basal cell adenocarcinoma 299f
   basal cell adenoma 286, 286f, 306f
   basaloid cells in 292
   benign 281, 286–287
   carcinoma 297f
     mucoepidermoid carcinoma *vs* 290
   carcinoma ex-pleomorphic adenoma 298,
     298f
   common types (WHO classification) 281
   cytological findings, mucoepidermoid
     carcinoma 290
   diffuse large B-cell lymphoma 299f
   epimyoepithelial carcinoma 298, 298f
   hyaline globules in 292
   intraduct papilloma 287, 287f
   lymphomas 299f
   malignant 281, 288
     rare 298
   MALT lymphoma 304, 305f
   metastatic 298
   metastatic squamous cell carcinoma 295,
     295f, 299f
   mucoepidermoid carcinoma 294f
     cytological findings 290, 290f–291f,
      307f
     differential diagnosis 290, 291f, 302f
     histology 290, 291f
   myoepithelial carcinoma 299f
   myoepithelioma 286, 286f, 299f
   nerve sheath tumour 299f
   oncocytic adenoma 287, 287f, 307f
   oncocytic carcinoma 307f
   oncocytoma 285f
   pleomorphic adenoma 282
     chrondroid stroma 283f
     cytological findings 281f–283f, 282
     differential diagnosis 282
     hyaline globules 306f
     myxoid stroma 281f–283f
     oncocytic metaplasia with atypia 298f
     parotid 282
     squamous metaplasia 294f
   polymorphous low-grade
     adenocarcinoma 296, 296f, 306f
   sebaceous adenoma 287, 287f
   squamous cell carcinoma 299f
     metastatic 295, 295f, 299f
   T-cell lymphoma 299f
sarcoidosis 98f, 179, 179f
   granulomatous lymphadenopathy 178–179,
     179f
   lung 98
   salivary gland 301f

sarcoma
   alveolar soft part 382, 382f
   breast 275
   childhood 352
   chromosomal translocations 407
   clear cell *see* clear cell sarcoma
   embryonal 324, 324f
   endometrial, metastasis to breast 276f
   Ewing's *see* Ewing's (sarcoma) family of
     tumours; Ewing's sarcoma (classic)
   fibromyxoid 378t
   histiocytic 242, 242f
   myeloid 241, 241f
   pleomorphic, differential diagnosis
     380
   polymerase chain reaction 405
   pulmonary 81
   small round cell 386t
   soft tissue, classification and grading
     386t
   spindle cell 386t
   synovial *see* synovial sarcoma
schistosomal species, cervical smears 12f
scleroid, cervical smears 12f
sclerosing haemangioma 81, 81f
sclerosing lymphocytic lobulitis 252, 252f
sebaceous adenoma, salivary gland 287,
   287f
seborrhoeic keratosis 368, 368f
secretory intracytoplasmic vacuoles 119t
seminal vesicle cells, in urine sample 136f
seminoma 86
   cystic, mediastinal 86f
serous cavities 103f
serous cystadenocarcinoma, ovary 56f
serous cystadenoma
   ovary 55, 55f
   pancreatic 344t, 346, 346f
     biochemical cyst fluid parameters 344t
     differential diagnosis 346
serous effusions 103–130
   benign reactive 104, 107f
     benign findings 108
     carcinoma *vs* 115
     causes 110
     cell types 108, 108f–109f
     immunocytochemistry 128
     infections causing 110
     macrophages in 108, 108f
     with specific features 110, 110f–111f
   carcinomatous 122t
     cell arrangements 114
     cytoplasmic features 114, 114f
     differential diagnosis 115, 127t
     further investigations 115
     metastatic 113–119, 113f–114f
     nuclear features 114, 114f
   chylous 104t, 120
   cirrhosis of liver causing 110, 110f
   clinicopathological significance 104
   cytomorphological features 122t
     adenocarcinoma *vs* 127t
   eosinophilic 111f
   gross appearance 104f
   haematolymphoid malignancies 120,
     120f–121f
     differential diagnosis 120
     low-grade lymphoma *vs* 128

immunocytochemistry 115, 128–130
   algorithm 128f
   immunomarkers 129t, 130f–131f
   recommended, routine diagnosis 128t
lung tumour 132f
macrophages 108, 108f–109f
malignant 104
   algorithm for second foreign population
     113, 113f
   carcinomatous *see above*
   dual population approach 107, 112–113,
     113f, 115f, 126f
   general diagnostic approach 112–120
   metastatic *see* serous effusions,
     metastatic
malignant squamous cells 116f
melanoma, *vs* carcinoma 115
mesothelial cells *see* mesothelial cell(s)
mesothelioma 112, 124
metastatic 112–119, 112f
   adenocarcinoma 112f, 130f
   bladder carcinoma 119f
   breast carcinoma 112f, 114f–116f, 116,
     130f, 134f
   carcinoma cells 112–119, 112f
   characteristic features 116
   cholangiocarcinoma 119f
   colon carcinoma 131f
   duodenal carcinoma 118f
   female genital tract carcinomas 117,
     117f
   gastric carcinoma 118f
   gastrointestinal tract carcinoma 118,
     118f
   immunomarkers for 130f, 134f
   lung carcinomas 116, 116f, 131f
   ovarian carcinomas 117, 117f, 130f
   pancreatic carcinoma 118f
   prostate carcinoma 119f
   renal carcinoma 119f
   small cell carcinoma of lung 131f
   unknown primary carcinoma 115
non-specific 107
   conditions causing 107
reactive
   benign *see* serous effusions, benign
     reactive
   malignant cells with 112
   non-specific, mesothelial cells 107, 107f
sampling method 392, 392f
therapeutic effects, carcinoma *vs* 115
types 104t
see also mesothelial cell(s)
serous fluid 103
serous lining 103f
Sezary cells 200, 200f
Sezary syndrome 200, 200f
sialadenitis
   acute 300, 300f
   calculi associated 300
   cholesterol crystals 301f
   chronic 285f, 294f, 300, 300f
     amylase crystals 301f
     foreign body giant cell reaction 301f
   mucoepidermoid carcinoma *vs* 290
   myoepithelial 280, 304
     cytological findings 304, 304f
   tuberculous 301f

sideroblasts
  abnormal, refractory cytopenia of childhood (RCC) 226f
  ring *see* ring sideroblasts
siderophage
  in CSF 362, 362f
  see also macrophage, haemosiderin-laden
signet cell carcinoma 142f
signet ring cell 118f, 122t
silicone, lymphadenopathy 180
silicone granuloma 251f
sinus histiocytosis with massive lymphadenopathy 178
Sjögren's syndrome 304
skeletal tumours 383
skin cytology 366–368
  infections 367
  normal 366, 366f
  primary cutaneous lymphoma 371, 371f
  sampling techniques 366, 366f
  scraping technique 392
skin tumours 371
  basal cell *see* basal cell carcinoma of skin
  melanoma *see* melanoma, malignant
  squamous cell *see* squamous cell carcinoma, skin
small blue cell neoplasms 371f
small cell carcinoma of lung 64–75
  cytological findings 69, 69f–70f
    'salt and pepper' pattern 69, 69f
  differential diagnosis 69, 70f, 365
    carcinoid tumour 78f
    lymphoma 70f
    metastatic breast carcinoma 70f
    neuroendocrine carcinoma 70f
  further investigations 69
  immunomarkers 131f
  lymph node metastases 207f
  metastatic, serous effusions 116f
small cell carcinoma of pancreas 343, 343f
small lymphocytic lymphoma (SLL) 185
  cytological findings 185, 185f–186f
  immunocytochemistry 191t
  lymphoplasmacytoid features 186f
  Reed–Sternberg-like cell 186f
small round cell sarcoma 386t
small round cell tumour 414, 414f
  desmoplastic 381t
  see also Ewing's sarcoma (classic)
smearing artefact 395, 395f
smoking, squamous cell carcinoma (SCC) 66
soft tissue
  normal cytology 373–374
  reactive, cytology 373
  see also adipose tissue; fibrous tissue; striated muscle
soft tissue lesions 372–386
  cytogenetics 372
  definitive cytological features 386t
  immunocytochemistry 372
soft tissue tumours 375–376
  benign 372, 375–376
    adipocytic 375, 375f, 375t
    miscellaneous types 378
  cytological report 386
  definitive cytological features 386t
  FNA cytology 372
  FNA cytology for management 372

leiomyoma 378f
  malignant 379–382
  myxoid background matrix 378t
  sarcoma, classification and grading 386t
solar keratosis 368, 368f, 370
solid pseudopapillary neoplasm (SPN), pancreas 340, 340f
solitary fibrous tumour, lung/pleura 81, 81f–82f
spermatozoa
  cervical smears 11, 11f
  urine sample 136f
spindle cell(s)
  fibroblastic reticular cell tumour 244, 244f
  inflammatory pseudotumour of liver 313f
  lipoma 375f
  malignant, phyllodes tumour 275f
  malignant peripheral nerve sheath tumours 380f
  squamous cell carcinoma of cervix 35f–36f
spindle cell carcinoma, lung 78f
spindle cell lipoma 375f, 375t
spindle cell sarcoma 386t
spindle cell thymoma 78f, 85f
spindle cell tumours, childhood 356b
spleen
  marginal zone lymphoma 187f
  primary myelofibrosis 213
sputum sample 60, 60f, 64, 392
  adenocarcinoma with lepidic growth pattern 73f, 78f
  adenosquamous carcinoma 72f
  asthma 97f
  bronchiectasis 96f
  COAD 96f
  inadequate/unsatisfactory sample 61f
  normal cytology 60
  small cell carcinoma of lung 69f
  squamous cell carcinoma differential diagnosis 68f
  viral infections of lung 90f
squamous cell(s)
  cervical transformation zone 6, 6f–7f
  'ghost' cells 371, 371f
  lung, dyskaryotic 67f
  mucoepidermoid carcinoma (salivary gland) 290, 290f
  oral 393f
  in serous effusions 116f
  skin 366, 366f
    dysplastic, actinic keratosis 368, 368f
  sputum sample 60, 60f
  thyroglossal cyst sample 152f
  urine cytology/specimen 135, 135f–136f, 145f
squamous cell carcinoma (SCC)
  bile ducts (extrahepatic) 331, 331f
  cervical *see* cervical carcinoma
  lung *see* lung tumours
  metastatic
    CSF in 364
    salivary gland 295, 295f, 299f
    squamous metaplasia (salivary gland) *vs* 285f
    respiratory tract reactive changes *vs* 62
  salivary gland 299f
  skin 370, 370f
    basal cell carcinoma *vs* 369
    diagnostic pitfalls 370

urinary tract 141
  vulval 49f
squamous epithelium, regenerative 370
squamous metaplasia
  cervical 4
  respiratory system 62, 62f
    atypical 62
  salivary glands *see* salivary gland
staghorn cluster, urothelial cells 138f
staining methods 396–397
  lymph node FNA samples 173
  rapid method 397, 397f
  routine 396
  special 397
steatosis (fatty liver) 311, 311f
steroids, synovial fluid 'wet prep' 387
striated muscle 373, 373f
  reactive changes 373, 373f
stroma, metachromatic, Riedel's thyroiditis 155f
Strongyloides infection, lung 95, 95f
subareolar abscess 250, 250f
subareolar papillomatosis 262–263
sublingual gland, anatomy 279f
submandibular gland, anatomy 279f
'sulphur granules' 312
surgery, cervical cytology changes 21, 21f
suture granuloma, differential diagnosis 180, 180f
swelling, tissue, childhood tumours 352t
synaptophysin, pancreatic endocrine neoplasms (PEN) 342f
synovial fluid 387–389
  cell types 388, 388f
  cytocentrifuge preparation 388
  diagnostic algorithms 389f
  'high cell count', diagnostic algorithm 389f
  'low cell count', diagnostic algorithm 389f
  microscopy, approach 387
  'wet prep' 387
    crystal identification 387, 387f
    particular material 388, 388f
synovial sarcoma 382, 382f
  chromosomal translocation detection 407
synoviocytes, synovial fluid 388f
systemic lupus erythematosus (SLE), effusions 110, 111f

T

tadpole cells
  cervical squamous cell carcinoma 35, 36f
  lung squamous cell carcinoma 66f
  squamous cell carcinoma of skin 370f
talc 12f
talc granuloma 101, 101f
talc lymphadenopathy 180
tamoxifen, cervical cytology changes 20
T-cell(s) *see* T-lymphocytes
T-cell lymphoma 182t
  angioimmunoblastic 201, 201f
  clonality analysis 406f
  peripheral *see* peripheral T-cell lymphoma
  primary cutaneous *see* primary cutaneous lymphoma
  salivary gland 299f
  sarcoidosis *vs* 179
T-cell prolymphocytic leukaemia 200f
T-cell receptor 406, 406f

techniques 391–414
    quality control 401
    routine procedures 392–397
    see also specific techniques
teratoma
    malignant, mediastinal 86, 87f
    mature cystic, ovarian 56, 57f
    mature mediastinal 86, 87f
thoracic mass, childhood tumours 352t
thrombocytes, essential thrombocythaemia 214, 214f
thrombocytopenia, refractory cytopenia with unilineage dysplasia 220, 220f
thrombomodulin 132f
thymic carcinoma 84, 85f
thymoma 84, 84f
    lymphoepithelial, metastasis to lung 85f
    spindle cell 78f, 85f
    types 84
thymus, lymphoblastic lymphoma 85f
thyroglossal cyst 152
    cytological findings 152, 152f
thyroid carcinoma
    anaplastic 168, 168f
        differential diagnosis 155f
        immunohistochemistry 168t
    follicular 158, 158f–161f
        cytological findings 160, 160f–161f
        follicular adenoma *vs* 160f
        minimally invasive 159f
    lymphoma 168
    medullary 166, 166f
        amyloid deposits 166f–167f
        cytological findings 166, 167f
        differential diagnosis 166f
        eccentric nuclei 167f
        immunocytochemistry 167f
    metastatic 168, 169f
    papillary 159f, 162
        colloid cyst *vs* 165f
        columnar cell variant 164
        cribriform-morula variant 164, 165f
        cystic neck metastases 163f
        cysts *vs* 151f
        cytological findings 162, 162f–163f
        differential diagnosis 161f, 162, 163f, 165f
        diffuse sclerosing variant 164, 165f
        follicular variant 164, 164f
        hyaline globules 164, 165f
        hyalinising trabecular adenoma *vs* 165f
        intranuclear inclusions 159f, 162, 162f–164f
        lymphocytic thyroiditis with 153f
        lymphoid infiltrated 164
        NF-like struma with 164
        nuclear grooves 159f, 163f–164f
        oncocytic tumour *vs* 161f
        oncocytic variant 165f
        papillary arrangement 162, 162f–163f
        psammoma bodies 162, 163f, 164
        special types 164
        tall cell variant 164, 164f
        warthin-like variant 164
thyroid cysts 150
    colloid, cystic papillary carcinoma *vs* 165f
    cytological findings 150, 150f–151f
    differential diagnosis 150, 151f

thyroid epithelium 148f–149f
    degenerative changes 151f
    follicular 148, 148f–149f
        thyroid hyperplasia 156f–157f
    follicular lesions 158f
    metastatic carcinoma of thyroid 169f
    subacute thyroiditis 154f
    thyroid cyst wall 151f
thyroid gland 147–170
    anatomy 147f
    cysts *see* thyroid cysts
    diffuse enlargement *see* goitre
    FNA cytology 147, 150
        indication 150
        malignancy risk, categories 170t
        management implications 171f
        nondiagnostic features 171f
        reporting categories 170, 170t
    follicular cells 148, 148f–149f
        degenerate 150f
    follicular lesions 158, 159f, 161f, 164f
        cytological features 158, 158f
        differential diagnosis 157f, 158
        follicular papillary carcinoma 164
        see also thyroid carcinoma, follicular
    hyperplasia 156
        cytological findings 156, 156f–157f
        differential diagnosis 156, 157f
        drug-induced changes 157f
        'fire flare' appearance 156f
        paravacuolar granules 156f
    inflammation *see* thyroiditis
    intranuclear inclusions, disorders with 162, 163f
    microfollicules 157f–158f
    nodules *see* thyroid nodules
    normal histology 147f
    swelling 147f, 150
thyroid gland neoplasms 160–168
    carcinoma *see* thyroid carcinoma
    follicular adenoma 158f–160f, 160
        carcinoma *vs* 160f
    non-Hodgkin's lymphoma 168, 169f
    oncocytic (Hürthle cell) 160, 161f
thyroid nodules 147
    benign 148–155
    colloid 147–148, 148f
    dominant 148
    hyperplastic 157f–158f
thyroiditis 153
    Hashimoto's 153
    lymphocytic and autoimmune 153, 153f
    Riedel's (Riedel's struma) 155, 155f
    subacute (De Quervain's) 154, 154f
tingible bodies 176
tingible body macrophages 34f, 176f, 353, 353f
T-lymphoblastic leukaemia (T-ALL) 183, 184f
    cytological findings 183, 184f
T-lymphocytes
    lymphoblastic leukaemia (T-ALL) 183
    lymphoma *see* T-cell lymphoma
    mature, neoplasms 182t, 198–204
        ALCL *see* anaplastic large cell lymphoma (ALCL)
        angioimmunoblastic T-cell lymphoma 201, 201f

hepatosplenic lymphoma *see* hepatosplenic T-cell lymphoma
mycosis fungoides/Sezary syndrome 200, 200f
peripheral lymphoma *see* peripheral T-cell lymphoma
receptor 406, 406f
touch imprint cytology 366
trachelectomy 46
training, cytopathology 1
transformation zone, cervical *see* cervix
transitional cell carcinoma (urothelial carcinoma), bladder 139
    carcinoma-in-situ, cytological findings 139
    differential diagnosis 143
        BK/human polyomavirus 143, 143f
        degenerative changes 143, 144f
        other infections 144, 145f
    grade I 141f
    high-grade 139, 139f
        differential diagnosis 144
    histology 140f–141f
    instrumental effects on cytology 144
    low-grade 141, 141f
    metastatic cells, lung 68f
    papillary (grade II) 140f
    recurrent 144f
    squamous differentiation, with 141f
    urine cytology 139, 139f
transport of samples 392, 393f
transudates 104t
Trichomonas vaginalis 16, 17f
tuberculosis, pulmonary 88
    histology 89f
tuberculous lymphadenitis 178, 178f
tuberculous mastitis 251f
tuberculous meningitis 362, 362f
tuberculous sialadenitis 301f
tubo-endometrioid metaplasia 21, 21f
    CGIN diagnostic pitfalls and 44, 45f
tubular adenoma 258, 258f
tumour suppressor genes 337

U

ulcers, regenerative squamous epithelium 370
uraemia, non-specific reactive mesothelial cells 111f
ureteric brush sample, urothelial malignancy 140f
urinary calculus, cytology 144, 145f
urinary symptoms, urinary tract malignancy 139
urinary tract malignancy 139–141
    adenocarcinoma 137, 141
        differential diagnosis 141, 142f
    ileal conduit samples 137, 138f
    metastatic 141
    squamous cell carcinoma 141
    transitional cell *see* transitional cell carcinoma
urine cytology 135–144
    appearance 135–137
    casts 135, 136f
    corpora amylacea 135f
    diagnosis and sensitivity 139
    epithelial granuloma 144f

instrumentation effects 144
   lithiasis/calculus formation 144, 145f
   papillaroid groups 144
   reactive conditions 144, 144f–145f
   instrumented sample 137, 137f–138f
   malignancy 139–141
      see also urinary tract malignancy
   normal 135, 135f–136f
   red blood cells 136f
   spermatozoa 136f
   squamous cells 135f, 145f
   urothelial cells 135, 135f–136f
urine specimens 135, 392
   ileal conduit samples 137, 138f
   instrumented samples 137, 137f–138f
   processing 135
   types 135–137
urothelial carcinoma *see* transitional cell
   carcinoma
urothelial cell(s)
   atypical 140f–141f, 144f
   benign, groups 138f, 145f
   columnar-shaped, instrumented
      sample 137f
   degenerative changes 139f, 143, 143f
   instrumented urine sample 137f–138f
   intermediate 145f
   in lithiasis 144, 145f
   malignant 139f–140f
      hyperchromasia 140f
      see also transitional cell carcinoma
   nuclei 138f, 144f–145f
   reactive, 'bubbly' cytoplasm 144f
   staghorn cluster 138f
   superficial, *vs* deep, instrumented sample
      137f
   in urine specimen 135, 135f–136f

uterine cytology 50–51
   endometrial cells 50, 50f
   non-neoplastic conditions 50
   normal, directly sampled 50
   stromal clusters 50, 50f

V

vacuoles
   degenerative *vs* secretory
      intracytoplasmic 119t
   metastatic ovarian neoplasms 117f
   mucin *see* mucin vacuoles
vaginal cytology 22, 47–49
   radiotherapy-induced changes 22, 22f
   'two cell population' 22
vaginal infections 16
   bacterial 15f–16f, 16
   fungal 16
   protozoa 16
   Trichomonas vaginalis 16, 17f
vaginal intraepithelial neoplasia 47
vaginal melanoma 49, 49f
vaginitis 14
   non-specific changes 14, 14f–15f
viral infections
   cervix *see* cervical infections
   CSF in 362, 362f
   lung *see* lung infections
vulva
   cytology 47–49
      hyperkeratosis 47f–48f
      inadequate scrape sample 47f
      scrape cytology 48f
      squamous hyperplasia 47f
   dyskaryosis 48f
   invasive cell carcinoma 49f

melanoma 49, 49f
   Paget's disease 49, 49f
vulval intraepithelial neoplasia (VIN) 47, 48f
   VIN I 48f
   VIN III 48f

W

Waldenström's macroglobulinaemia, differential
   diagnosis 186f
Warthin–Finkeldey giant cell 180, 180f
Warthin's tumour (adenolymphoma) 281f,
   284
   cytological findings 281f, 284, 284f–285f,
      307f
   differential diagnosis 284, 285f
      mucoepidermoid carcinoma *vs*
         290
   squamous metaplasia 294f
Wilm's tumour *see* nephroblastoma
World Health Organization (WHO)
   classification
   breast tumours 266b
   lymphoproliferative disease 182t
   malignant adipose tissue tumours
      379–380
   myeloid neoplasms 209t
   salivary gland tumours 281

X

xanthogranulomatous reaction, liver 313f

Z

Ziehl–Neelsen stain 88, 89f, 178
   leprosy 367, 367f